DIABETES

DIABETES

Oxidative Stress and Dietary Antioxidants

Edited by

VICTOR R. PREEDY BSc, PhD, DSc, CBiol, FSB, FRSH, FRIPH, FRSPH, FRCPath, FRSC

Department of Nutrition and Dietetics, School of Medicine, King's College London, London, UK

ELSEVIER

AMSTERDAM • BOSTON • HEIDELBERG • LONDON
NEW YORK • OXFORD • PARIS • SAN DIEGO
SINGAPORE • SAN FRANCISCO • SYDNEY • TOKYO
Academic Press is an imprint of Elsevier

Academic Press is an imprint of Elsevier
32 Jamestown Road, London NW1 7BY, UK
225 Wyman Street, Waltham, MA 02451, USA
525 B Street, Suite 1800, San Diego, CA 92101-4495, USA

British Library Cataloguing-in-Publication Data
A catalogue record for this book is available from the British Library

Library of Congress Cataloging-in-Publication Data
A catalog record for this book is available from the Library of Congress

ISBN: 978-0-12-405885-9

Typeset by TNQ Books and Journals Pvt Ltd
www.tnq.co.in

Printed and bound in United States of America

14 15 16 17 18   10 9 8 7 6 5 4 3 2 1

Contents

II

Antioxidants and Diabetes

7. α-Tocopherol Supplementation, Lipid Profile, and Insulin Sensitivity in Diabetes Mellitus Type 2

LIANIA ALVES LUZIA, PATRICIA HELEN RONDO

8. Effect of *Salvia miltiorrhiza* on Antioxidant Enzymes in Diabetic Patients

QINGWEN QIAN, SHUHONG QIAN, VINOOD B. PATEL

9. Antioxidant Spices and Herbs Used in Diabetes

ROBERTA CAZZOLA, BENVENUTO CESTARO

10. Resveratrol and Oxidative Stress in Diabetes Mellitus

PÁL BRASNYÓ, BALÁZS SÜMEGI, GÁBOR WINKLER, ISTVÁN WITTMANN

11. Vitamin D, Oxidative Stress and Diabetes: Is There a Link?

TIRANG R. NEYESTANI

12. Glutamine and Antioxidant Potential in Diabetes

SUNG-LING YEH, YU-CHEN HOU

13. The Anti-Oxidative Component of Docosahexaenoic Acid (DHA) in the Brain in Diabetes

EMMA ARNAL, MARÍA MIRANDA, SIV JOHNSEN-SORIANO, FRANCISCO J. ROMERO

14. Diabetic Nephropathy and Tocotrienol

KANWALJIT CHOPRA, VIPIN ARORA, ANURAG KUHAD

Preface

In the past few decades there have been major advances in our understanding of the etiology of disease and its causative mechanisms. Increasingly it is becoming evident that free radicals are contributory agents: either to initiate or propagate the pathology or to add to an overall imbalance. Furthermore, reduced dietary antioxidants can also lead to specific diseases and preclinical organ dysfunction. On the other hand, there is abundant evidence that dietary and other naturally occurring antioxidants can be used to prevent, ameliorate or impede such diseases. The science of oxidative stress and free radical biology is rapidly advancing and new approaches include the examination of polymorphism and molecular biology. The more traditional sciences associated with organ functionality continue to be explored but their practical or translational applications are now more sophisticated.

However, most textbooks on dietary antioxidants do not have material on the fundamental biology of free radicals, especially their molecular and cellular effects on pathology. They also fail to include material on the nutrients and foods which contain anti-oxidative activity. In contrast, most books on free radicals and organs disease have little or no text on the usage of natural antioxidants.

The series ***Oxidative Stress and Dietary Antioxidants*** aims to address the aforementioned deficiencies in the knowledge base by combining in a single volume the science of oxidative stress and the putative therapeutic usage of natural antioxidants in the diet, its food matrix or plants. This is done in relation to a single organ, disease or pathology. These include cancer, addictions, immunology, HIV, ageing, cognition, endocrinology, pregnancy and fetal growth, obesity, exercise, liver, kidney, lungs, reproductive organs, gastrointestinal tract, oral health, muscle, bone, heart, kidney and the CNS.

In the present volume, ***Diabetes: Oxidative Stress and Dietary Antioxidants,*** holistic information is imparted within a structured format of two main sections:

I. Oxidative Stress and Diabetes.
II. Antioxidants and Diabetes.

The first section, Oxidative Stress and Diabetes, covers the basic biology of oxidative stress from molecular biology to physiological pathology. Topics include mitochondria, iron, neuropathy, cerebral ischemia, cardiomyopathy and retinopathy. The second section, Antioxidants and Diabetes, covers spices and herbs, including red sage, chrysanthemi flos, *Ginkgo biloba*, pomegranate juice, polyphenols, alpha-tocopherol and tocotrienols, lutein, Vitamin D, taurine, glutamine, statins, docosahexaenoic acid, resveratrol, micronutrients and many other antioxidants. Both preclinical and clinical studies are embraced using an evidence-based approach. An important cautionary note is required as in many cases more in-depth clinical studies are required to determine safety and therapeutic efficacy. However, the science of oxidative stress is not described in isolation but in concert with other processes such as apoptosis, cell signalling, receptor mediated responses and so on. This approach recognizes that diseases are often multifactorial and that oxidative stress is a single component of this.

The series is designed for dietitians and nutritionists, and food scientists, as well as health care workers and research scientists. Contributions are from leading national and international experts including those from world renowned institutions.

Professor Victor R Preedy, King's College London

Contributors

Amanda I. Adler Wolfson Diabetes & Endocrine Clinic, Cambridge University Hospitals NHS Foundation Trust, Addenbrooke's Treatment Centre, Cambridge, United Kingdom

Emma Arnal Fundación Oftalmológica del Mediterráneo, Valencia, Spain

Vipin Arora Pharmacology Research Laboratory, University Institute of Pharmaceutical Sciences, UGC Center of Advanced Study, Panjab University, Chandigarh, India

Denise M. Arrick Department of Cellular Biology and Anatomy, and Center of Excellence in Cardiovascular Diseases and Sciences, Louisiana State University Health Sciences Center-Shreveport, Shreveport, LA, USA

Somasundaram Arumugam Dept. of Clinical Pharmacology, Niigata University of Pharmacy and Applied Life Sciences, Niigata Shi, Japan

Maria Luisa Balestrieri Department of Biochemistry, Biophysics and General Pathology, Second University of Naples, Naples, Italy

Arpita Basu Department of Nutritional Sciences, Oklahoma State University, Stillwater, OK, USA

Pál Brasnyó Second Department of Medicine and Nephrological Center, Faculty of Medicine, University of Pécs, Pécs, Hungary

Alecia L. Bryant Department of Nutritional Sciences, Oklahoma State University, Stillwater, OK, USA

Maria Carmela Capoluongo Department of Geriatrics and Metabolic Diseases, Naples, Italy

Roberta Cazzola Department of Biomedical and Clinical Sciences 'L. Sacco', University of Milan, Milan, Italy

Benvenuto Cestaro Department of Biomedical and Clinical Sciences 'L. Sacco', University of Milan, Milan, Italy

Kanwaljit Chopra Pharmacology Research Laboratory, University Institute of Pharmaceutical Sciences, UGC Center of Advanced Study, Panjab University, Chandigarh, India

Zafer Cukurova Bakirkoy Dr. Sadi Konuk Training and Research Hospital, Department of Anaesthesiology and Intensive Care, Istanbul, Turkey

Nunzia D'Onofrio Department of Biochemistry, Biophysics and General Pathology, Second University of Naples, Naples, Italy

Joydeep Das Division of Molecular Medicine, Bose Institute, Kolkata, India

Kunjan R. Dave The Cerebral Vascular Disease Research Laboratories, Department of Neurology Leonard M. Miller School of Medicine, University of Miami, Miami, FL, USA

Monica del-Rio-Vellosillo Department of Anesthesiology, University Hospital La Arrixaca, El Palmar, Murcia, Spain

Mala Dharmalingam Department of Endocrinology, M.S. Ramaiah Medical College, MSRIT Post, Bangalore, India

Gulay Eren Bakirkoy Dr. Sadi Konuk Training and Research Hospital, Department of Anaesthesiology and Intensive Care, Istanbul, Turkey

Perry Fuchs The Cerebral Vascular Disease Research Laboratories, Department of Neurology Leonard M. Miller School of Medicine, University of Miami, Miami, FL, USA

Roberto Gallego-Pinazo Department of Ophthalmology, University and Polytechnic Hospital La Fe, Valencia, Spain

Jose Javier Garcia-Medina Department of Ophthalmology, University General Hospital Reina Sofía and Department of Ophthalmology and Optometry, School of Medicine, University of Murcia, Murcia, Spain

Manuel Garcia-Medina Department of Ophthalmology, Torrecardenas Hospital, Almeria, Spain

Hagit Goldenstein The Ruth and Bruce Rappaport Faculty of Medicine, Technion-Israel Institute of Technology, Haifa, Israel

Oya Hergunsel Bakirkoy Dr. Sadi Konuk Training and Research Hospital, Department of Anaesthesiology and Intensive Care, Istanbul, Turkey

Yu-Chen Hou School of Nutrition and Health Sciences, Taipei Medical University, Taipei, Taiwan

Siv Johnsen-Soriano Fundación Oftalmológica del Mediterráneo, Valencia, Spain

Vengadeshprabhu Karuppagounder Dept. of Clinical Pharmacology, Niigata University of Pharmacy and Applied Life Sciences, Niigata Shi, Japan

Sung-Jin Kim Department of Pharmacology and Toxicology, School of Dentistry, Kyung Hee University, Seoul, Republic of Korea

Anurag Kuhad Pharmacology Research Laboratory, University Institute of Pharmaceutical Sciences, UGC Center of Advanced Study, Panjab University, Chandigarh, India

Christine Lee Department of Nutritional Sciences, University of Toronto, Toronto, ON, Canada

Andrew P. Levy The Ruth and Bruce Rappaport Faculty of Medicine, Technion-Israel Institute of Technology, Haifa, Israel

Soo Lim Department of Internal Medicine, Seoul National University College of Medicine, Seoul, South Korea, Seoul National University Bundang Hospital, Seoul, Republic of Korea

Liania Alves Luzia Department of Nutrition, Public Health School, University of Sao Paulo, Sao Paulo, Brazil

Timothy J. Lyons Section of Endocrinology and Diabetes, University of Oklahoma Health Sciences Center, Oklahoma City, OK, USA

Sara Rani Marcus MSU-GEF International Medical School, MSRIT Post, Bangalore, India

Raffaele Marfella Department of Geriatrics and Metabolic Diseases, Naples, Italy

William G. Mayhan Department of Cellular Biology and Anatomy, and Center of Excellence in Cardiovascular Diseases and Sciences, Louisiana State University Health Sciences Center-Shreveport, Shreveport, LA, USA

María Miranda Universidad CEU Cardenal Herrera, Moncada, Spain

Jonathan R. Murrow Georgia Regents University – University of Georgia Medical Partnership, Athens, GA, USA

Tirang R. Neyestani National Nutrition and Food Technology Research Institute (NNFTRI) and Faculty of Nutrition Science and Food Technology, Shahid Beheshti University of Medical Sciences, Tehran, Iran

Yoko Ozawa Laboratory of Retinal Cell Biology, Department of Ophthalmology, Keio University School of Medicine, Tokyo, Japan

Giuseppe Paolisso Department of Geriatrics and Metabolic Diseases, Naples, Italy

Yongsoo Park Department of Internal Medicine and Bioengineering, Hanyang University, Seoul, Republic of Korea

Kyong Soo Park Department of Internal Medicine, Seoul National University College of Medicine, Seoul, South Korea

Vinood B. Patel Department of Biomedical Science, Faculty of Science & Technology, University of Westminster, London, UK

Miguel A. Perez-Pinzon The Cerebral Vascular Disease Research Laboratories, Department of Neurology Leonard M. Miller School of Medicine, University of Miami, Miami, FL, USA; Neuroscience Program, Department of Neurology Leonard M. Miller School of Medicine, University of Miami, Miami, FL, USA

Maria Dolores Pinazo-Duran Ophthalmology Research Unit 'Santiago Grisolia' and Department of Surgery, School of Medicine, University of Valencia, Valencia, Spain

Vigneshwaran Pitchaimani Dept. of Clinical Pharmacology, Niigata University of Pharmacy and Applied Life Sciences, Niigata Shi, Japan

Qingwen Qian Department of Medicine, First Affiliated Hospital, Zhengzhou University, Zhengzhou, China

Shuhong Qian Department of Clinical Laboratory, First Affiliated Hospital, Zhengzhou University, Zhengzhou, China

Maria Rosaria Rizzo Department of Geriatrics and Metabolic Diseases, Naples, Italy

Francisco J. Romero Fundación Oftalmológica del Mediterráneo, Valencia, Spain, Facultad de Medicina, Universidad Católica de Valencia 'San Vicente Mártir', Valencia, Spain

Patricia Helen Rondo Department of Nutrition, Public Health School, University of Sao Paulo, Sao Paulo, Brazil

Mariko Sasaki Laboratory of Retinal Cell Biology, Department of Ophthalmology, Keio University School of Medicine, Tokyo, Japan

Luigi Servillo Department of Biochemistry, Biophysics and General Pathology, Second University of Naples, Naples, Italy

Parames C. Sil Division of Molecular Medicine, Bose Institute, Kolkata, India

Ivana Sirangelo Department of Biochemistry, Biophysics and General Pathology, Second University of Naples, Naples, Italy

Hirohito Sone Dept. of Internal Medicine, Division of Hematology, Endocrinology and Metabolism, Niigata University Faculty of Medicine, Niigata, Japan

Balázs Sümegi Department of Biochemistry and Medical Chemistry, Faculty of Medicine, University of Pécs, Pécs, Hungary

Rajarajan A. Thandavarayan Dept. of Clinical Pharmacology, Niigata University of Pharmacy and Applied Life Sciences, Niigata, Japan

Victor M. Victor Fundacion para la Investigacion Sanitaria y Biomedica de la Comunidad Valenciana FISABIO, University Hospital Doctor Peset, Endocrinology Service, Avda Gaspar Aguilar, Valencia, Spain, Fundacion para la Investigación (INCLIVA), Department of Pharmacology and CIBER CB06/04/0071 Research Group, CIBER Hepatic and Digestive Diseases, and Department of Physiology, University of Valencia, Valencia, Spain

John Ward The Ruth and Bruce Rappaport Faculty of Medicine, Technion-Israel Institute of Technology, Haifa, Israel

Kenichi Watanabe Dept. of Clinical Pharmacology, Niigata University of Pharmacy and Applied Life Sciences, Niigata, Japan

Gábor Winkler Second Department of Internal Medicine-Diabetology, St. John's Hospital, Budapest, Hungary

István Wittmann Second Department of Medicine and Nephrological Center, Faculty of Medicine, University of Pécs, Pécs, Hungary

Sung-Ling Yeh School of Nutrition and Health Sciences, Taipei Medical University, Taipei, Taiwan

Vicente Zanon-Moreno Genetic and Molecular Epidemiology Unit, Department of Preventive Medicine and Public Health, School of Medicine, University of Valencia and CIBER Fisiopatología de la Obesidad y Nutrición, Valencia, Spain

SECTION I

OXIDATIVE STRESS AND DIABETES

CHAPTER

1

Oxidative Stress and Diabetic Neuropathy

Yongsoo Park

Department of Internal Medicine and Bioengineering, Hanyang University, Seoul, Republic of Korea

List of Abbreviations

AGE Advanced glycation end product
ATPase Adenosine triphosphatase
DCCT Diabetes Control and Complications Trial
DN Diabetic neuropathy
DPN Diabetic peripheral neuropathy
DTR Deep tendon reflex
DSP Distal symmetric polyneuropathy
ER Endoplasmic reticulum
MAPK Mitogen-activated protein kinases
MT Metallothionein
NADPH Nicotinamide adenine dinucleotide phosphate
NATHAN Neurological Assessment of Thioctic Acid in Diabetic Neuropathy
NCV Nerve conduction velocity
NF-κB Nuclear factor kappa
OLETF rats Otsuka Long-Evans Tokushima fatty rats
PKC Protein kinase C
QST Quantitative sensory testing
ROS Reactive oxygen species
SOD Superoxide dismutase
STZ Streptozotocin
TPT Thermal perception threshold
VPT Vibration perception threshold

INTRODUCTION AND EPIDEMIOLOGY

Diabetic neuropathy (DN) is a chronic, heterogeneous condition that encompasses a wide range of dysfunction and whose development might be attributable to diabetes mellitus *per se* or to factors associated with the disease. DN is a chronic complication of diabetes, present in both major phenotypes, T1DM and T2DM. Diabetic peripheral neuropathy (DPN) is a chronic microvascular complication affecting both somatic and autonomic peripheral nerves. It may be defined as the presence of symptoms and/or signs of peripheral nerve dysfunction in people with diabetes, after the exclusion of other causes of neuropathy. The most common form of DPN is distal symmetric polyneuropathy (DSP), which can affect somatic sensory or motor nerves and the autonomic nervous system. DSP is usually characterized by a number of neural symptoms including numbness, sensory loss, and stabbing or burning pain typically experienced in the hands and feet. These sensory symptoms are thought to be associated with the progressive loss or damage to sensory nerve fibers. Focal or multifocal forms of DN are asymmetric, and affect cranial, trunk, or limb innervations. Most often, DPN represents an insidious and progressive disorder which begins with a long asymptomatic stage. Ultimately, late stage DPN may lead to serious consequences, such as foot ulceration, gangrene, amputation, and neuropathic pain. The loss of sensation predisposes diabetic patients to ulceration, infection, and ultimately limb loss, accounting for the high morbidity and mortality.

DPN is a complex disorder in which the disease process may affect different sets of nerve fibers to different degrees in different individuals [1]. The signs, symptoms, and neurological deficits vary depending on the classes of nerve fibers involved. Thus, one individual may have an abnormality of large-fiber sensory function, which could be detected by measuring the vibration perception threshold (VPT), while another may have a predominantly small-fiber neuropathy that can only be detected by measuring the thermal perception threshold (TPT) (Figure 1.1). This feature of neuropathy can cause problems in the selection of a single test with which to screen a population. This issue of measurement of neurological function is further complicated by the subjectivity of the quantitative sensory testing (QST) comprising of different psychophysical tests, in which the subject is required to interpret the nature of an external stimulus. Thus, to determine if a given subject is affected by DPN, several different tests should be performed and DN should only be diagnosed when more than one test is abnormal [1].

Diabetes: Oxidative Stress and Dietary Antioxidants.
http://dx.doi.org/10.1016/B978-0-12-405885-9.00001-2

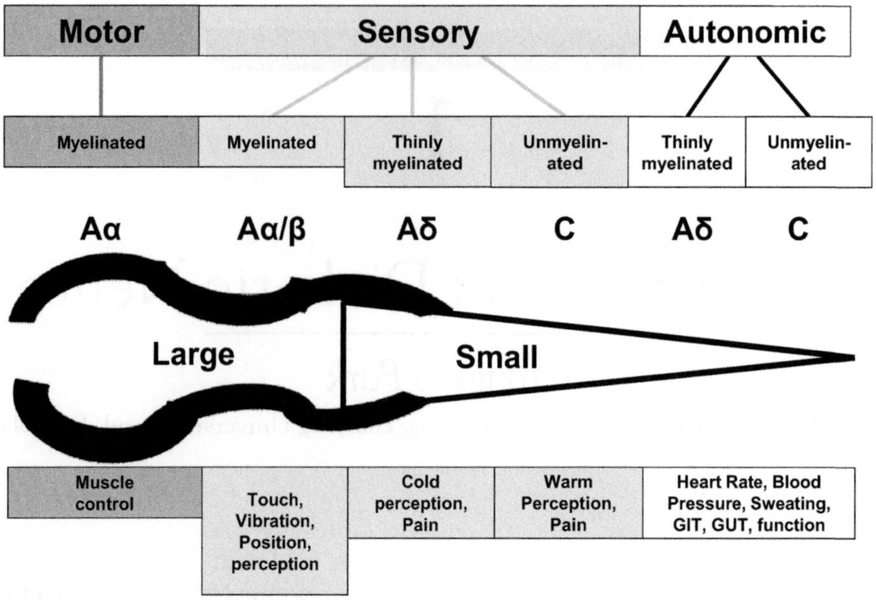

FIGURE 1.1 **A schematic presentation of the peripheral nervous system indicating relative fiber diameter, the degree of myelination, and function of each component.**

The impact of varying the diagnostic testing procedure can be seen in the Diabetes Control and Complications Trial (DCCT) data, where the prevalence of DSP at baseline in the conventional therapy cohort varied from 0.3% (abnormalities of reflexes, sensory examination, and neuropathic symptoms) to 21.8% (abnormal nerve conduction in at least two nerves) [2]. Therefore, multiple testing of different neurological functions is recommended as the gold standard [1], although it can be difficult and expensive. Complex patterns of sensation in DSP with decreased VPT (hypoesthesia) and heat stimulus-induced hyperesthesia (low TPT thresholds) are known to be characteristic of mild DSP as they correlate with neuropathic symptoms and deficits, whereas panmodality hypoesthesia is typical of severe DSP [3].

However, the influence of test selection on our understanding of the etiological factors associated with neuropathy is likely to be considerably smaller than that on its prevalence. The major confirmed risk factors are poor glycemic control, diabetes duration and height, with possible roles for hypertension (probably only in T1DM), age, smoking, hypoinsulinemia, and dyslipidemia. Additional risk factors for DPN are represented by increasing age, alcohol consumption or other drug abuse, and classic cardiovascular risk factors including obesity and albuminuria. There is a long way to go in finding a universal definition of neuropathy that can be widely used, although it is clearly needed for accurate epidemiological study.

DN in a clinical setting is considered a common complication affecting more than half of T2DM patients in their lifetime [4]. Neurological abnormalities affecting the distal lower extremities are known to appear in the early stages of T2DM and even in patients with prediabetes and abnormal glucose tolerance [5]. Although it is difficult to determine the prevalence of DN with any precision, several large studies have examined the prevalence in hospital-based populations and found prevalences of DSP in T2DM at approximately 30%, among both European and African populations [6,7]. DN is also one of the most frequently encountered complications in T1DM, occurring in about 60% of diabetic patients in a cumulative sense [8].

NATURAL HISTORY AND PROGNOSIS

It is difficult to describe the natural history of DN as a whole, since the signs, symptoms, and neurological deficits found in a diabetic patient may vary depending on the types of nerve fibers impaired. Neuropathies may be either sensory or motor, and may involve primarily small or large nerve fibers (Figure 1.1). Small nerve fiber damage usually (although not always) precedes large nerve fiber damage and is manifested first in the lower limbs, with pain and hyperalgesia, followed by a loss of thermal sensitivity and reduced light touch and pinprick sensation. When pain occurs, nerve conduction velocity (NCV) is often normal or minimally reduced [9]. However, slowing of NCVs is one of the earliest neuropathic abnormalities in diabetes and is often present even at diagnosis [10,11], especially in patients with T2DM. After diagnosis, slowing of NCV usually progresses at a steady rate by approximately 1 m/s/yr, and level of impairment is positively correlated with duration of diabetes [12]. Sensory fibers are usually affected first, followed by motor fibers, testifying the need for multiple measures of sensory function if early intervention is to be possible [13]. Although slowing of NCV is common in diabetes and often occurs early in the course of the disease, there is considerable uncertainty as to the relevance of these abnormalities to the future development of either subclinical manifestations or clinically apparent DN. Although symptomatic patients are more likely to have slower NCVs than patients without symptoms [13,14], NCV does not appear to be related to the severity of symptoms [15]. Symptoms referable to one fiber tract may not relate to those of other tracts. Progressive reduction of VPT and loss of DTR, characteristics of which implies large nerve fiber damage have been observed in patients who at the same time reported an improvement in pain symptoms.

Symmetrical neuropathies of the sensory and autonomic nervous systems affect an increasing proportion of diabetic patients as their disease progresses [16,17]. The incidence and severity of neuropathy are increased by poor control of glycemia [16,18], indicating that excess glucose may be the biochemical trigger in pathogenesis. Characteristic morphological changes are aspects of primary segmental demyelination of long axons, axonal degeneration, decreased density of small unmyelinated fibers, paranodal anarchic regeneration processes and Wallerian degeneration. After 20 years of diabetes, the cumulative incidence of neuropathy may be as high as 50% of the T1DM population [19]. Although symptomatic somatic sensorimotor neuropathy usually precedes the development of symptomatic autonomic neuropathy, signs of parasympathetic autonomic neuropathy sometimes appear before other signs of neuropathy. Although the relationship with sensorimotor neuropathy is variable, autonomic and sensory motor abnormalities usually coexist. Of people with DPN, 50% have asymptomatic autonomic neuropathy. When symptoms of autonomic neuropathy are present, the anticipated mortality rate is 15% to 40% within five years [20].

One might therefore ask whether DN is a condition which predisposes to clinical endpoints such as foot ulceration and amputation, in which case QST should suffice, or if it is a condition in which neurological function differs from that in a healthy population, in which case diagnosis may require a more detailed assessment. There is still considerable uncertainty as to the relevance of the abnormalities found in patients with T2DM to the future development of either clinical manifestation of foot ulceration and amputation, or mortality associated with DN. Nevertheless, there is accumulating evidence to suggest that not only surrogate markers of microangiopathy such as albuminuria, but also those used for polyneuropathy such as NCV and VPT may predict mortality in diabetic patients [19], but clearly further studies are needed to assess the prognostic role of polyneuropathy in diabetes. In diabetic patients with ultimate clinical endpoints of neuropathy such as foot ulcers, the risk of death was increased to 12 per 100 person-years of follow-up, compared to 5 per 100 person-years in those without foot ulcers [21].

HYPERGLYCEMIA AS A CRUCIAL CAUSE OF DIABETIC NEUROPATHY

Both T1DM and T2DM are characterized by a slow progression towards the generation of some specific lesions of the blood vessels affecting both small (microangiopathy) and larger (macroangiopathy) vessels. The classical microvascular complications of diabetes are diabetic retinopathy (the main cause of blindness in adults), diabetic renal disease representing currently the main cause of renal substitution therapy (dialysis or renal transplantation) in developed countries, and DN, our main topic. Major epidemiological and interventional studies have shown that chronic hyperglycemia is the main contributor to diabetic tissue damage in these complications, especially in microangiopathy [22,23]. By the same token, the main contributor to DPN development is the cumulative effect of chronic hyperglycemia – duration of diabetes and level of metabolic control. Increasing evidence suggests that consequent oxidative stress and endothelial dysfunction may be the key mediators of the deleterious effects of hyperglycemia. If hyperglycemia remains the main risk factor for the development of diabetic chronic complications, an important contribution can be attributed to genetic risk factors, some of them being common to all microvascular complications (diabetic retinopathy, DN, and renal disease) and some being specific for each of them. Additional factors are represented by some accelerators, such as hemodynamic (hypertension) and metabolic (insulin resistance, dyslipidemia) components.

However, despite the substantial progresses which have been made in unveiling the epidemiologic associations characterizing the natural history of DPN, the molecular pathogenesis and development mechanisms are still incompletely understood. Current data suggest that DPN results from the damage of the vasa nervorum (microvessels responsible for the irrigation of neural tissue) suggesting the role of microangiopathy, associated with the direct damage of neuronal components. Both are the result of the interaction between metabolic (chronic hyperglycemia, dyslipidemia, oxidative stress), hemodynamic/ischemic (microangiopathy of the nerve blood vessels) factors and impairment of the nerve fiber repair mechanisms [24]. The vascular and metabolic mechanisms act simultaneously and have an additive

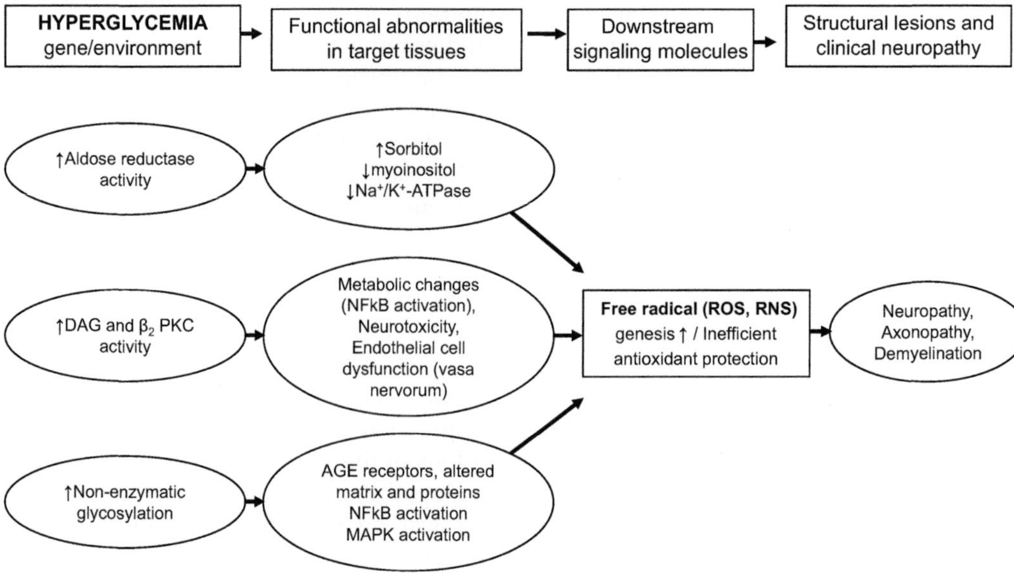

FIGURE 1.2 **How chronic hyperglycemia may lead to diabetic neuropathy.**

effect. The presence of neuronal microangiopathy is the main reason for considering DPN as one of the chronic microvascular complications of diabetes.

As the primary crucial factor, the persistent hyperglycemia (duration of diabetes and level of metabolic control) is the main contributor to the DPN development [16,22,23,25]. Chronic hyperglycemia contributes to the development of DPN by the same mechanism involved in all other diabetic microvascular complications. A unifying mechanism was proposed by Brownlee et al., suggesting that the key element is the hyperglycemia induced overproduction of superoxide (O_2^-) anions by the mitochondrial electron transport chain during the process of oxidative phosphorylation [26,27]. It was postulated that hyperglycemia induces increased mitochondrial production of reactive oxygen species (ROS) followed by nuclear DNA strand breaks that, in turn, activate the enzyme poly ADP-ribose polymerase and may associate with and lead to a cascade of processes that finally activate four major pathways of diabetic complications (Figure 1.2). These pathways are as follows:

(1) Increased aldose reductase activity and activation of the polyol pathway leading to increased sorbitol accumulation with osmotic effects, including neuronal edema, impaired nerve conduction and, finally, apoptosis [24]. Persistent hyperglycemia increases polyol pathway activity with accumulation of sorbitol and fructose in nerves, damaging them by as yet unknown mechanisms in real sense. This is accompanied by decreased myoinositol uptake and inhibition of Na^+/K^+-adenosine triphosphatase (ATPase) activity, resulting in Na^+ retention, edema, myelin swelling, axoglial dysjunction and nerve degeneration.

(2) Activation of protein kinase C (PKC) with subsequent activation of the NF-κB pathway. Hyperglycemia is known to stimulate the formation of diacylglycerol, which leads to the activation of PKC [25]. PKC then activates the transcription factor NF-κB, which is responsible for the modification the expression of many genes [28]. NF-κB is a transcription factor that is activated by a number of stimuli and is responsible for initiating the transcription of a number of different inflammatory and immune mediators.

(3) Intracellular advanced glycation end product (AGE) generation [26]. AGEs are a heterogeneous group of molecules formed from the non-enzymatic reaction of reducing sugars with free amino groups of proteins, lipids, and nucleic acids. Hyperglycemia induces a non-enzymatic glycation of proteins and AGEs which in turn activate NF-κB. Local generation of superoxide also occurs by the interaction of the residues of L-lysine (and probably other amino acids) of the protein with α-ketoaldehydes, and results in oxidative modification of proteins and other biomolecules. Non-enzymatic superoxide generation might be an element of the autocatalytic intensification of the pathophysiological action of carbonyl stress. Glycation of cytoskeletal proteins through structural or functional changes of the nerve fibers has also been involved in the pathogenesis of DN.

(4) Activation of the hexosamine pathway [26].

As for DPN, several studies have shown that enhanced oxidative stress in peripheral nerves and vasa nervorum leads to neural dysfunction and impaired neurotrophic support, as well as characteristic neuropathic morphologic nerve alterations [29]. Most morphological, histological and electrophysiological studies show that DN is accompanied by nerve structural changes (characteristic segmental demyelination and axonal degeneration) and functional changes (assessed by NCV) in diabetic patients [30]. Since glucose uptake by the Schwann cells of nerves is independent of insulin, glucose enters and accumulates in neurons initiating the aldose reductase pathway. This metabolic pathway leads to the accumulation of sorbitol and fructose, to the depletion of myo-inositol, and compromises the glutathion cycle and Na^+/K^+-ATPase activity. However, although inhibitors of aldose reductase act very efficiently on functional impairment due to diabetes in rats, they are much less efficient in diabetic patients. The difference is probably related to the relative importance of the polyol pathway in rodents compared to humans.

Excess glucose in neurons is responsible for the increase of oxidative stress by a combination of free radical genesis and inefficient antioxidant protection systems. Most ROS (O_2^-, OH, H_2O_2) produced by the mitochondrial respiratory chain, NADPH oxidase and xanthine reductase, as well as reactive species of nitrogen (nitric oxide NO, peroxynitrite, $ONOO^-$) produced by the NO synthesis enzyme NO-synthase, have been shown to be involved in the development of DPN in streptozotocin (STZ)-treated rats [31]. In these rats it was shown that free radicals exerted their deleterious effects on Schwann cells as well as on neuronal cells. Chain reactions of ROS are always neutralized by superoxide dismutase (SOD), catalase and glutathione peroxidase, the tissue levels of which are not enough to circumvent increased oxidative stress in diabetic patients [31,32].

Apart from the major role of hyperglycemia, additional risk factors for DPN are represented by increasing age, alcohol consumption or other drug abuse and classic cardiovascular risk factors including hypertension, dyslipidemia, obesity, cigarette smoking and albuminuria [25]. In addition, genetic susceptibility has an important contribution in determining the global risk for DPN. Moreover, several cardiovascular risk factors reported to be associated with DPN are also markers of insulin resistance. The potential link between insulin resistance and diabetic microvascular complications including DPN is their association with oxidative stress and endothelial dysfunction. Furthermore, one of the most important links between the metabolic and vascular mechanisms of DPN was reported to be the depletion of nitric oxide and failure of antioxidant protection, both resulting in increased oxidative stress [24,28,33].

In summary, the incidence and severity of neuropathy are increased by poor control of glycemia, indicating that excess glucose may be the biochemical trigger in pathogenesis. Damage of the vasa nervorum as well as that of neurons resulting from metabolic and vascular mechanisms cause DN. Therefore, the pathology of neuropathies is multifocal, with changes in axons, Schwann cells, microvascular elements in the endoneurium, and extracellular matrix [16,30,32,34]. However, there is generic component of these events, as the change in the phenotype of each of the above cells is induced by hyperglycemia. Thus, a critical feature of the etiology of neuropathies is the mechanism by which raised extracellular glucose alters the pattern of gene expression that constitutes the cell phenotype. The effects of glucose may be primary or secondary; via the polyol pathway, oxidative stress, protein glycation, or other unidentified consequences of hyperglycemia [24,26,27,29,31,32]. As a unifying mechanism, increase oxidative stress might be an important mediator representing the influence of hyperglycemia on the development of DN.

OXIDATIVE STRESS AND DIABETIC NEUROPATHY

Numerous population studies of diabetes and its long-term complications support the idea that there is an association between diabetes and oxidative stress [4,7,30,31]. However, it is less certain whether oxidative stress contributes to the development of long-term complications, or merely reflects associated processes that are affected by diabetes. In any case, DN, one of chronic microvascular's complications, is among the complications recognized to be associated with increased oxidative stress. An increase in oxidative stress may occur because of either an increase in free radical production, or a reduction in antioxidant defenses [31,32,35]. There are many hypotheses regarding the origins of oxidative stress in diabetes, beside the inevitable oxidative phosphorylation, including free radical accumulation related to glycation of proteins [26], consumption of NADPH through the polyol pathway [24,36], glucose autoxidation [37], hyperglycemia-induced pseudohypoxia [38], or activation of PKC [25,28,39]. Monocytes found in patients with diabetes also have an increased capacity to produce superoxide anion [40]. In addition, SOD, which has the important role of neutralizing superoxide radicals, is reduced in peripheral nerve tissue in diabetes patients, thus aggravating any enhancement of free radical formation [35]. Although several pathways contribute to the development of DN, including increased activation of the polyol pathway, oxidative stress, AGE formation, nerve hypoxia/ischemia, protein kinase C and reduction of nerve growth factor support (Figure 1.2, Figure 1.3), oxidative stress is the main important underlying factor which is found in various tissues under diabetic conditions, and is involved in the development of this diabetic complication.

The potential for a pivotal role for oxidative stress in the etiology of DN was indicated some time ago from differences in functional changes, or from phenotype measures associated with antioxidant treatment [41,42]. Therefore,

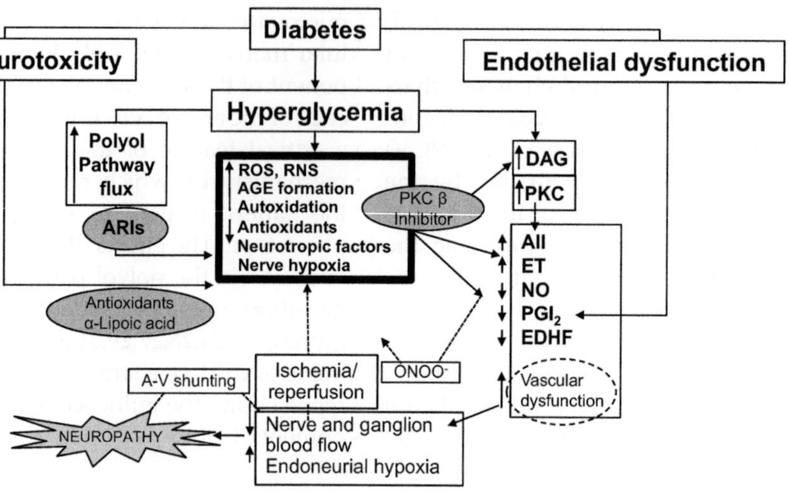

FIGURE 1.3 **Therapeutic interventions for diabetic neuropathy based on pathogenetic mechanisms.**

the alteration in cellular phenotype oxidative stress induces is certainly a feature of these neuropathies and may be the critical stage in this complication. Activation of the mitogen-activated protein kinases (MAPK) offers a link between these events [43]. All three groups of MAPK can be activated by osmotic perturbations derived from glucose itself or from the polyol pathway, by oxidative stress, and AGE via the receptors for AGE (RAGE) [32,43–45].

There are several sources of ROS in cells; such as high glucose, hypoxia and AGEs. Neuropathy is especially characterized by an activation of MAPK in different neuronal and Schwann cells induced by overproduction of ROS, which then leads to mitochondrial dysfunction, neuronal damage, and finally apoptosis of these cells. Under diabetic conditions, endoplasmic reticulum (ER) stress is also increased in various tissues including neuronal cells [45,46]. The ER is another crucial place where oxidative stress is generated. Increased production of ROS and decreased antioxidant defense in DN has been reported. Actually, ER stress and oxidative stress are closely linked events, although the molecular pathways that couple these processes are poorly understood. Recent studies have raised the possibility that the ER also plays an important role in maintaining neurons in neuropathological situations [46,47]. Important roles for ER stress and ER stress-induced cell death have been demonstrated in various pathological situations, including brain ischemia and neurodegeneration [48], as well as in DN.

OXIDATIVE STRESS AND ANTIOXIDANT TREATMENT IN DIABETIC NEUROPATHY

There is no accepted consensus on the treatment of neurological abnormalities in patients with diabetes. No drugs have been widely approved for patients with DN. Pharmacological interventions aimed at normalizing plasma glucose and A1C level have remained a mainstay treatment for DN [22–25]. The involvement of chronic hyperglycemia in the development and aggravation of DN in humans has been confirmed by the DCCT performed on 1,441 patients followed during 6.5 years [22]. In this study, the prophylactic use of glycemic control reduced the progression of DN by 60%. Other viable pharmacological options are pain management (tricyclic antidepressants, serotonin or epinephrine reuptake inhibitors, α2δ ligands, antiepileptics, opioids) and anti-inflammatory drugs [49]. Although innovative treatment modalities (gene therapy, stem cell therapy, use of neurotrophic and growth factors) are under development, their introduction into routine clinical practice is likely to take some time [50]. Practically, neurotrophic factors, the proteins that promote the survival of specific neuronal populations, which could be used to promote the regeneration of peripheral nervous system have been developed and used on an experimental basis. Although symptomatic treatment always produces some temporary improvements, the etiology- and mechanism-oriented treatment of DN is still not available, because of the lack of precise knowledge about the pathophysiological mechanisms underlying neurological defects in T2DM (Figure 1.4).

However, it has been shown clearly that DN is a direct consequence of abnormal glucose turnover, mirroring improvements and deteriorations in glucose homeostasis. Chronic hyperglycemia in T2DM leads to up to a four-fold increase in the neuronal glucose level which cannot be neutralized by anaerobic and glycolytic burst. Glucose neurotoxicity develops due to the unique oxidative biochemistry of glucose, leading to accumulation of free radicals in the neuronal tissue via non-enzymatic, enzymatic and mitochondrial mechanisms [51]. Hyperglycemia promotes the formation of superoxide through

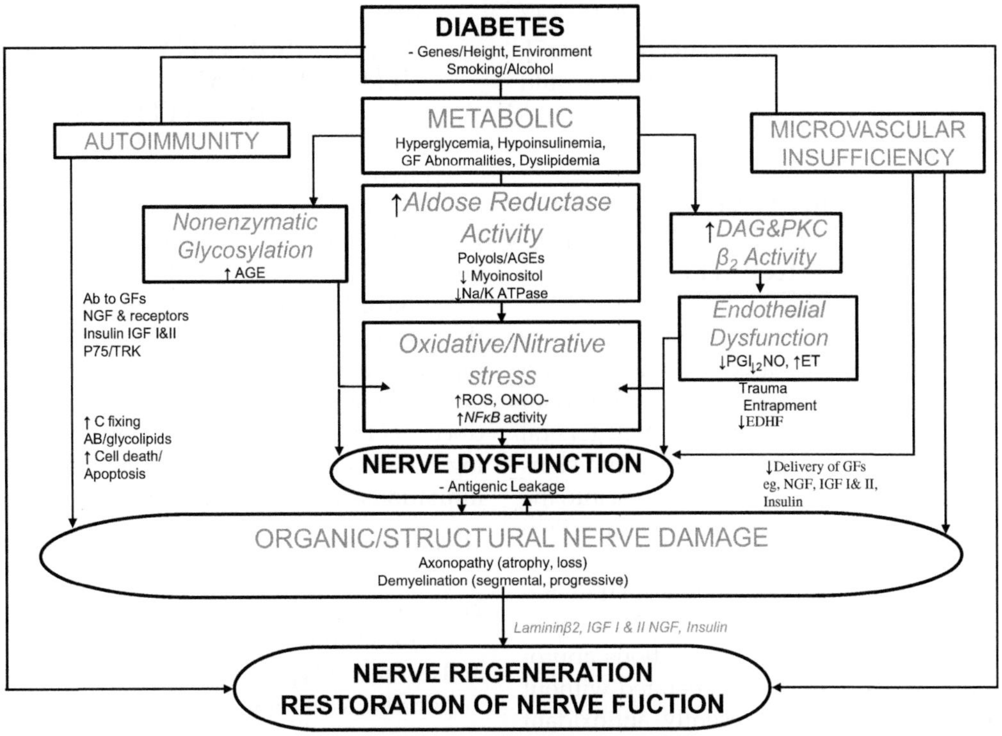

FIGURE 1.4 Theoretic framework for the pathogenesis and treatment of diabetic neuropathy.

the polyol pathway, which is accompanied by the nonenzymatic generation of Amadori products and subsequent formation of AGEs [24,26,36]. Moreover, ROS have been shown to be generated in the nitric oxide synthase, NADPH oxidase and xanthine oxidase systems [31]. It is now believed that oxidative damage is a primary pathogenetic mechanism causing impaired axonal transport, structural breakdown of Schwann cells and subsequent abnormalities in the propagation of action potentials [32,34,45,46]. Thanks to advances in the understanding of the mechanisms of oxidative stress in the development of DN, it may become feasible to target oxidative stress by applying various forms of medicine with antioxidant properties [52–56] (Figure 1.4). This leads to an important novel strategy in the treatment of DN. The recently published multicenter randomized double blind parallel trial, Neurological Assessment of Thioctic Acid in Diabetic Neuropathy (NATHAN) 1, which involved 460 patients with mild to moderate DSP is a good example. Four year treatment with α-lipoic acid (®thioctic acid) appeared to improve neurological function, as evaluated by seven nerve function tests in patients with DN [55]. Although α-lipoic acid treatment did not affect NCV directly in patients with T2DM, the Neuropathy Impairment Score of the lower limbs was improved in the α-lipoic acid treatment group and worsened in the placebo group. Similar improvements in neurological functions were also shown on a smaller scale in comparable clinical settings [56] and animal studies [57,58], recently. In spite of several limitations, the results of the NATHAN 1 trial represent the first systematic and crucial evidence that reveals the therapeutic effect of an antioxidant on DN at the clinical level. Since several prior trials looking for clinically measurable effects of antioxidants in different clinical settings have failed for decades, α-lipoic acid has proved to be an orthomolecular medicine with extremely potent free radical scavenging capabilities [59]. Besides reducing lipid peroxidation, α-lipoic acid has been shown to normalize microcirculation and insulin sensitivity, enhance endogenous SOD, reduce ischemia-reperfusion syndrome and prevent apoptosis [60]. The implications of the NATHAN 1 trial go far beyond the therapeutic use of α-lipoic acid in diabetes care. It has been shown recently that the effect of α-lipoic acid in DN can be enhanced by other antioxidants, in particular SOD [61]. It is plausible to assume that the effect of α-lipoic acid is unlikely to be caused by its particular chemical nature, but is rather related to the antioxidant properties of the compound.

In addition, many other nutrients (resveratrol, lycopene, soy isoflavones) with antioxidant properties have been shown in both *in vitro* and *in vivo* systems to have a significant positive influence on this complication of T2DM [62]. New clinical trials along with NATHAN 1 may unveil the possible benefits of antioxidant use in T2DM. However, there will be multiple challenges to clinical use of these nutrients with antioxidant properties. Unlike α-lipoic acid, many of them are susceptible to auto-oxidation [63], have limited absorption [64] and/or can be rapidly metabolized by the gut microbiota [65]. Therefore, stabilized formulations of antioxidants would be required for new clinical research trials.

THERAPEUTIC POTENTIAL OF A NEW ANTIOXIDANT PROTEIN DELIVERY IN DIABETIC NEUROPATHY

Since diabetes and/or its long-term complications have been shown to associate with increased oxidative stress, a different way of delivering medicines having antioxidant properties has also been studied. If antioxidants in general are to improve the pathophysiology, symptoms and signs of DN, steady delivery at required concentrations into the cells or into the cellular compartment which generates ROS would be most important. As already mentioned above, developments in the experimental and clinical strategies for treatment of DN would become possible if the antioxidant could be given in cellular concentrations appropriate to tackle ROS levels as they are generated without significant toxicity [45,66–68]. Until recently, antioxidant therapy has been extensively explored for the prevention and treatment of DN, but the results have been inconsistent because of factors such as the difficulty in maintaining a consistent circulating antioxidant level, inadequate tissue distribution, and lack of suitable exogenous antioxidants. Therefore, a strategy to induce an endogenous and nonspecific antioxidant, or to deliver one in a more efficient way could be a more effective approach. As diabetic complications may result from oxidative stress in various tissues and organs (including neuronal tissues) due to glucotoxicity, hypoxia, and AGE accumulation, endogenous nonspecific antioxidant treatment may improve tissue repair (neuronal repair) in patients with T2DM (especially DN), nonspecific antioxidants such as metallothionein (MT), SOD and catalase have been exploited as a possible way to combat increased ROS in various (neuronal) tissues, by applying intracellular delivery [45,66]. Taking advantage of the recently developed cell-penetrating peptide technologies [67,68], it was seen that each of the antioxidants and their combinations inhibited various oxidative stresses and had the potential to protect cells and tissues against diabetes and diabetic complications due to their anti-apoptotic and antioxidant effects, either *in vitro* or *in vivo*. Tat-MT and Tat-SOD given in combination intraperitoneally at regular intervals were protective against various injuries, and protected against attenuation of NCV under diabetic condition in OLETF rats [45]. This result is in accordance with other reports [69], wherein a similar delay in reduction of motor NCV by antioxidant in streptozotocin-induced diabetic rats is reported. Moreover, Tat-MT and Tat-SOD decreased ER stress-induced apoptosis against various injuries.

FROM EXPERIMENTAL EVIDENCE OF NEUROPATHY IN ANIMALS TO THE TREATMENT OF DIABETIC NEUROPATHY IN MAN

Although DN is a common clinical complication of diabetes mellitus, the exact neurological impairment is insufficiently understood and treatments are still empirical and inefficient. Rodent models as a surrogate for clinical DN offer a powerful tool for understanding the mechanisms of diabetes-mediated peripheral nerve injury. The majority of studies which have investigated DN in rodents used the STZ-induced rat, which reproduces metabolic lesions and may share the same pathologic mechanisms as T1DM in man. There are some limitations on the clinical relevance of this model due to:

1) A high prevalence of T2DM compared to T1DM in man,
2) The important alteration of the general clinical state of the animals, and
3) The lack of typical morphological changes in peripheral nerves.

However, many studies performed with the STZ-induced rat model have contributed to a better pathophysiological and pharmacological understanding of DPN. As a surrogate model for T2DM, OLETF rats are also frequently used.

Until recently, the exact pathogenetic mechanisms of sensory neuropathy in man have remained unproven, although several explanations have arisen from experimental works in diabetic rats. Several mechanisms underlying glucotoxicity in peripheral nerve fibers have been proposed, including an enzymatic mechanism involving the polyol pathway, protein glycation and expression of advanced glycation end product receptors, as well as oxidative stress. Treatment of STZ rats with antioxidants not only prevents or suppresses functional impairment [70] but also pain-related behaviors [71]. Conversely, treatment of healthy rats with a pro-oxidant agent (premaquine) induces functional changes similar to those observed after the induction of diabetes [72]. Some signaling pathways involving MAPK were found to be activated in sensory neurons exposed to increased glucose *in vitro* and *in vivo* in rats before the studies in humans with diabetes [43].

Although extensive accumulation of AGEs has been described in peripheral nerves of diabetic patients [73], the functional effects of AGE deposition and AGE-mediated cellular signaling on neuronal dysfunction in man have not been defined. Based on studies in the STZ-induced rat model, neuronal dysfunction was found to be closely associated with activation of NF-κB [74] and expression of proinflammatory cytokines including IL-6 and TNF-α [74,75]. Antioxidants which suppress activation of NF-κB *in vitro* [76] and in diabetic animals *in vivo* [77] attenuate symptoms in somatic and autonomous neuropathies and ameliorate blood flow in man [78,79]. The ligation of the RAGE with various ligands including AGEs results in sustained activation of NF-κB [80], and the RAGE-ligand interaction might contribute to neuronal dysfunction and, ultimately to clinical neuropathy. As an initial signaling molecule, hyperglycemia-induced overproduction of mitochondrial superoxide would result in AGE formation [81,82]. A two hour period of hyperglycemia would be sufficient to form intracellular AGEs and activate NF-κB and subsequent NF-κB-dependent gene expression in mononuclear blood cells [83]. Expression of the RAGE itself increases in an environment rich in RAGE ligands, especially AGEs [84]. As the blood-nerve barrier displays increased permeability to glycated species [85], AGE-modified adducts formed in the periphery, outside of as well as in the nerve itself have easy access to the vasculature (such as the vasa nervorum) and neurons, potentially causing vascular and neuronal dysfunction, respectively. The impact of the RAGE-mediated activation of NF-κB was revealed in neuronal dysfunction in human sural nerve biopsies and animal models of diabetes in which the RAGE gene was deleted [86].

CONCLUSION

We have reviewed the basic pathophysiology of DN thoroughly from the epidemiology to the treatment, with special emphasis on the role of oxidative stress. In patients with DN, the most frequent clinical form is diabetic DSP or sensorimotor polyneuropathy, affecting 30% of community-based people with diabetes. Sensory polyneuropathy presents a typical distribution 'in glove and stocking', and can sometimes be asymptomatic but usually causes abnormal sensations (paresthesia and dysesthesia) and/or pain. The longest fibers are first affected, which explains the distal distribution. Neuropathy occurs in both T1DM and T2DM, suggesting that hyperglycemia is the primary etiological factor. DN might be a direct consequence of abnormal glucose turnover resulting from protean diurnal changes in glucose homeostasis found in patients with diabetes. A number of mechanisms, which include increased activation of the polyol pathway, oxidative stress, AGE formation, nerve hypoxia/ischemia, protein kinase C and reduction of nerve growth factor support, have been proposed to link chronic hyperglycemia to the development of DN. As a central integrative mechanism, overproduction of ROS in peripheral nerves leads to oxidative stress, mitochondrial dysfunction, neuronal damage and finally apoptosis. That is to say that DN might result from oxidative stress in neuronal and endoneurial tissues due to glucotoxicity, hypoxia, and AGE accumulation. Oxidative stress would explain an increase in substrate for AGEs, an increase in precursors for glycoxidation and lipoxidation products, and an acceleration of the free radical formation that may be accompanied or caused by a deficiency of antioxidant and detoxification pathways. Oxidative stress is accompanied by the activation of the NF-κB, and then MAPK in Schwann cells as well as in neurons, which will lead to the activation of various inflammatory cytokines. Oxidative stress is found in various tissues under diabetic conditions, and is involved in the development of diabetic complications. Therefore, antioxidant treatment delivered in a proper way may improve neuronal repair in patients with DN.

SUMMARY POINTS

- Diabetic neuropathy is a serious and popular complication found in both type 1 and type 2 diabetes mellitus.
- Diabetic patients with neuropathy often have foot ulcers as ultimate clinical endpoints, and the risk of death also increases significantly. Therefore, surrogate markers of polyneuropathy may predict mortality in diabetic patients.
- The incidence and severity of diabetic neuropathy are increased by poor control of glycemia, indicating that excess glucose may be the biochemical trigger in pathogenesis.
- Increased oxidative stress might be an important mediator representing the influence of hyperglycemia to the development of diabetic neuropathy.
- Antioxidant treatment in a proper way may improve neuronal repair in patients with diabetic neuropathy.

Acknowledgments

This research was supported by the Basic Science Research Program through the National Research Foundation of Korea (NRF) funded by the Ministry of Education, Science and Technology (2010–0010898) and the Korea Health 21 R&D Project, Ministry of Health and Welfare, Republic of Korea (A102065–1011–1070100).

References

[1] Statement C. Report and recommendations of the San Antonio Conference on diabetic neuropathy. Diabetes Care 1988;37:1000–4.

[2] The Diabetes Control and Complications Trial Research Group. The effect of intensive diabetes therapy on the development and progression of diabetic neuropathy. Ann Intern Med 1995;122:561–8.

[3] Dyck PJ, Dyck PJB, Velosa JA, Larson TS, O'Brien PC and The Nerve Growth Factor Study Group. Patterns of quantitative sensation testing of hypoesthesia and hyperalgesia are predictive of diabetic polyneuropathy. A study of three cohorts. Diabetes Care 2000;23:510–7.

[4] Vincent AM, Callaghan BC, Smith AL, Feldman EL. Diabetic neuropathy: cellular mechanisms as therapeutic targets. Nat Rev Neurol 2011;7:573–83.

[5] Basić-Kes V, Zavoreo I, Rotim K, Bornstein N, Rundek T, Demarin V. Recommendations for diabetic polyneuropathy treatment. Acta Clin Croat 2011;50:289–302.
[6] Fedele D, Comi G, Coscelli C, Cucinotta D, Feldman EL, Ghirlanda G, et al. A multicenter study on the prevalence of diabetic neuropathy in Italy. Italian Diabetic Neuropathy Committee. Diabetes Care 1997;20:836–43.
[7] Tesfaye S, Stevens LK, Stephenson JM, Fuller JH, Plater M, Ionescu-Tirgoviste C, et al. Prevalence of diabetic peripheral neuropathy and its relation to glycemic control and potential risk factors: the EURODIAB IDDM Complications study. Diabetologia 1996;39:1377–84.
[8] Dyck PJ, Kratz KM, Karnes JL, Litchy WJ, Klein R, Pach JM, et al. The prevalence by staged severity of various types of diabetic neuropathy, retinopathy, and nephropathy in a population-based cohort: the Rochester Diabetic Neuropathy Study. Neurology 1993;43:817–24.
[9] Archer AG, Watkins PJ, Thomas PK, Sharma AK, Payan J. The natural history of acute painful neuropathy in diabetes mellitus. J Neurol Neurosurg Psychiatry 1983;46:491–9.
[10] Fraser DM, Campbell IW, Ewing DJ, Murray A, Neilson JM, Clarke BF. Peripheral and autonomic nerve function in newly diagnosed diabetes mellitus. Diabetes 1997;26:546–50.
[11] Ward JD, Barnes CG, Fisher DJ, Jessop JD, Baker RW. Improvement in nerve conduction following treatment in newly diagnosed diabetics. Lancet 1971;1:428–30.
[12] Gregersen G. Diabetic neuropathy: influence of age, sex, metabolic control, and duration of diabetes on motor conduction velocity. Neurology 1867;17:972–80.
[13] Lamontagne A, Buchthal F. Electrophysiological studies in diabetic neuropathy. J Neurol Neurosurg Psychiatry 1970;33: 442–52.
[14] Boulton AJ, Knight G, Drury J, Ward JD. The prevalence of symptomatic diabetic neuropathy in an insulin-treated population. Diabetes Care 1985;8:125–8.
[15] Mayne N. The short-term prognosis in diabetic neuropathy. Diabetes 1968;17:270–3.
[16] Vinik AI, Park TS, Stansberry K, Pittenger GL. Diabetic neuropathies. Diabetologia 2000;43:957–73.
[17] Feldman EL, Stevens MJ, Russell JW. Diabetic peripheral and autonomic neuropathy. In: Sperling MA, editor. Contemporary endocrinology. Totowa, NJ: Humana Press; 2002. p. 437–61.
[18] Coppini DV, Bowtell PA, Weng C, Young PJ, Sonksen PH. Showing neuropathy is related to increased mortality in diabetic patients – a survival analysis using an accelerated failure time model. J Clin Epidemiol 2000;53:519–23.
[19] Thomas PK. Diabetic peripheral neuropathies: Their cost to patient and society and the value of knowledge of risk factors for development of interventions. Eur Neurol 1999;41:35–43.
[20] Ewing DJ, Campbell IW, Clarke BF. Mortality in diabetic autonomic neuropathy. Lancet 1976;1:601–3.
[21] Boyko EJ, Ahroni JH, Smith DG, Davignon D. Increased mortality associated with diabetic foot ulcer. Diabet Med 1996;13:967–72.
[22] DCCT Research Group. The effect of intensive treatment of diabetes on the development and progression of long-term complications in insulin-dependent diabetes mellitus. The Diabetes Control and Complications Trial Research Group. N Engl J Med 1993;329:977–86.
[23] UK Prospective Diabetes Study (UKPDS) Group. Intensive blood glucose control with sulphonylureas or insulin compared with conventional treatment and risk of complications in patients with type 2 diabetes (UKPDS 33). Lancet 1998;352:837–53.
[24] Boulton AJ. Diabetic neuropathy: classification, measurement and treatment. Curr Opin Endocrinol Diabetes Obes 2007;14:141–5.
[25] Tesfaye S, Chaturvedi N, Eaton SE, Ward JD, Manes C, Ionescu-Tirgoviste Cand EURODIAB Prospective Complications Study Group, et al. Vascular risk factors and diabetic neuropathy. N Engl J Med 2005;352:341–50.
[26] Brownlee M. The pathobiology of diabetic complications. An unifying mechanism. Diabetes 2005;54:1615–25.
[27] Nishikawa T, Edelstein D, Du XL, Yamagishi S, Matsumura T, Kaneda Y, et al. Normalizing mitochondrial superoxide production blocks three pathways of hyperglycaemic damage. Nature 2000;404:787–90.
[28] Cameron NE, Cotter MA. Pro-inflammatory mechanisms in diabetic neuropathy: focus on the nuclear factor kappa B pathway. Curr Drug Targets 2008;9:60–7.
[29] Hounsom L, Corder R, Patel J, Tomlinson DR. Oxidative stress participates in the breakdown of neuronal phenotype in experimental diabetic neuropathy. Diabetologia 2001;44:424–8.
[30] Said G. Diabetic neuropathy – a review. Nat Clin Pract Neurol 2007;3:331–40.
[31] Vincent AM, Russell JW, Low P, Feldman EL. Oxidative stress in the pathogenesis of diabetic neuropathy. Endocr Rev 2004;25:612–28.
[32] Bierhaus A, Haslbeck KM, Humpert PM, Liliensiek B, Dehmer T, Morcos M, et al. Loss of pain perception in diabetes is dependent on a receptor of the immunoglobulin superfamily. J Clin Invest 2004;114:1741–51.
[33] Yamagishi S, Matsui T. Nitric oxide, a janus-faced therapeutic target for diabetic microangiopathy – Friend or foe? Pharmacol Res 2011;64:187–94.
[34] Dyck PJ, Giannini C. Pathologic alterations in the diabetic neuropathies of humans: a review. J Neuropathol Exp Neurol 1996;55:1181–93.
[35] Maxwell SR, Thomason H, Sandler D, Leguen C, Baxter MA, Thorpe GH, et al. Antioxidant status in patients with uncomplicated insulin-dependent and non-insulin-dependent diabetes mellitus. Eur J Invest 1997:27,484–90.
[36] Lee AY, Chung SS. Contributions of polyol pathway to oxidative stress in diabetic cataract. FASEB J 1999;13:23–30.
[37] Wolff SP, Dean RT. Glucose autoxidation and protein modification. The potential role of 'autoxidative glycosylation' in diabetes. Biochem J 1987;245:243–50.
[38] Williamson JR, Chang K, Frangos M, Hasan KS, Ido Y, Kawamura T, et al. Hyperglycemic pseudohypoxia and diabetic complications. Diabetes 1993;42:801–13.
[39] Koya D, King GL. Protein kinase C activation and the development of diabetic complications. Diabetes 1998;47:859–66.
[40] Nourooz-Zadeh J, Tajaddini-Sarmadi J, McCarthy S, Betteridge DJ, Wolff SP. Elevated levels of authentic plasma hydroperoxides in NIDDM. Diabetes 1995;44:1054–8.
[41] Karasu C, Dewhurst M, Stevens EJ, Tomlinson DR. Effects of antioxidant treatment on sciatic nerve dysfunction in streptozotocin-diabetic rats, comparison with essential fatty acids. Diabetologia 1995;38:129–34.
[42] Ziegler D. Current concepts in the management of diabetic polyneuropathy. Curr Diabetes Rev 2011;7:208–20.
[43] Purves T, Middlemas A, Agthong S, Jude E, Boulton A, Fernyhough P, et al. A role for mitogen-activated protein kinases in the etiology of diabetic neuropathy. FASEB J 2001;15:2508–14.
[44] Schiekofer S, Andrassy M, Chen J, Rudofsky G, Schneider J, Wendt T, et al. Acute hyperglycemia causes intracellular formation of CML and activation of ras, p42/44 MAPK, and nuclear factor kappaB in PBMCs. Diabetes 2003;52:621–33.
[45] Min D, Kim H, Park L, Kim TW, Hwang S, Kim MJ, et al. Improvement of diabetic neuropathy applying TAT-mediated enhanced delivery of metallothionein and SOD. Endocrinology 2012;153:81–91.

[46] Kaneto H, Matsuoka TA, Nakatani Y, Kawamori D, Miyatsuka T, Matsuhisa M, et al. Oxidative stress, ER stress, and the JNK pathway in type 2 diabetes. J Mol Med 2005;83:429–39.
[47] Takano K, Kitao Y, Tabata Y, Miura H, Sato K, Takuma K, et al. A dibenzoylmethane derivative protects dopaminergic neurons against both oxidative stress and endoplasmic reticulum stress. Am J Physiol Cell Physiol 2007;293:C1884–94.
[48] Bossy-Wetzel E, Schwarzenbacher R, Lipton SA. Molecular pathways to neurodegeneration. Nat Med 2004;10:S2–9.
[49] Smith HS, Argoff CE. Pharmacological treatment of diabetic neuropathic pain. Drugs 2011;71:557–89.
[50] Kim H, Kim JJ, Yoon YS. Emerging therapy for diabetic neuropathy: Cell therapy targeting vessels and nerves. Endocr Metab Immune Disord Drug Targets 2012;12:168–78.
[51] Tomlinson DR, Gardiner NJ. Glucose neurotoxicity. Nat Rev Neurosci 2008;9:36–45.
[52] Firuzi O, Miri R, Tavakkoli M, Saso L. Antioxidant therapy: current status and future prospects. Curr Med Chem 2011;18:3871–88.
[53] Miranda-Massari JR, Gonzalez MJ, Jimenez FJ, Allende-Vigo MZ, Duconge J. Metabolic correction in the management of diabetic peripheral neuropathy: improving clinical results beyond symptom control. Curr Clin Pharmacol 2011;6:260–73.
[54] Golbidi S, Badran M, Laher I. Diabetes and alpha lipoic Acid. Front Pharmacol 2011;2:69.
[55] Ziegler D, Low PA, Litchy WJ, Boulton AJ, Vinik AI, Freeman R, et al. Efficacy and safety of antioxidant treatment with α-lipoic acid over 4 years in diabetic polyneuropathy: the NATHAN 1 trial. Diabetes Care 2011;34:2054–60.
[56] Mijnhout GS, Kollen BJ, Alkhalaf A, Kleefstra N, Bilo HJG. Alpha lipoic Acid for symptomatic peripheral neuropathy in patients with diabetes: a meta-analysis of randomized controlled trials. Int J Endocrinol 2012;45:62–79.
[57] Morgado C, Pereira-Terra P, Tavares I. α-Lipoic acid normalizes nociceptive neuronal activity at the spinal cord of diabetic rats. Diabetes Obes Metab 2011;13:736–41.
[58] Skalská S, Kucera P, Goldenberg Z, Stefek M, Kyselová Z, Jariabka P, et al. Neuropathy in a rat model of mild diabetes induced by multiple low doses of streptozotocin: effects of the antioxidant stobadine in comparison with a high dose alpha-lipoic acid treatment. Gen Physiol Biophys 2010;29:50–8.
[59] Gorąca A, Huk-Kolega H, Piechota A, Kleniewska P, Ciejka E, Skibska B. Lipoic acid - biological activity and therapeutic potential. Pharmacol Rep 2011;63:849–58.
[60] Papanas N, Maltezos E. α-Lipoic acid, diabetic neuropathy, and Nathan's prophecy. Angiology 2012;63:81–3.
[61] Bertolotto F, Massone A. Combination of alpha lipoic acid and superoxide dismutase leads to physiological and symptomatic improvements in diabetic neuropathy. Drugs R D 2012;12:29–34.
[62] Golbidi S, Ebadi SA, Laher I. Antioxidants in the treatment of diabetes. Curr Diabetes Rev 2011;7:106–25.
[63] Xianquan S, Shi J, Kakuda Y, Yueming J. Stability of lycopene during food processing and storage. J Med Food 2005;8:413–22.
[64] Kwon DY, Daily 3rd JW, Kim HJ, Park S. Antidiabetic effects of fermented soybean products on type 2 diabetes. Nutr Res 2010;30:1–3.
[65] Selma MV, Espín JC, Tomás-Barberán FA. Interaction between phenolics and gut microbiota: role in human health. J Agric Food Chem 2009;57:6485–501.
[66] Park L, Min D, Kim H, Chung HY, Lee CH, Park IS, et al. TAT-enhanced delivery of metallothionein can partially prevent the development of diabetes. Free Radic Biol Med 2011;51:1666–74.
[67] Grdisa M. The delivery of biologically active (therapeutic) peptides and proteins into cells. Curr Med Chem 2011;18:1373–9.
[68] Johnson RM, Harrison SD, Maclean D. Therapeutic applications of cell-penetrating peptides. Methods Mol Biol 2011;683:535–51.
[69] Nakamura J, Hamada Y, Sakakibara F, Hara T, Wakao T, Mori K, et al. Physiological and morphometric analyses of neuropathy in sucrose-fed OLETF rats. Diabetes Res Clin Pract 2001;51:9–20.
[70] Cameron NE, Cotter MA, Maxfield EK. Anti-oxidant treatment prevents the development of peripheral nerve dysfunction in streptozotocin-diabetic rats. Diabetologia 1993;36:299–304.
[71] Jolivalt CG, Mizisin LM, Nelson A, Cunha JM, Ramos KM, Bonke D, et al. B vitamins alleviate indices of neuropathic pain in diabetic rats. Eur J Pharmacol 2009;612:41–7.
[72] Cameron NE, Cotter MA, Archibald V, Dines KC, Maxfield EK. Anti-oxidant and pro-oxidant effects on nerve conduction velocity, endoneurial blood flow and oxygen tension in non-diabetic and streptozotocin-diabetic rats. Diabetologia 1994;37:449–59.
[73] Vlassara H, Brownlee M, Cerami A. Nonenzymatic glycosylation of peripheral nerve protein in diabetes mellitus. Proc Natl Acad Sci USA 1981;78:5190–2.
[74] Mattson MP, Camandola S. NF-κB in neuronal plasticity and neurodegenerative disorders. J Clin Invest 2001;107:247–54.
[75] Okamoto K, Martin DP, Schmelzer JD, Mitsui Y, Low PA. Pro- and antiinflammatory cytokine gene expression in rat sciatic nerve chronic constriction injury model of neuropathic pain. Exp Neurol 2001;169:386–91.
[76] Bierhaus A, Chevion S, Chevion M, Hofmann M, Quehenberger P, Illmer T, et al. Advanced glycation end product-induced activation of NF-κB is suppressed by α-lipoic acid in cultured endothelial cells. Diabetes 1997;46:1481–90.
[77] Haak ES, Usadel KH, Kohleisen M, Yilmaz A, Kusterer K, Haak T. The effect of alpha-lipoic acid on the neurovascular reflex in patients with diabetic neuropathy assessed by capillary microscopy. Microvasc Res 1999;58:28–34.
[78] Ziegler D, Hanefeld M, Ruhnau KJ, Hasche H, Lobisch M, Schütte K, et al. Treatment of symptomatic diabetic polyneuropathy with the antioxidant alpha-lipoic acid: a 7-month multicenter randomized controlled trial (ALADIN III study). ALADIN III Study Group. Alpha-Lipoic Acid in Diabetic Neuropathy. Diabetes Care 1999;22:1296–301.
[79] Ametov AS, Barinov A, Dyck PJ, Hermann R, Kozlova N, Litchy WJ, et al. The sensory symptoms of diabetic polyneuropathy are improved with alpha-lipoic acid: the SYDNEY trial. Diabetes Care 2003;26:770–6.
[80] Bierhaus A, Schiekofer S, Schwaninger M, Andrassy M, Humpert PM, Chen J, et al. Diabetes-associated sustained activation of the transcription factor nuclear factor-κB. Diabetes 2001;50:2792–808.
[81] Nishikawa T, Edelstein D, Du XL, Yamagishi S, Matsumura T, Kaneda Y, et al. Normalizing mitochondrial superoxide production blocks three pathways of hyperglycemic damage. Nature 2000;404:787–90.
[82] Brownlee M. Biochemistry and molecular cell biology of diabetic complications. Nature 2001;414:813–20.
[83] Schiekofer S, Andrassy M, Chen J, Rudofsky G, Schneider J, Wendt T, et al. Acute (2h) hyperglycemic clamp causes intracellular formation of carboxymethyllysine, activation of Ras, p42/p44 MAPK and NF-κB in peripheral blood mononuclear cells. Diabetes 2003;52:621–33.
[84] Schmidt AM, Yan SD, Yan SF, Stern DM. The multiligand receptor RAGE is a progression factor amplifying immune and inflammatory responses. J Clin Invest 2001;108:949–55.
[85] Poduslo JF, Curran G. Increased permeability across the blood-nerve barrier of albumin glycated *in vitro* and *in vivo* from patients with diabetic polyneuropathy. Proc Natl Acad Sci USA 1992;89:2218–22.
[86] Constien R, Forde A, Liliensiek B, Gröne HJ, Nawroth P, Hämmerling G, et al. Characterization of a novel EGFP reporter mouse to monitor Cre recombination as demonstrated by a Tie2 Cre mouse line. Genesis 2001;30:36–44.

CHAPTER

2

Cerebral Ischemia in Diabetics and Oxidative Stress

Perry Fuchs, Miguel A. Perez-Pinzon*†*, Kunjan R. Dave**

*The Cerebral Vascular Disease Research Laboratories, Department of Neurology Leonard M. Miller School of Medicine, University of Miami, Miami, FL, USA, †Neuroscience Program, Department of Neurology Leonard M. Miller School of Medicine, University of Miami, Miami, FL, USA

List of Abbreviations

AGE Advanced glycation end products
ALS Amyotrophic Lateral Sclerosis
APE Apurinic/apyrimidinic endonuclease
ATP Adenosine-5'-triphosphate
CuZnSOD Copper-zinc superoxide dismutase
DHBA 2,5- and 2,3-dihydroxybenzoic acid
DNA Deoxyribonucleic acid
eNOS Endothelial nitric oxide synthase
FADH Reduced flavin adenine dinucleotide
HNE 4-hydroxynonenal
H_2O_2 Hydrogen peroxide
iNOS Inducible nitric oxide synthase
MDA Malondialdehyde
MnSOD Manganese mitochondrial superoxide dismutase
NAD^+ Nicotinamide adenine dinucleotide
NADH Reduced nicotinamide adenine dinucleotide
NADPH Reduced nicotinamide adenine dinucleotide phosphate
NF-κB Nuclear factor-κB
nNOS Neuronal nitric oxide synthase
NO Nitric oxide
NOS Nitric oxide synthase
OH· Hydroxyl radical
$ONOO^-$ Peroxynitrite
PARP Poly(ADP-ribose) polymerase
PDH Pyruvate dehydrogenase
RNS Reactive nitrogen species
ROS Reactive oxygen species
TCA Total antioxidant capacity
tPA Tissue plasminogen activator
USA United States of America

INTRODUCTION – DIABETES AND CEREBRAL ISCHEMIA

Diabetes mellitus is a chronic disease in which the body does not produce or properly utilize insulin, resulting in disturbed blood glucose balance in the body. The World Health Organization estimates that 347 million people have diabetes worldwide [1]. Long-term diabetes is often associated with secondary complications, including cerebral ischemia, heart disease, high blood pressure, blindness, kidney and nervous system diseases, dental disease, and complications of pregnancy, among others [2]. Cerebral ischemia and heart disease account for 84% of mortality among diabetics in the USA alone [3,4]. Epidemiological studies suggest that diabetes increases the risk of cerebral ischemia by 2–4 fold over non-diabetic populations, and also exacerbates cerebral ischemic damage [5–7]. These epidemiological studies are also confirmed in studies of experimental cerebral ischemia in animal models of diabetes [8–11]. Free radicals play an important role in cerebral ischemic damage in diabetics.

This chapter aims to provide an overview of the implications of free radicals for cerebral ischemia in diabetics. We first provide a brief overview of the roles of free radicals in pathophysiology, and then in oxidative stress generating pathways in diabetes. These pathways are not described in detail as they are covered by other chapters in this book. In the second part, we review the literature describing how oxidative stress participates in cerebral ischemia-induced cell death. Toward the end of this chapter we review how increased oxidative stress in diabetes exacerbates cerebral ischemic damage.

PATHOPHYSIOLOGICAL ROLES OF FREE RADICALS

Free radicals are atoms or groups of atoms that contain an unpaired electron in their valence shell. Reactive

Diabetes: Oxidative Stress and Dietary Antioxidants.
http://dx.doi.org/10.1016/B978-0-12-405885-9.00002-4

oxygen species (ROS) and reactive nitrogen species (RNS) are chemically reactive metabolites classified as free radicals owing to the presence of one unpaired electron in an oxygen atom and a nitrogen atom, respectively [12,13]. In biological systems, free radicals are produced naturally and are essential in certain cellular and homeostatic functions. The majority of ROS are produced during mitochondrial respiration. With an abundance of oxidation-reduction reactions occurring at each complex of the electron transport chain, individual electrons will occasionally diffuse from these complexes, and if one is accepted by molecular oxygen, it becomes the superoxide anion ($O_2{\cdot}^-$) [14]. $O_2{\cdot}^-$ serves as the precursor for almost all other ROS, which include hydrogen peroxide (H_2O_2), and the hydroxyl radical (OH·) [15]. Nitric oxide (NO·) is the foundation for most RNS, which include the highly oxidative free radical peroxynitrite ($ONOO^-$). More complex organisms have evolved ways to use these ROS and RNS as signaling molecules in a wide variety of physiological functions [16]. They serve integral roles in the normal functioning of cells by performing tasks that include signal transduction, defense against bacteria, and vasodilatation [16].

Antioxidants comprise a type of defense mechanism against free radicals, as they protect cells by behaving like scavengers of free radicals and thus neutralize their damaging oxidative capacity. The entire spectrum of antioxidants can be divided into two different classes based upon their mechanism of action. These are the enzyme antioxidants and the non-enzyme antioxidants. Enzyme antioxidants include superoxide dismutase, catalase, and glutathione peroxidase among others, which scavenge free radicals by converting them into less reactive molecules which later may be easily metabolized. Non-enzyme antioxidants cover a wider range of compounds, such as the antioxidant Vitamins A, C, and E and glutathione, which compete for oxidation by free radicals with other substrates in order to delay or inhibit the oxidation of molecules that should not otherwise undergo oxidation [16].

Normally, the cell's antioxidant defense system prevents oxidative damage by neutralizing free radicals effectively, and the resultant products are then metabolized by the complementary antioxidant enzymes. However, in numerous pathological states that include, but are not limited to, ALS, Parkinson's disease, Alzheimer's disease, certain cancers, heart attack, stroke, and diabetes, a variety of mechanisms lead to the overwhelming generation of free radicals, which causes saturation of the antioxidant defense system, and finally results in increased oxidative stress [17,18]. Below we provide mechanisms by which oxidative stress plays a role in diabetes and cerebral ischemia.

DIABETES AND FREE RADICALS

Hyperglycemia caused by diabetes mellitus (both type 1 and type 2) is a major cause of oxidative stress. Research has shown that there are numerous pathways by which hyperglycemia can lead to greater free radical production, and these include mitochondrial respiration, glucose autoxidation, activation of the polyol pathway, and the formation of advanced glycation end products. Below we provide a brief description of oxidative stress generating pathways in diabetes.

Larger amounts of NADH and FADH are produced in hyperglycemic conditions owing to glucose autoxidation. Because of this increased concentration of electron donors, the mitochondrial proton gradient is increased, resulting in leakage of electrons to facilitate the formation of superoxide radicals [19]. Hyperglycemia also results in a depletion of NADPH due to the increased rate of sorbitol synthesis via the polyol pathway. This depletion of NADPH impairs the rate of regeneration of reduced glutathione from oxidized glutathione, as NADPH is used as a co-factor in this reaction resulting in impaired cellular antioxidant capacity [19,20]. Advanced glycation end product (AGE) formation occurs during hyperglycemia. AGE formation is irreversible and is shown to promote ROS production by multiple mechanisms, including AGE-induced protein cross-linking, resulting in structural and functional alterations of proteins [19,20].

Besides hyperglycemia, hypoglycemia, which is a common side effect of glucose lowering drugs in either type 1 or type 2 diabetes mellitus patients, also increases oxidative stress. An earlier study reported that insulin-induced hypoglycemia in mice resulted in increased lipid peroxidation [21]. In an *in vitro* study, Liu et al. observed that glucose deprivation resulted in increased ROS production [22]. Hypoglycemia is shown to increase hydrogen peroxide production and decrease the activity of mitochondrial superoxide dismutase (MnSOD) [23]. Several other studies have also demonstrated increased oxidative stress following hypoglycemia in normal and diabetic conditions [21,24–26]. In a recent study we also observed that recurrent hypoglycemia results in increased mitochondrial ROS production [27]. The mechanisms by which hypoglycemia increases oxidative stress are not well explored. However, calcium-dependent pathways are suggested to play a role in hypoglycemia-induced ROS production [28]. It is also believed that imbalance between substrates and oxygen tension during hypoglycemia may be responsible for increased ROS production [29]. These studies suggest that hypoglycemia may also contribute to increased oxidative stress in diabetics.

Diabetes not only increases the rate of ROS production, but also lowers cellular antioxidant capacity. For example, earlier studies demonstrated impaired antioxidant capacity in brains of streptozotocin-diabetic rats [30]. Mooradian observed that streptozotocin-induced diabetes reduced the antioxidative potential of cerebral microvessels [31]. It should be noted that functioning of cerebral microvessels plays a crucial role in cerebral ischemic damage [32]. Overall, the literature suggests an imbalance between oxidative stress and antioxidant pathways leading to an increased oxidative stress in diabetics.

CEREBRAL ISCHEMIA

Cerebral ischemia, depending upon the amount of brain to which blood flow is interrupted, may be classified as focal, affecting only a portion of the brain, or global, affecting the entire brain. Cardiac arrest results in global cerebral ischemia, while stroke results in focal cerebral ischemia owing to interruption in cerebral blood flow in both cases. Approximately 87% of all stroke cases are ischemic, which is caused by an arterial blood clot in the brain [33]. Hemorrhagic stroke is caused by an arterial hemorrhage in the brain and accounts for 13% of all strokes (10% intracerebral hemorrhagic strokes, whereas 3% are subarachnoid hemorrhagic strokes) [34]. Cardiac arrest can result from numerous conditions such as ventricular fibrillation, cardiomyopathy, arrhythmias, coronary abnormalities, aortic rupture, and myocardial infarctions [35].

When cerebral blood flow is halted, the supply of both oxygen and glucose to the brain is also halted, and these events cause the initiation of many molecular cascades that may result in cell necrosis and/or apoptosis in ischemic tissues. There are various cell death pathways after cerebral ischemia that are both individually and concertedly damaging. However, one of the most important mechanisms of cerebral ischemic cell damage is the oxidative stress placed on cells through increased free radical production and suppression of the innate antioxidant defense [36] (Figure 2.1).

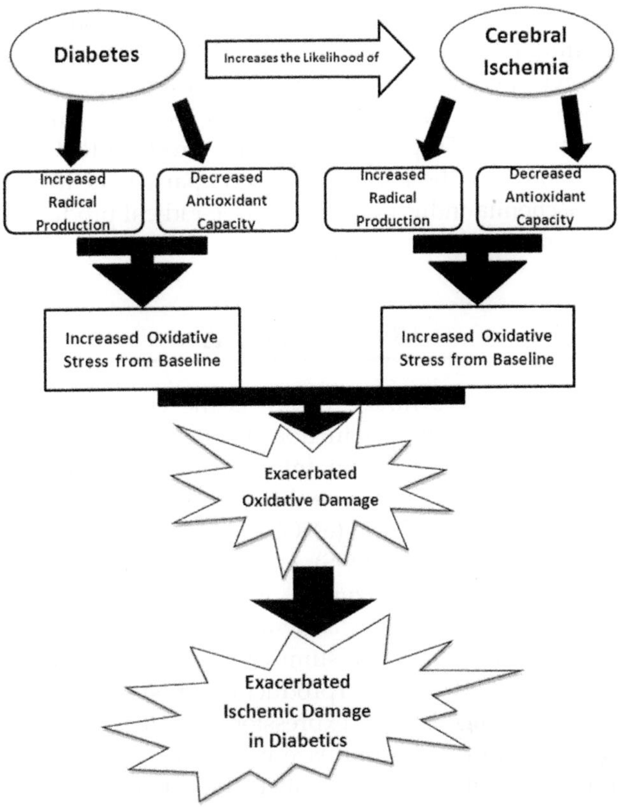

FIGURE 2.1 A summary of the causes of exacerbated ischemic damage in diabetics as pertaining to oxidative stress. In diabetes, literature has shown that there are increases in baseline radical production and decreases in antioxidant capacity that result in an overall increased level of oxidative stress. With a cerebral ischemic event, many studies have observed that the activation of many different cellular pathways results in increased radical production as well as inhibition of antioxidant defenses that also result in increased oxidative stress from baseline levels. We have surmised that these increases in oxidative stress are independent and additive in nature, and therefore, would lead to exacerbated oxidative damage and overall ischemic damage in diabetics over non-diabetics.

FREE RADICAL PRODUCTION DURING ISCHEMIA/REPERFUSION

The production of free radicals during stroke is the result of a sequence of events in the cycle of ischemia and reperfusion that begins as soon as brain cells start experiencing ischemia. After neurons can no longer produce ATP owing to lack of oxygen and glucose, the ATP-dependent ion channels are unable to function. This causes cellular membranes to depolarize and in turn causes an increase in intracellular calcium. This influx of calcium is associated with the excessive release of the neurotransmitter glutamate, which stimulates a greater influx of calcium into the cell, leading to even higher intracellular calcium levels [37]. These high levels of calcium in the cell have been shown to increase levels of ROS and RNS by the activation of numerous free radical production pathways during ischemia, both in cytosol and in the mitochondria. It has also been observed that there are calcium-independent pathways that lead to increased ROS production during both ischemia, and reperfusion.

In the cytosol, large amounts of intracellular calcium cause the activation of enzymes that stimulate pathways towards production of free radicals such as the calcium-dependent nitric oxide synthase (NOS) pathways, and also the dissociation and cellular uptake of iron. There are minor pathways (not discussed in this chapter) in the cytosol including the NADPH (reduced nicotinamide adenine dinucleotide) oxidase pathway and the cytochrome P450 pathway that also produce ROS. The ways in which these major pathways participate in cerebral ischemia-induced increased free radical production is summarized below.

NOS PATHWAY

Nitric oxide synthase (NOS) is the enzyme that is responsible for the production of nitric oxide in cells. NOS converts L-arginine into L-citrulline and nitric oxide (NO). There are three different isozymes of NOS, namely endothelial NOS (eNOS), inducible NOS (iNOS) and neuronal NOS (nNOS). eNOS and nNOS are both calcium-dependent enzymes, while iNOS is calcium independent. Following ischemia, the increased intracellular calcium levels stimulate calcium-dependent NOSs leading to the overproduction of NO [38]. Using transgenic mice lacking expression of nNOS, eNOS, or iNOS and *in vivo* and *in vitro* models of cerebral ischemia, Samdani et al. determined the role of each NOS isozyme in cerebral ischemic damage [39]. They concluded that overproduction of NO by nNOS is harmful to neurons and plays an important role in damage following cerebral ischemia. However, stimulation of eNOS leads to vasodilatation and maintenance of cerebral blood flow, resulting in the prevention of neuronal injury. iNOS, which is not normally present but is induced (transcriptional activation) following cerebral ischemia, participates in cerebral ischemic damage in the late post-ischemia phase. In summary, cerebral ischemia-induced activation of nNOS and iNOS are detrimental while activation of eNOS is protective. For further reading on this topic refer to earlier published review articles [40,41] (Table 2.1).

THE ROLE OF IRON

Iron, the most plentiful transition metal in the brain, has an integral role in the normal functioning of brain cells. The majority of the brain's iron is bound to transport proteins, specifically to the oxygen-carrying heme proteins and hemoglobin [42]. However, the remaining iron in the brain is bound to storage proteins such as intracellular ferritin (found mainly in glial cells) and circulating transferritin. During ischemia, iron can become disassociated from either of its storage proteins. Ferritin-bound iron's dissociation is caused by the reduction of ferric iron to ferrous iron, which is expedited by the presence of superoxide, acidosis, and nitric oxide, all of which are common outcomes of ischemia [43]. Transferritin bound iron becomes dissociated when conditions become acidic. Neuronal uptake of this unbound (ferrous) iron is mediated by intracellular calcium. After ischemia, once inside the neuron, ferrous iron can then become involved in the production of hydroxyl free radicals through the iron-catalyzed, superoxide-driven Haber-Weiss Reaction [44]. In this reaction, ferrous iron converts hydrogen peroxide into the extremely oxidizing hydroxyl radical [45]. In summary, cerebral ischemia-induced release of iron from its transport proteins contributes to further ROS production following cerebral ischemia (Table 2.1).

TABLE 2.1 Production of and Damage Caused by Free Radicals Following Cerebral Ischemia

Production of free radicals during ischemia/reperfusion	Increased cytosolic calcium	[37]
	Nitric oxide synthase (NOS)	[38–41]
	Dissociation of Iron	[44,45]
	Mitochondrial production	[45–47]
	Reperfusion	[48,49]
Cell death pathways post-ischemia	DNA oxidation	[14,38,54–56]
	Protein oxidation	[14,54,57–59]
	Lipid peroxidation	[14,60–62]
Disruption of cell signaling pathways	Apurinic/apyrimidinic endonuclease (APE)	[36]
	Nuclear factor-κB (NF-κB)	[36]

MITOCHONDRIAL PRODUCTION OF FREE RADICALS

Superoxide radicals are the major initial form of ROS produced by mitochondria. Superoxide radicals produced by mitochondria are converted into hydrogen peroxide (H_2O_2) by mitochondrial superoxide dismutase. Mitochondrial respiratory chain complexes I and III are considered major sources of ROS in the mitochondria. There are two major mechanisms by which mitochondrial ROS production is exacerbated by cerebral ischemia, the first being the increasing rate of mitochondrial respiration. Cerebral ischemia leads to increased calcium concentration in mitochondria as mitochondria attempt to buffer cerebral ischemia-induced increased cytosolic calcium. An increased calcium level in the mitochondria stimulates activities of several enzymes, namely pyruvate dehydrogenase, isocitrate dehydrogenase, and α-ketoglutarate dehydrogenase. This in turn leads to an increase in flux of electrons to complex I of the mitochondrial respiratory chain and thus to an increased rate of mitochondrial respiration. This increased rate of electron transfer is speculated to be the initiator of mitochondrial ROS. Secondly, the cerebral ischemia-induced increase in mitochondrial calcium concentration results in mitochondrial swelling which is consistent with opening of the mitochondrial permeability transition pore and release of cytochrome *c* into the cytosol. This release of cytochrome *c* from the mitochondria results in inhibition of the mitochondrial electron transport chain and maximal reduction of redox sites proximal to cytochrome *c*. This leads to increased mitochondrial ROS production from complexes I and III. Overall, mitochondria are the major source of ROS following cerebral ischemia, primarily producing superoxide radicals [45–47] (Table 2.1).

REPERFUSION

The reperfusion/reoxygenation phase is considered a major contributor of ROS. Using a global cerebral ischemia/reperfusion model in gerbils, Cao et al. observed that ischemia alone leads to a marginal increase in ROS, while ischemia and reperfusion together lead to massive increase in ROS [48]. ROS were quantified by measuring conversion of salicylate, a relatively non-toxic but highly effective hydroxyl radical trap. Upon oxidation, salicylate converts into 2,5- and 2,3-dihydroxybenzoic acid (DHBA) [48] . A similar study by Piantadosi and Zhang in a rat model of global cerebral ischemia also confirmed production of ROS during post-ischemia reperfusion [49]. These authors observed that ROS production during ischemia and reperfusion was inhibited in presence of rotenone (an inhibitor of mitochondrial electron transport chain complex I). However, ROS production was restored when rotenone was delivered along with succinate (substrate for mitochondrial electron transport chain complex II). This study suggests that complex I of the mitochondrial electron transport chain is a major source of ROS during ischemia/reperfusion. The abrupt availability of oxygen during reperfusion to highly reduced mitochondrial electron transport chain components and accumulated free electrons is believed to induce the release of free radicals during post-ischemia reperfusion [50]. Post-ischemia reperfusion induces overload of the cellular antioxidant defense capacity, resulting in the depletion of all endogenous antioxidants, which inhibits cells from restoring antioxidant concentrations and leads to exacerbated oxidative stress [51,52]. Overall, the literature indicates that reperfusion/reoxygenation following cerebral ischemia also contributes to ROS generation [46,47] (Table 2.1).

FREE RADICALS AND CEREBRAL ISCHEMIA-INDUCED CELL DEATH PATHWAYS

Oxidative stress has been known to affect cell viability and survival through several modalities of direct and intense damage. It is believed that cerebral ischemia-induced oxidative stress plays an important role in activating both necrotic and apoptotic pathways of cell death [53]. Necrosis is defined by premature cell death due to trauma, while apoptosis is known as programmed cell death caused internally by the cell. After ischemia, the resultant damage to cells by free radical release can directly lead to necrosis of the neuron and/or indirectly cause the initiation of apoptotic cell death pathways. The cell death pathway that predominates is dependent upon many factors, such as the severity and the location of the ischemia. It is important to note that although these mechanisms cause cell damage, any of these types of damage to a high enough degree can result in cell death. Neuronal damage by DNA oxidation, protein oxidation, and lipid peroxidation are major mechanisms for ROS-induced cell death [45]. These mechanisms are described below (Table 2.1).

DNA Oxidation

The production of free radicals from the numerous reactions discussed previously has a detrimental effect on the nucleic acids of DNA. Most commonly, the resultant damage to DNA is a strand break, however, DNA base modification products (e.g., 8-hydroxy-2'-deoxyguanosine) may also be formed [54]. This damage to DNA occurs when ROS reacts with iron or copper molecules located on or close to the DNA strand to produce the hydroxyl radical [14]. The hydroxyl radical extracts the hydrogen from the backbone of the deoxysugar of DNA and causes the strand breakage [55]. Additionally, the RNS peroxynitrite has been implicated in DNA damage after ischemia. Peroxynitrite has been shown to cause single strand breaks in DNA. Excessive DNA damage activates the DNA repair protein poly(ADP-ribose) polymerase (PARP) which leads to depletion of cellular stores of NAD^+ and ultimately ATP. This stimulation of PARP has been shown to add to brain damage after ischemia [38]. A study by Takahashi et al. demonstrated that a PARP inhibitor leads to decreased infarct size in focal cerebral ischemia in a rat model [56]. These studies demonstrate the role of oxidative stress-induced DNA damage in cerebral ischemic damage (see Figure 2.2).

Protein Oxidation

Similar to DNA, the oxidation of proteins can occur through the combined action of free radicals and the trace metals iron and copper. A large variety of proteins

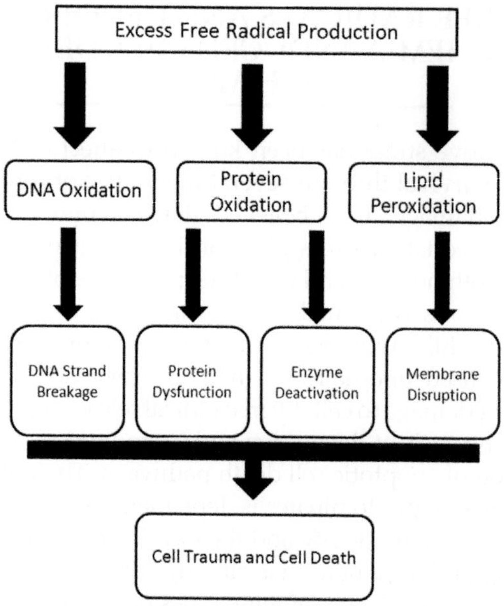

FIGURE 2.2 **A summary of the primary causes of cell trauma and death due to the excess production of free radicals.** The oxidative stress presented by the excess free radicals has been shown to adversely affect the three major macromolecules. In the case of DNA, when oxidized by free radicals, the most common result is DNA strand breakage. When proteins are oxidized, literature has shown that, in addition to protein dysfunction, many enzyme proteins may also be inactivated. Finally, oxidative stress to lipids may initiate the cycle of lipid peroxidation and perturb the lipid membrane of cells. All of these outcomes of oxidative stress lead to cell trauma, and if severe enough, may lead to cell death.

are susceptible to oxidative damage, with membrane proteins potentially losing their receptor capabilities, and enzyme proteins evincing a rapid loss of enzymatic activity (Figure 2.2) [14,54]. One of the most important enzymes in cellular energy production, pyruvate dehydrogenase (PDH), is believed to lose its function owing to oxidative stress. The PDH complex is the link between anaerobic and aerobic metabolism, taking pyruvate and converting it to acetyl-CoA to be utilized in the Krebs cycle for energy production. This oxidative inactivation of PDH is evidenced by the marked decrease in the activity of the PDH complex in the time following reperfusion – a time, as discussed above, in which there is a dramatic rise in the production of free radicals [57,58]. Another important enzyme that may experience a loss in activity from oxidative stress is glutamine synthase: responsible for glutamate metabolism [14,59]. Inactivation of glutamine synthase contributes to cerebral ischemia-induced excitotoxicity by inhibiting the recycling of released glutamate following cerebral ischemia [59]. The oxidation of proteins inhibits the function of the affected proteins, resulting in deficits in cellular function that can lead to cellular death.

Lipid Peroxidation

Lipid peroxidation is the process in which free radicals attack unsaturated fatty acids in a lipid membrane. The radical extracts a hydrogen atom from the lipid leaving behind a lipid radical and setting off an oxygen-mediated chain reaction that leaves the membrane riddled with lipid hydroperoxides (non-radical intermediates of lipid peroxidation) [60]. These lipid hydroperoxides severely hamper membrane functionality, by way of increased rigidity and allowing ions like calcium to leak across the membrane [14]. The brain is particularly susceptible to lipid peroxidation because it contains high levels of unsaturated fatty acids [61]. Certain byproducts of lipid peroxidation, such as 4-hydroxynonenal (HNE), can be toxic to neurons. Earlier, McCracken et al. undertook a study to determine the effect of cerebral ischemia-induced accumulation of HNE on white matter damage. Using *in vivo* and *in vitro* model systems they observed that exogenous delivery of HNE leads to axonal damage and oligodendrocyte cell death [62]. As is the case with all macromolecule oxidation, if the damage to the lipid membrane is severe enough, it may result in the activation of necrotic or apoptotic neuronal death pathways (Figure 2.2).

Effect of Free Radicals on Cell Signaling Pathways

Apart from directly affecting macromolecules, free radicals can also affect cell survival by influencing cell signaling pathways. For example, apurinic/apyrimidinic endonuclease (APE) which is involved in DNA base excision repair is inactivated following cerebral ischemia; this inactivation can be prevented by reducing cerebral ischemia-induced oxidative stress by overexpression of the antioxidant enzyme CuZnSOD (see review for details) [36]. Nuclear factor-κB (NF-κB), a transcription factor that is regulated by the redox state of the cell, is another example of a cell signaling molecule affected by ROS. Post-cerebral ischemia oxidative stress-induced activation of NF-κB has been shown to play a role in cerebral ischemic damage (see review for details) [36]. These studies shed light on the critical role of cellular signaling altered by ROS on cerebral ischemic damage (Table 2.1).

OXIDATIVE STRESS IN DIABETIC CEREBRAL ISCHEMIA

It is believed that increased oxidative stress in diabetic patients contributes to the secondary complications of diabetes, including cerebral ischemia. Since the baseline level of oxidative stress is higher in diabetic patients, and oxidative stress plays a key role in cerebral ischemia-induced brain damage, we surmise that higher baseline oxidative stress in diabetics will lead to increased cerebral ischemic damage (see Figure 2.1). A clinical study aimed to determine oxidative stress in diabetic patients with and without cerebral ischemia observed that plasma levels of malondialdehyde (MDA), a measure of lipid peroxidation, were higher in diabetics without cerebral ischemia compared to non-diabetic controls [63]. MDA levels were further increased in diabetic patients with cerebral ischemia. This study suggests that, owing to increased baseline oxidative stress, cerebral ischemia in diabetics will further exacerbate oxidative stress – which may be responsible for increased cerebral damage in diabetics [63]. In a similar study, Guldiken et al. compared total antioxidant capacity (TCA) and oxidative stress in acute stroke patients with and without diabetes [64]. They observed that TCA and levels of nitric oxide were significantly elevated in diabetic acute stroke patients compared to non-diabetic acute stroke patients. They concluded that oxidative stress and TCA ('counterbalancing antioxidant capacity') are significantly higher in diabetic stroke patients. As mentioned in the 'NOS Pathway' section above, NO production by eNOS is beneficial while NO production by nNOS and iNOS is detrimental.

In a rat model of type 1 diabetes (streptozotocin-diabetic rats) Aragone and colleagues determined the effect of cerebral ischemia on oxidative state and antioxidant balance in isolated nerve terminals ('synaptosomes') [64]. They observed that the levels of hydrogen peroxide, hydroxyl radicals and ROS (measured by 2′,7′-dichlorofluorescin diacetate) were significantly higher following cerebral ischemia/reperfusion in diabetic rats compared to non-diabetic rats. They also observed that dehydroepiandrosterone treatment reduced cerebral ischemia-induced oxidative stress and neuronal damage in diabetic rats.

In a rat model of focal cerebral ischemia, hyperglycemia resulted in an increased incidence of tissue plasminogen activator (tPA)-induced cerebral hemorrhage [65]. Treatment of rats with apocynin (a blocker of superoxide production by NADPH oxidase) was able to attenuate the damaging effects of hyperglycemia. This study concluded that the increased risk of hemorrhagic transformation following tPA treatment in hyperglycemic rats is mediated by increased superoxide production. Streptozotocin-induced hyperglycemia in rats is also shown to increase astrocyte death following cerebral ischemia. This increase in astrocyte damage was observed to coincide with increased ROS production [66]. In summary, the literature demonstrates exacerbated ROS production and damage from these ROS following cerebral ischemia in diabetics.

CONCLUSION

In conclusion, the literature indicates that oxidative stress plays a key role in cerebral ischemic damage by activating cell death pathways (Figure 2.1). Owing to increased baseline oxidative stress in diabetics, it appears that cerebral ischemia-induced oxidative stress is exacerbated in diabetics. This exacerbated oxidative stress may be responsible for increased cerebral ischemic damage in diabetics (Figure 2.1). Therapies targeted at reducing oxidative stress in diabetics may help lower the incidence of cerebral ischemia as well as lowering cerebral ischemic damage.

SUMMARY POINTS

- Free radicals in excess are the cause of oxidative stress to tissues, and it is the role of antioxidants to combat this oxidative stress.
- Diabetes has been shown to increase free radical production through many pathways as well as to decrease antioxidant capacity, leading to increased oxidative stress.
- Cerebral ischemia and reperfusion cause increased oxidative stress through the induction of many free radical generating pathways.
- Cell damage and death due to increased oxidative stress from cerebral ischemia primarily occurs via DNA oxidation, protein oxidation, and/or lipid peroxidation.
- Cerebral ischemic damage in diabetics is exacerbated compared to non-diabetics owing to the increased baseline oxidative stress caused by diabetes.

References

[1] Diabetes, http://www.who.int/mediacenter/factsheets/fs312/en/ World Health Organization. Retrieved on 6/7/13.
[2] National Diabetes Statistics, 2011 http://diabetes.niddk.nih.gov/dm/pubs/statistics/index.aspx#Complications. National Diabetes Information Clearinghouse (NDIC). Retrieved on 6/7/13.
[3] Diabetes Statistics. American Diabetes Association. http://www.diabetes.org/diabetes-basics/diabetes-statistics/. Retrieved on 12/29/2012.
[4] National Diabetes Fact Sheet, 2011: Centers for Disease Control and Prevention. http://www.cdc.gov/diabetes/pubs/pdf/ndfs_2011.pdf: Retrieved on 6/13/2011.
[5] Evans BA, Sicks JD, Whisnant JP. Factors affecting survival and occurrence of stroke in patients with transient ischemic attacks. Mayo Clin Proc Mayo Clin 1994;69(5):416–21.
[6] Biller J, Love BB. Diabetes and stroke. Med Clin North Am 1993;77(1):95–110.
[7] Jorgensen H, Nakayama H, Raaschou HO, Olsen TS. Stroke in patients with diabetes. The Copenhagen Stroke Study. Stroke 1994;25(10); 1977–84.
[8] Martini SR, Kent TA. Hyperglycemia in acute ischemic stroke: a vascular perspective. J Cereb Blood Flow Metab 2007;27(3):435–51.

[9] Kagansky N, Levy S, Knobler H. The role of hyperglycemia in acute stroke. Arch Neurol 2001;58(8):1209–12.
[10] Auer RN. Insulin, blood glucose levels, and ischemic brain damage. Neurology 1998;51(3 Suppl. 3):S39–43.
[11] Helgason CM. Blood glucose and stroke. Stroke 1988;19(8): 1049–53.
[12] Thannickal VJ, Fanburg BL. Reactive oxygen species in cell signaling. Am J Physiol Lung Cell Mol Physiol 2000;279(6):L1005–28.
[13] Valko M, Leibfritz D, Moncol J, Cronin MT, Mazur M, Telser J. Free radicals and antioxidants in normal physiological functions and human disease. Int J biochem cell biol 2007;39(1):44–84.
[14] Halliwell B. Reactive oxygen species and the central nervous system. J neurochem 1992;59(5):1609–23.
[15] Turrens JF. Mitochondrial formation of reactive oxygen species. J physiol 2003;552(Pt 2):335–44.
[16] Droge W. Free radicals in the physiological control of cell function. Physiol Rev 2002;82(1):47–95.
[17] Janda E, Isidoro C, Carresi C, Mollace V. Defective autophagy in Parkinson's disease: role of oxidative stress. Mol Neurobiol 2012;46(3):639–61.
[18] Jovanovic Z. Mechanisms of neurodegeneration in Alzheimer's disease. Med Pregl 2012;65(7–8):301–7.
[19] Jay D, Hitomi H, Griendling KK. Oxidative stress and diabetic cardiovascular complications. Free Radic Biol Med 2006; 40(2):183–92.
[20] Bonnefont-Rousselot D. Glucose and reactive oxygen species. Curr Opin Clin Nutr Metab Care 2002;5(5):561–8.
[21] Patockova J, Marhol P, Tumova E, et al. Oxidative stress in the brain tissue of laboratory mice with acute post insulin hypoglycemia. Physiol Res 2003;52(1):131–5.
[22] Liu Y, Song XD, Liu W, Zhang TY, Zuo J. Glucose deprivation induces mitochondrial dysfunction and oxidative stress in PC12 cell line. J Cell Mol Med 2003;7(1):49–56.
[23] Cardoso S, Santos MS, Seica R, Moreira PI. Cortical and hippocampal mitochondria bioenergetics and oxidative status during hyperglycemia and/or insulin-induced hypoglycemia. Biochim Biophys Acta 2010;1802(11):942–51.
[24] Fioramonti X, Marsollier N, Song Z, et al. Ventromedial hypothalamic nitric oxide production is necessary for hypoglycemia detection and counterregulation. Diabetes 2010;59(2):519–28.
[25] Singh P, Jain A, Kaur G. Impact of hypoglycemia and diabetes on CNS: correlation of mitochondrial oxidative stress with DNA damage. Mol Cell Biochem 2004;260(1–2):153–9.
[26] Winiarska K, Malinska D, Szymanski K, Dudziak M, Bryla J. Lipoic acid ameliorates oxidative stress and renal injury in alloxan diabetic rabbits. Biochimie 2008;90(3):450–9.
[27] Dave KR, Tamariz J, Desai KM, et al. Recurrent hypoglycemia exacerbates cerebral ischemic damage in streptozotocin-induced diabetic rats. Stroke 2011;42(5):1404–11.
[28] Paramo B, Hernandez-Fonseca K, Estrada-Sanchez AM, Jimenez N, Hernandez-Cruz A, Massieu L. Pathways involved in the generation of reactive oxygen and nitrogen species during glucose deprivation and its role on the death of cultured hippocampal neurons. Neuroscience 2010;167(4):1057–69.
[29] McGowan JE, Chen L, Gao D, Trush M, Wei C. Increased mitochondrial reactive oxygen species production in newborn brain during hypoglycemia. Neurosci Lett 2006;399(1–2):111–4.
[30] Maritim AC, Sanders RA, Watkins 3rd JB. Diabetes, oxidative stress, and antioxidants: a review. J Biochem Mol Toxicol 2003;17(1):24–38.
[31] Mooradian AD. The antioxidative potential of cerebral microvessels in experimental diabetes mellitus. Brain Res 1995; 671(1):164–9.
[32] del Zoppo GJ, Mabuchi T. Cerebral microvessel responses to focal ischemia. J Cereb Blood Flow Metab 2003;23(8):879–94.
[33] American Heart Association. Ischemic Stroke. http://www.strokeassociation.org/STROKEORG/AboutStroke/TypesofStroke/IschemicClots/Ischemic-Strokes-Clots_UCM_310939_Article.jsp: Retrieved on 12/31/2012.
[34] American Heart Association. Hemorrhagic Stroke. http://www.strokeassociation.org/STROKEORG/AboutStroke/TypesofStroke/HemorrhagicBleeds/Hemorrhagic-Strokes-Bleeds_UCM_310940_Article.jsp Retrieved on 12/31/2012.
[35] Neumann JT, Cohan CH, Dave KR, Wright CB, Perez-Pinzon MA. Global Cerebral Ischemia: Synaptic and Cognitive Dysfunction. Curr Drug Targets 2012.
[36] Chan PH. Reactive oxygen radicals in signaling and damage in the ischemic brain. J Cereb Blood Flow Metab 2001;21(1): 2–14.
[37] Crack PJ, Taylor JM. Reactive oxygen species and the modulation of stroke. Free Radic Biol Med 2005;38(11):1433–44.
[38] Love S. Oxidative stress in brain ischemia. Brain pathol 1999;9(1):119–31.
[39] Samdani AF, Dawson TM, Dawson VL. Nitric oxide synthase in models of focal ischemia. Stroke 1997;28(6):1283–8.
[40] Matsui T, Nagafuji T, Kumanishi T, Asano T. Role of nitric oxide in pathogenesis underlying ischemic cerebral damage. Cell Mol Neurobiol 1999;19(1):177–89.
[41] Moro MA, Cardenas A, Hurtado O, Leza JC, Lizasoain I. Role of nitric oxide after brain ischaemia. Cell Calcium 2004;36 (3–4):265–75.
[42] Moos T. Brain iron homeostasis. Dan Med Bull 2002;49(4): 279–301.
[43] Palmer C, Menzies SL, Roberts RL, Pavlick G, Connor JR. Changes in iron histochemistry after hypoxic-ischemic brain injury in the neonatal rat. J Neurosci Res 1999;56(1):60–71.
[44] Selim MH, Ratan RR. The role of iron neurotoxicity in ischemic stroke. Ageing Res Rev 2004;3(3):345–53.
[45] Lewen A, Matz P, Chan PH. Free radical pathways in CNS injury. J Neurotrauma 2000;17(10):871–90.
[46] Niizuma K, Yoshioka H, Chen H, et al. Mitochondrial and apoptotic neuronal death signaling pathways in cerebral ischemia. Biochim Biophys Acta 2010;1802(1):92–9.
[47] Starkov AA, Chinopoulos C, Fiskum G. Mitochondrial calcium and oxidative stress as mediators of ischemic brain injury. Cell Calcium 2004;36(3–4):257–64.
[48] Cao W, Carney JM, Duchon A, Floyd RA, Chevion M. Oxygen free radical involvement in ischemia and reperfusion injury to brain. Neurosci Lett 1988;88(2):233–8.
[49] Piantadosi CA, Zhang J. Mitochondrial generation of reactive oxygen species after brain ischemia in the rat. Stroke 1996;27(2): 327–31; discussion 32.
[50] Won SJ, Kim DY, Gwag BJ. Cellular and molecular pathways of ischemic neuronal death. J Biochem Mol Biol 2002;35(1): 67–86.
[51] Saito A, Maier CM, Narasimhan P, et al. Oxidative stress and neuronal death/survival signaling in cerebral ischemia. Mol Neurobiol 2005;31(1–3):105–16.
[52] Chan PH. Role of oxidants in ischemic brain damage. Stroke 1996;27(6):1124–9.
[53] Sugawara T, Chan PH. Reactive oxygen radicals and pathogenesis of neuronal death after cerebral ischemia. Antioxid Redox Signal 2003;5(5):597–607.
[54] Floyd RA, Carney JM. Free radical damage to protein and DNA: mechanisms involved and relevant observations on brain undergoing oxidative stress. Ann Neurol 1992;32(Suppl):S22–7.
[55] Juurlink BH. Response of glial cells to ischemia: roles of reactive oxygen species and glutathione. Neurosci Biobehav Rev 1997;21(2):151–66.

[56] Takahashi K, Greenberg JH, Jackson P, Maclin K, Zhang J. Neuroprotective effects of inhibiting poly(ADP-ribose) synthetase on focal cerebral ischemia in rats. J Cereb Blood Flow Metab 1997;17(11):1137–42.
[57] Martin E, Rosenthal RE, Fiskum G. Pyruvate dehydrogenase complex: metabolic link to ischemic brain injury and target of oxidative stress. J Neurosci Res 2005;79(1–2):240–7.
[58] Bogaert YE, Rosenthal RE, Fiskum G. Postischemic inhibition of cerebral cortex pyruvate dehydrogenase. Free Radic Biol Med 1994;16(6):811–20.
[59] Oliver CN, Starke-Reed PE, Stadtman ER, Liu GJ, Carney JM, Floyd RA. Oxidative damage to brain proteins, loss of glutamine synthetase activity, and production of free radicals during ischemia/reperfusion-induced injury to gerbil brain. Proc Natl Acad Sci U S A 1990;87(13):5144–7.
[60] Girotti AW. Lipid hydroperoxide generation, turnover, and effector action in biological systems. J Lipid Res 1998;39(8):1529–42.
[61] Margaill I, Plotkine M, Lerouet D. Antioxidant strategies in the treatment of stroke. Free Radic Biol Med 2005;39(4):429–43.
[62] McCracken E, Valeriani V, Simpson C, Jover T, McCulloch J, Dewar D. The lipid peroxidation by-product 4-hydroxynonenal is toxic to axons and oligodendrocytes. J Cereb Blood Flow Metab 2000;20(11):1529–36.
[63] Cojocaru IM, Cojocaru M, Musuroi C, Botezat M, Lazar L, Druta A. Lipid peroxidation and catalase in diabetes mellitus with and without ischemic stroke. Rom J Intern Med 2004;42(2):423–9.
[64] Guldiken B, Demir M, Guldiken S, Turgut N, Turgut B, Tugrul A. Oxidative stress and total antioxidant capacity in diabetic and nondiabetic acute ischemic stroke patients. Clin Appl Thromb Hemost 2009;15(6):695–700.
[65] Won SJ, Tang XN, Suh SW, Yenari MA, Swanson RA. Hyperglycemia promotes tissue plasminogen activator-induced hemorrhage by Increasing superoxide production. Ann Neurol 2011;70(4):583–90.
[66] Muranyi M, Ding C, He Q, Lin Y, Li PA. Streptozotocin-induced diabetes causes astrocyte death after ischemia and reperfusion injury. Diabetes 2006;55(2):349–55.

CHAPTER

3

Diabetic Cardiomyopathy and Oxidative Stress

Somasundaram Arumugam, Vengadeshprabhu Karuppagounder*, Rajarajan A. Thandavarayan*, Vigneshwaran Pitchaimani*, Hirohito Sone†, Kenichi Watanabe**

*Dept. of Clinical Pharmacology, Niigata University of Pharmacy and Applied Life Sciences, Niigata, Japan, †Dept. of Internal Medicine, Division of Hematology, Endocrinology and Metabolism, Niigata University Faculty of Medicine, Niigata, Japan

List of Abbreviations

ADP Adenosine diphosphate
AGEs Advanced glucation end products
ATP Adenosine triphosphate
cAMP cyclic adenosine monophosphate
CM Cardiomyopathy
DM Diabetes mellitus
DNA Deoxyribonucleic acid
FADH Flavin adenine dinucleotide
GLUT Glucose transporter
GSH Reduced glutathione
HF Heart failure
NADH Nicotinamide adenine dinucleotide
NADPH Nicotinamide adenine dinucleotide phosphate
NOS Nitric oxide synthase
Nox4 NADPH oxidase 4
p22phox p22 phagocyte oxidase
PARP Poly(ADP-ribose) polymerases
RNA Ribonucleic acid
RNS Reactive nitrogen species
ROS Reactive oxygen species
UDP Uridine diphosphate

INTRODUCTION

Diabetes mellitus (DM) is a metabolic disorder characterized by hyperglycemia and insufficient secretion of or receptor insensitivity to endogenous insulin. This disease affects both the duration and the quality of life, as it can produce various complications affecting the cardiovascular, renal, and nervous systems. DM has a marked influence on cardiac metabolism due to altered substrate supply, impaired insulin action, and metabolic maladaptations in the diabetic heart [1]. This syndrome markedly potentiates the risk of heart failure (HF), and its increased incidence is the major cause of morbidity and mortality in patients with DM [2]. The association between DM and HF are stronger in patients aged 65 years or less, being four-fold and eight-fold higher in male and female patients, respectively, than in non-diabetic subjects [3]. The high incidence and poor prognosis of HF in diabetic patients have been linked in part to the presence of an underlying diabetic cardiomyopathy characterized by myocellular hypertrophy and myocardial fibrosis [4]. The worsening of glycemic control increases lipid and lipoprotein abnormalities, leading to cardiovascular complications [5]. Several molecular mechanisms have been proposed as contributors to the pathogenesis of diabetic cardiomyopathy. In this chapter we focus on the involvement of oxidative stress in the pathophysiology of diabetic cardiomyopathy.

DIABETIC CARDIOMYOPATHY

Epidemiology

Cardiovascular diseases are the primary cause of death in diabetic patients, not only from diabetic complications, but also because of the direct adverse effects of hyperglycemia on the heart [6]. A study has reported echocardiographic evidence for the existence of diabetic cardiomyopathy, using data from 4,515 patients of both genders [7]. In addition, the Uppsala Longitudinal study, using 1,187 elderly diabetic men, suggests that insulin resistance predicted HF incidence independently

Diabetes: Oxidative Stress and Dietary Antioxidants.
http://dx.doi.org/10.1016/B978-0-12-405885-9.00003-6

of established risk factors. The association between obesity and subsequent HF may also be mediated largely by insulin resistance [8]. The Atherosclerosis Risk in Communities Study reported that elevated hemoglobin-a1c was associated with the incidence of HF in a middle-aged population, suggesting that chronic hyperglycemia prior to the development of DM contributes to development of HF [9]. From these clinical study reports and various other studies we can be reasonably certain that there is a strict association between factors like chronic hyperglycemia and insulin resistance and cardiovascular complications.

HALLMARKS OF DM

DM is a complex disorder characterized by multiple metabolic disturbances with the symptoms of a metabolic syndrome. They include hyperglycemia, insulin resistance, high blood pressure, weight loss/obesity, uricosuria, polyphagia, polydipsia, and polyuria (shown in Figure 3.1). Glucose utilization becomes impaired through the changes in insulin level or function, leading to changes in several subcellular organelles such as myofibrils, sarcoplasmic reticulum, mitochondria and sarcolemma, as well as in heart function in long-term DM. Varying degrees of defects in cardiac contractile proteins, sarcoplasmic reticulum Ca^{2+} pumps, sarcolemmal membranes, mitochondria and their interaction with Ca^{2+} (which leads to improper contratile-relaxation processes in the cardiac tissue) are observed in long-term DM conditions [10]. The improper utilization of glucose, leading to the generation of reactive oxygen species (ROS), and accompanying oxidative stress are hallmarks of the molecular mechanisms responsible for cardiovascular disease [11].

OXIDATIVE STRESS

There is a definite relation between oxidative stress and diabetic cardiovascular complications, but it is debatable which precedes the other. Several reports suggest that hyperglycemia can induce the production of free radicals and thereby causes oxidative stress. Thus we can predict that chronic hyperglycemia and improper lipid metabolism in diabetic individuals increases the production of free radicals which overrides the innate antioxidant defense system leading to the diabetic complications of heart and various other tissue systems.

Normal physiological processes in living tissues produce several free radicals (any atom or molecule capable of independent existence that contains one or more unpaired electrons), and these fall in the category of either ROS or reactive nitrogen species (RNS). These species, which include various derivatives of oxygen and nitrogen such as superoxide, hydroxyl, peroxide and peroxynitrite, are highly reactive and can damage the structure of protein, RNA and DNA. Recently, highly reactive electrophiles such as 4-hydroxynonenal, RNS including nitric oxide, and other endo- and xenobiotic-metabolites have also been included in this category. Some reactive compounds responsible for the oxidative stress *in vivo* are listed in Table 3.1. In healthy individuals with normal physiological conditions, these molecules are quenched by innate antioxidant defense mechanisms, comprising various enzymes and compounds which take part in a cascade of

TABLE 3.1 List of the reactive oxygen and nitrogen species

Type	Radicals	Non-Radicals
Reactive oxygen species	Superoxide ($O_2^{\cdot -}$)	Hydrogen peroxide (H_2O_2)
	Hydroxyl ($^{\cdot}OH$)	Hypochlorous acid ($HOCl^-$)
	Peroxyl ($RO_2^{\cdot}$)	Ozone (O_3)
	Alkoxyl ($RO^{\cdot}$)	Singlet oxygen ($^1O_2$)
	Hydroperoxyl ($HO_2^{\cdot}$)	
Reactive nitrogen species	Nitric Oxide ($NO^{\cdot}$)	Alkyl peroxynitrite (ROONO)
	Nitrogen dioxide ($NO_2^{\cdot}$)	Dinitrogen trioxide (N_2O_3)
		Dinitrogen tetroxide (N_2O_4)
		Nitronium anion (NO_2^+)
		Nitrosyl cation (NO^+)
		Nitrous acid (HNO_2)
		Nitroxyl anion (NO^-)
		Nitryl chloride (NO_2Cl)
		Peroxynitrite ($ONOO^-$)

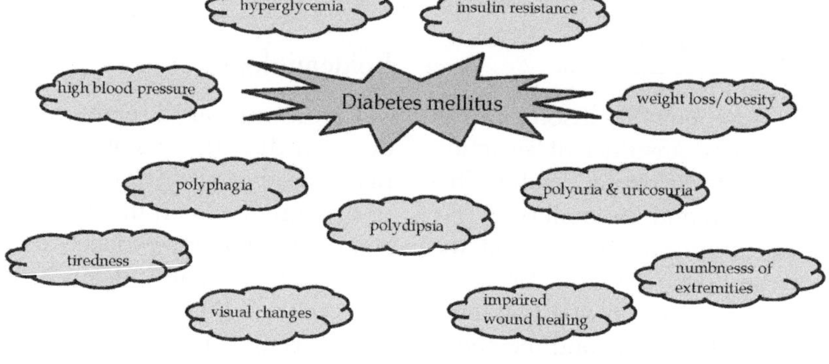

FIGURE 3.1 **Various hallmarks of diabetes mellitus.**

reactions. This process prevents these reactive molecules having deleterious effects on the normal structure and functions of cells. Any malfunction in this antioxidant defense system, or excessive production of free radicals in the tissues, leads to a condition called oxidative stress. For example, chronic hyperglycemia affects the normal turnover of free radicals by triggering the production of reactive superoxide radicals and inactivating the enzymes involved in their scavenging process by glycation [12], leading to oxidative stress and tissue damage. Observation of the excessive production of free radicals during diabetic complications has generated an interest in searching for the mechanism by which they lead to cardiomyopathy in DM. It is hoped to develop treatment strategies by targeting them.

HYPERGLYCEMIA

DM is a condition in which acute as well as chronic alterations in blood glucose concentrations are encountered, and these affect cellular metabolic processes (Figure 3.2). As glucose is the major fuel used by most of the living cells to produce energy, changes in the blood glucose concentration lead to alterations in the metabolic reactions which use it [1]. Hyperglycemia and prolonged cellular exposure to high glucose concentrations increases mitochondrial superoxide production in human coronary artery endothelial cells [13]. This affects not only the vascular endothelium and beta cells of the islets of pancreas, but also the myocardium. There are several proposed mechanisms for the effect of hyperglycemia on mitochondrial function, which include [14]:

1) Mitochondrial ROS production is central in the signaling pathway of harmful effects of hyperglycemia.
2) AMP activated protein kinase activation is a major regulator of both glucose and lipid metabolism connected with cellular energy status.
3) Hyperglycemia, by inhibiting glucose-6-phosphate dehydrogenase by a cAMP mechanism, plays a crucial role in NADPH/NADP ratio and thus in the pro-oxidant/antioxidant cellular status.
4) Via ROS induction, hyperglycemia causes oxidation of cardiolipin and releasing cytochrome c into the cytosol. The cytosolic cytochrome c forms apoptosome, thereby causing activation of caspase 9 followed by other caspases (such as 3, 6 and 7) leading to apoptotic cell death (Figure 3.3).

Discussion of the role of hyperglycemia in triggering ROS and oxidative stress will be essential for understanding the involvement of oxidative stress in the pathogenesis of diabetic cardiomyopathy. Most of the hyperglycemia

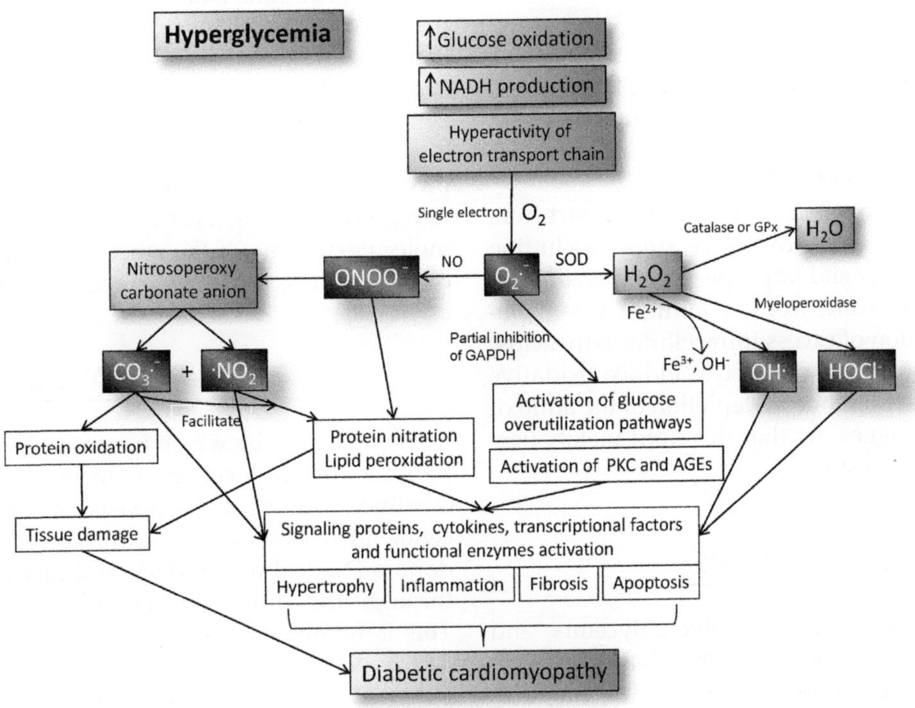

FIGURE 3.2 Hyperglycemia mediated diabetic cardiomyopathy. Chronic hyperglycemia causes hyperactivity of electron transport chain in the mitochondria, which causes leakage of superoxide radical ($O_2\cdot^-$) formed by single electron reduction of molecular oxygen. $O_2\cdot^-$ can either be dismutated by superoxide dismutase (SOD) to form hydrogen peroxide (H_2O_2) or react with nitric oxide (NO) to form peroxynitrite ($OONO^-$). H_2O_2 is converted to hydroxyl radical (OH·) or hypochlorite ($HOCl^-$). Similarly $OONO^-$ can be converted to carbonate radical ($CO_3\cdot^-$) or nitrogen dioxide radical ($\cdot NO_2$). All of these reactive species are involved in the signaling leading to inflammation, hypertrophy, fibrosis and apoptosis resulting in diabetic cardiomyopathy.

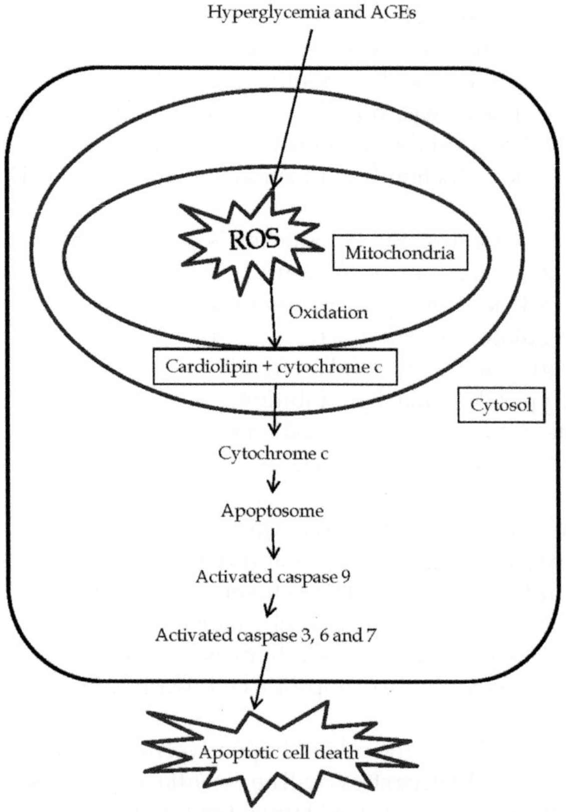

FIGURE 3.3 **Apoptosis mediated by mitochondria.** One of the possible mechanisms of hyperglycemia and AGEs induced apoptosis with the involvement of mitochondrial cytochrome c and caspases.

mediated cardiac damage reported during DM is indirect, via its action on vascular endothelium; however, similar reactions in cardiomyocytes are possible, which would directly affect their function.

There are other factors in diabetic patients apart from hyperglycemia which cause oxidative stress, including abnormal insulin levels and improper lipid metabolism. Diabetic patients also suffer from a condition called lipotoxicity (accumulation of excess intracellular fatty acids) and hypercholesterolemia, which can induce oxidative stress in the myocardium due to depletion of the antioxidant reserve [15], suggesting that this lipid metabolism could induce oxidative stress.

LIPOTOXICITY

Biochemical changes such as hyperglycemia and hypoinsulinemia, which occur in the diabetic condition, decrease cardiac glucose oxidation. The products of glucose metabolism inhibit the expression of theglucose transporter (GLUT), leading to insulin resistance as the GLUT mediated importing of glucose is an insulin-mediated process. The reduction in glucose supply further shifts the cardiac energy provision to the β-oxidation of fatty acids. The supply of fatty acids is maintained by lipoprotein lipase, which hydrolyzes circulatory lipoproteins. Increased fatty acid oxidation promotes acidosis and generation of free radicals, leading to the aggravation of myocardial injury. In addition, the non-oxidative metabolism of fatty acids induces ceramide and nitric oxide formation, damages mitochondrial membrane, and further potentiates oxidative stress. Excess intracellular fatty acid can cause caspase-mediated apoptosis of cardiomyocytes, and fatty acids can directly impair mitochondrial function via uncoupling of oxidative phosphorylation [16]. The major routes via which lipotoxicity leads to diabetic cardiomyopathy are depicted in Figure 3.4.

Thus, either alone or in combination with increased fatty acid availability and metabolism, hyperglycemia triggers oxidative stress, thereby causing damage to the myocardium and leading to diabetic cardiomyopathy. We have discussed the conditions that can trigger oxidative stress in cardiomyocytes, but it is also important to understand the types of reactive species produced, along with their actions and fate.

ROS AND RNS IN DIABETIC CARDIOMYOPATHY

Potential sources of cardiac ROS/RNS include mitochondria, xanthine oxidases, uncoupled nitric oxide synthases and NADPH oxidases [17]. The mitochondrion is the major source of ROS production, especially in tissues with high rates of respiration such as cardiomyocytes and this is potentially significant in the setting of hyperglycemia. There are two kinds of reactive species produced during oxidative stress; oxygen containing and nitrogen containing reactive species (free radicals, ions, or molecules). Some of the reactive species responsible for oxidative stress and their sources are listed in Table 3.2.

SUPEROXIDE

The pathway by which increased levels of superoxide radicals are produced by mitochondria in the diabetic condition can be hypothesized as follows: hyperglycemia increases the concentration of electron transfer donors (NADH and FADH) and increases electron flux through the mitochondrial electron transport chain. This is followed by an increase in the ATP/ADP ratio and hyperpolarization of the mitochondrial membrane potential. This high electrochemical potential difference generated by the proton gradient leads to partial inhibition of the electron transport in complex III, resulting in an accumulation of electrons to coenzyme Q. In turn, this drives a partial reduction of molecular oxygen to generate the free radical anion superoxide [1]. A study

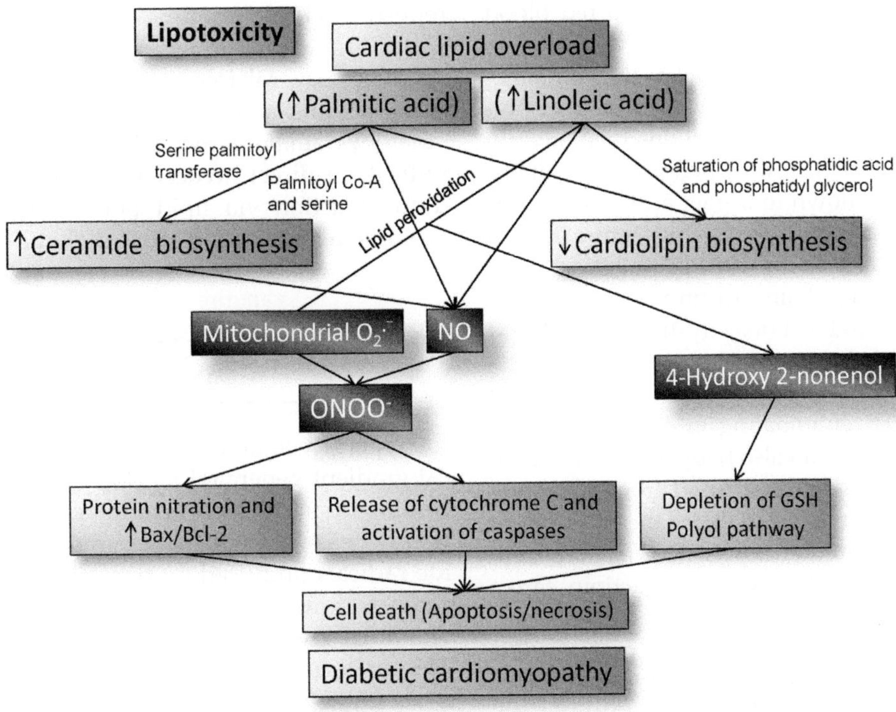

FIGURE 3.4 **Lipotoxicity is involved in the pathogenesis of diabetic cardiomyopathy.** Altered lipid metabolism in chronic diabetes mellitus leads to cardiac lipid overload, which increases the intracellular palmitic and linoleic acid levels. These alterations result in increased ceramide biosynthesis and reduced cardiolipin biosynthesis. It causes lipid peroxidation and increased production of reactive species like superoxide radical, nitric oxide and peroxynitrite leading to reduced antioxidant capacity as well as cardiomyocytes apoptosis via caspases or BCl_2 family proteins.

TABLE 3.2 Intracellular sources of some important reactive species

Reactive species	Source
Superoxide ($O_2^{\cdot-}$)	**Mitochondrial** – NADH dehydrogenase, succinate dehydrogenase, ubiquinol-cytochrome C reductase, glycerol phosphate dehydrogenase, dehydroorotate dehydrogenase, mono amino oxidase **Endoplasmic reticulum** – cytochrome p-450 **Peroxisomal** – xanthine oxidase **Cell membrane** – NAD(P)H oxidase
Nitric oxide ($NO^{\cdot}$)	**Peroxisomal and cytoplasmic** – Nitric oxide synthase
Nitrogen dioxide ($NO_2^{\cdot}$)	**Lysosomal** – Myeloperoxidase
Hydrogen peroxide (H_2O_2)	**Peroxisomal** – Acyl CoA oxidases, D-amino acid oxidase, D-aspartate oxidase, α-hydroxy acid oxidase, pipecolic acid oxidase, polyamine oxidase and urate oxidase **Microsomal** – cytochrome p-450 containing monooxidases
Hydroxyl ($^{\cdot}OH$)	From H_2O_2 in presence of Fe^{2+} or direct action of Fe^{3+} on OH^-
Singlet oxygen ($^1O_2$)	Peroxidase and lipoxygenase

using vascular smooth muscle cells reported that hyperglycemia induced the activation of NADPH oxidase 4 (Nox4) and p22 phagocyte oxidase (p22phox), a subunit of NADPH oxidase leading to increased ROS generation [18]. NADPH oxidases appear to be the only enzymes whose primary function is ROS generation; they also appear to be especially important for redox signaling. Furthermore, ROS derived from NADPH oxidases can induce NOS uncoupling (through oxidation of tetrahyrdrobiopterin) as well as xanthine oxidase activation, so that they serve as priming sources for the amplification of ROS production [17].

NITRIC OXIDE AND PEROXYNITRITE

Nitric oxide is an omnipresent intercellular messenger in all vertebrates, modulating blood flow, thrombosis, and neural activity. The involvement of nitric oxide in diabetic cardiovascular complications has been reported by many researchers. Calcium dependent nitric oxide synthases are responsible for the generation of nitric oxide in cardiomyocytes and endothelium. When present alone, neither nitric oxide nor superoxide can be toxic *in vivo*, as efficient means are available to minimize their accumulation. Superoxide is removed by the enzyme superoxide dismutase, whereas nitric oxide diffuses into red blood cells and gets converted to nitrate. However, oxidative stress increases their availability, as well as the spontaneous combination of both leading to the formation of peroxynitrite. Most of the pathological actions mediated by nitric oxide are related to the production of peroxynitrite. Peroxynitrite has been shown to trigger apoptosis in cardiomyocytes, to decrease the spontaneous contraction of cardiomyocytes and to cause irreversible inhibition of the mitochondrial respiratory chain. An important pathway of peroxynitrite-mediated cellular dysfunction in DM involves activation of the nuclear enzyme poly (ADP-ribose) polymerases (PARP enzymes) consuming NAD^+ and consequently ATP, culminating in cell dysfunction, apoptosis or necrosis. This can also happen via the activation of matrix metalloproteinases. Apart from activating these pathways, peroxynitrite can cause the nitration of several cellular proteins and enzymes, such as myofibrillar creatine kinase, myocardial aconitase, α-actinin, sarcoplasmic reticulum Ca^{2+}-ATPase, voltage gated and Ca^{2+} activated potassium channels and vascular prostacycline synthase. As it can cause nitration of the tyrosine residues of the cellular proteins, they lose their structural and functional integrity and the effect of damage can be measured by estimation of the nitrotyrosine levels. Thus in chronic diabetic conditions, hyperglycemia activates superoxide as well as nitric oxide production, thereby causing cardiovascular damage by the association product peroxynitrite, ultimately leading to diabetic cardiomyopathy [19,20].

HYDROXYL RADICAL

The formation of hydroxyl radicals influences platelet activation and thrombosis in the blood vessels, thereby increasing the risk of cardiovascular disease. Hyperglycemia activates the production of superoxide radicals, which can react with hydrogen peroxide (formed by the action of superoxide dismutase) to form hydroxyl radicals (Figure 3.2). In the circulation, in the presence of Fe^{2+} the hydroxyl radical can further activate platelets and cause aggregation and thrombus formation, leading to vascular abnormalities and so indirectly affecting cardiac function. In the cardiomyocytes, the increased fatty acid levels can cause transport of iron into the mitochondria [21], which causes the generation of hydroxyl radicals from hydrogen peroxide. Thus hydroxyl radicals, apart from platelet aggregation, can activate arachidonic acid metabolism and promote lipid peroxidation and athereosclerosis via the activation of protein kinase C [22]. Similarly, they can also modify immunoglobulin G resulting in the generation of new epitopes, and they act as potent immunogens, inducing the autoantibodies found in type 2 DM [23]. In addition, the hydroxyl radical modified glutamic acid decarboxylase-65 has been reported to be an immunological marker for type 1 DM [24]. Chronic, hyperglycemia-induced, oxidative stress produces several free radicals and reactive species in many organs and tissues including the myocardium –thereby damaging them. The involvement of hydroxyl radicals in direct myocardial damage, as well as their indirect action via lipid peroxidation and abnormal immune response, can cause diabetic cardiomyopathy.

THE MODULATION OF CELL SIGNALING PATHWAYS

Hyperglycemia increases the proton electrochemical gradient generated by the electron transport chain, leading to single electron reduction of molecular oxygen which generates superoxide radicals. Excess superoxide radicals produced by the mitochondrial respiratory chain and increased glucose levels cause partial inactivation of glyceraldehyde 3-phosphate dehydrogenase. This in turn causes accumulation of the intermediate molecules of the glycolysis pathway, which then triggers the activation of glucose overutilization pathways such as polyol, hexosamine, protein kinase C and advanced glycation end products [25].

1) Activation of the polyol pathway, which converts excess glucose to sorbital via aldose reductase, utilizes more NADPH (a co-factor for aldose reductase). This reaction reduces the regeneration of reduced glutathione, because glutathione peroxidase also depends on the NADPH for its reaction. This chain of events finally leads to the depletion of intracellular reduced glutathione levels, thereby strengthening oxidative stress [26].

2) Similarly, activation of the hexosamine biosynthetic pathway causes accumulation of its end product UDP-N-acetylglucosamine thereby interfering with the serine/threonine phosphorylation of various cytosolic and nuclear proteins [27].

3) Hyperglycemia can also stimulate the non-enzymatic reaction between glucose and amino acids in the proteins to form glycation products, and their degradation produces advanced glycation end products. These compounds can activate their specific receptors to alter cellular signaling and produce further free radicals [28].

4) Hyperglycemia and augmented superoxides can increase diacylglycerol synthesis or phosphatidylcholine hydrolysis and causes chronic activation of protein kinase C, a family of serine/threonine-related protein kinase involved in controlling the function of other proteins, thereby affecting many cellular functions and signal transduction pathways [29].

Most of these signaling pathways mediate the cardiomyocyte death via either apoptosis or necrosis, leading to structural and functional changes in the myocardium, which in turn results in diabetic cardiomyopathy. We have previously reviewed the involvement of various cell signaling pathways mediated by oxidative stress during the development of diabetic cardiomyopathy [30]. In addition there are several signal transduction molecules regulating normal cellular biochemistry, among which mammalian 14-3-3 dimeric phosphoserine binding proteins play important roles in preventing the development of diabetic cardiomyopathy. These proteins modulate the actions of other signaling molecules, such as p38 mitogen activated protein kinase and apoptosis regulating kinase, which are seen to be involved in the myocardial apoptosis, hypertrophy and fibrosis during chronic DM in animals. We have performed several studies on 14-3-3 protein to investigate its protective effects against pathological cardiac complications using transgenic mouse models [31–34]. These studies confirm its beneficial effects against oxidative stress during DM using various signaling proteins, but as yet the exact mechanism remains to be identified.

CONCLUSION

DM is a common chronic illness causing patient mortality mostly via cardiovascular malfunction [35]. Various studies and trials have been conducted to relate the DM to cardiovascular disorders, and those reports suggest several theories to explain the development of DM-linked cardiovascular defects. Among them, the theories of Dr. Brownlee provide us with an insight into the involvement of ROS in the development of cardiovascular complications in DM [25]. ROS produced within the mitochondria initiate the development of diabetic cardiac complications. The heart is the organ which works throughout the lifetime maintaining adequate contractility and rhythmicity, for which it requires a continuous source of substrate and optimal mitochondrial metabolism to meet its high-energy demands. During DM, the substrate supply for the cardiomyocytes' mitochondrial metabolism switches between glucose and fatty acids irregularly. Thus a high glucose and fatty acid supply causes an increase in the workload of the mitochondrial electron transport chain, which further worsens its leaky nature. The leakage produces superoxide radicals by single electron reduction of oxygen molecules. This excess superoxide radical is the source of most other free radicals and reactive species, which cause oxidative stress followed by cardiomyocytes dysfunction, because of several cell signaling changes involved in apoptosis, necrosis and other cardiac remodeling processes.

SUMMARY POINTS

- Most of the pathological remodeling occurring in diabetic cardiomyopathy has oxidative stress as the prerequisite for its development.
- Hyperglycemia and lipotoxicity are the major metabolic disturbances leading to the development of diabetic cardiomyopathy.
- Oxidative stress in diabetic cardiomyopathy involves the excess production of mitochondrial superoxide radical followed by several other reactive species which are not counter-balanced by the innate antioxidant defense system.
- Several cellular signaling pathways are activated by oxidative stress or vice versa, and both can serve as important targets for the treatment of diabetic cardiomyopathy.
- Reports suggest mixed effectiveness of antioxidants against the cardiac effects of DM. The individual properties of the particular antioxidant, its mechanism of action, the concentration reached at the site of action, is likely to determine its effectiveness.

References

[1] Rolo AP, Palmeira CM. Diabetes and mitochondrial function: role of hyperglycemia and oxidative stress. Toxicol Appl Pharmacol 2006;212:167–78.

[2] Bell DSH. Heart failure: the frequent, forgotten, and often fatal complication of diabetes. Diabetes Care 2003;26:2433–41.

[3] Kannel WB, McGee DL. Diabetes and cardiovascular disease: the Framingham study. JAMA 1979;241:2035–8.

[4] Factor SM, Minase T, Sonnenblick EH. Clinical and morphological features of human hypertensive-diabetic cardiomyopathy. Am Heart J 1980;99:446–58.

[5] Laakso M. Dyslipidemia, morbidity, and mortality in non-insulin-dependent diabetes mellitus. Lipoproteins and coronary heart disease in non-insulin-dependent diabetes mellitus. J Diabetes Complications 1997;11:137–41.

[6] Ernande L, Derumeaux G. Diabetic cardiomyopathy: myth or reality? Arch Cardiovasc Dis 2012;105:218–25.

[7] Galderisi M, Anderson KM, Wilson PW, Levy D. Echocardiographic evidence for the existence of a distinct diabetic cardiomyopathy (the Framingham Heart Study). Am J Cardiol 1991;68:85–9.

[8] Ingelsson E, Sundstrom J, Arnlov J, Zethelius B, Lind L. Insulin resistance and risk of congestive heart failure. JAMA 2005;294:334–41.

[9] Matsushita K, Blecker S, Pazin-Filho A, Bertoni A, Chang PP, Coresh J, et al. The association of hemoglobin a1c with incident heart failure among people without diabetes: the atherosclerosis risk in communities study. Diabetes 2010;59:2020–6.

[10] Takeda N, Dixon IM, Hata T, Elimban V, Shah KR, Dhalla NS. Sequence of alterations in subcellular organelles during the development of heart dysfunction in diabetes. Diabetes Res Clin Pract 1996;30:S113–22.

[11] Selvaraju V, Joshi M, Suresh S, Sanchez JA, Maulik N, Maulik G. Diabetes, oxidative stress, molecular mechanism, and cardiovascular disease – an overview. Toxicol Mech Methods 2012;22:330–5.

[12] Nishikawa T, Edelstein D, Du XL, Yamagishi S, Matsumura T, Kaneda Y, et al. Normalizing mitochondrial superoxide production blocks three pathways of hyperglycaemic damage. Nature 2000;404:787–90.

[13] Mukhopadhyay P, Rajesh M, Yoshihiro K, Haskó G, Pacher P. Simple quantitative detection of mitochondrial superoxide production in live cells. Biochem Biophys Res Commun 2007;358:203–8.
[14] Leverve XM, Guigas B, Detaille D, Batandier C, Koceir EA, Chauvin C, et al. Mitochondrial metabolism and type-2 diabetes: a specific target of metformin. Diabetes Metab 2003;29; 6S88–6S94.
[15] Prasad K, Mantha SV, Kalra J, Lee P. Hypercholesterolemia-induced oxidative stress in heart and its prevention by vitamin E. Int J Angiol 1997;6:13–7.
[16] Ghosh S, Rodrigues B. Cardiac cell death in early diabetes and its modulation by dietary fatty acids. Biochimica et Biophysica Acta 2006;1761:1148–62.
[17] Xi G, Shen X, Maile LA, Wai C, Gollahon K, Clemmons DR. Hyperglycemia enhances IGF-I-stimulated Src activation via increasing Nox4-derived reactive oxygen species in a PKCζ-dependent manner in vascular smooth muscle cells. Diabetes 2012;61:104–13.
[18] Murdoch CE, Grieve DJ, Cave AC, Looi YH, Shah AM. NADPH oxidase and heart failure. Curr Opin Pharmacol 2006;6:148–53.
[19] Pacher P, Beckman JS, Liaudet L. Nitric oxide and peroxynitrite in health and disease. Physiol Rev 2007;87:315–424.
[20] Son SM. Reactive oxygen and nitrogen species in pathogenesis of vascular complications of diabetes. Diabetes Metab J 2012;36:190–8.
[21] Yao D, Shi W, Gou Y, Zhou X, Yee Aw T, Zhou Y, et al. Fatty acid-mediated intracellular iron translocation: a synergistic mechanism of oxidative injury. Free Radic Biol Med 2005;39:1385–98.
[22] Pratico D, Pasin M, Barry OP, Ghiselli A, Sabatino G, Iuliano L, et al. Iron-dependent human platelet activation and hydroxyl radical formation: involvement of protein kinase C. Circulation 1999;99:3118–24.
[23] Tripathi T, Rasheed Z. The oxidative by-product, hydroxyl radical, damaged immunoglobulin-G in patients with non-insulin dependent diabetes mellitus. Bratisl Lek Listy 2010;111:477–84.
[24] Khan MW, Sherwani S, Khan WA, Ali R. Characterization of hydroxyl radical modified GAD65: a potential autoantigen in type 1 diabetes. Autoimmunity 2009;42:150–8.
[25] Brownlee M. Biochemistry and molecular cell biology of diabetic complications. Nature 2001;414:813–20.
[26] Chung SS, Ho EC, Lam KS, Chung SK. Contribution of polyol pathway to diabetes-induced oxidative stress. J Am Soc Nephrol 2003;14:S233–6.
[27] McNulty PH. Hexosamine biosynthetic pathway flux and cardiomyopathy in type 2 diabetes mellitus. Focus on 'Impact of type 2 diabetes and aging on cardiomyocyte function and O-linked N-acetylglucosamine levels in the heart'. Am J Physiol Cell Physiol 2007;292:C1243–4.
[28] Yan SD, Schmidt AM, Anderson GM, Zhang J, Brett J, Zou YS, et al. Enhanced cellular oxidant stress by the interaction of advanced glycation end products with their receptors/binding proteins. J Biol Chem 1994;269:9889–97.
[29] Geraldes P, King GL. Activation of protein kinase C isoforms and its impact on diabetic complications. Circ Res 2010;106:1319–31.
[30] Watanabe K, Thandavarayan RA, Harima M, Sari FR, Gurusamy N, Veeraveedu PT, et al. Role of differential signaling pathways and oxidative stress in diabetic cardiomyopathy. Curr Cardiol Rev 2010;6:280–90.
[31] Gurusamy N, Watanabe K, Ma M, Zhang S, Muslin AJ, Kodama M, et al. Inactivation of 14-3-3 protein exacerbates cardiac hypertrophy and fibrosis through enhanced expression of protein kinase C beta 2 in experimental diabetes. Biol Pharm Bull 2005;28:957–62.
[32] Thandavarayan RA, Giridharan VV, Sari FR, Arumugam S, Veeraveedu PT, Pandian GN, et al. Depletion of 14-3-3 protein exacerbates cardiac oxidative stress, inflammation and remodeling process via modulation of MAPK/NF-κB signaling pathways after streptozotocin-induced diabetes mellitus. Cell Physiol Biochem 2011;28:911–22.
[33] Thandavarayan RA, Watanabe K, Ma M, Gurusamy N, Veeraveedu PT, Konishi T, et al. Dominant-negative p38alpha mitogen-activated protein kinase prevents cardiac apoptosis and remodeling after streptozotocin-induced diabetes mellitus. Am J Physiol Heart Circ Physiol 2009;297:H911–9.
[34] Thandavarayan RA, Watanabe K, Ma M, Veeraveedu PT, Gurusamy N, Palaniyandi SS, et al. 14-3-3 protein regulates Ask1 signaling and protects against diabetic cardiomyopathy. Biochem Pharmacol 2008;75:1797–806.
[35] Desai AS, O'Gara PT. Diabetes and heart failure: epidemiology, pathophysiology and management. Indian Heart J 2005;57: 295–303.

CHAPTER

4

Diabetic Retinopathy and Oxidative Stress

Jose Javier Garcia-Medina[*], *Monica del-Rio-Vellosillo*[†], *Manuel Garcia-Medina*[**], *Vicente Zanon-Moreno*[‡], *Roberto Gallego-Pinazo*[***], *Maria Dolores Pinazo-Duran*[§]

*Department of Ophthalmology, University General Hospital Reina Sofía and Department of Ophthalmology and Optometry, School of Medicine, University of Murcia, Murcia, Spain, †Department of Anesthesiology, University Hospital La Arrixaca, El Palmar, Murcia, Spain, **Department of Ophthalmology, Torrecardenas Hospital, Almeria, Spain, ‡Genetic and Molecular Epidemiology Unit, Department of Preventive Medicine and Public Health, School of Medicine, University of Valencia and CIBER Fisiopatología de la Obesidad y Nutrición, Valencia, Spain, ***Department of Ophthalmology, University and Polytechnic Hospital La Fe, Valencia, Spain, §Ophthalmology Research Unit 'Santiago Grisolia' and Department of Surgery, School of Medicine, University of Valencia, Valencia, Spain

List of Abbreviations

AGEs Advanced glycation end products
ATP Adenosine triphosphate
Bax BCL2-associated X protein
DR Diabetic retinopathy
ETC Electron transport chain
FRs Free radicals
GSH Gluthatione
iBRB Inner blood retina barrier
IL Interleukin
MMP Matrix metalloproteinases
mtDNA Mitochondrial DNA
NF-κB Nuclear factor kappa B
NO Nitric oxide
oBRB Outer blood retina barrier
OS Oxidative stress
PKC Protein kinase C
RPE Retinal pigment epithelium
SOD Superoxide dismutase
TAS Total antioxidant status
TNF Tumor necrosis factor
VEGF Vascular endothelial growth factor

HISTOPATHOLOGY OF DR

The retina is located on the inner surface of the ocular globe between the choroid and the vitreous. It is made up of four main kinds of cells:

- vascular cells (pericytes and endothelial cells),
- macroglia (Müller cells and astrocytes),
- neurons (photoreceptors, second-order neurons and ganglion cells), and
- microglia.

We ought to remember that blood cells circulate in vessels and that an ongoing functional integration among these cells continuously takes place.

The retina has dual circulation. Retinal blood vessels provide nourishment to the inner retinal layers and carry off waste products from them. Outer retinal layers are avascular and are supplied by diffusion from the choroid. In the retinal capillaries, endothelial cells and pericytes, which seem to possess endothelial cell-regulating properties, share a common basement membrane [1] (Figure 4.1).

Endothelial cell membranes are likewise interfused by tight junctions responsible for the inner blood retina barrier (iBRB) [2]. This barrier constitutes a tight seal between the cells controlling the flux of fluids, proteins, and even ions, across tissue barriers. Hence molecular exchange is mainly transcellular, and is not due to passive diffusion. Thus, the extracellular stable environment required for adequate neural activity is achieved [3] (Figure 4.1). Otherwise the outer blood retina barrier (oBRB) is formed by the retinal pigment epithelium (RPE). It also regulates fluids and molecular movement, and prevents macromolecules and other potentially harmful agents from leaking into the retina.

Diabetes: Oxidative Stress and Dietary Antioxidants.
http://dx.doi.org/10.1016/B978-0-12-405885-9.00004-8

Endothelial cells play a key role in the control of vascular tone and hemostasis, and are involved in several immunological processes [4]. In addition, these cells also synthesize compounds for basement membrane formation, such as fibronectine, collagen IV or laminin [5], and they produce growth factors [6]. There is a continuous ongoing functional interaction between endothelial cells and neighboring cells (pericytes, astrocytes, Müller cells and circulating blood cells).

Pericytes provide vascular stability and control endothelial proliferation [7]. They seem to perform a similar contractile function to that of smooth muscle cells in regulating vascular flow [8]. They also participate in basement membrane formation [9].

In the retinas of diabetic patients, changes apparently occur early at the molecular level. Diabetic retinopathy (DR) develops in stages, and various pathophysiological processes can be identified during the course of this disease, which are described below (Figure 4.2). One initial measurable sign is dysfunctional autoregulation, which results in diminished blood flow [10].

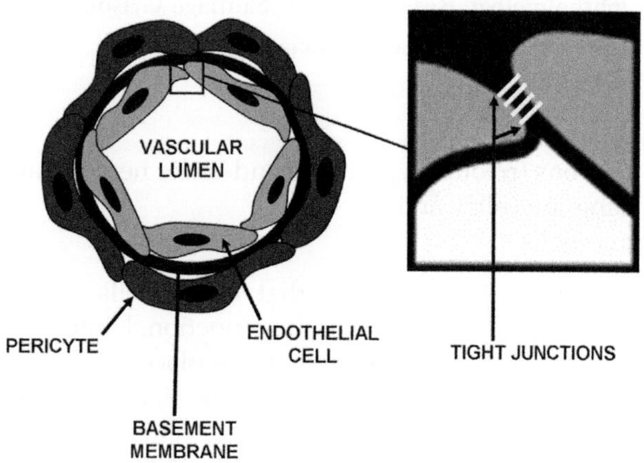

FIGURE 4.1 Structure of retinal capillary wall.

Loss of pericytes is a main early finding in DR [7] (Figure 4.2). Pericytes normally occur in a 1:1 ratio with endothelial cells. However in diabetics, the endothelial cell to pericyte ratio alters to become 4:1 [11]. This fact is detectable only by histological examination and cannot be seen clinically.

Pericyte loss leads to both altered vascular tone and phenotypic changes in endothelial cells [7]. Dilatations of the capillary wall, called microaneurysms, appear in areas where supporting pericytes have been lost, and localized increases in hydrostatic pressure take place, and are surrounded by non-perfused areas [12]. Microaneurysms are the earliest clinically observable lesion of DR, and are clinically identified by ophthalmoscopy as red dots mainly in the posterior pole (Figures 4.2 and 4.3).

As pericytes die, endothelial cells attempt to repair the damaged vessel by proliferating on the inner side of the vessel wall [13]. As the disease progresses, it results in a blockade of capillaries (capillary occlusion), leading to local ischemia (Figure 4.2). This is followed by loss of retinal capillary endothelial cells, resulting in the formation of acellular capillaries (also known as ghost capillaries) [14] (Figure 4.2).

In parallel, endothelial cell tight junctions disrupt and alter the iBRB. Thus capillaries become leaky and allow fluids, macromolecules, and even blood cells, to seep out into the retina. All these elements also interfere with the normal diffusion of nutrients to retinal cells. Yellow deposits (hard exudates), retinal edema (due to fluid diffusion) and small hemorrhages can be ophthalmoscopically observed [2] (Figures 4.2 and 4.3). If the edema is located in the macula (Figure 4.3), it is known as macular edema. This is one of the clinical features that best correlates with the degree of vision loss in diabetic patients. Otherwise the common basement membrane of endothelial cells and pericytes thickens (Figure 4.2), leading to increased vessel wall rigidity, which interferes with

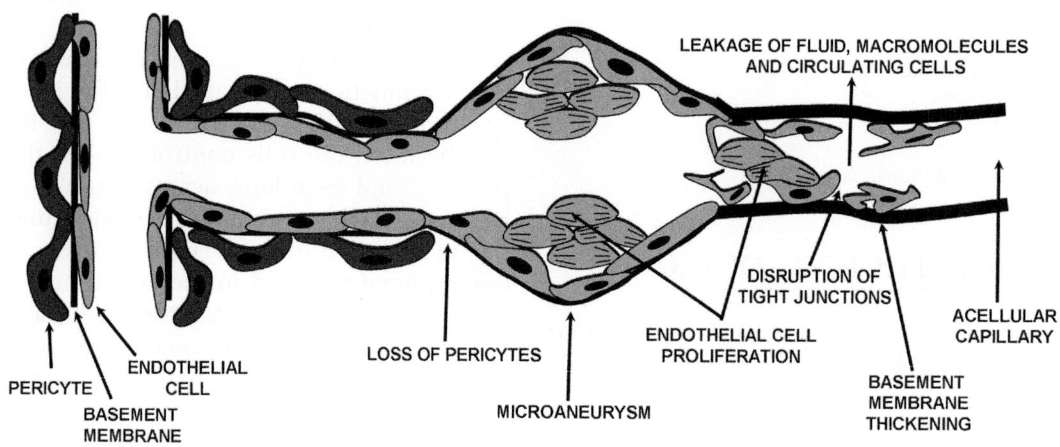

FIGURE 4.2 Vascular microscopic changes in diabetic retinopathy.

pericyte-endothelial cell interaction and makes the diffusion of nutrients through it difficult [15].

Basement membrane thickening, disruption of the iBRB, loss of pericytes and endothelial cells, and transformation of the remaining endothelial cells into a more prothrombotic phenotype can all lead to local tissue ischemia. This local ischemia is further aggravated by the formation of micro-occlusions, believed to be caused by leukostasis, platelet aggregation and endothelial dysfunction [1].

Other associated findings are fluffy white patches, known as cotton wool spots (Figure 4.3), which represent localized arrest during the axoplasmic transport of retinal nerve fibers due to retinal nerve fiber layer infarction.

Non-proliferative DR proceeds to proliferative DR. When perfusion is sufficiently low, hypoxia stimulates the development of new vessels from existing ones by the sprouting and migration of endothelial cells, endothelial cell proliferation and tube formation [1]. All these changes are mediated by growth factors such as VEGF. These newly formed blood capillaries (neovessels) are fragile and tend to break, causing vitreous hemorrhaging and subsequent loss of vision (Figure 4.4). The extension of these new vessels into the vitreous of eyes, and their fibrous proliferation on the retina, may scar the vitreous body, leading to tractional retinal detachment, and ultimately to blindness [15].

Besides cellular retinal vascular alterations, diabetes also damages non-vascular retinal cells, such as neuron cells and glial cells, and neuronal degeneration may occur. Moreover, new insights into retinal physiology suggest that diabetes-associated retinal dysfunction may be viewed as a change in the retinal neurovascular unit. The neurovascular unit refers to the physical and biochemical relationship among neurons, glia and vascular cells [16]. Müller cells and astrocytes (macroglia) are the interface between neurons and vascular cells, and provide neurons with nourishment and regulatory support. Macroglial cells are also required for the specialized differentiation of the endothelial cells required to form the iBRB. Microglial cells are resident macrophages that monitor the local environment and provide immunomodulatory functions [17].

Most retinal neurons and glial cells alter concomitantly with the development of microvascular lesions, and are progressively impaired with worsening retinopathy. From early DR phases, apoptotic loss of photoreceptors and ganglionar cells occurs [18]. In accordance with neuronal loss, disturbances in functional tests, such as automated perimetry, electroretinogram, color vision and contrast sensitivity, have been found in diabetic patients [19].

Since the communication and interdependence between the retinal vascular system and the neuronal network is intense, neuronal retina degeneration may well initiate or aggravate diabetic vascular disturbances [19].

OXIDATIVE STRESS MECHANISMS

Free radicals (FRs) can be defined as atoms or molecules containing one or more unpaired electrons, which makes them unstable and highly reactive. It is a

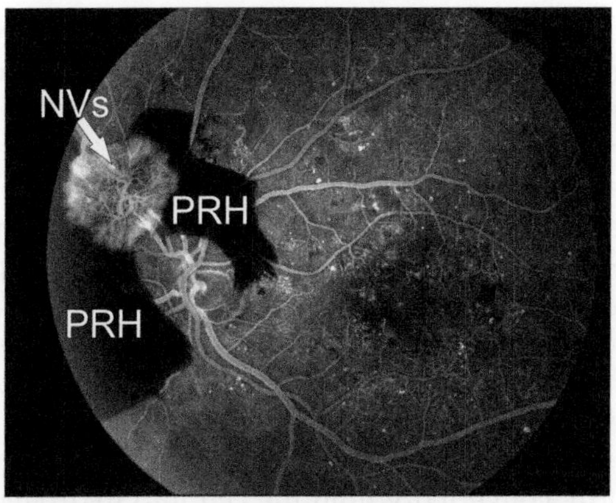

FIGURE 4.4 Angiographic photograph of proliferative diabetic retinopathy showing parapapillary newly formed vessel (NVs) and adjacent areas of preretinal hemorrhage (PRH).

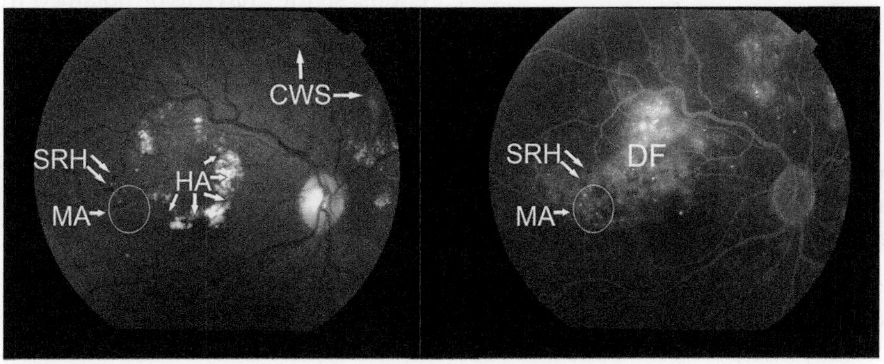

FIGURE 4.3 Corresponding images showing microaneurysms (MA), small retinal hemorrhages (SRH), cotton wool spots (CWS), hard exudates (HA) and diffusion (DF) in red-free (left) and angiographic (right) photographs.

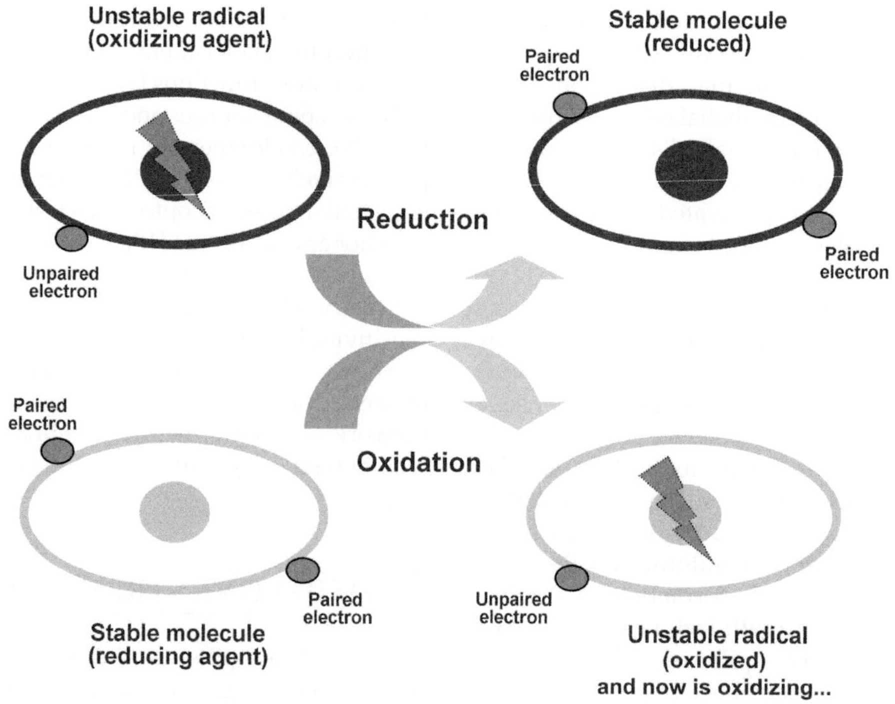

FIGURE 4.5 **An oxidation process is always associated with another reduction process.**

reaction-prone molecule given its desire to gain an electron from neighboring molecules [20]. An oxidation process is always associated with another reduction process (Figure 4.5).

FRs are produced continuously in all cells to support normal cellular functions, but those derived from oxygen (ROS) are the most important type of such species generated in living systems [21].

Under physiological conditions, approximately 0.1–5% of the oxygen entering the mitochondrial electron transport chain (ETC) is reduced to superoxide, while the rest is used in metabolic processes [21]. Superoxide is rapidly converted within the cell into hydrogen peroxide by superoxide dismutases. Then excess hydrogen peroxide is converted into water by the action of catalase, glutathione peroxidase and other peroxidases. Hydrogen peroxide can react with reduced transition metals or with superoxide in the presence of metal iron or copper to produce the highly damaging molecule known as reactive hydroxyl radical. In addition to forming hydrogen peroxide, superoxide radicals can rapidly react with nitric oxide (NO) to generate cytotoxic peroxynitrite anions, which are more reactive than superoxide [22].

Besides mitochondria, there are other cellular sources of ROS, these being:

1) NAD(P)H oxidase(s);
2) phagocytic cell activation, including neutrophils eosinophils and macrophages;
3) NO synthases;
4) cytochrome P450 metabolism;
5) peroxisomes;
6) xanthine oxidases related to the hypoxia-reperfusion mechanism;
7) the auto-oxidation of glucose [23].

The effect of ROS is neutralized by the antioxidant action of enzymatic and non-enzymatic antioxidants. Non-enzymatic antioxidants include α-tocopherol (vitamin E), ascorbic acid (vitamin C), natural flavonoids, uric acid, bilirubin, albumin, thiol antioxidants (α-lipoic acid, glutathione and thioredoxin), melatonin and other compounds [24]. Enzymatic antioxidants include intracellular catalase, superoxide dismutase, and glutathione peroxidase [25]. Another classification is established according to origin: endogenous or exogenous. Glutathione, SOD, catalase and glutathione peroxidase are endogenous, so they are synthesized by the organism. Vitamins C and E, and flavonoids are, for example, exogenous, so they have to be obtained from the diet.

Under normal physiological conditions, ROS are effectively eliminated by these antioxidant systems. However, if this balance is disrupted by excess ROS production, which cannot be neutralized by antioxidant defenses, oxidative stress (OS) appears.

ROS are able to oxidize proteins, lipids (lipoxidation), carbohydrates (glycoxidation) and cause mitochondrial DNA (mtDNA) strand breakage. The resulting molecules are capable of causing further oxidative damage to cellular organelles, giving functional and structural alterations when oxidized molecules accumulate in the cell [23]. ROS can also modulate many cellular functions and can alter gene expressions by stimulating signal transduction pathways [26].

OXIDATIVE STRESS AND DR

Before considering oxidative stress in the DR context, it is interesting to remark that the retina is a peculiar tissue in the human body [27]. It is rich in polyunsaturated fatty acids. The specific susceptibility of these molecules to damage by lipid peroxidation is due to the large quantity of double bonds that they contain. Each double bond is a source of an atom of hydrogen that contains an electron. This electron is captured by FRs and the lipid peroxidation cascade is initiated.

Chronic exposure to blue light occurs at between 10 and 100 times higher than skin exposure due to the corneal and lens focusing of light (loupe effect). Blue light stimulates the production of FRs such as singlet oxygen.

Otherwise the retina has the highest oxygen uptake and glucose oxidation of any tissue. As it is highly active in metabolic terms, it also presents one of the highest densities of mitochondria, which are concentrated mostly in the RPE and in the outer segments of the rods. All these phenomena make the retina more susceptible to OS than other tissues [27].

ROS overproduction in the mitochondria has been considered to play a major role in the pathophysiology of DR. The mitochondria constitute a important organelle for cell survival and their main functions include the production of chemical energy and the regulation of programd cell death. Under high glycemic conditions, the mitochondrial ETC is in charge of energy formation through ATP production. Electron flow through the mitochondrial ETC proceeds via four enzyme complexes; I, II, III, and IV; which are bound to the inner mitochondrial membrane. Electron transfer among these complexes is accomplished by the coenzymes ubiquinone (from complexes I and II to complex III) and cytochrome *c* (from complex III to complex IV). The energy from the electron transfer through these complexes serves to extrude protons outwardly across the inner membrane to generate a proton or voltage gradient. The energy from this voltage gradient is used for the synthesis of ATP [28].

However, more glucose is oxidized under hyperglycemic conditions, which means that more electron donors enter the ETC. Consequently, the gradient across the mitochondrial membrane increases to the extent that complex III is blocked, causing electrons to accumulate in coenzyme Q, which donates electrons to the molecular oxygen to generate superoxide [29,30].

ROS overproduction by the mitochondrial ETC is not the only source of ROS, but is considered the first step in initiating superoxide production by other sources.

Other sources of ROS production in diabetes include an increased flux of glucose and other sugars through the polyol pathway, increased intracellular formation of advanced glycation end products (AGEs), increased expression of the receptor for advanced glycation end products and its activating ligands, activation of protein kinase C (PKC) isoforms, and overactivity of the hexosamine pathway. The vast majority of publications on the mechanisms underlying hyperglycemia-induced diabetic damage focus on the aforementioned mechanisms. However, the results of clinical studies in which only one of these pathways is blocked have proved disappointing. This has led to the unifying hypothesis that all these mechanisms are activated by a single event: overproduction of ROS [31] (Figure 4.6).

To make the situation worse, antioxidant defenses, such as SOD, catalase, glutathione peroxidase and intracellular antioxidant GSH levels, are also impaired in diabetes [32,33].

Increased superoxide formation leads to the oxidative damage of mtDNA, proteins and lipid membranes. On the one hand, the alteration of ETC proteins and mtDNA-encoded genes induces a vicious cycle of damage to macromolecules by amplifying more ROS production. Initially, the insult can be compensated by protective mechanisms, but these mechanisms are overwhelmed with sustained insult, and mtDNA and ETC proteins become increasingly damaged [34]. Thus, ROS can indirectly induce apoptosis by changing cellular redox potentials, by altering mtDNA, by depleting GSH, and by reducing ATP levels [35,36].

On the other hand, the damage that ROS does to the mitochondrial lipid membrane increases organelle permeability, which causes the mitochondria to swell. Then the release of mitochondrial cytochrome c into the cytoplasm can result in caspase-9 activation, which triggers a cascade of events that activates caspase-3, a pro-apoptotic factor [36b]. Otherwise the translocation of pro-apototic protein Bax (BCL2-associated X protein) from the cytoplasm into the mitochondria also activates apoptotic mechanisms in retinal and capillary cells in diabetes [37].

A number of studies support a role for ROS in the activation of signal transduction pathways that results in increased production of cytokines and growth factors. For example, ROS activate nuclear transcription factor NF-κB, which is known to activate downstream of inflammatory cytokines, NO and prostaglandins. NF-κB has been linked to retinal capillary cell apoptosis, vascular inflammation, and neovascularization [38]. Levels of cytokines, including IL-1β, IL-6 and IL-8, increase in the vitreous fluid of patients with proliferative DR and in the retinas of diabetic rodent models [39]. Besides, redox stress has been correlated with increased VEGF production under *in vitro* conditions and is thought to be involved in the up-regulation of the VEGF expression in DR [39]. VEGF is produced by hypoxic tissue, and promotes both vascular permeability and angiogenesis. In diabetic rats, the retinal VEGF levels increase, which can be blocked by antioxidant treatment [40]. Positive correlations have also been found between the potential antioxidant and VEGF levels, and between the lipid peroxide and VEGF concentrations in the vitreous of patients with proliferative DR [41].

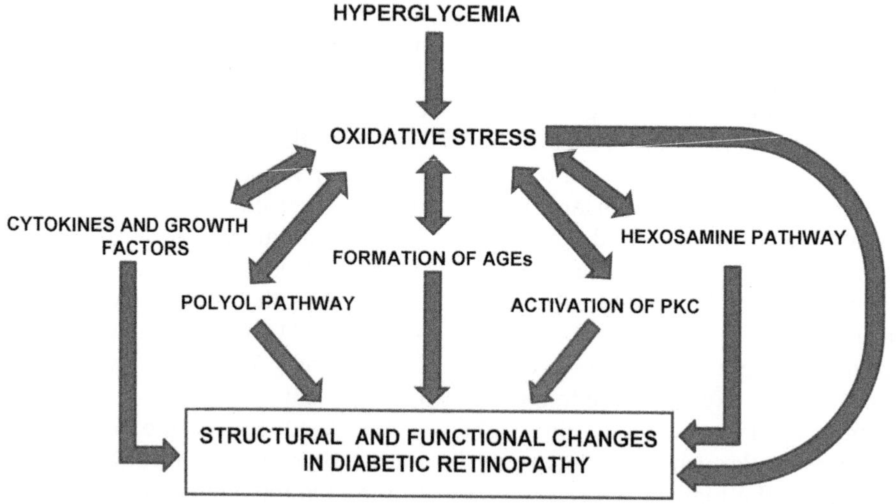

FIGURE 4.6 Schematic representation of the proposed unifying theory of how hyperglycemia results in the pathophysiology of diabetes via the generation of ROS and the subsequent oxidative stress. ROS can also inflict damage directly.

In addition, matrix metalloproteinases (MMPs) are sensitive to oxidative stress, and are induced by an increase in ROS [42]. MMPs are generally associated with the degradation of extracellular matrix proteins, but have also been found to be present within the cells in nuclear, mitochondrial and cytoplasmic compartments [43]. MMPs contribute to disease pathophysiology via a number of different pathways in both the non-proliferative and proliferative stages of DR.

MMP-2 and MMP-9 are involved in the damage of retinal mitochondria in diabetes [44–45]. The activation of MMPs is shown to accelerate the apoptosis process in diabetes [46]. Increased retinal MMPs facilitate enhanced vascular permeability via the proteolytic degradation of the tight junction protein and the subsequent disturbance of the iBRB in DR [47]. Increased MMP-9 has been observed in the human retina, where active neovascularization was revealed over two decades ago [48]. MMPs may degrade the capillary basement membrane before new vessels form, to facilitate the tissue availability of bound VEGF, and may alternatively act as angiogenesis agonists [49].

Otherwise oxidative stress has been related to metabolic memory. This phenomenon in DR defines some basic causes of chronic damage in diabetic vasculopathy that cannot be reversed, not even by subsequent, good control of blood glucose [50]. Studies conducted with type 1 diabetic patients have indicated that increased levels of plasma oxidative stress markers persist in those with poor glycemic control (glycated hemoglobin over 7%) for the first five years of the disease, even if normoglycemia is achieved [51].

In a study with diabetic rats, reinstitution of good glyacaemic control for seven months after only a two month poor glycemic control was found to inhibit increases in retinal lipid peroxides, inducible nitric oxide synthase and NO levels. However, these retinal oxidative and nitrative modifications were not reversed secondarily to the reinstitution of normoglycemia after six months of hyperglycemia [52].

Another study in diabetic rats, with a poor six month metabolic control, also showed that the nitrotyrosine concentration in retinal capillaries failed to reverse when normoglycemia was reinstituted [53].

In vitro studies with retinal cells have concluded that ROS overproduction mediates cellular hyperglycemia memory after glucose normalization. In addition, it also has been shown that glucose fluctuation further enhances ROS production, oxidative stress, and DNA damage, and that it induces a more adverse hyperglycemia memory effect than constant high glucose [54].

In short, ROS not only contribute to the development of DR, but also play a role in its progression when hyperglycemic insult is controlled.

During the pathogenesis of DR, retinal capillary cells and other non-capillary cells are affected by accelerated apoptosis before clinical manifestations of retinopathy are observed, as explained above. OS has been associated with pericyte and endothelial loss [39]. Tight junctions between endothelial cells are also damaged by ROS in DR. In the normal state, neural retina cells, including glial cells and pericytes, produce pro-barrier factors that contribute to maintain tight junction integrity and the iBRB. However in hyperglycemia, pro-barrier factors decrease, while perycites and glial cells respond to excessive ROS production by secreting cytokines (TNF-a, IL-1b) or growth factors (VEGF) that disturb tight junctions, thus increasing permeability and allowing vascular leakage of liquid and molecules into retinal parenchyma. Tight junction damage by a direct mechanism is also feasible [55].

However, retinal non-capillary cells are also affected by excess free radicals. Recently it has been shown that angiotensin II type I receptor blockade by losartan acts as a neuroprotective treatment to prevent the apoptosis of neural and glial cells in DR by re-establishing oxidative redox and mitochondrial functions [56].

Both structural and functional changes have been related to OS in DR, such as decreased retinal blood flow [57]. In fact, vitamin E, an antioxidant agent, supplemented over an eight month period in short-duration diabetic patients with little or no retinopathy has been reported to lead to normalized retinal blood flow [57].

Several biomarkers of oxidative stress and antioxidant capacity can be measured not only in ocular tissues or cells under hyperglycemic conditions, but also in blood. Antioxidant enzymes levels are usually measured together as the total antioxidant status (TAS). Reports on the status of antioxidants and antioxidant enzymes in diabetic patients prove somewhat contradictory, as both increases and decreases in antioxidant activity have been reported. In general terms, TAS has been shown to be significantly lower in patients with proliferative DR than in diabetics who do not develop retinopathy [38].

Moreover, diabetes induces the generation of oxidative-related damage in DNA, lipids and proteins. The serum biomarkers of these processes, such as malondialdehyde, thiobarbituric acid reacting substances, conjugated diene, advanced oxidation protein products, protein carbonyl, 8-hydroxydeoxyguanosin, nitrotyrosine, and F(2) isoprostanes, have been found to be higher in patients or animals with DR than in diabetic patients/animals without DR [38].

In conclusion, OS plays a pivotal role in the development of DR, but the relative contribution of each oxidative-induced alteration in DR remains to be clarified and to be more precisely integrated into the remaining metabolic ways in the physiopathology of this disease. FR summarizes some possible issues associated with OS in DR. Biomarkers of both OS and antioxidant status may be indicative of diabetic subjects' susceptibility to develop DR. However more studies along these lines are required. Finally, treatment with antioxidants seems to be a promising strategy to partially halt the progression of DR (see Chapter 22, 'Antioxidant Supplements and Diabetic Retinopathy' in this book).

SUMMARY POINTS

- Biochemical abnormalities in DR contribute to both the microscopic structural and functional changes in the retina.
- All these alterations result in macroscopic retinal damage and vision loss.
- Oxidative stress is considered a causal link between elevated glucose and other biochemical abnormalities.
- Mitochondrial electron transport chain is not the only source of ROS, but is considered the first step to initiate superoxide production by other sources.
- Oxidative stress may activate several biochemical pathways involved in the pathophysiology of DR.
- These pathways, in turn, can induce ROS overproduction, resulting in a vicious cycle.
- Antioxidant defenses are impaired in diabetes.
- ROS increase the production of cytokines and growth factors.
- Oxidative stress has been related to metabolic memory.

References

[1] Khan ZA, Chakrabarti S. Cellular signaling and potential new treatment targets in diabetic retinopathy. Exp Diabetes Res 2007;2007:31867.

[2] Madsen-Bouterse SA, Kowluru RA. Oxidative stress and diabetic retinopathy: pathophysiological mechanisms and treatment perspectives. Rev Endocr Metab Disord 2008;9:315–27.

[3] Gardner TW, Antonetti DA, Barber AJ, Lieth E, Tarbell JA. The molecular structure and function of the inner blood-retinal barrier. Penn State Retina Research Group. Doc Ophthalmol 1999;97:229–37.

[4] Demuth K, Myara I, Moatti N. Biology of the endothelial cell and atherogenesis. Ann Biol Clin 1995;53:171–91.

[5] Mandarino LJ, Sundarraj N, Finlayson J, Hassell HR. Regulation of fibronectin and laminin synthesis by retinal capillary endothelial cells and pericytes *in vitro*. Exp Eye Res 1993;57:609–21.

[6] Brooks RA, Burrin JM, Kohner EM. Characterization of release of basic fibroblast growth factor from bovine retinal endothelial cells in monolayer cultures. Biochem J 1991;276:113–20.

[7] Ejaz S, Chekarova I, Ejaz A, Sohail A, Lim CW. Importance of pericytes and mechanisms of pericyte loss during diabetes retinopathy. Diabetes Obes Metab 2008;10:53–63.

[8] Ruggiero D, Lecomte M, Michoud E, Lagarde M, Wiernsperger N. Involvement of cell-cell interactions in the pathogenesis of diabetic retinopathy. Diabetes Metab 1997;23:30–42.

[9] Yamagishi S, Kobayashi K, Yamamoto H. Vascular pericytes not only regulate growth, but also preserve prostacyclin-producing ability and protect against lipid peroxide-induced injury of co-cultured endothelial cells. Biochem Biophys Res Commun 1993;190:418–25.

[10] Lorenzi M, Gerhardinger C. Early cellular and molecular changes induced by diabetes in the retina. Diabetologia 2001;44:791–804.

[11] Robison Jr WG, Kador PF, Kinoshita JH. Early retinal microangiopathy: prevention with aldose reductase inhibitors. Diabet Med 1985;2:196–9.

[12] Aguilar E, Friedlander M, Gariano RF. Endothelial proliferation in diabetic retinal microaneurysms. Arch Ophthalmol 2003;121:740–1.

[13] Hofman P, van Blijswijk BC, Gaillard PJ, Vrensen GF, Schlingemann RO. Endothelial cell hypertrophy induced by vascular endothelial growth factor in the retina: new insights into the pathogenesis of capillary nonperfusion. Arch Ophthalmol 2001;119:861–6.

[14] Mizutani M, Kern TS, Lorenzi M. Accelerated death of retinal microvascular cells in human and experimental diabetic retinopathy. J Clin Invest 1996;97:2883–90.

[15] Durham JT, Herman IM. Microvascular modifications in diabetic retinopathy. Curr Diab Rep 2011;11:253–64.

[16] Antonetti DA, Klein R, Gardner TW. Diabetic retinopathy. N Engl J Med 2012;366:1227–39.

[17] Coorey NJ, Shen W, Chung SH, Zhu L, Gillies MC. The role of glia in retinal vascular disease. Clin Exp Optom 2012;95:266–81.
[18] Barber AJ, Gardner TW, Abcouwer SF. The significance of vascular and neural apoptosis to the pathology of diabetic retinopathy. Invest Ophthalmol Vis Sci 2011;52:1156–63.
[19] Gardner TW, Antonetti DA, Barber AJ, LaNoue KF, Levison SW. Diabetic Retinopathy: more than meets the eye. Surv Ophthalmol 2002;47:S253–62.
[20] Halliwell B, Gutteridge JM. Lipid peroxidation, oxygen radicals, cell damage and antioxidant therapy. Lancet 1984;1:1396–7.
[21] Kowluru RA, Chan PS. Oxidative stress and diabetic retinopathy. Exp Diabetes Res 2007:43603.
[22] Dröge W. Free radicals in the physiological control of cell function. Physiol Rev 2002;82:47–95.
[23] Garcia-Medina JJ, Garcia-Medina M. Estrés oxidativo. Mecanismos moleculares al alcance del oftalmólogo. Barcelona: Domènech Pujades; 2007.
[24] McCall MR, Frei B. Can antioxidant vitamins materially reduce oxidative damage in humans? Free Radic Biol Med 1999;26:1034–53.
[25] Mates JM, Perez-Gomez C, Nuez de Castro I. Antioxidant enzymes and human diseases. Clin Biochem 1999;32:595–603.
[26] Cutler RG. Oxidative stress profiling: part I. Its potential importance in the optimization of human health. Ann N Y Acad Sci 2005;1055:93–135.
[27] Garcia-Medina JJ, Garcia-Medina M, Pinazo-Duran MD. Estrés oxidativo y retinopatía diabética. Barcelona: Domènech Pujades; 2007.
[28] Wallace DC. Disease of the mitochondrial DNA. Annu Rev Biochem 1992;61:1175–212.
[29] Korshunov SS, Skulachev VP, Starkov AA. High protonic potential actuates a mechanism of production of reactive oxygen species in mitochondria. FEBS Lett 1997;416:15–8.
[30] Paradies G, Petrosillo G, Pistolese M, Ruggiero FM. Reactive oxygen species generated by the mitochondrial respiratory chain affect the complex III activity via cardiolipin peroxidation in beef-heart submitochondrial particles. Mitochondrion 2001:1,151–59.
[31] Giacco F, Brownlee M. Oxidative stress and diabetic complications. Circ Res 2010;107:1058–70.
[32] Madsen-Bouterse SA, Mohammad G, Kanwar M, Kowluru RA. Role of mitochondrial DNA damage in the development of diabetic retinopathy, and the metabolic memory phenomenon associated with its progression. Antioxid Redox Signal 2010;13:797–805.
[33] Madsen-Bouterse SA, Zhong Q, Mohammad G, Ho YS, Kowluru RA. Oxidative damage of mitochondrial DNA in diabetes, and its protection by manganese superoxide dismutase. Free Radic Res 2010;44:313–21.
[34] Santos JM, Tewari S, Kowluru RA. A compensatory mechanism protects retinal mitochondria from initial insult in diabetic retinopathy. Free Radic Biol Med 2012;53:1729–37.
[35] Hancock JT, Desikan R, Neill SJ. Does the redox status of cytochrome C act as a fail-safe mechanism in the regulation of programd cell death? Free Radical Biol Med 2001;31:697–703.
[36] Madsen-Bouterse SA, Zhong Q, Mohammad G, Ho YS, Kowluru RA. Oxidative damage of mitochondrial DNA in diabetes and its protection by manganese superoxide dismutase. Free Radic Res Mar 2010;44:313–21.
[36b] Phaneuf S, Leeuwenburgh C. Cytochrome c release from mitochondria in the aging heart: a possible mechanism for apoptosis with age. Am J Physiol Regul Integr Comp Physiol 2002;282:R423–30.
[37] Santos JM, Mohammad G, Zhong Q, Kowluru RA. Diabetic retinopathy, superoxide damage and antioxidants. Curr Pharm Biotechnol 2011;12:352–61.
[38] Al-Shabrawey M, Smith S. Prediction of diabetic retinopathy: role of oxidative stress and relevance of apoptotic biomarkers. EPMA J 2010;1:56–72.
[39] Yang Y, Hayden MR, Sowers S, Bagree SV, Sowers JR. Retinal redox stress and remodeling in cardiometabolic syndrome and diabetes. Oxid Med Cell Longev 2010;3:392–403.
[40] Obrosova IG, Minchenko AG, Marinescu V, Fathallah L, Kennedy A, Stockert CM, et al. Antioxidants attenuate early up regulation of retinal vascular endothelial growth factor in streptozotocin-diabetic rats. Diabetologia 2001;44:1102–10.
[41] Izuta H, Matsunaga N, Shimazawa M, Sugiyama T, Ikeda T, Hara H. Proliferative diabetic retinopathy and relations among antioxidant activity, oxidative stress, and VEGF in the vitreous body. Mol Vis 2010;16:130–6.
[42] Hasebe Y, Egawa K, Shibanuma M, Nose K. Induction of matrix metalloproteinase gene expression in an endothelial cell line by direct interaction with malignant cells. Cancer Sci 2007;98: 58–67.
[43] Klein T, Bischoff R. Physiology and pathophysiology of matrix metalloproteases. Amino Acids 2011;41:271–90.
[44] Mohammad G, Kowluru RA. Novel role of mitochondrial matrix metalloproteinase-2 in the development of diabetic retinopathy. Invest Ophthalmol Vis Sci 2011;52:3832–41.
[45] Kowluru RA, Zhong Q, Santos JM. Matrix metalloproteinases in diabetic retinopathy: potential role of MMP-9. Expert Opin Investig Drugs 2012;21:797–805.
[46] Ovechkin AV, Tyagi N, Rodriguez WE, Hayden MR, Moshal KS, Tyagi SC. Role of matrix metalloproteinase-9 in endothelial apoptosis in chronic heart failure in mice. J Appl Physiol 2005;99: 2398–405.
[47] Navaratna D, McGuire PG, Menicucci G, Das A. Proteolytic degradation of VE cadherin alters the blood-retinal barrier in diabetes. Diabetes 2007;56:2380–7.
[48] Das A, McGuire PG, Eriqat C, Ober RR, DeJuan Jr E, Williams GA, et al. Human diabetic neovascular membranes contain high levels of urokinase and metalloproteinase enzymes. Invest Ophthalmol Vis Sci 1999;40:809–13.
[49] Siefert SA, Sarkar R. Matrix metalloproteinases in vascular physiology and disease. Vascular 2012;20:210–6.
[50] Holman RR, Paul SK, Bethel MA, Matthews DR, Neil HA. 10-year follow-up of intensive glucose control in type 2 diabetes. N Engl J Med 2008;359:1577–89.
[51] Ceriello A, Esposito K, Ihnat M, Thorpe J, Giugliano D. Long-term glycemic control influences the long-lasting effect of hyperglycemia on endothelial function in type 1 diabetes. J Clin Endocrinol Metab 2009;94:2751–6.
[52] Kowluru RA. Effect of reinstitution of good glycemic control on retinal oxidative stress and nitrative stress in diabetic rats. Diabetes 2003;52:818–23.
[53] Kowluru RA, Kanwar M, Kennedy A. Metabolic memory phenomenon and accumulation of peroxynitrite in retinal capillaries. Exp Diabetes Res 2007;2007:21976.
[54] Ola MS, Nawaz MI, Siddiquei MM, Al-Amor S, Abu El-Asrar AM. Recent advances in understanding the biochemical and molecular mechanism of diabetic retinopathy. J Diabetes Complications 2012;26:56–64.
[55] Frey T, Antonetti DA. Alterations to the blood-retinal barrier in diabetes: cytokines and reactive oxygen species. Antioxid Redox Signal 2011;15:1271–84.
[56] Silva KC, Rosales MA, Biswas SK, Lopes de Faria JB, Lopes de Faria JM. Diabetic retinal neurodegeneration is associated with mitochondrial oxidative stress and is improved by an angiotensin receptor blocker in a model combining hypertension and diabetes. Diabetes 2009;58:1382–90.
[57] Bursell SE, Clermont AC, Aiello LP, Aiello LM, Schlossman DK, Feener EP, et al. High-dose vitamin E supplementation normalizes retinal blood flow and creatinine clearance in patients with type 1 diabetes. Diabetes Care 1999;22:1245–51.

CHAPTER

5

Mitochondrial Oxidative Stress in Diabetes

Victor M. Victor

Fundacion para la Investigacion Sanitaria y Biomedica de la Comunidad Valenciana FISABIO, University Hospital Doctor Peset, Endocrinology Service, Avda Gaspar Aguilar, Valencia, Spain, Fundacion para la Investigación (INCLIVA), Department of Pharmacology and CIBER CB06/04/0071 Research Group, CIBER Hepatic and Digestive Diseases, and Department of Physiology, University of Valencia, Valencia, Spain

List of Abbreviations

AGE Advanced glycation endproducts
AMPK AMP-activated protein kinase
CL Cardiolipin
CVD Cardiovascular diseases
CAT Catalase
COX Cytochrome c oxidase
eNOS Endothelial nitric oxide synthase
FFAs Free fatty acids
GPx GSH peroxidase
HOMA Homeostasis Model Assessment
H_2O_2 Hydrogen peroxide
·HO Hydroxyl radicals
HIFα Hypoxia inducible factor alpha
iNOS Inducible nitric oxide synthase
NADH Nicotinamide adenine dinucleotide
NADPH Nicotinamide adenine dinucleotide phosphate
NO Nitric oxide
NO_2 Nitrogen dioxide
N_2O Nitrous oxide
NF-κB Nuclear factor kappa B
PPARγ Peroxisome proliferator-activated receptor gamma
$ONOO^-$ Peroxynitrite
RNS Reactive nitrogen species
ROS Reactive oxygen species
$O_2{\cdot}^-$ Superoxide
SOD Superoxide dismutase
VCAM-1 Vascular cell adhesion molecule-1
XO Xanthine oxidase

INTRODUCTION

In normal physiological conditions there is a homeostatic control which ensures a balance between the generation of reactive oxygen species (ROS) and their scavenging by endogenous antioxidants. Oxidative stress is produced when there is excessive production of ROS, and this has been implicated in many of the diseases that affect humans. These species include, among others, superoxide ($O_2{\cdot}^-$), hydroxyl radicals (HO·), hydrogen peroxide (H_2O_2) and peroxynitrite ($ONOO^-$) (Table 5.1). Oxidative stress is also associated with endothelial and mitochondrial dysfunction, both of which are related to risk factors of cardiometablic diseases, including diabetes.

The mitochondrion is the principal source of ROS, though they are also produced in other locations. In addition, there are various types of antioxidants that exert beneficial effects on the mitochondrial electron transport chain. The damaging effects of ROS affect carbohydrates, proteins, lipids, DNA and enzymes, leading to cellular dysfunction. Therefore, mitochondria are more susceptible to accumulative oxidative damage than the rest of the cell [1].

Mitochondrial impairment and damage may be involved in a large number of cellular pathologies. In this context, several studies have demonstrated that the deleterious effects of ROS are counteracted by antioxidants such as α-tocopherol, ascorbic acid, N-acetylcysteine and ubiquinol, all of which are capable of reducing mitochondrial oxidative damage [2]. However, given that these substances do not accumulate in the mitochondria, their effectiveness may be limited [3].

OXIDATIVE STRESS: ROS AND REACTIVE NITROGEN SPECIES (RNS)

The deleterious effect of ROS-mediated damage is evident in different disorders [4]. Oxidative stress can occur when there is an imbalance between ROS production and antioxidant defenses [4], and is associated with

Diabetes: Oxidative Stress and Dietary Antioxidants.
http://dx.doi.org/10.1016/B978-0-12-405885-9.00005-X

risk factors for multiple conditions, including diabetes, atherosclerosis, hypercholesterolaemia and cancer [4].

Levels of ROS depend on the pathophysiological and physiological state of the organism; for example, under physiological conditions, there is a homeostatic balance between the production of ROS and their elimination by antioxidants [5]. ROS are secondary messengers generated in response to different forms of stress, and very slight changes in their intracellular levels can alter cell communication and activate signal transduction pathways. ROS and RNS have a seriously damaging property in common; both exert an effect on the mitochondrial lipid cardiolipin (CL) by which mitochondrial cytochrome c is released, leading to activation of the intrinsic cell death pathway.

TABLE 5.1 Reactive Species: Sources and Antioxidant Defenses

Reactive Species	Source	Antioxidant Defense
$O_2{\cdot}^-$	ETC, peroxisoma, NOx, Lipoxigenase, Xanthine oxidase NADPHoxidase, NOS	Mn-SOD CuZn-SOD
OH·	Fenton reaction	Trx, Prdx
H_2O_2	From $O_2{\cdot}^-$ (in mitochondria by Mn-SOD) From $O_2{\cdot}^-$ (in cytosol by Mn-SOD)	GPx Catalase
RNS NO ONOO⁻	NOS NO+ $O_2{\cdot}^-$ Radicals	Carboxyl/hydroxyl Radicals

$O_2{\cdot}^-$ superoxide anion; ETC electron transport chain; NOx reduced nicotinamide adenine dinucleotide phosphate oxidase; NOS nitric oxide synthase; Mn-SOD mitochondrial superoxide dismutase; CuZn-SOD cytosolic superoxide dismutase; OH· hydroxyl radical; GPx glutathione peroxidase; RNS reactive nitrogen species; NO nitric oxide.

ROS

ROS are generated by biochemical reactions in organisms (Figure 5.1). One of its main sources is the leakage of electrons from the mitochondrial electron transport chain, as a result of which $O_2{\cdot}^-$ is the first ROS to be released [6]. $O_2{\cdot}^-$ can be converted to H_2O_2 by different kind of enzymes, including superoxide dismutase (SOD) and α-ketoglutarate dehydrogenase, and the pyruvate dehydrogenase complex generates both $O_2{\cdot}^-$ and H_2O_2 via the oxidation pathway [7]. Although not itself a free radical, H_2O_2 is an important biological marker of oxidative stress due to its ability to cross cellular membranes. Indeed, it can act as an intracellular messenger that activates redox pathways. Excess H_2O_2 is converted to H_2O through a harmless action exerted by catalase (CAT), GSH peroxidase (GPx) and other enzymes. OH· is synthesized through the reaction of $O_2{\cdot}^-$ with H_2O_2 in the presence of metal ions and is more reactive than $O_2{\cdot}^-$, which makes it highly deleterious for cellular

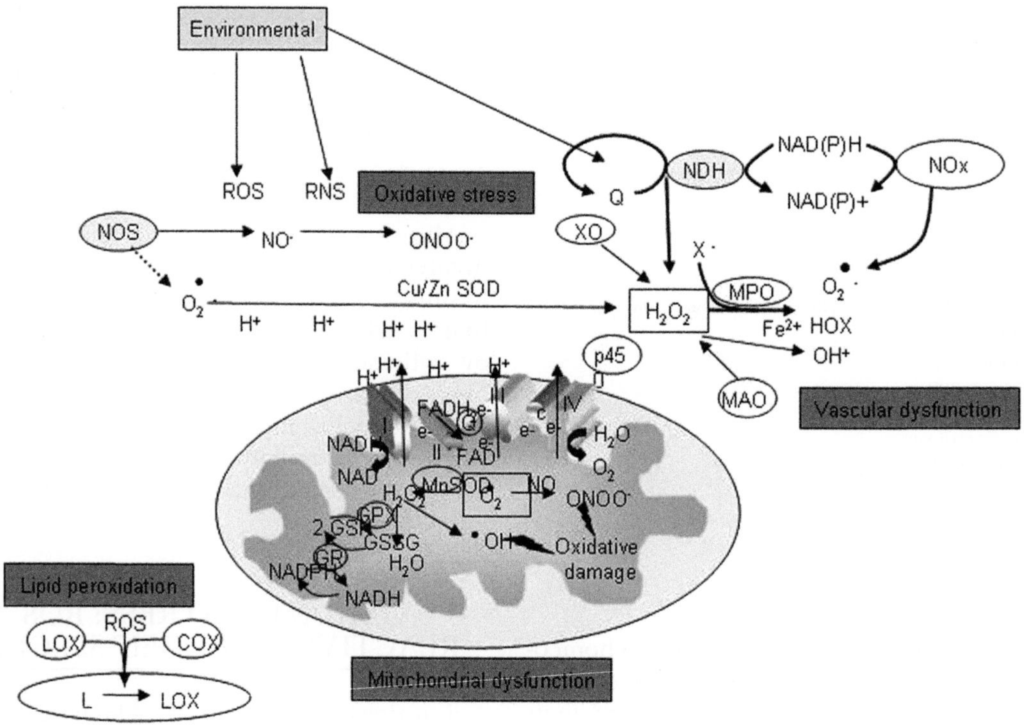

FIGURE 5.1 There are different cellular sources of reactive oxygen species (ROS), including the mitochondrial electron transport chain, trycarboxilic acid (TCA) cycle, monoamine oxidase (MAO), xanthine oxidase (XO), cytochrome p450 reductases, NADPH oxidases, myeloperoxidase (MPO), nitric oxide synthase (NOx) and cytochrome P450.

membranes and molecules and an inducer of oxidative stress. Iron-catalyzed OH· generation requires Fe in its reduced, ferrous form (Fe^{2+}), whereas the majority of Fe present in the organism is that of the oxidized form (Fe^{3+}). $O_2\cdot^-$ can also reduce Fe^{3+} to Fe^{2+}, thereby promoting the production of OH·.

In physiological conditions, the majority of ROS are released from the electron transport chain and the membrane NADPH oxidase in phagocytic cells (macrophages and neutrophils) during the inflammatory response.

In diabetes, there are several potential sources of ROS, including endothelial cells, muscle cells, nitric oxide synthase, myeloperoxidase, release of iron and copper ions, metalloproteins, vascular damage caused by ischemia reperfusion, the mitochondrial respiratory electron transport chain, xanthine oxidase (XO) activation, the respiratory burst associated with immune cell activation, and arachidonic acid metabolism. NAD(P)H oxidase, which catalyzes the production of $O_2\cdot^-$ by one-electron reduction of O_2 using NADPH or NADH as the electron donor, is present mainly in leukocytes, particularly in phagocytes but also in non-phagocytes (epithelial cells, fibroblasts, chondrocytes and mesangial cells), and in microglial, endothelial and vascular smooth muscle cells [8]. This enzyme plays an important role in the development of diabetes due to the damage it causes to the endothelium by generating hypertension and vascular dysfunction.

Importantly, as oxidants produced by immune cells, ROS and RNS have a dual function. On the one hand, they function as potent antimicrobicidal molecules by killing pathogens, while on the other they can act as signaling molecules that modulate different nuclear transcription factors and physiological signaling pathways in cells. In the latter role, ROS and RNS are modulators of key enzymes, including proteins, lipid kinases and phosphatases, transporters, membrane receptors, ion channels and transcription factors including nuclear factor kappa B (NF-κB) and hypoxia inducible factor alpha (HIFα). In addition, they regulate pro-inflammatory cytokines, such as interleukin 6 (IL-6) and tumour necrosis factor alpha (TNFα), and chemokines, thus controlling the inflammatory response, during which ROS and, in turn, RNS modulate the different functions of immune cells (adhesion, migration and phagocytosis) as well as secretion, gene expression, autophagy and apoptosis. Under pathological circumstances, excess production of ROS can affect vicinal cells such as those found in the endothelium or epithelium, thereby contributing to inflammatory tissue injury and damage [9]. In this context cells faced with oxidative stress usually undergo alterations in different immune functions, such as an increase in adherence, ROS production and phagocytosis and a decrease in chemotaxis [2].

RNS

Currently, research regarding nitric oxide (NO) and the oxides of nitrogen is of considerable biomedical interest due to the pathophysiological implications of these molecules. NO, nitrous oxide (N_2O) and nitrogen dioxide (NO_2) can be homeostatic or deleterious. NO_2 is an environmental pollutant which is also produced *in vivo* in response to reactions against NO, and it is implicated in lipid peroxidation, cellular membrane damage and apoptotic processes. NO reacts slowly with the majority of molecules in the human body (non-radicals); as a free radical, on the other hand, it reacts quickly with other molecules, including ROS (e.g., $O_2\cdot^-$), transition metals and amino acid radicals. NO and $O_2\cdot^-$ react to produce peroxynitrite ($ONOO^-$) [10], which is implicated in a large number of human diseases; in fact, diminished availability of NO and increased ROS formation may constitute key events in the development of cardiovascular diseases (CVD), including atherosclerosis.

Inducible nitric oxide synthase (iNOS) expression is triggered as a consequence of the activation of macrophages, monocytes and endothelial cells, and induces the transformation of L-arginine into NO, which combines with $O_2\cdot^-$ to form $ONOO^-$. NO stimulates ROS – for example, H_2O_2 and $O_2\cdot^-$ – production by the mitochondria [11] – possibly by inhibiting cytochrome c oxidase (COX), which promotes the leakage of electrons from the respiratory chain, and through irreversible inhibition of mitochondrial complex I. H_2O_2, in turn, is involved in the up-regulation of iNOS expression via nuclear transcription factors such as NF-κB. In tissue damage, inflammatory reactions play a key role which is mediated by the adhesion and migration of leukocytes through the vessel, generation of RNS and ROS, and the production of several pro-inflammatory cytokines and chemokines by monocytes/macrophages. In addition, local generation of RNS can contribute to tissue damage.

DIABETES

Diabetes is one of the major health problems worldwide. In addition, it is associated with a series of comorbidities that affect the life expectancy and quality of life of patients. Currently, 270 million people around the world live with diabetes, and this figure is expected to rise to 400 million over the coming years. The link between diabetes and cancer has been studied in great depth, and the majority of the evidence obtained suggests that diabetes enhances the risk of developing different types of cancer, which obviously magnifies the clinical implications of the former disease. However, there are contradictory data that deserve careful interpretation, as diabetes is a complex disease in which multiple metabolic pathways and nuclear transcription factors are affected. Taking this into account, the different existing types of diabetes produce an array of metabolic and hormonal abnormalities that can affect patients in varying ways. As a consequence, it is necessary to study diabetic patients as a heterogeneous cohort. In addition, there are numerous parameters which may hold the key to understanding the relationship between cancer and diabetes, including metabolic controls, diet, population, obesity, statistical methods, diet and sex. Nevertheless, it is already well demonstrated that oxidative stress is linked to diabetes, that the latter is characterized by mitochondrial impairment (Figure 5.2) [4], and that both conditions are related to cancer.

DIABETES, INFLAMMATION AND OXIDATIVE STRESS

Diabetes is associated with oxidative stress and inflammation, which are related to a high production of adhesion molecules and pro-inflammatory cytokines, including IL-6 and TNFα. Diabetes is, therefore, a chronic pro-inflammatory state that gradually reduces intracellular antioxidant stores, leaving cells vulnerable to damage. In fact, ROS at high concentrations can damage cell DNA by direct oxidation or by interfering with cell repair mechanisms [12]. ROS can also impair lipids and proteins, releasing molecules that alter cellular homeostasis and promote the accumulation of key mutations, which eventually contributes to cancer [13]. Mitochondrial activity is crucial for DNA repair, as the impairment of mitochondria not only results in a low, insufficient energy supply, but also increases ROS production and, consequently, oxidative stress [14]. In addition, there are factors which correlate with insulin resistance, such as the pro-inflammatory cytokine TNFα released by adipose tissue, or the accumulation of free fatty acids (FFA) [15]. TNFα can trigger the progression and development of different tumors [16] by activating transcription factors such as NF-κB (Figure 5.3), which is involved in the pro-tumoral effects of cytokines. In conclusion, diabetes promotes the biological aging processes that can induce cancerogenesis through mechanisms specific to both diabetes and other chronic degenerative diseases.

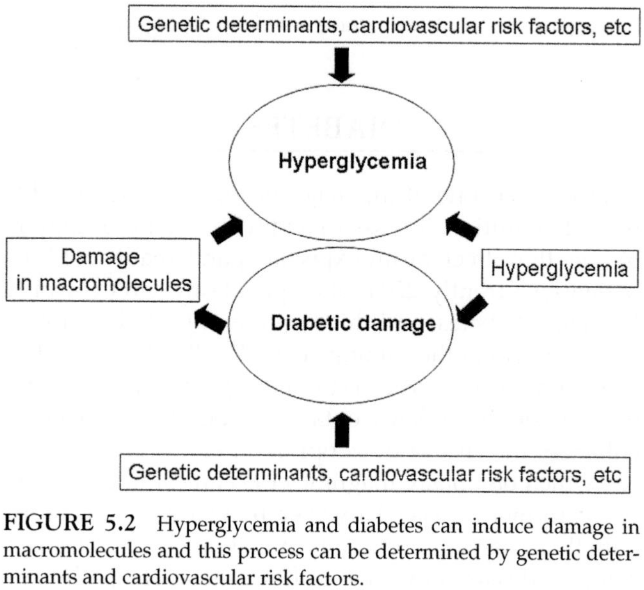

FIGURE 5.2 Hyperglycemia and diabetes can induce damage in macromolecules and this process can be determined by genetic determinants and cardiovascular risk factors.

ROS PRODUCTION AND DIABETIC COMPLICATIONS

There is a wealth of evidence to suggest that oxidative stress plays a key role in the development and progression of diabetic complications such as nephropathy, retinopathy, neuropathy, silent myocardial ischemia, or coronary artery disease. The use of different agents to modulate ROS generation can reduce the cellular uptake of glucose and subsequently delay the feeding of glucose metabolites during oxidative phosphorylation. Nevertheless, oxidative phosphorylation and mitochondrial function are considered to be key targets in the modulation of the aforementioned diabetic complications, among which nephropathy is very important. High levels of glucose can induce mitochondrial ROS, which activates different biochemical pathways, hexosamine, increased flux through the polyol, enhanced formation of advanced glycation endproducts (AGE) and activation of protein kinase C isoforms (Figure 5.3) [17]. However, there are other important pathways, including NADPH oxidase, the uncoupling of endothelial nitric oxide synthase (eNOS) and myeloperoxidase, which require further investigation in order to determine their relative importance in progressive diabetic complications such as renal disease.

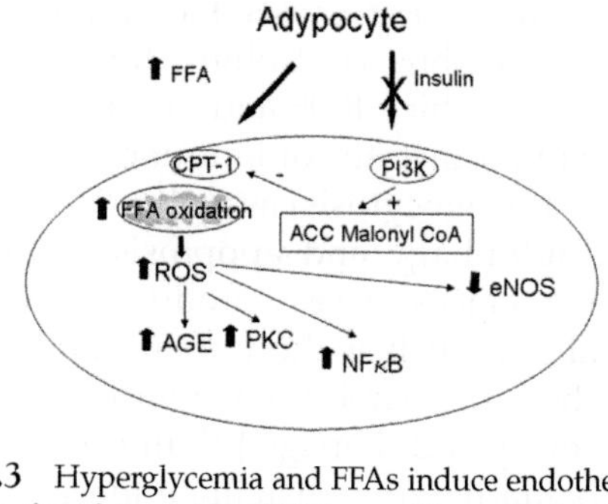

FIGURE 5.3 Hyperglycemia and FFAs induce endothelial ROS production. FFA, free fatty acids; CPT-1, carnitine palmitoyltransferase 1; ROS, reactive oxygen species; AGE, advanced glycation endproducts; PKC, protein kinase C; NF-κB, nuclear factor κB; PI3K, phosphoinositide 3 kinase; ACC, acetylcoA; eNOS, endothelial nitric oxide.

ANTIOXIDANTS AND DIABETES

Organisms have numerous antioxidant systems designed to ameliorate the deleterious effects of ROS production and oxidative stress. SOD is one of the most important of these antioxidant enzymes. SOD has three isoenzymes – CuZn-SOD (SOD1), Mn-SOD (SOD2) and extracellular (SOD3) – whose main function is the detoxification of $O_2^{\cdot -}$ to H_2O_2 and water. Catalase and GPx are other antioxidant enzymes that catalyze the conversion of H_2O_2 to H_2O. In addition, many of the antioxidants present in cells, such as vitamins and glutathione, play a homeostatic role. However, studies have shown that these antioxidants have no real beneficial effects in the treatment of diabetic complications. In one study, it was demonstrated that overexpression of CuZn-SOD countered organ impairment in models of type 2 diabetic nephropathy [18]. In another, MnTBAP (Mn-SOD mimetic) was shown to be effective in preventing ROS-induced injury *in vitro* [17], although the *in vivo* use of such drugs has produced controversial data [19] that do not confirm any substantial beneficial effects. It should be mentioned that some polymorphisms of the Mn-SOD gene are related to the development of diabetic nephropathy [20]. Interestingly, in an animal model of GPx-1-deficient mice, diabetic nephropathy and microvascular disease were not found to be more pronounced [21]. Overexpression of other antioxidant enzymes, such as catalase, in several models of type 2 diabetic nephropathy seems to be beneficial [22], suggesting the importance of eradicating high levels of ROS. In human studies, however, no relationship has been detected between the incidence of nephropathy in diabetes and catalase gene polymorphisms [23].

DIETARY ANTIOXIDANTS

As mentioned previously, an excessive energy intake owing to saturated fatty acids and high glycemic index foods is an important source of oxidative stress. In order to counteract this, there are several antioxidants (carotenoids, vitamin E, ascorbic acid, tocopherols and flavonoids) which protect against oxidative damage and its complications, including diabetes and insulin resistance (Figure 5.4).

Different *in vitro* and animal studies have shown that dietary antioxidants have beneficial effects on glucose metabolism and can help to prevent diabetes or related diseases. Polyphenols are one of the most studied of these antioxidants and have produced interesting and beneficial results. For example, quercetin, one of the most consumed flavonoids in the human diet, has demonstrated beneficial effects on glucose metabolism by attenuating TNFα–mediated inflammation and insulin resistance in primary human adipocytes [24]. Cyanidin-3-O-β-glucoside has been shown to have insulin-like activities by activating peroxisome proliferator-activated receptor gamma (PPARγ) in human adipocytes [25]. Other flavonoids, such as hesperetin and naringenin, inhibit TNFα-stimulated free fatty acid secretion in cultured mouse adipocytes [26], as well as increasing glucose uptake by AMPK in cultured skeletal muscle cells [27] and enhancing insulin sensitivity by increasing tyrosine phosphorylation in fructose-fed rats. In one study, the flavonoid luteolin was shown to increase insulin sensitivity by activating PPARγ transcriptional activity in 3T3-L1 adipocytes [28]. Caffeic acid phenethyl ester stimulates glucose uptake into cultured skeletal muscle cells through the AMPK pathway [29] and glucose

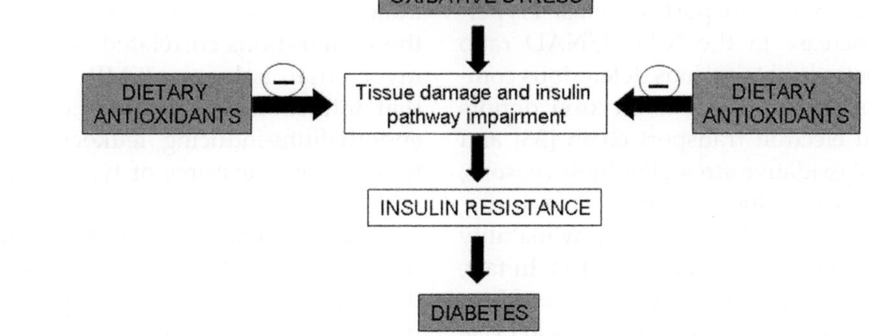

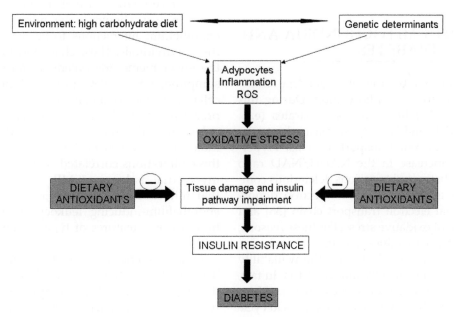

FIGURE 5.4 Dietary antioxidants can avoid tissue damage and insulin pathway impairment induced by hyperglycemia.

uptake into insulin-resistant mouse hepatocytes, as does cinnamic acid [30]. Resveratrol improves mitochondrial activity and energy balance, protecting mice against diet-induced obesity and insulin resistance. Therefore, resveratrol may have an important role to play in the prevention of metabolic diseases and diabetes. In addition to its antioxidant capacity, glucose metabolism exerts its actions through other molecules, such as sirtuin 1 [31].

The beneficial effects of dietary antioxidants in cells and animal models have been well demonstrated, but few intervention studies have been carried out to directly assess the effects of antioxidants on diabetes and glucose metabolism in humans. Some studies have reported positive effects of α-lipoic acid and vitamin E and C supplementation, alone or in association with other antioxidants [32], though others have failed to detect any benefits.

Other research has demonstrated that a high dose of *trans*-resveratrol has favorable effects on glucose homeostasis in obese subjects by improving their Homeostasis Model Assessment (HOMA) index, thus exerting a positive effect on insulin sensitivity.

Epidemiologic studies have reported that diets rich in antioxidants such as α-tocopherol [33], vitamin C [34], vitamin E [35] or β-carotene [33] are beneficial in that they prevent diabetes and improve glucose metabolism. Two meta-analyses have evaluated the association between intake of fruit, vegetables and antioxidants and the risk of diabetes. One concluded that consumption of antioxidants but not that of fruits and vegetables produced a 13% decrease in the risk of diabetes that was attributed mainly to vitamin E [36]. In the other, intake of green leafy vegetables was associated with a 14% decrease in the risk of developing diabetes [37].

ANTIOXIDANTS, MITOCHONDRIA AND DIABETES

Glucose is employed by the mitochondrial transport chain via oxidative phosphorylation. During this process, it is converted into various substrates (e.g., pyruvate) and NADH and $FADH_2$ are released into the mitochondria via different transport systems. Hyperglycemia and the increase in the NADH/NAD ratio associated with diabetes lead to serious deleterious complications. NADH is one of the main electron donors to the mitochondrial electron transport chain [38] and favors the presence of oxidative stress. For these reasons, it is of great importance to reduce hyperglycemia during diabetic complications [39] by decreasing the availability of the substrate fuel consumed by mitochondria. In fact, mitochondria consume other substrates, such as FFAs, as fuel, and their oxidation in the tricarboxylic acid cycle generates $FADH_2$ and NADH. Therefore, the presence of high levels of FFAs mimics the effects of hyperglycemia on mitochondrial impairment.

Oxidative stress and ROS production are recognized as key mediators of the development of diabetic complications [17], and mitochondria are their main source. Therefore, therapies which use molecules to ameliorate mitochondrial ROS could be of benefit in the management of diabetic comorbidities. During oxidative phosphorylation, electrons from different substrates are transferred to O_2 via the electron transport chain. Protons are then pumped across the mitochondrial membrane and the resulting voltage gradient generates ATP. Complex I and III of the electron transport chain are the two main sites of electron leakage. In diabetes, the excessive production of ROS as a consequence of high levels of glucose is believed to play an important role in mitochondrial membrane potential and, as a consequence, in apoptosis [17]. However, the majority of studies which have explored this aspect have been carried out in tissues, so *in vivo* investigation is now necessary. In this context, it has been hypothesized that mitochondrial dysfunction and damage of the mitochondrial respiratory chain contribute to many pathologies; indeed, patients with deleterious genetic mutations that reduce the activity of different mitochondrial complexes display high levels of mitochondrial ROS [40]. Recently, diabetic patients have been reported to develop mitochondrial complex I dysfunction, which is followed by an increase in ROS production and decrease in membrane potential and antioxidant levels [41]. In relation to this idea, an impairment of mitochondrial complex I [42] and a subsequent rise in oxidative stress have also been described in pathologies characterized by insulin resistance, such as polycystic ovary syndrome.

In a recent study of diabetic patients, mitochondrial function was shown to be impaired and leukocyte-endothelium interactions to be more frequent among these individuals. These characteristics were evident in the lower membrane potential, mitochondrial O_2 consumption, GSH/GSSG ratio and polymorphonuclear cell rolling velocity, and in the higher mitochondrial ROS production and rolling flux, leukocyte adhesion and vascular cell adhesion molecule-1 (VCAM-1) and E-selectin molecules observed in these subjects [43]. In addition, these alterations correlated with the presence of silent myocardial ischemia (SMI). The authors concluded that mitochondrial dysfunction, oxidative stress and endothelium-inducing leukocyte-endothelium interactions are key features of type 2 diabetes and correlate with SMI.

Other evidence is available for the role of mitochondrial oxidative stress as one of the main factors in the development of diabetic complications such as Friedreich's ataxia, a genetic disorder caused by mutations implicated in the down-regulation of mitochondrial

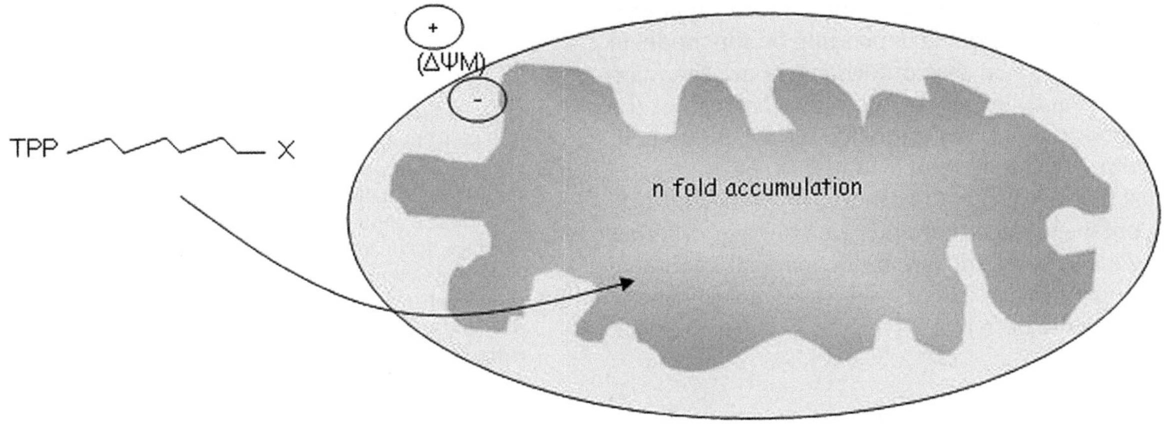

FIGURE 5.5 Mitochondria-targeted antioxidants can be accumulated in mitochondria.

complex I and highly mitochondrial ROS generation [44]. In one study, mitochondria were shown to play a key role in diabetic nephropathy, as renal diseases were detected in around 45% of a child population with mitochondrial dysfunction [45]. In addition, renal disease is the primary pathology in patients with oxidative phosphorylation defects [46]. These results highlight mitochondrial impairment as a priority for research into future therapies. In this sense, mitochondria-targeted antioxidants are a potential tool for the treatment of diabetes.

As mentioned previously, mitochondrial ROS production can lead to a wide range of deleterious reactions that can damage several structures or molecules, including proteins, lipids and nucleic acids. Apart from being a source of ROS, mitochondria possess multiple enzymes that are susceptible to damage by ROS, which results in alterations of the membrane potential, impairment of cellular calcium storage and a diminution of ATP production (all related to reticulum stress, autophagy and the development of apoptosis or necrosis).

Idebenone is a mitochondrial antioxidant that is highly available inside many organs. This kind of antioxidant is efficient and safe for protecting mitochondrial function from oxidative damage in humans with Friedreich's ataxia [47]. Idebenone has been shown to reduce cardiomyopathy in these subjects, unlike dietary antioxidants such as vitamin E and α-tocopherol [47].

MitoQ is a mitochondria-targeted antioxidant that is selectively taken into mitochondria due to the covalent attachment to the lipophilic triphenylphosphonium cation. This antioxidant can accumulate in mitochondria 1000-fold (Figure 5.5) [48]. Although the efficacy of these mitochondria-targeted antioxidants in the treatment of insulin resistance and diabetes is yet to be determined, their targeted specificity for mitochondria makes them potential therapeutic agents in cardiometabolic diseases and diabetes. In this sense, it has been reported that MitoQ administered orally over a 12-week period improves tubular and glomerular function in Ins2($^{+/-}$) (AkitaJ) mice (an animal model of diabetes). In the study in question, MitoQ did not have a notable effect on plasma creatinine levels, but reduced urinary albumin levels to those of non-diabetic controls. Furthermore, treatment with MitoQ significantly reduced glomerular damage and interstitial fibrosis, and prevented the nuclear accumulation of β-catenin and the transcription factor phospho-Smad2/3 in Ins2($^{+/-}$) (AkitaJ) mice. These results support the hypothesis that mitochondrially-targeted treatments can be beneficial in the treatment of diabetic nephropathy [49].

CONCLUSIONS

Although experimental data have been obtained in different cellular and animal models regarding the role of oxidative stress in insulin resistance and diabetes and the positive effects of dietary antioxidants, research carried out in humans until now has provided contradictory results.

The poor outcome of trials with antioxidants is comprehensible if we bear in mind the magnitude and variety of oxidative events caused by ROS, rather than focusing on classic antioxidants that are effective only against oxidative reactions. In this context, it is of vital importance to obtain future experimental evidence regarding the protection that scavengers of ROS offer against disease.

There are several possible reasons for the discrepancies found among the data reported in the literature. First, the antioxidant actions of dietary antioxidants may be modified by environmental conditions such as metal ions and pH, and by their concentration and location. Indeed, they can even become pro-oxidant at high doses. Second, ROS are capable of acting as secondary messengers and are necessary for the transduction of insulin signals, which means that their excessive neutralization can be harmful. Third, the efficiency of dietary supplements and natural products is not restricted to their antioxidative capability, which can be highly variable depending on the model in question. Fourth, given that mitochondria are the main source of ROS and are key to the redox balance of the cell, mitochondria-targeted antioxidants are fundamental tools with which to control oxidative stress.

We trust that work over the coming years will indicate in which organs these compounds are effective, whether they alleviate disease-related mitochondrial oxidative damage, and to what extent their use can positively affect the outcome of treatments.

SUMMARY POINTS

- Diabetes is related to oxidative stress and, as a consequence, to overproduction of ROS.
- Dietary antioxidants, such as vitamin E or vitamin C, polyphenols and flavonoids, can modulate the oxidative stress created in diabetes.
- Until now, clinical trials have been contradictory with respect to the beneficial effects of antioxidant treatment, perhaps as a consequence of the targets selected and/or design of the studies in question.
- The antioxidant actions of dietary antioxidants may be modified by environmental conditions.
- Given that mitochondria are the main source of ROS and are key to the redox balance of the cell, mitochondria-targeted antioxidants could be fundamental tools with which to control oxidative stress.

Acknowledgements

We thank B Normanly for his editorial assistance.

This study was financed by grants PI10/1195, PI12/1984, CIBERehd CB06/04/0071 and PROMETEO 2010/060. V.M.V. is the recipient of a contract from the Ministry of Health of the Valencian Regional Government and Carlos III Health Institute (CES10/030).

References

[1] Kowaltowski AJ, Vercesi AE. Mitochondrial damage induced by conditions of oxidative stress. Free Radic Biol Med 1999;26:463–71.

[2] Victor VM, Rocha M, De la Fuente M. Immune cells: free radicals and antioxidants in sepsis. Int Immunopharmacol 2004;4:327–47.

[3] Kagan VE, Serbinova EA, Stoyanovsky DA, Khwaja S, Packer L. Assay of ubiquinones and ubiquinols as antioxidants. Methods Enzymol 1994:234,343–54.

[4] Victor VM, Apostolova N, Herance R, Hernandez-Mijares A, Rocha M. Oxidative stress and mitochondrial dysfunction in atherosclerosis: mitochondria-targeted antioxidants as potential therapy. Curr Med Chem 2009;16:4654–67.

[5] Gutteridge JM, Mitchell J. Redox imbalance in the critically ill. Br Med Bull 1999;55:49–75.

[6] Boveris A, Cadenas E. Cellular sources and steady-state levels of reactive oxygen species. In: Clerch LB, Massaro DJ, editors. Oxygen, gene expression, and cellular function. New York: Marcel Dekker; 1997. p. 1–25.

[7] Satarkov AA, Fiskum G, Chinopoulos C, Lorenzo BJ, Browne SE, Patel MS, et al. Mitochondrial α-ketoglutarate dehydrogenase complex generates reactive oxygen species. J Neurosci 2004;24:7779–88.

[8] Rains JL, Jain SK. Oxidative stress, insulin signaling, and diabetes. Free Radic Biol Med 2011;50:567–75.

[9] Fialkow L, Wang Y, Downey GP. Reactive oxygen and nitrogen species as signaling molecules regulating neutrophil function. Free Radic Biol Med 2007;42:153–64.

[10] Huie RE, Padmaja S. The reaction of NO with superoxide. Free Radic Res Commun 1993;18:195–9.

[11] Poderoso JJ, Carreras MC, Lisdero C, Riobó N, Schöpfer F, Boveris A. Nitric oxide inhibits electron transfer and increases superoxide radical production in rat heart mitochondria and submitochondrial particles. Arch Biochem Biophys 1996;328:85–92.

[12] Federico A, Morgillo F, Tuccillo C, Ciardiello F, Loguercio C. Chronic inflammation and oxidative stress in human carcinogenesis. Int J Cancer 2007;121:2381–6.

[13] Ohshima H, Tatemichi M, Sawa T. Chemical basis of inflammation-induced carcinogenesis. Arch Biochem Biophys 2003;417:3–11.

[14] Cebioglu M, Schild HH, Golubnitschaja O. Diabetes mellitus as a risk factor for cancer: stress or viral etiology? Infect Disord Drug Targets 2008;8:76–87.

[15] Kern PA, Ranganathan S, Li C, Wood L, Ranganathan G. Adipose tissue tumour necrosis factor and interleukin- 6 expression in human obesity and insulin resistance. Am J Physiol 2001;280:745–51.

[16] Szlosarek P, Charles KA, Balkwill FR. Tumour necrosis factor-alpha as a tumour promoter. Eur J Cancer 2006;42:745–50.

[17] Nishikawa T, Edelstein D, Du XL, Yamagishi S, Matsumura T, Kaneda Y, et al. Normalizing mitochondrial superoxide production blocks three pathways of hyperglycaemic damage. Nature 2000;404:787–90.

[18] DeRubertis FR, Craven PA, Melhem MF. Acceleration of diabetic renal injury in the superoxide dismutase knockout mouse: effects of tempol. Metabolism 2007;56:1256–64.

[19] Asaba K, Tojo A, Onozato ML, Goto A, Fujita T. Double-edged action of SOD mimetic in diabetic nephropathy. J Cardiovasc Pharmacol 2007;49:13–9.

[20] Mollsten A, Marklund SL, Wessman M, Svensson M, Forsblom C, Parkkonen M, et al. A functional polymorphism in the manganese superoxide dismutase gene and diabetic nephropathy. Diabetes 2007;56:265–9.

[21] de Haan JB, Stefanovic N, Nikolic-Paterson D, Scurr LL, Croft KD, Mori TA, et al. Kidney expression of glutathione peroxidase-1. is not protective against streptozotocin-induced diabetic nephropathy. Am J Physiol Renal Physiol 2005;289:F544–51.

[22] Brezniceanu ML, Liu F, Wei CC, Tran S, Sachetelli S, Zhang SL, et al. Catalase overexpression attenuates angiotensinogen expression and apoptosis in diabetic mice. Kidney Int 2007;71:912–23.

[23] dos Santos KG, Canani LH, Gross JL, Tschiedel B, Souto KE, Roisenberg I. The catalase-262C/T promoter polymorphism and diabetes complications in Caucasians with type 2 diabetes. Dis Markers 2006;22:355–9.

[24] Chuang CC, Martinez K, Xie G, Kennedy A, Bumrungpert A, Overman A, et al. Quercetin is equally or more effective than resveratrol in attenuating tumor necrosis factor-α–mediated inflammation and insulin resistance in primary human adipocytes. Am J Clin Nutr 2010;92:1511–21.

[25] Scazzocchio B, Var R, Filesi C, D'Archivio M, Santangelo C, Giovannini C, et al. Cyanidin-3-O-β-glucoside and protocatechuic acid exert insulin-like effects by upregulating PPARγ activity in human omental adipocytes. Diabetes 2011;60:2234–44.

[26] Yoshida H, Takamura N, Shuto T, Ogata K, Tokunaga J, Kawai K, et al. The citrus flavonoids hesperetin and naringenin block the lipolytic actions of TNF-alpha in mouse adipocytes. Biochem Biophys Res Commun 2010;394:728–32.

[27] Zygmunt K, Faubert B, MacNeil J, Tsiani E. Naringenin, a citrus flavonoid, increases muscle cell glucose uptake via AMPK. Biochem Biophys Res Commun 2010;398:178–83.
[28] Ding L, Jin D, Chen X. Luteolin enhances insulin sensitivity via activation of PPARg transcriptional activity in adipocytes. J Nutr Biochem 2010;21:941–7.
[29] Eid HM, Vallerand D, Muhammad A, Durst T, Haddad PS, Martineau LC. Structural constraints and the importance of lipophilicity for the mitochondrial uncoupling activity of naturally occurring caffeic acid esters with potential for the treatment of insulin resistance. Biochem Pharmacol 2010;79:444–54.
[30] Huang DW, Shen SC, Wu JSB. Effects of caffeic acid and cinnamic acid on glucose uptake in insulin-resistant mouse hepatocytes. J Agric Food Chem 2009;57:7687–92.
[31] de Kreutzenberg SV, Ceolotto G, Papparella I, Bortoluzzi A, Semplicini A, Dalla Man C, et al. Downregulation of the longevity-associated protein sirtuin 1 in insulin resistance and metabolic syndrome: potential biochemical mechanisms. Diabetes 2010;59:1006–15.
[32] Bisbal C, Lambert K, Avignon A. Antioxidants and glucose metabolism disorders. Curr Opin Clin Nutr Metab Care 2010;13:439–46.
[33] Arnlöv J, Zethelius B, Riserus U, Basu S, Berne C, Vessby B, et al. Uppsala Longitudinal Study of Adult Men Study. Serum and dietary beta-carotene and alpha-tocopherol and incidence of type 2 diabetes mellitus in a community-based study of Swedish men: report from the Uppsala Longitudinal Study of Adult Men (ULSAM) study. Diabetologia 2009;52:97–105.
[34] Harding AH, Wareham NJ, Bingham SA, Khaw K, Luben R, Welch A, et al. Plasma vitamin C level, fruit and vegetable consumption, and the risk of new-onset type 2 diabetes mellitus: the European prospective investigation of cancer-Norfolk Prospective Study. Arch Intern Med 2008;168:1493–9.
[35] Costacou T, Ma B, King IB, Mayer-Davis EJ. Plasma and dietary vitamin E in relation to insulin secretion and sensitivity. Diabetes Obes Metab 2008;10:223–8.
[36] Carter P, Gray LJ, Troughton J, Khunti K, Davies MJ. Fruit and vegetable intake and incidence of type 2 diabetes mellitus: systematic review and meta-analysis. BMJ 2010;341:4229.
[37] Hamer M, Chida Y. Intake of fruit, vegetables, and antioxidants and risk of type 2 diabetes: systematic review and meta-analysis. J Hypertens 2007;25:2361–9.
[38] Kabat A, Ponicke K, Salameh A, Mohr FW, Dhein S. Effect of a beta 2-adrenoceptor stimulation on hyperglycemia-induced endothelial dysfunction. J Pharmacol Exp Ther 2004;308:564–73.
[39] Hipkiss AR. Does chronic glycolysis accelerate aging? Could this explain how dietary restriction works? Ann N Y Acad Sci 2006;1067:361–8.
[40] Verkaart S, Koopman WJ, van Emst-de Vries SE, Nijtmans LG, van den Heuvel LW, Smeitink JA, et al. Superoxide production is inversely related to complex I activity in inherited complex I deficiency. Biochim Biophys Acta 2007;1772:373–81.
[41] Hernandez-Mijares A, Rocha M, Apostolova N, Borras C, Jover A, Bañuls C, et al. Mitochondrial complex I impairment in leukocytes from type 2 diabetic patients. Free Radic Biol Med 2011;50:1215–21.
[42] Victor VM, Rocha M, Bañuls C, Sanchez-Serrano M, Sola E, Gomez M, et al. Mitochondrial complex I impairment in leukocytes from polycystic ovary syndrome patients with insulin resistance. J Clin Endocrinol Metab 2009;94:3505–12.
[43] Hernandez-Mijares A, Rocha M, Rovira-Llopis S, Bañuls C, Bellod L, de Pablo C, et al. Human leukocyte/endothelial cell interactions and mitochondrial dysfunction in type 2 diabetic patients and their association with silent myocardial ischemia. Diabetes Care 2013;36:1695–702.
[44] Rotig A, de Lonlay P, Chretien D, Foury F, Koenig M, Sidi D, et al. Aconitase and mitochondrial iron-sulphur protein deficiency in Friedreich ataxia. Nat Genet 1997;17:215–7.
[45] Martin-Hernandez E, Garcia-Silva MT, Vara J, Campos Y, Cabello A, Muley R, et al. Renal pathology in children with mitochondrial diseases. Pediatr Nephrol 2005;20:1299–305.
[46] Diomedi-Camassei F, Di Giandomenico S, Santorelli FM, Santorelli FM, Caridi G, Piemonte F, et al. COQ_2 nephropathy: a newly described inherited mitochondriopathy with primary renal involvement. J Am Soc Nephrol 2007;18:2773–80.
[47] Hausse AO, Aggoun Y, Bonnet D, Sidi D, Munnich A, Rötig A, et al. Idebenone and reduced cardiac hypertrophy in Friedreich's ataxia. Heart 2002;87:346–9.
[48] Green K, Brand MD, Murphy MP. Prevention of mitochondrial oxidative damage as a therapeutic strategy in diabetes. Diabetes 2004;53:S110–8.
[49] Chacko BK, Reily C, Srivastava A, Johnson MS, Ye Y, Ulasova E, et al. Prevention of diabetic nephropathy in Ins2(+/)$^{-}$(AkitaJ) mice by the mitochondria-targeted therapy MitoQ. Biochem J 2010;432:9–19.

CHAPTER

6

Iron, Oxidative Stress and Diabetes

Sara Rani Marcus, Mala Dharmalingam*†

*MSU-GEF International Medical School, MSRIT Post, Bangalore, India, †Department of Endocrinology, M.S.Ramaiah Medical College, MSRIT Post, Bangalore, India

List of Abbreviations

AGE Advanced glycation end product
ALA 5-amino levulinate
ATP Adenosine triphosphate
DMT Divalent metal transporter
Fe^{2+}-O Ferryl species
Fe^{2+}-O_2 Perferryl species
FRDA Friedreich's ataxia
GSH-Px Glutathione peroxidase
HbA_{1C} Glycated hemoglobin
HCV Hepatitis C virus
HFE Hemochromatosis gene
HH Hereditary hemochromatosis
HO Heme oxygenase
IL Interleukin
IRE Iron response element
IRP Iron regulatory proteins
ISC Iron-sulfur cluster
LDL Low density lipoprotein
LIP Labile iron pool
NAPDH Nicotinamide adenine dinucleotide phosphate (reduced)
NF-κB Nuclear factor κB
NO˙/NO Nitric oxide
NOS Nitric oxide synthase
Nox NAD(P)H oxidase
NTBI Non-transferrinbound iron
$O_2^{\cdot -}$ Superoxide anion
OH˙ Hydroxyl radical
$ONOO^-$ Peroxynitrite ion
RAGE Receptor for AGE
RAS Renin-angiotensin system
RO˙ Alkoxyl radical
ROO˙ Peroxyl radical
ROS Reactive oxygen species
RS˙ Thiyl radical
RSOO˙ Thiyl-peroxyl radical
SOD Superoxide dismutase
sTfR Soluble extracellular domain of TfR
TBARS Thiobarbituric acid reactive substances
Tf Transferrin
TfR Transferrin receptor
Tf-TfR Transferrin-transferrin receptor complex
TNFα Tumor necrosis factor α
UTR Untranslated regions

INTRODUCTION

Iron, a d-block transition metal, predominantly found in biological systems in the bivalent ferrous (Fe^{2+}) and trivalent ferric (Fe^{3+}) oxidation states, is indispensable for the metabolic activities of the cell. The easy and reversible switching between the Fe^{2+} and Fe^{3+} species and its ability to form coordination complexes with organic ligands provide the basis for the biological functions of iron [1].

Iron can associate with proteins and enzymes as either heme or non-heme iron. Hemoproteins are involved in several vital functions, including oxygen transport (hemoglobin in erythroid tissue), oxygen storage (muscle myoglobin), oxygen metabolism (catalases and peroxidases), cellular respiration (cytochromes), nitric oxide (NO) synthesis (nitric oxide synthases [NOS]), NO sensing (guanylate cyclase), and detoxification reactions (cytochrome P450 system) [1]. The predominant non-heme iron proteins are the iron-sulfur clusters (ISC) (e.g., 2Fe-2S, 3Fe-4S, 4Fe-4S clusters) which have diverse functions, such as electron transport in the respiratory chain, transcriptional regulation, structural stabilization and catalysis [1]. Other catalytically active forms include iron-oxo clusters (e.g., ribonucleotide reductase for DNA synthesis) and mononuclear iron centers (e.g., cyclooxygenase and lipooxygenase, involved in the inflammatory response) [2]. Non-heme iron also has a role in oxygen sensing, via the hypoxia-inducible factor, which controls the transcription of several genes involved in erythropoiesis, angiogenesis, cell proliferation and survival, glycolysis and iron metabolism, depending upon the availability of oxygen [3].

Another iron pool exists called the labile iron pool (LIP), which is also known as 'exchangeable', 'regulatory' or 'chelatable' iron pool, and is found mainly within cells [2]. The LIP contains either Fe^{2+} or Fe^{3+}, is a low molecular

Diabetes: Oxidative Stress and Dietary Antioxidants.
http://dx.doi.org/10.1016/B978-0-12-405885-9.00006-1

weight pool of weakly chelated iron, and represents a small fraction (3–5%) of the cellular iron [4]. It is thought to be in steady state equilibrium and bound to low molecular weight chelates like organic anions (phosphates, citrates and carboxylates) and polyfunctional ligands [2]. The LIP links cellular iron uptake with iron utilization, storage, or export and is biologically active in intracellular metabolism via oxidation-reduction reactions, cell proliferation and cell signaling, but toxic in large amounts [4,5].

Serum iron levels exceeding the binding capacity of transferrin contribute to the non-transferrin bound iron (NTBI) [5]. This NTBI does not correspond to iron bound to heme or ferritin and is seen in chronic iron overload diseases (hemochromatosis) and certain other diseases which are not primarily due to iron overload conditions (alcoholic liver disease, acute or chronic liver failure, diabetes and end-stage renal failure) [6]. NTBI is potentially toxic due to its propensity to induce reactive oxygen species (ROS) and is responsible for both cellular and intracellular damage [6].

DISTRIBUTION OF IRON IN THE BODY

The body contains ~3–5 g of iron, most of which is present in hemoglobin (>2 g) and myoglobin (~300 mg). Macrophages of spleen, liver and bone marrow maintain a small fraction of iron (~600 mg), while the excess is stored in the form of ferritin in liver parenchyma (~1000 mg). The other iron-containing proteins and enzymes together contain ~ 8 mg of iron [2] (Figure 6.1).

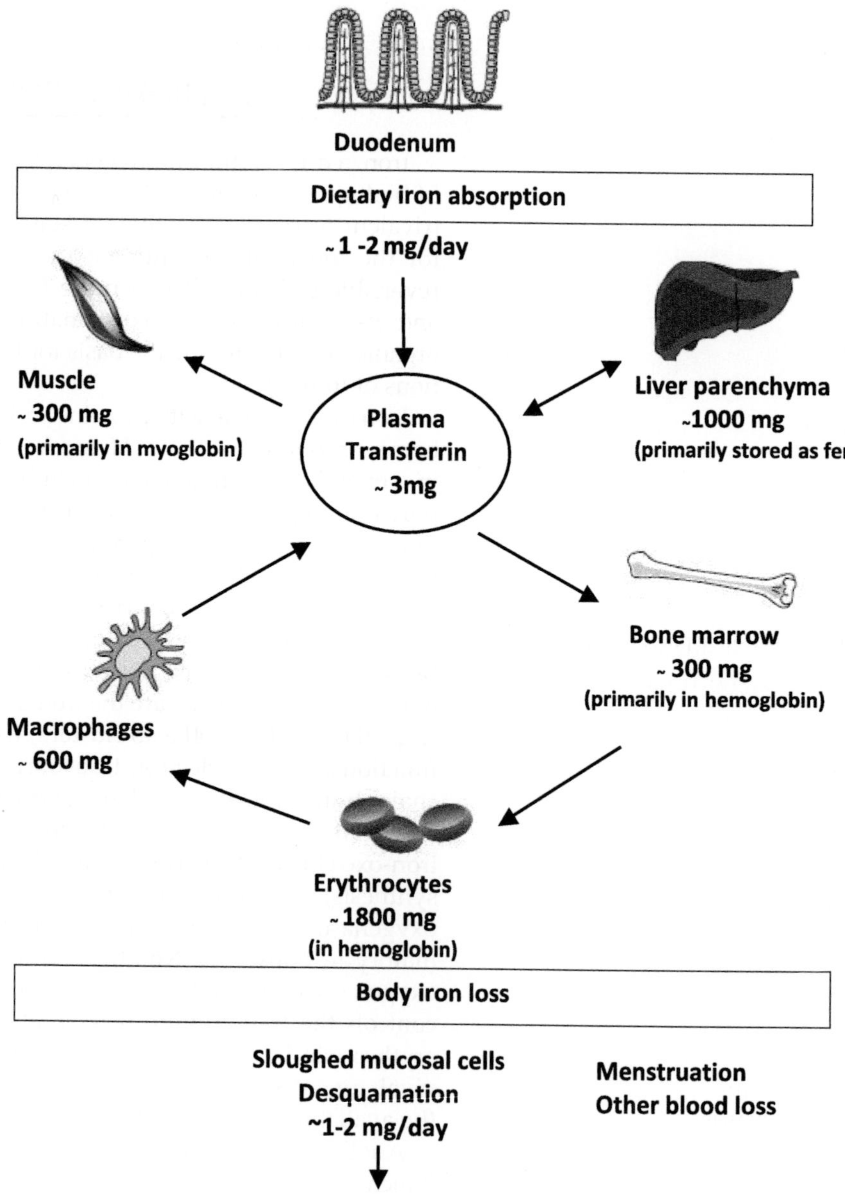

FIGURE 6.1 **Distribution of iron in the body.** The absorption, distribution and recycling of iron in the body. *(Reproduced from Reference 1 with copyright permission from Elsevier Inc.)*

Iron is essentially a 'one way element' and a healthy individual absorbs about 1–2 mg of iron from the diet to replenish the non-specific iron losses by cell desquamation in the skin and intestine, and the physiological loss of iron by menstruating women and other forms of bleeding. Erythropoiesis requires about 30 mg of iron per day, and this is obtained by recycling iron by the macrophages of the reticuloendothelial system [1]. Hence, the transferrin-bound iron pool is very dynamic and undergoes recycling > 10 times a day to supply iron for erythropoiesis [1].

Iron deficiency is one of the most common nutritional deficiencies worldwide, especially among women and children. This deficiency is associated with many disorders including increased risk of poor pregnancy outcomes and impaired cognitive development in young children [7]. Conversely, iron overload (hemochromatosis) or accumulation of excess iron occurs due to a lack of mechanisms for iron secretion, excessive absorption of dietary iron or through multiple blood transfusions. Iron overload may be hereditary (Hereditary hemochromatosis [HH]) or secondary due to chronic blood transfusion and ineffective erythropoiesis [8].

IRON HOMEOSTASIS

In the redox couple, Fe^{2+}/Fe^{3+}, at physiological pH, Fe^{3+} is the relatively insoluble and less active species, whereas Fe^{2+} is the more soluble and potentially toxic form especially under aerobic conditions [2]. Therefore, it is necessary to sequester free Fe^{2+} to limit its bioavailability. The human body has developed mechanisms to make iron available for physiological functions, yet at the same time conserve and handle iron to avoid its deleterious effects. Iron homeostasis is controlled at two different levels of regulation: iron uptake and synthesis of iron binding proteins like transferrin receptor and ferritin, and other proteins involved in iron homeostasis like divalent metal transporter 1 (DMT1) and 5-amino levulinate synthase [9].

Dietary iron consists of both non-heme iron and heme, and the amount absorbed depends on the amount excreted from the body; hence, a balance is maintained by regulation of the amount of iron absorbed in the duodenum [10]. The absorption of dietary iron involves the reduction of Fe^{3+} to Fe^{2+} by ferric reductases such as duodenual cytochrome b, and/or reducing agents such as ascorbic acid, in the intestinal lumen. The Fe^{2+} is then transported across the apical membrane of enterocytes by DMT1 [10]. The mechanism of transport of dietary heme into the enterocyte is not yet clear and may be receptor dependent [2]. Heme, within the enterocyte, is degraded by heme oxygenase-1 (HO-1) to release Fe^{2+} in the endosome or lysosome (Figure 6.2). The Fe^{2+} thus obtained in the enterocyte is either exported to the plasma or stored within the cell after incorporation into ferritin. Fe^{2+} export across the basolateral membrane of the enterocyte occurs with the help of ferroportin, the transmembrane transporter, together with the reoxidation of Fe^{2+} to Fe^{3+} by hephaestin (from the basolateral membrane of enterocytes) or by plasma ceruloplasmin [2].

Splenic reticuloendothelial macrophages recycle iron derived from senescent erythrocytes. Within the macrophages, the heme of hemoproteins is cleaved by HO-1 to release Fe^{2+} into the circulation by ferroportin. Plasma ceruloplasmin reoxidizes Fe^{2+} to Fe^{3+} and the Fe^{3+} is then transferred to apotransferrin [10].

The export of iron is regulated by hepcidin (an iron regulatory hormone produced by the liver) [2]. The release of hepcidin by the liver is also highly regulated [2]. Hepcidin binds ferroportin, brings about its internalization and degradation, and thereby reduces the release of iron into the circulation. However, in iron deficiency, the release of hepcidin by the liver is reduced, while in iron overload the release of hepcidin is stimulated [2]. Hepcidin is considered as a negative regulator which inhibits both intestinal iron absorption and release of iron by the macrophages of the reticuloendothelial system [5].

The exported iron (from enterocytes and macrophages) is scavenged by apotransferrin to form

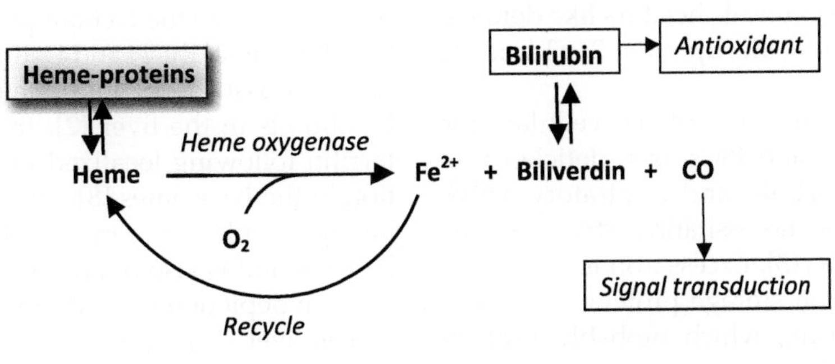

FIGURE 6.2 **Heme oxygenase reaction.** The degradation of heme, derived from mainly hemoglobin and myoglobin, catalyzed by heme oxygenase in the microsomes forms biliverdin and releases Fe^{2+} and carbon monoxide (CO). The biliverdin is enzymatically reduced to bilirubin, an antioxidant; CO probably functions in signal transduction, and the released Fe^{2+} is recycled and incorporated into heme for hemoprotein synthesis.

transferrin (Tf) which maintains the iron in the inert Fe^{3+} state and delivers iron to the tissues. This small, but highly dynamic, Tf pool maintains erythropoiesis [10]. Tf is a glycoprotein, produced mainly by the liver, and also by the lymph nodes, thymus, spleen, salivary gland, bone marrow and testes [2]. Tf can bind two Fe^{3+} ions and the binding or release of iron is accomplished by a pH-dependent conformational change in the protein [2]. The interaction between Fe^{3+} and Tf is very strong at the physiological pH of plasma but, at pH <5, the binding is essentially very weak [2].

Although Tf has two high affinity binding sites for Fe^{3+}, it is only partially saturated (30%) with Fe^{3+} under physiological conditions. Thus, Tf provides a reservoir for the uptake of more iron under conditions of iron overload in the plasma and prevents the build-up of NTBI [2]. This free NTBI, if present in the plasma, is taken up essentially by the liver, endocrine pancreas and heart with the help of carrier molecules, like DMT1 and Zrt-IRt-like protein 14 (ZIP 14) [11]. Increased levels of NTBI can promote oxidative injury both at the cell surface and intracellularly [6]. In conditions like HH and other iron overload states, the Tf is fully saturated and the excess iron spills into the plasma [6].

In mammalian cells, the uptake of iron from Tf is mostly by the binding to transferrin receptor 1 (TfR1) forming the Tf-TfR1 complex which gains entry into the cells. The TfR1 is a transmembrane glycoprotein homodimer, each monomer capable of binding a Tf molecule. The receptor preferentially binds Tf containing two Fe^{3+} ions compared to monoferric Tf or apotransferrin [2]. The Tf-TfR1 complex is taken up by an energy-dependent endocytosis via clathrin coated pits [10]. After the release of Fe^{3+} from the TfR1-Tf complex, the transferrin receptor complex returns to the cell surface where Tf dissociates from TfR1. The ferrireductase, STEAP 3 (six-transmembrane epithelial antigen of prostate-3), reduces Fe^{3+} to Fe^{2+} which is then exported from the endosome by DMT1 to the cytosol to enter the LIP [2]. This LIP is readily available for utilization and probably contributes to the adverse side-effects of redox active iron [4]. LIP functions as a mediator of apoptosis: cellular iron deficiency or treatment with chemical chelators like deferoxamine or biological chelators like lipocalin 24p3 leads to apoptosis [12].

The mitochondria utilize most of the cellular iron for the synthesis of heme and ISCs: iron deficiency or overload impairs the metabolic and respiratory activities of the mitochondria, necessitating strict maintenance of iron homeostasis [13]. Excess iron is stored in a mitochondrion-specific iron storage protein, mitochondrial ferritin or mitoferritin, which probably protects against oxidative stress. The expression of mitoferritin in most cells is low; however, overexpression of mitoferritin significantly affects intracellular homeostasis by the transport of iron from the cytosol and deposition in the mitochondria and rendering it ineffective for metabolic use [13].

The first and last steps of heme synthesis occur in the mitochondria. First, the condensation of succinyl CoA and glycine to form 5-amino levulinate (ALA) catalyzed by the erythroid specific ALA synthase 2 or the housekeeping ALA synthase 1 in non-erythroid cells, occurs in the mitochondrial matrix. The ALA is then transported to the cytosol and subsequently undergoes several reactions to form protoporphyrinogen IX. The final step of incorporation of iron into protoporphyrin also occurs in the mitochondria, and is catalyzed by mitochondrial ferrochelatase to form heme [10].

ISCs are essential and highly adaptable enzyme cofactors required for a wide range of cellular reactions [14]. Although they are distributed in mitochondria and cytosol, their synthesis primarily occurs in the mitochondrial matrix utilizing iron present in the mitochondria [14]. ISCs are assembled on scaffold proteins and then targeted to specific proteins via the sulfur of cysteine residues. In mammals, the scaffold protein is 'ISC assembly protein U' and iron is donated by frataxin [14]. Thus, defects in frataxin/ ISC synthesis are associated with dysregulation of cellular iron homeostasis, resulting in an accumulation of mitochondrial iron and depletion of cytosolic iron; which can promote oxidative stress [14].

Cells can eliminate excess intracellular iron by secretion of Fe^{2+} by ferroportin or by secretion of heme using the putative heme exporter FLVCR1 (feline leukemia virus subgroup C receptor 1) from hematopoietic cells [15]. Cells also store and thereby detoxify excess iron in the cytosol within ferritin, a conserved protein consisting of 24 H (Heavy) and L (Light) subunits. Ferritin assembly provides a shell-like structure with a cavity that can store 4,500 Fe^{3+} ions in the form of ferric oxy-hydroxide phosphate. This prevents iron from catalyzing Fenton type reactions. The mechanism of incorporation of iron into ferritin is not clear; it is probably brought about by the iron chaperone PCBP1 poly(RC)- binding protein 1) [10]. Iron is incorporated into ferritin in the Fe^{3+} state and this requires the ferroxidase activity of the H chain of ferritin while the L chain provides the nucleation center. The ratio of the H and L subunits vary in ferritin from different tissues – H subunits predominate in heart and L subunits in the liver [2]. Iron can be mobilized from ferritin following localized protein unfolding, degradation in the lysosomes [8], and, in the presence of reducing agents like vitamin C and superoxide anion ($O_2^{\cdot-}$) [16]. Ferritin is also degraded in the proteasome following iron depletion or oxidation [8].

The liver is the major storage organ for iron and the uptake of iron by the hepatocyte is by both TfR1 and TfR2; while TfR1 is found in most cells, TfR2 is found exclusively in the hepatocytes and differentiated erythroblasts

[2]. Iron is stored in the liver as ferritin and hemosiderin. Hemosiderin is a structure consisting of degradation products of ferritin and iron oxide clusters [10].

The expression of TfR1 and ferritin are coordinately regulated post-transcriptionally by the binding of iron regulatory proteins-1 (IRP1) and -2 (IRP2) to iron response elements (IRE) in the untranslated regions (UTR) of the respective mRNAs. TfR1 mRNA contains multiple IREs within its long 3'-UTR, whereas mRNAs encoding H- and L-ferritin contain only a single IRE in their 5'-UTRs. In an iron deficient cell, IRPs bind with high affinity to the cognate IREs [10]. The IRE-IRP stabilize TfR1 mRNA and, impose a steric blockade for the translation of ferritin mRNA. The increased TfR1 levels stimulate the uptake of iron from the plasma to counteract the deficiency; ferritin synthesis is inhibited resulting in decreased iron storage. However, in iron excess, the IRPs are inactivated causing degradation of TfR1 mRNA and translation of ferritin mRNA; thus, the IRE-IRP switch minimizes further iron uptake through the TfR1 channel and promotes storage of excess iron in newly synthesized ferritin [10]. mRNAs encoding other proteins of iron transport (DMT1 and ferroportin), erythroid heme synthesis (ALA synthase-2) and mitochondrial aconitases also contain functional IREs [10]. Additional mechanisms for regulation of ferritin gene expression at the level of transcription have been reported. Ferritin gene expression is altered by pro-inflammatory cytokines like TNFα (Tumor necrosis factor α) and IL-1α (Interleukin -1α) [10], and activated by oxidative stress by an upstream antioxidant response element in the promoter region of the ferritin gene [17]. However, extracellular hydrogen peroxide (H_2O_2) inhibits ferritin translation by activating the IRE-IRP regulatory system [2]. Therefore, by sequestering redox active iron, ferritin functions as an antioxidant and protects the cell.

OXIDATIVE STRESS

ROS are highly reactive, short-lived derivatives of oxygen, generated during the course of normal cellular processes and quenched by the antioxidant defense systems of the body in order to maintain a stable intracellular milieu [8].

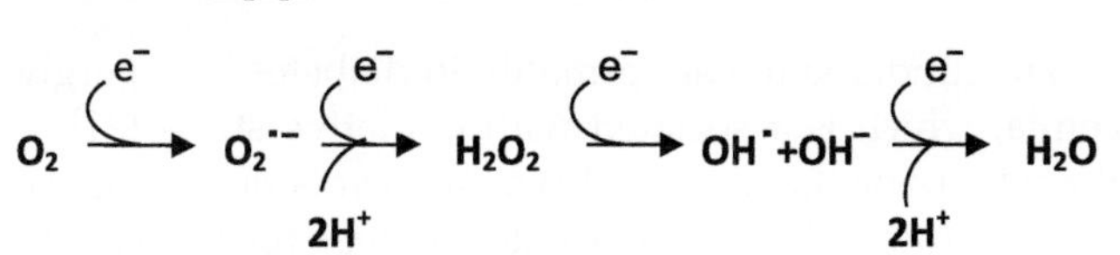

(1)

Superoxide anion ($O_2^{\cdot-}$), the first ROS formed (Eq. 1), is moderately reactive; it liberates iron from proteins containing ISCs (especially 4Fe-4S clusters) and inactivates the proteins. $O_2^{\cdot-}$ also reacts with $NO^{\cdot}$ (nitric oxide) to form highly reactive peroxynitrite ($ONOO^-$) [18] which nitrate proteins and DNA [8]. $O_2^{\cdot-}$ is dismutated by the superoxide dismutases (SODs) present in all aerobic cells. (Eq. 2) [8].

$$O_2{\cdot}^- + O_2{\cdot}^- \rightarrow H_2O_2 + O_2 \qquad (2)$$

H_2O_2, a moderately active ROS, derived from the two-electron reduction of oxygen (Eq. 1) and the dismutation of $O_2^{\cdot-}$ (Eq. 2), is reduced to water by the action of catalases, glutathione peroxidases (GSH-Px) and peroxyredoxins using H_2O_2, GSH and thioredoxin, respectively [8]. This prevents the formation of the highly reactive hydroxyl radical ($OH^{\cdot}$), especially in the presence of iron. Thus, $O_2^{\cdot-}$ and H_2O_2 are produced in an intracellular steady state depending on the cell type and cell compartment; and they are continuously removed by specific enzymes [8]. However, these ROS are also necessary for certain biochemical processes such as signal transduction, cellular differentiation, growth arrestment, apoptosis, immunity and defense against microorganisms [19].

In order to combat the action of free radicals, the body has developed antioxidant defense systems. These are: the free radical scavenging enzymes (like SOD, catalase and GSH-Px) and the non-enzymatic compounds (like vitamin C, GSH, uric acid, vitamin E, β-carotene and bilirubin) [19].

Oxidative stress occurs when the net amount of ROS exceeds the antioxidant capacity: a consequence of overproduction of ROS, decreased levels of antioxidants, or both [19]. Free radicals, like ROS, are highly reactive species that can lead to lipid peroxidation, protein oxidation and damage and nucleic acid modifications. Similarly, reactive nitrogen species such as peroxynitrite can damage proteins by nitration [19]. If these oxidative and nitrosative reactions are not counter-balanced by the antioxidant defense systems, it can contribute to the development of many pathological conditions [19,20].

IRON AND OXIDATIVE STRESS

The transition between Fe^{2+} (electron donor) and Fe^{3+} (electron acceptor) in the cellular environment is responsible for several biochemical reactions and also for its toxicity. Catalytic amounts of Fe^{2+} can result in the propagation of highly reactive ROS species like the $OH^{\cdot}$ radical, especially under aerobic conditions [10].

The toxicity of iron is mainly based on Fenton and Haber Weiss chemistry (Figure 6.3).

$$Fe^{2+} + H_2O_2 \rightarrow Fe^{3+} + OH^- + OH^{\cdot} \text{ (Fenton reaction)} \qquad (3)$$

$$Fe^{3+} + O_2{\cdot}^- \rightarrow Fe^{2+} + O_2 \qquad (4)$$

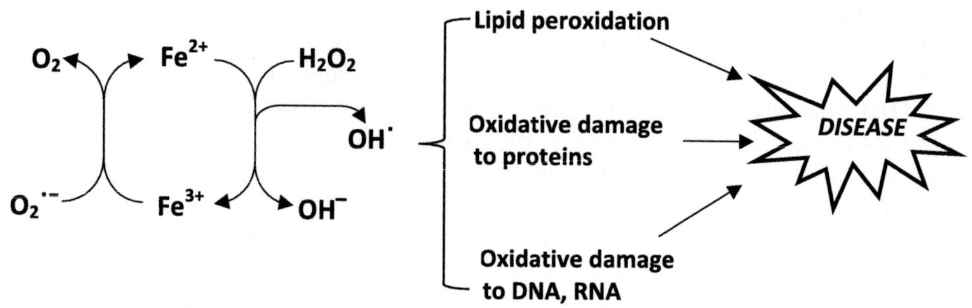

FIGURE 6.3 **The Fenton/Haber Weiss reactions.** The Fenton/Haber Weiss reactions and its effect on biomolecules. $O_2^{\cdot-}$ = superoxide anion; $OH^{\cdot}$ = hydroxyl radical; OH^- = hydroxyl ion.

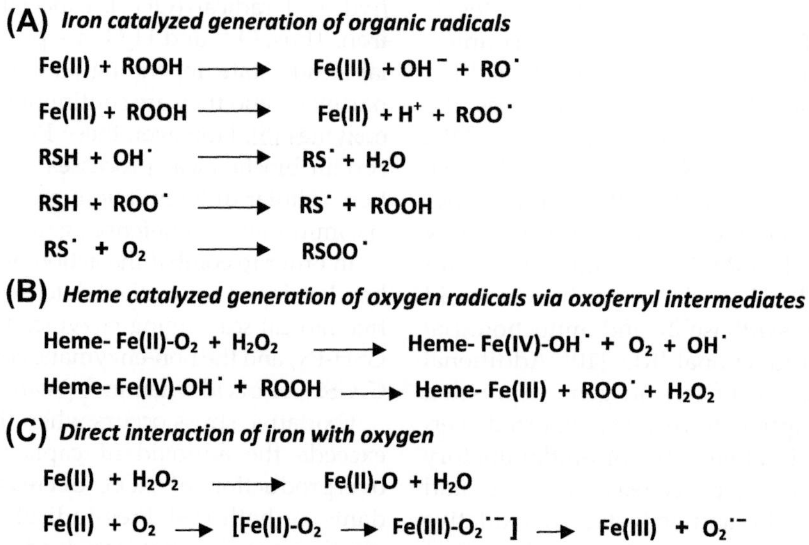

FIGURE 6.4 **The role of iron in the generation of reactive oxygen species.** The generation of free radicals by (A) iron (B) heme (C) iron as a substrate. $RO^{\cdot}$ = alkoxyl radical; $ROO^{\cdot}$ = peroxyl radical; $RS^{\cdot}$ = thiyl radical; $RSOO^{\cdot}$ = thiyl-peroxyl radical; Fe^{2+}-O = ferryl species; Fe^{2+}-O_2 = perferryl species. *(Reproduced from Ref. 1 with copyright permission from Elsevier Inc.)*

Net reaction

$$H_2O_2 + O_2^{\cdot-} \rightarrow OH^- + OH^{\cdot} + O_2 \text{ (Haber Weiss reaction)} \quad (5)$$

Cellular reactions generate ROS during normal metabolism. For example, the mitochondrial electron transport chain and NADPH oxidase generate $O_2^{\cdot-}$, xanthine oxidase and other oxidases release H_2O_2, the dismutation of $O_2^{\cdot-}$ by SODs also releases H_2O_2. Both $O_2^{\cdot-}$ and H_2O_2 participate in the Fenton/Haber Weiss reactions to produce the more potent hydroxyl radical ($OH^{\cdot}$) [1]. However, while $OH^{\cdot}$ interacts with biomolecules in the vicinity of its generation, $O_2^{\cdot-}$ and H_2O_2 diffuse away from their sites of formation. Hence the site of availability of catalytic iron also controls the generation of the $OH^{\cdot}$ [8].

Redox active iron also catalyzes the generation of organic reactive species such as peroxyl ($ROO^{\cdot}$), alkoxyl ($RO^{\cdot}$), thiyl ($RS^{\cdot}$) or thiyl-peroxyl ($RSOO^{\cdot}$) radicals [1] (Figure 6.4A). Heme iron (either as free heme or as hemoprotein) catalyzes the generation of free radicals resulting in oxoferryl intermediates [1] (Figure 6.4B). In addition, the Fe^{2+} ion functions as a reactant and interacts directly with oxygen to generate free radicals resulting in ferryl (Fe^{2+}-O) or perferryl (Fe^{2+}-O_2) iron intermediates [1] (Figure 6.4C). Therefore, excessive amounts of redox active iron can aggravate oxidative stress and precipitate tissue damage as observed in hereditary and secondary iron overload disorders [1].

OXIDATIVE STRESS IN DIABETES

The fundamental abnormality in diabetes is hyperglycemia, which is associated with oxidative stress [21]. In diabetic patients, increased plasma levels of ROS markers like thiobarbituric acid reactive substances (TBARS) [22,23], 8α- isoprotanes, oxidized LDL, protein oxidation products [19], 8-oxo-deoxyguanosine and 8-oxoguanosine [24] along with decreased antioxidant defenses, such as total antioxidant capacity [16], bilirubin, SOD, and antioxidant vitamins have been reported [25]. The sources

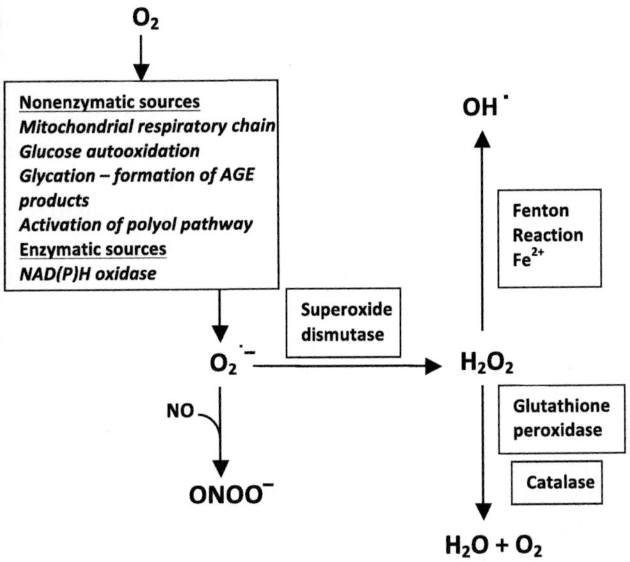

FIGURE 6.5 **Sources of reactive oxygen and nitrogen species in diabetes.** Oxygen is converted to $O_2^{\cdot-}$ (superoxide anion) by the activation of non-enzymatic or enzymatic sources. $O_2^{\cdot-}$ is dismutated by superoxide dismutase to H_2O_2 (hydrogen peroxide) or reacts with NO (nitric oxide) to form peroxynitrite ($ONOO^-$). H_2O_2 can be converted to water by glutathione peroxidase using GSH (glutathione) or by catalase or to highly reactive $OH^{\cdot}$ (hydroxyl radical) by the Fenton reaction in the presence of Fe^{2+} . *(Reproduced from Ref. 18.)*

of oxidative stress in diabetes include non-enzymatic, enzymatic, and mitochondrial pathways [18] (Figure 6.5).

Nonenymatic sources: The non-enzymatic mechanisms include: generation of $OH^{\cdot}$ by the auto-oxidation of glucose [18]; the non-enzymatic glycation of proteins followed by a series of reactions and rearrangements resulting in the formation of advanced glycation end products (AGEs). These mechanisms, together with the interaction of the AGEs with their receptors (RAGE), induce ROS production [18]. Glycated transferrin has decreased ability to bind Fe^{3+} and thus induces the pool of free iron to stimulate ferritin synthesis. Glycated holo-transferrin also serves as a source of ROS [26]. Low anti-oxidant levels facilitate the rapid release of iron from ferritin, down-regulate the ferroxidase activity of the H chain of ferritin and decrease the incorporation of Fe^{3+} into ferritin, resulting in an increase in the free iron pool and concomitant oxidative stress. However, free iron and oxidative stress also promote the synthesis of ferritin which can serve as a protective mechanism against iron toxicity [27].

Besides protein glycation, high levels of glucose have been reported to destroy the heme groups of hemoglobin and myoglobin *in vitro*, probably initiated by H_2O_2, and resulting in the release of Fe^{2+}. The released iron can promote AGE formation [28]. The enhanced metabolism of glucose through the polyol pathway produces $O_2^{\cdot-}$ and the stimulation of the renin-angiotensin system (RAS) in diabetes also promotes the formation of ROS [18].

Enzymatic sources: The enzymatic sources of ROS generation in diabetes include NOS, NAD(P)H oxidase (Nox) and xanthine oxidase [18]. The three isoforms of NOS (endothelial NOS [eNOS], neuronal NOS [nNOS], and inducible NOS [iNOS]) require five cofactors/prosthetic groups (FAD, FMN, heme, 5,6,7,8-tetrahydrobiopterin and Ca-calmodulin) in order to convert L-arginine to NO. If NOS lacks any of the cofactors or the substrate, it switches from the coupled state of NO production to the uncoupled state of $O_2^{\cdot-}$ generation [29]. The resulting $O_2^{\cdot-}$ reacts with preformed NO to form peroxynitrite ($ONOO^-$), an extremely potent oxidizing agent. This peroxynitrite, in turn, can oxidize the cofactor of eNOS, namely 5,6,7,8-tetrahydrobiopterin to 7,8-dihydrobiopterin, thus further uncoupling NO generation [29]. In addition, the increased pro-oxidant activity can facilitate the oxidation of LDL to oxidized LDL particles, which in turn, can limit the availability of L-arginine and enhance uncoupling of NOS, and contribute to both increased ROS generation and decreased availability of NO in diabetes [29].

NAD(P)H oxidase (Nox) is a membrane-associated, heme-containing enzyme complex consisting of several subunits and is a major source of $O_2^{\cdot-}$ production in diabetes. Nox is activated by a variety of stimuli, including hyperglycemia, AGEs, RAS, inflammatory factors (TNFα, IL-6), growth factors (TGF-β [Transforming growth factor-β]) and shear stress [29]. The $O_2^{\cdot-}$ and other ROS formed, in turn, can stimulate the signaling pathways associated with cell growth, inflammation, apoptosis, and fibrosis which eventually lead to the development of the complications of diabetes [30]. Xanthine oxidase mediates the last two reactions of purine metabolism and generates significant amounts of ROS [29].

Mitochondrial sources: The mitochondrial respiratory chain can generate ROS under physiological and pathological conditions. In diabetes, the persistent hyperglycemia elevates the free fatty acid levels which are metabolized to produce increased levels of reduced coenzymes, NADH and $FADH_2$. These reduced coenzymes enter the respiratory chain, and consequently, in order to combat the flux of electrons, this leads to increased production of $O_2^{\cdot-}$ [29]. In diabetes, this mitochondrial $O_2^{\cdot-}$ stimulates the production of more ROS and reactive nitrogen species by activation of nuclear factor-κB (NF-κB)-mediated cytokines, protein kinase C and Nox [18]. Further, oxidative stress of the ISCs found in association with the mitochondrial enzymes also release iron [31]. The β-cells of the pancreas normally respond to enhanced metabolic stress by increasing in mass and thus synthesizing and secreting more insulin. However, in type 2 diabetes, the accumulation of ROS (H_2O_2 and $OH^{\cdot}$ generated in the presence of Fe^{2+}) results in a progressive reduction in β-cell mass by apoptosis

[32]. The peroxidation of the mitochondrial membrane phospholipids by these ROS causes loss of membrane integrity and the release of cytochrome c into the cytosol, where it initiates apoptosis [32]. Hence, oxidative stress results in mitochondrial dysfunction, which is associated with insulin resistance and the development of type 2 diabetes and its complications [18].

The outer mitochondrial membrane contains an integral protein (mitoNEET) with a pH labile redox active ISC which controls the respiratory rate of the mitochondria [33]. Overexpression of mitoNEET preserves insulin sensitivity in the adipose tissue, inhibits the transport of iron into the mitochondrial matrix, and lowers the activity of the respiratory chain. Conversely, decreased expression of mitoNEET protein enhances the respiratory capacity by increasing the iron content of the matrix, heightening oxidative stress and glucose intolerance [34].

Antioxidants: A whole range of defense mechanisms, in the form of antioxidants, are present in the body to counteract oxidative stress. They include the enzymes like SOD, catalase (lysosomes) and GSH-Px (mitochondria) and the fat- and water-soluble antioxidants such as vitamins A, C and E, GSH, trace elements like copper, selenium and zinc, coenzyme Q, bilirubin, uric acid, albumin, etc. A general reduction in these defense mechanisms has been observed in diabetes [16,18].

IRON AND DIABETES

There is a close association between the metabolisms of iron and glucose. Insulin is required for the cellular uptake of iron: an *in vitro* study reported that the uptake of iron by adipose tissue and liver occurred by the redistribution of TfR to the cell surface [35]. In the liver, iron influences glucose metabolism by interfering with the inhibition of glucose production and the uptake and metabolism of insulin [27].

Generally, iron stores have been represented by serum ferritin levels. Serum ferritin levels may not completely reflect an elevation in iron stores since it is an acute phase reactant influenced by factors like inflammation. However, after adjustment for these factors, an increase was still observed in ferritin levels indicating high iron stores [36]. Serum levels of the soluble extracellular domain of TfR (sTfR), derived by the proteolytic cleavage of the receptor during endocytosis of the Tf-TfR complex, are directly proportional to tissue TfR concentration and are regulated by cellular iron stores. Serum ferritin positively correlates with NTBI and inversely with sTfR [36]. The sTfR: ferritin ratio or sTfR index is another good estimate of iron stores, independent of inflammation, and inversely proportional to the iron stores [36].

The increased incidence of type 2 diabetes in iron overload conditions and its reversal or improvement following reduction of the iron load by phlebotomy or iron chelation suggests a potential role of iron in the etiopathogenesis of diabetes [27]. Although the mechanism of iron-induced diabetes is unclear, the oxidative stress due to the pro-oxidant role of iron contributes to tissue damage and increases the risk for diabetes.

The $OH^{\cdot}$ generated by iron may also contribute to type 2 diabetes by causing insulin to become more hydrophobic [37]. Insulin circulates in the blood in a monomeric form which binds to its receptor under physiological conditions; but there is impairment in the interaction of the receptor with the hydrophobically bonded dimer [37]. This probably explains the inactivity of the hormone in hyperinsulinemic patients [37].

The interaction of AGE with its receptor (RAGE) besides causing oxidative stress also induces HO-1 [38]. The formation of bilirubin by this reaction contributes to the antioxidant pool (Figure 6.2). This effect is only observed in the early stages of diabetes, but in the later stages, the expression of the enzyme is reduced due to a dyscompensative effect [38]. Thus, HO-1 helps to maintain iron homeostasis and also prevents diabetes and its complications [38].

IRON OVERLOAD STATES

Idiopathic Hemochromatosis: An increase in the total body iron stores is related to a high risk of the development of type 2 diabetes [27]. Type 2 diabetes is a common manifestation of hemochromatosis, a group of iron overload disorders. In HH, a genetic iron overload disorder characterized by increased iron stores (increased levels of serum ferritin), there is a high prevalence of diabetes [39]. Hemochromatosis is characterized by increased transferrin saturation and the presence of NTBI in the plasma which is taken up by cells using DMT1 [40].

HH is a group of autosomal recessive disorders mostly arising due to two missense mutations (C282Y and H63D) in the hemochromatosis gene (HFE) located on the short arm of chromosome 6 [1]. The product of the gene, HFE protein, normally binds to TfR and reduces its affinity for transferrin; however, due to a mutation in the gene, the repressor function of the protein is lost, resulting in an enhanced uptake of iron by some tissues [39]. Also, in HH, the increased absorption of iron is probably due to a deficiency of hepcidin [39]. About 25–60% of HH patients develop secondary type 2 diabetes and this may be due to insulin resistance and β-cell failure caused by increased iron deposition [39]. In other genetic iron overload syndromes like ferroportin disease, hemojuvelin disease, or hereditary aceruloplasminemia a high incidence of type 2 diabetes has been reported [41]. The mechanisms that are proposed to explain the development of diabetes in HH are iron overload in the liver causing insulin resistance, and iron accumulation in pancreatic β-cells, resulting in cell damage [38].

Iron overload due to transfusions: Transfusional iron overload, a common cause of acquired iron overload, is also associated with impaired glucose tolerance and diabetes [41]. In a group of transfusion-dependent β-thalassemic patients with diabetes or impaired glucose tolerance, it was found that the risk factors for these conditions were elevated serum ferritin and hepatitis C infection (HCV) [42]. The deposition of iron in the interstitial pancreatic cells resulted in insulin deficiency together with excess collagen deposition and defective microcirculation [1]. Treatment with intravenous or oral iron chelation therapy improved the glucose tolerance in some of these patients, suggesting a causal role for iron [41].

Dietary overload: Dietary iron overload has been described among South African tribals, who eat acidic cereal cooked in iron pots, which enhances the absorption of iron. Type 2 diabetes has also been reported in this population, as a late manifestation [41]. A high meat diet and increased dietary heme intake have also been associated with type 2 diabetes [43]. In patients with porphyria cutanea tarda, where iron overload is present, there was a high incidence of glucose intolerance. In HCV infection, iron accumulates in the liver parenchyma, and many patients with chronic HCV infection were found to have elevated serum iron, transferrin saturation and ferritin levels, and in some instances even severe iron overload [41]. This suggests the probable link between HCV infection and accelerated end-organ damage in diabetes [41].

Mitochondrial overload: In mitochondrial iron overload conditions, like Friedreich's ataxia, type 2 diabetes has been reported. Friedreich's ataxia (FRDA) is an inherited neurodegenerative disorder due to a defect in the FRDA gene which results in reduced levels of frataxin (product of the FRDA gene); and therefore, decreased synthesis of ISC, accumulation of iron in the mitochondria and cellular iron dysregulation, probably enhancing oxidative stress [14]. Diabetes develops in these individuals after the first decade of life [14]. The disruption of the FRDA gene causes cellular growth arrest and apoptosis of pancreatic β-cells, together with an increase in ROS in islets. This also leads to progressive damage in both mitochondrial and nuclear DNA [44].

Thus, iron stores have been correlated with insulin sensitivity, insulin secretion, and type 2 diabetes. Frequent blood donation by healthy volunteers reduced the iron storage and postprandial hyperinsulinemia, improved insulin sensitivity and provided protection against the development of type 2 diabetes [27]. Similarly, the use of iron chelators and phlebotomy in iron overload patients also decreased iron levels and improved glycemia [27]. These studies imply a causal role of iron in diabetes.

The mechanisms underlying the association of iron and diabetes are not yet clearly defined. Both iron and diabetes promote oxidative stress, the impact of which varies from tissue to tissue; and, the vulnerability of the tissue depends on the expression of its antioxidant defense systems [45]. In diabetes, the secretion and metabolism of insulin by the pancreatic β-cell and the hepatocytes, respectively, are affected by the ROS [27]. In the presence of iron overload, the increased sensitivity of

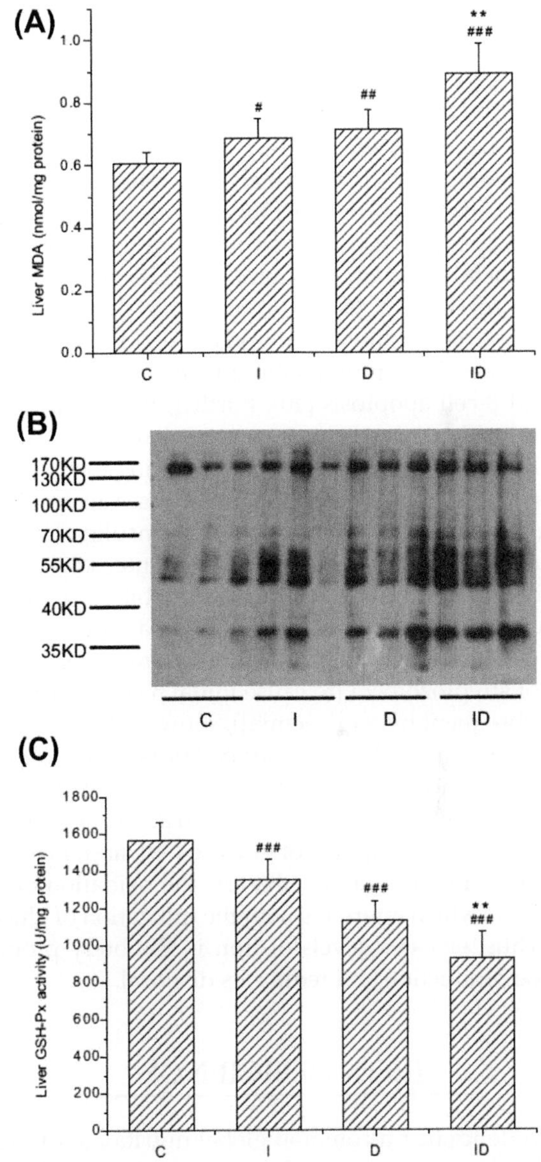

FIGURE 6.6 **Oxidative stress parameters in the livers of differently treated rats.** (A) Malondialdehyde (MDA) levels, (B) protein oxidation status, and (C) glutathione peroxidase (GSH-Px) activities in the liver of control rats and animals subjected to iron and/or high fat diet/streptozotocin administration. C = control, I = iron overload, D = high fat diet/streptozotocin-induced diabetes, ID = iron overload & high fat diet/ streptozotocin-induced diabetes. Values are means ± SD obtained from 7 or 8 rats per experimental group. # $P < 0.05$, ##$P < 0.01$, ### $P < 0.001$ vs. C group, **$P < 0.01$ vs. D group. *(Figure reproduced from Ref. 47 with copyright permission from Elsevier Inc.)*

TABLE 6.1 Iron Profile and Oxidative Stress Parameters in Asian Indian type 2 Diabetics with Iron Deficiency

Parameter	Group I N=30	*P* Value I vs. II	Group II N=30	*P* Value II vs. III	Group III N=30	*P* Value I vs. III
Hemoglobin (g/L)	79.6 ± 16.22	0.000	128.0 ± 9.25	–	130.1 ± 11.91	0.000
Serum iron (μmole/L)	7.73 ± 3.73	0.000	14.75 ± 4.67	–	13.00 ± 4.28	0.000
Serum ferritin (μg/L)	62.03 ± 46.25	0.000	132.47 ± 67.44	0.040	96.28 ± 50.79	–
Malondialdehyde (nmol/L)	454.25 ± 88.47	0.000	212.80 ± 93.80	–	165.67 ± 85.03	0.000
Uric acid (μmol/L)	211.22 ± 69.03	0.006	281.25 ± 102.58	–	300.13 ± 81.22	0.000

Data is presented as mean ± SD of Group I (11 male/19 female) diabetics with iron deficiency; Group II (11 male/19 female) diabetics without iron deficiency; and, Group III (12 male/18 female) non-diabetic, without iron deficiency, healthy control subjects. $P < 0.05$ is statistically significant.
(Reproduced from Ref. 23).

the β-cell to iron is not completely understood: a plausible explanation for the build-up of iron in the β-cell compared to other cells is the enhanced expression of DMTs in the β-cell probably to facilitate the uptake of zinc for the packaging of insulin in secretory granules [46]. The β-cells mainly rely on the mitochondrial metabolism of glucose for insulin secretion: oxidative damage to the mitochondria resulting from iron overload will therefore impair the secretion of insulin, together with β-cell failure and β-cell apoptosis [40]. Further, the expression of the antioxidant scavenging enzymes like SOD, catalase and GSH-Px is decreased thus augmenting the oxidative stress [24]. Iron overload in the liver causes an amplification of oxidative stress and results in insulin resistance because of its reduced capacity for the internalization of insulin and also impairment in the inhibition of glucose production [39]. A study conducted on a type 2 diabetic rat model (high fat diet [to elicit insulin resistance] + low dose of streptozotocin [to cause initial β-cell dysfunction and subsequent hyperglycemia]), showed that iron overload enhanced the diabetes-induced pro-oxidant/antioxidant imbalance facilitating liver injury [47] (Figure 6.6). In the adipocytes, iron impairs insulin action and thereby interferes with the uptake of glucose [39]; and, increased iron stores in the muscle enhances the oxidation of free fatty acids which interferes with the utilization of glucose [39]. Thus, elevated levels of iron in the body promote glucose production and reduce its disposal.

IRON DEFICIENCY

Iron deficiency, a common global nutritional disorder, may be due to an increased demand, increased loss, or decreased uptake of iron or due to factors like inflammation and chronic disease [38]. In diabetic patients, the major glycated hemoglobin (HbA_{1C}), which normally reflects glycemic control, is abnormally elevated. Iron deficiency in both diabetics and non-diabetics resulted in a marked increase in HbA_{1C} levels, which decreased on iron supplementation [48]. Iron deficiency is associated with increased levels of lipid peroxidation [23] (Table 6.1), and it has been suggested that lipid peroxidation increases HbA_{1C} levels which are reversed by antioxidants [38].

There are conflicting results regarding whether blood donation can improve insulin sensitivity by causing a transient iron deficiency. A comparison of male blood donors (who donated blood between six months and five years previously) and non-donors matched for age, body mass index and cardiovascular risk profile revealed that frequent blood donors had significantly increased insulin sensitivity, insulin secretion and reduced iron stores [49]. In another study of type 2 diabetics with high ferritin levels, blood donors had decreased HbA_{1C} levels, altered insulin secretion, and insulin resistance in comparison with matched subjects who were not blood donors [50]. In contrast, no appreciable association between the frequency of blood donation and the risk of diabetes has also been reported [51].

Iron deficiency affects the production of hemoglobin (and erythrocyte proliferation), and also the synthesis of other iron-containing proteins like cytochromes, myoglobin, catalase and peroxidase [20,52]. The deficiency of iron also affects mitochondrial oxidative phosphorylation leading to decreased ATP production and causes loss of structural and functional integrity of the cell [18]. In iron deficiency, there is oxidative stress due to both increased free radical generation and impairment in the antioxidant defense systems, decreased cellular immunity and decreased myeloperoxidase activity [52] (Figure 6.7). Thus, the deficiency of iron causes tissue hypoxia and also affects the production of iron-containing antioxidant proteins which tilts the balance to the oxidative side [53] (Figure 6.8).

THE ROLE OF IRON IN DIABETES WITHOUT OVERT IRON OVERLOAD

Higher serum ferritin levels (but below the range for hemochromatosis) have also been reported in diabetic patients compared to non-diabetics [23], and altered body iron levels have been observed in high risk diabetic conditions like obesity, metabolic syndrome, polycystic ovarian

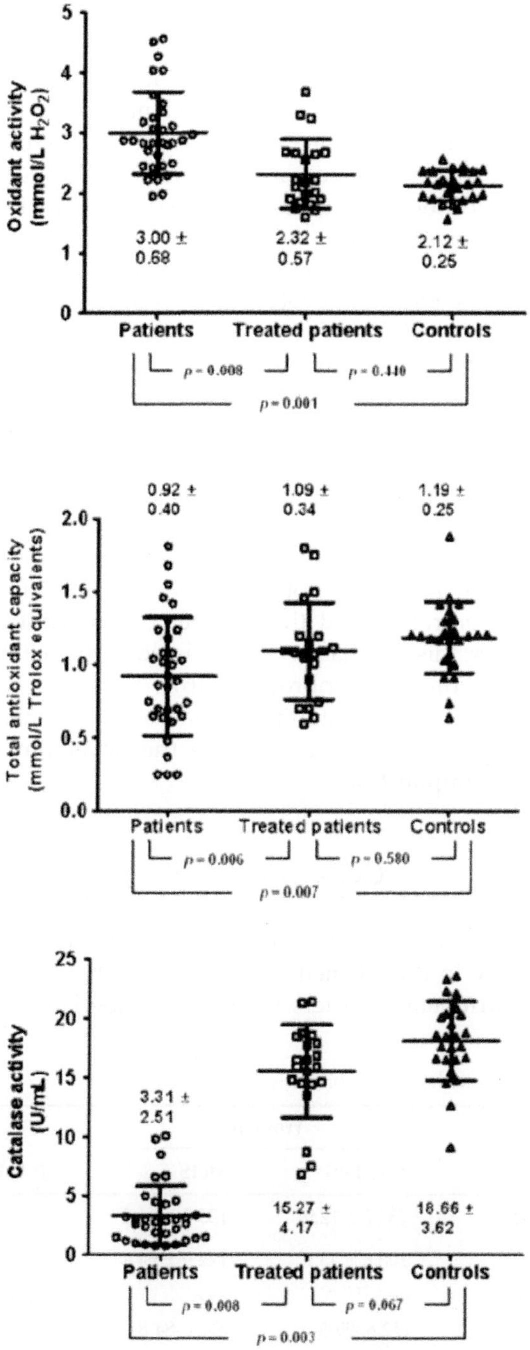

FIGURE 6.7 **Oxidative stress in iron deficiency anemia patients and treated patients.** Data is presented as mean ± SD of 33 iron deficiency anemia patients, 21 treated patients (oral administration of 160 mg bid ferrous sulfate for a period of 4 months) and 25 normal controls. $P < 0.05$ is statistically significant. *(Reproduced from Ref. 20 with copyright permission from Wiley Inc.)*

syndrome, gestational diabetes, and in the pre-diabetic state [39]. A study of the adult offspring of diabetic and non-diabetic parents revealed an elevated iron nutritional status (higher ferritin, total body iron and lower TfR) and altered oxidative stress parameters in the offspring (although normoglycemic) of diabetic parents (Table 6.2); these results were similar to their parents [54]. The reported positive correlation between serum ferritin and basal insulin levels suggest the pre-diabetic state of the offspring of diabetic parents and indicate a causal relationship between iron metabolism and diabetes [54]. In another study on subjects with and without metabolic syndrome, increased oxidative stress parameters (oxidized LDL, TBARS, HO) and iron storage (high ferritin, total body iron and low TfR) have been reported to be associated with metabolic syndrome [55] (Table 6.3). The increased iron levels cause oxidative stress which could lead to tissue damage and enhance the risk of developing diabetes [39].

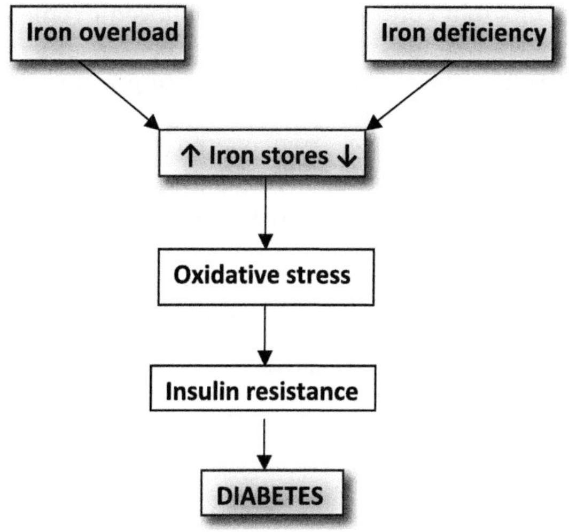

FIGURE 6.8 **The role of iron in diabetes.** The effects of iron overload and deficiency on diabetes. Iron overload causes oxidative stress which leads to pancreatic β-cell damage and decreased insulin secretion and hepatic dysfunction. Iron deficiency also enhances the oxidative stress by increased ROS formation and decreased levels of antioxidant systems.

THE ROLE OF IRON IN COMPLICATIONS OF DIABETES

The generation of highly reactive free radicals by both iron and hyperglycemia aggravate the development and progression of diabetes and its complications. The hyperglycemia and hyperlipidemia associated with diabetes impairs most of the protective mechanisms, resulting in increased susceptibility of tissues and organs to oxidative stress [38]. Oxidative stress causes damage to membrane lipids, proteins and nucleic acids resulting in tissue damage and endothelial dysfunction, which further promotes the development of diabetic complications. Substantial evidence emphasizes the role of free iron as a trigger for metabolic derangements and its contribution to the pathogenesis of diabetes and its complications including microvascular and macrovascular disorders. Elevated serum ferritin levels in conditions that contribute to metabolic syndrome (such as obesity, diabetes, hypercholesterolemia and hypertension) have been reported, implicating a function for iron in the development of cardiovascular diseases [56]. Higher iron stores have also been linked to a greater frequency of coronary heart disease in female type 2 diabetic patients [36]. The vascular endothelium is a major target for oxidative stress – ROS enhance vascular endothelial permeability and promote leukocyte adhesion; impaired NO action, consequent to its inactivation by ROS, decreases endothelium-dependent vasodilation in diabetics. The abnormal NO metabolism is associated with advanced diabetic microvascular complications [57]. In addition, oxidation of LDL also enhances the atherogenic potential [58].

Increased iron levels have also been implicated in kidney disease. Elevated levels of iron in the kidneys of an animal model of diabetes [59], increased urinary catalytic iron in diabetic nephropathy, and the beneficial effects of iron chelators and iron-free diets have been reported [60]. In streptozotocin diabetic rats, the accumulation of iron in proximal tubular lysosomes is related independently with proteinuria and transferrin excretion, suggesting greater cellular uptake of iron from the tubular fluid [61]. In humans with diabetic nephropathy, there was also an increase in both proximal tubular lysosomal iron concentration and the number of iron-containing lysosomes: this iron has been associated with the tubular damage of diabetic nephropathy [61]. Thus iron, by virtue of its role in potentiating oxidative stress, enhances tissue/organ damage resulting in the development of diabetic complications.

TABLE 6.2 Hematological and Oxidative Stress Parameters of Offsprings of Diabetic and Non-Diabetic Parents

	Controls	Diabetics	*T*-Test
Serum iron (μmol/L)	16.11 ± 6.41	17.77 ± 6.91	NS
Serum Ferritin (pmol/L)*	52.6 (19.9–139.1)	70.1 (25.8–190.5)	<0.01
Transferrin receptor (μg/mL)	4.92 ± 2.16	3.52 ± 2.96	<0.008
Total body iron (mg/kg)	4.11 ± 3.86	8.01 ± 5.39	<0.001
HO (nmole bilirubin/mg protein/hr)*	2.27 (0.69–7.46)	5.69 (1.77–18.27)	<0.001
SOD (pg/mL)	3.29 ± 0.42	3.85 ± 0.64	<0.002
GSH (μmol/L)	56.5 ± 12.5	42.0 ± 15.5	<0.002
TBARS (nmoles/mL)	1.11 ± 0.80	1.51 ± 1.18	<0.01
E vitamin (μmol/L)	6.50 ± 3.25	6.04 ± 3.48	NS

The data of normoglycemic adult offsprings (35 male/36 female) of diabetic parents and offsprings (19 male/32 female) of non-diabetic, healthy parents (controls) are presented as means ± SD. * Geometric means ± 1 SE range. NS = not significant. $P < 0.05$ statistically significant.

(Reproduced from Table No.4 of Ref. 54, ©Springer Science+Business Media LLC, with kind permission from Springer Science+Business Media B.V.)

CONCLUSIONS

Iron is an essential micronutrient for cellular reactions: deficiency in this element causes one of the most common nutritional disorders worldwide, especially among

TABLE 6.3 Iron Nutrition and Oxidative Stress Parameters in Subjects with and without Metabolic Syndrome

	Men			Women		
Variable	No MetS	MetS	*P* Value[a]	No MetS	MetS	*P* Value[a]
Hemoglobin (g/L)	152.2 ± 10.3	145.2 ± 13.2	<0.02	133.7 ± 12.9	135.7 ± 14.2	NS
Serum iron (μg/dL)	142.3 ± 44.3	141.0 ± 51.0	NS	108.8 ± 43.1	122.9 ± 54.4	<0.03
Ferritin (μg/dL)[b]	55.4 (35.6–96.3)	72.4 (46.8–111.5)	<0.001	27.4 (12.6–59.5)	53.9 (34.1–84.8)	<0.001
Transferrin receptor (μg/mL)	5.8 ± 1.0	4.8 ± 2.1	<0.03	7.2 ± 2.9	6.0 ± 1.8	<0.004
Total body iron (mg/kg)	7.0 ± 2.1	8.3 ± 2.8	<0.04	4.1 ± 2.8	6.3 ± 2.3	<0.001
HO activity[b]	0.25 (0.09–0.75)	0.79 (0.34–1.85)	<0.001	0.21 (0.07–0.64)	0.96 (0.41–2.23)	<0.001
Oxidized LDL (U/L)[b]	41.6 (24.4–71.2)	65.4 (40.9–101.9)	<0.002	45.6 (27.7–75.0)	62.4 (41.9–93.0)	<0.001
TBARS (nmol/mL)[b]	1.27 (0.93–1.73)	1.65 (1.26–2.17)	<0.002	1.33 (1.08–1.64)	1.65 (1.28–2.12)	<0.001

Values are presented as mean ± SD of 22 men and 48 women without metabolic syndrome (No MetS) and 26 men and 59 women with metabolic syndrome (MetS).
[a]P values represent differences between no MetS and MetS by sex.
[b]Values are expressed as geometric mean and range.
(Reproduced from Table No. 2 of Ref. 55, ©Springer Science+Business Media N.Y., with kind permission from Springer Science+Business Media B.V.).

women and children; and, in excess, iron is highly toxic. Diabetes, on the other hand, is a chronic metabolic disorder and a major global health problem. Both diabetes and redox active iron are individually known to enhance oxidative stress. The proposed mechanisms for the role of iron in the pathogenesis of diabetes are: insulin deficiency, insulin resistance, and hepatic dysfunction together with decreased antioxidant defense systems [41]. Diabetes alters the availability of redox active Fe^{2+}, either from excessive iron stores or from alterations in the protective mechanisms which normally prevent the release of free iron [16]. Both iron overload and deficiency result in oxidative stress: besides increased free radical generation there is also impairment in antioxidant defense mechanisms. The observed increase in lipid peroxidation, protein oxidation and nitration, oxidation and damage to nucleic acids are the result of oxidative stress involving free iron together with an ineffective antioxidant system; this probably plays an important role in the prognosis and development of complications of diabetes. Hence, monitoring free iron levels could protect against the deleterious implications of iron on diabetes and its complications.

SUMMARY POINTS

- Iron is an essential micronutrient, which easily switches between the Fe^{3+} and Fe^{2+} states, a requisite for cellular metabolism; but in excess, it is highly toxic.
- In the body, iron is mainly present bound to proteins – hemoproteins or in non-heme iron proteins; however, under physiological conditions, the toxic Fe^{2+} is found in minute amounts.
- Iron homeostasis is maintained by regulation of the dietary uptake and gene expression of proteins required for iron sequestration.
- Catalytically active redox species Fe^{2+} generates highly reactive hydroxyl radicals by the Fenton/Haber Weiss reactions, which results in oxidative stress.
- Diabetes is a metabolic disorder characterized by hyperglycemia and oxidative stress.
- The proposed mechanisms for the effect of iron on diabetes are: insulin deficiency, insulin resistance, hepatic dysfunction and decreased antioxidant defense systems.
- Both iron overload and deficiency result in enhanced oxidative stress; however, in iron deficiency there is impairment in the antioxidant system also.
- Iron and diabetes thus enhance oxidative stress and this could contribute to the development of diabetic complications.
- Hence, it is necessary to maintain iron homeostasis in the body to prevent the deleterious effects on diabetes and its complications.

References

[1] Papanikolaou G, Pantopoulos K. Iron metabolism and toxicity. Toxicol Appl Pharmacol 2005;202:199–211.

[2] Pantopoulos K, Porwal SK, Tartakoff A, Devireddy L. Mechanisms of mammalian iron homeostasis. Biochemistry 2012;51:5705–24.

[3] Bruick RK. Oxygen sensing in the hypoxic response pathway: regulation of the hypoxia-inducible transcription factor. Genes Dev 2003;17:2614–23.

[4] Kruszewski M. Labile iron pool: The main determinant of cellular response to oxidative stress. Mutat Res 2003;531:81–92.

[5] Kohgo Y, Ikuta K, Ohtake T, Torimoto Y, Kato J. Body iron metabolism and pathophysiology of iron overload. Int J Hematol 2008;88:7–15.

[6] Brissot P, Ropert M, Lan CL, Loréal O. Non-transferrin bound iron: A key role in iron overload and iron toxicity. Biochimica et Biophysica Acta 2012;1820:403–10.

[7] Walter PB, Knutson MD, Paler-Martinez A, Lee S, Xu Y, Viteri FE, et al. Iron deficiency and iron excess damage mitochondria and mitochondrial DNA in rats. Proc Natl Acad Sci U S A 2002;99:2264–9.

[8] Galaris D, Pantopoulos K. Oxidative stress and iron homeostasis: mechanistic and health aspects. Crit Rev Clin Lab Sci 2008;45:1–23.

[9] Hinzmann R. Iron metabolism, iron deficiency and anemia. From diagnosis to treatment and monitoring. Sysmex Journal International 2003;13:65–74.

[10] Wang J, Pantopoulos K. Regulation of cellular iron metabolism. Biochem J 2011;434:365–81.

[11] Liuzzi JP, Aydemir F, Nam H, Knutson MD, Cousins RJ. Zip14 (Slc39a14) mediates non-transferrin-bound iron uptake into cells. Proc Natl Acad Sci U S A 2006;103:13612–7.

[12] Devireddy LR, Gazin C, Zhu X, Green MR. A cell-surface receptor for lipocalin 24p3 selectively mediates apoptosis and iron uptake. Cell 2005;123:1293–305.

[13] Tandara L, Salamunic I. Iron metabolism: current facts and future directions. Biochemia Medica 2012;22:314–31.

[14] Vaubel RA, Isaya G. Iron–sulfur cluster synthesis, iron homeostasis and oxidative stress in Friedreich ataxia. Mol Cell Neurosci 2013;55:50–61.

[15] Keel SB, Doty RT, Yang Z, Quigley JG, Chen J, Knoblaugh S, et al. A heme export protein is required for red blood cell differentiation and iron homeostasis. Science 2008;319:825–8.

[16] Campenhout AV, Campenhout CV, Lagrou AR, Abrams P, Moorkens G, Gaal LV, et al. Impact of diabetes mellitus on the relationship between iron-, inflammatory- and oxidative stress status. Diabetes Metab Res Rev 2006;22:444–54.

[17] Cozzi A, Corsi B, Levi S, Santambrogio P, Biasiotto G, Arosio P. Analysis of the biologic functions of H- and L-ferritins in HeLa cells by transfection with siRNAs and cDNAs: evidence for a proliferative role of L-ferritin. Blood 2004;103:2377–83.

[18] Johansen JS, Harris AK, Rychly DJ, Ergul A. Oxidative stress and the use of antioxidants in diabetes: linking basic science to clinical practice. Cardiovasc Diabetol 2005;4:5.

[19] Roberts CK, Sindhu KK. Oxidative stress and metabolic syndrome. Life Sci 2009;84:705–12.

[20] Yoo J-H, Maeng H-Y, Sun Y-K, Kim Y-A, Park D-W, Park TS, et al. Oxidative status in iron-deficiency anemia. J Clin Lab Anal 2009:23,319–23.

[21] Grattagliano I, Palmieri VO, Portincasa P, Moschetta A, Palasciano G. Oxidative stress-induced risk factors associated with the metabolic syndrome: a unifying hypothesis. J Nutr Biochem 2008;19:491–504.

[22] Kalaivanam KN, Dharmalingam M, Marcus SR. Lipid peroxidation in type 2 Diabetes mellitus. Int J Diab Dev Ctries 2006;26:30–2.

[23] Ganesh S, Dharmalingam M, Marcus SR. Oxidative stress in type 2 diabetes with iron deficiency in Asian Indians. J Med Biochem 2012;30:115–20.

[24] Poulsen HE, Specht E, Broedbaek K, Henriksen T, Ellervik C, Mandrup-Poulsen T, et al. RNA modifications by oxidation: a novel disease mechanism? Free Radic Biol Med 2012;52:1353–61.

[25] Chang CM, Hsieh CJ, Huang JC, Huang IC. Acute and chronic fluctuations in blood glucose levels can increase oxidative stress in type 2 diabetes mellitus. Acta Diabetol 2012;49(Suppl. 1):171–7.

[26] Fujimoto S, Kawakami N, Ohara A. Non-enzymatic glycation of transferrin: decrease of iron-binding capacity and increase of oxygen radical production. Biol Pharm Bull 1995;18:396–400.

[27] Fernández-Real JM, López-Bermejo A, Ricart W. Cross-talk between iron metabolism and diabetes. Diabetes 2002;51:2348–54.

[28] Cussimanio BL, Booth AA, Todd P, Hudson BG, Khalifah RG. Unusual susceptibility of heme proteins to damage by glucose during non-enzymatic glycation. Biophys Chem 2003:105,743–55.

[29] Mehta JL, Rasouli N, Sinha A, K., Molavi B. Oxidative stress in diabetes: a mechanistic overview of its effects on atherogenesis and myocardial dysfunction. Int J Biochem Cell Biol 2006;38:794–803.

[30] Sedeek M, Montezano AC, Hebert RL, Gray SP, Marco ED, Jha JC, et al. Oxidative stress, Nox isoforms and complications of diabetes – potential targets for novel therapies. J Cardiovasc Transl Res 2012;5:509–18.

[31] Bulteau AL, Ikeda-Saito M, Szweda LI. Redox-dependent modulation of aconitase activity in intact mitochondria. Biochemistry 2003;42:14846–55.

[32] Ma ZA. The role of peroxidation of mitochondrial membrane phospholipids in pancreatic β-cell failure. Curr Diabetes Rev 2012;8:69–75.

[33] Wiley SE, Murphy AN, Ross SA, van der Geer P, Dixon JE. MitoNEET is an iron-containing outer mitochondrial membrane protein that regulates oxidative capacity. Proc Natl Acad Sci U S A 2007;104:5318–23.

[34] Kusminski CM, Holland WL, Sun K, Park J, Spurgin SB, Lin Y, et al. MitoNEET-driven alterations in adipocyte mitochondrial activity reveal a crucial adaptive process that preserves insulin sensitivity in obesity. Nat Med 2012;18:1539–49.

[35] Davis RJ, Corvera S, Czech MP. Insulin stimulates cellular iron uptake and causes the redistribution of intracellular transferrin receptors to the plasma membrane. J Biol Chem 1986;261:8708–11.

[36] Mojiminiyi OA, Marouf R, Abdella NA. Body iron stores in relation to the metabolic syndrome, glycemic control and complications in female patients with type 2 diabetes. Nutr Metab Cardiovasc Dis 2008;18:559–66.

[37] Lipinski B, Pretorius E. Novel pathway of iron–induced blood coagulation: implications for diabetes mellitus and its complications. Pol Arch Med Wewn 2012;122:115–22.

[38] Liu Q, Sun L, Tan Y, Wang G, Lin X, Cai L. Role of Iron Deficiency and Overload in the Pathogenesis of Diabetes and Diabetic complications. Current Medicinal Chemistry 2009;16:113–29.

[39] Rajpathak SN, Crandall JP, Wylie-Rosett J, Kabat GC, Rohan TE, Hu FB. The role of iron in type 2 diabetes in humans. Biochim Biophys Acta 2008;1790:671–81.

[40] Cooksey RC, Jouihan HA, Ajioka RS, Hazel MW, Jones DL, Kushner J, et al. Oxidative stress, beta-cell apoptosis, and decreased insulin secretory capacity in mouse models of hemochromatosis. Endocrinology 2004;145:5305–12.

[41] Swaminathan S, Fonseca VA, Alam MG, Shah SV. The role of iron in diabetes and its complications. Diabetes Care 2007;30:1926–33.

[42] Chern JP, Lin KH, Lu MY, Lin DT, Lin KS, Chen JD, et al. Abnormal glucose tolerance in transfusion-dependent beta-thalassemic patients. Diabetes Care 2001;24:850–4.

[43] Rajpathak S, Ma J, Manson J, Willett WC, Hu FB. Iron intake and the risk of type 2 diabetes in women: a prospective cohort study. Diabetes Care 2006;29:1370–6.

[44] Ristow M, Mulder H, Pomplun D, Schulz TJ, Müller-Schmehl K, Krause A, et al. Frataxin deficiency in pancreatic islets causes diabetes due to loss of beta cell mass. J Clin Invest 2003;112:527–34.

[45] Silva M, Bonomo L d-F, Oliveira R d-P, de Lima WG, Silva ME, Pedrosa ML. Effects of the interaction of diabetes and iron supplementation on hepatic and pancreatic tissues, oxidative stress markers, and liver peroxisome proliferator activated receptor α expression. J Clin Biochem Nutr 2011;49:102–8.

[46] Pietrangelo A. Hereditary hemochromatosis. Annu Rev Nutr 2006;26:51–70.

[47] Li X, Li H, Lu N, Feng Y, Huang Y, Gao Z. Iron increases liver injury through oxidative/nitrosative stress in diabetic rats: involvement of nitrotyrosination of glucokinase. Biochimie 2012;94: 2620–7.

[48] Tarim O, Küçükerdoğan A, Günay U, Eralp O, Ercan I. Effects of iron deficiency anemia on hemoglobin A_{1c} in type 1 diabetes mellitus. Pediatr Int 1999;41:357–62.

[49] Fernandez-Real JM, Lopez-Bermejo A, Ricart W. Iron Stores, Blood Donation, and Insulin Sensitivity and Secretion. Clin Chem 2005;51:1201–5.

[50] Fernández-Real JM, Peñarroja G, Castro A, García-Bragado F, Hernández-Aguado I, Ricart W. Blood letting in high-ferritin type 2 diabetes: effects on insulin sensitivity and beta-cell function. Diabetes 2002;51:1000–4.

[51] Jiang R, Ma J, Ascherio A, Stampfer MJ, Willett WC, Hu FB. Dietary iron intake and blood donations in relation to risk of type 2 diabetes in men: a prospective cohort study. Am J Clin Nutr 2004;79:70–5.

[52] Acharya J, Punchard NA, Taylor JA, Thompson RPH, Pearson TC. Red cell lipid peroxidation and antioxidant enzymes in iron deficiency. Eur J Hematol 1991;42:287–91.

[53] Toxqui L, De Piero A, Courtois V, Bastida S, Sánchez-Muniz FJ, Cowboy MP. Iron deficiency and overload. Implications in oxidative stress and cardiovascular health. Nutr Hosp 2010;25:350–65.

[54] Blanc SL, Villarroel P, Candia V, Gavilan N, Soto N, Perez-Bravo F, et al. Type 2 diabetic patients and their offspring show altered parameters of iron status, oxidative stress and genes related to mitochondrial activity. Biometals 2012;25:725–35.

[55] Leiva E, Mujica V, Sepulveda P, Guzman L, Nunez S, Orrego R, et al. High levels of iron status and oxidative stress in patients with metabolic syndrome. Biol Trace Elem Res 2013;151:1–8.

[56] Wrede CE, Buettner R, Bollheimer LC, Scholmerich J, Palitzsch K-D, Hellerbrand C. Association between serum ferritin and the insulin resistance syndrome in a representative population. Eur J Endocrinol 2006;154:333–40.

[57] Hadi HAR, Suwaidi JA. Endothelial dysfunction in diabetes mellitus. Vasc Health Risk Manag 2007;3:853–76.

[58] Satchell L, Leake DS. Oxidation of Low-Density Lipoprotein by Iron at Lysosomal pH: Implications for Atherosclerosis. Biochemistry 2012;51:3767–75.

[59] Johnson WT, Evans GW. Effects of the interrelationship between dietary protein and minerals on tissue content of trace metals in streptozotocin-diabetic rats. J Nutr 1984;114:180–90.

[60] Rajapurkar MM, Hegde U, Bhattacharys A, Alam MG, Shah SV. Effect of deferiprone, an oral iron chelator, in diabetic and non-diabetic glomerular disease. Toxicol Mech Methods 2013;23: 5–10.

[61] Nankivell BJ, Tay YC, Boadle RA, Harris DC. Lysosomal iron accumulation in diabetic nephropathy. Ren Fail 1994;16:367–81.

SECTION II

ANTIOXIDANTS AND DIABETES

CHAPTER

7

α-Tocopherol Supplementation, Lipid Profile, and Insulin Sensitivity in Diabetes Mellitus Type 2

Liania Alves Luzia, Patricia Helen Rondo

Department of Nutrition, Public Health School, University of Sao Paulo, Sao Paulo, Brazil

List of Abbreviations

α-TTP Alpha-tocopherol transfer protein
AT Alpha-tocopherol
ATBC Alpha-tocopherol, beta-carotene cancer prevention
ATP Adenosine triphosphate
CAM Cell adhesion molecule
CoQ10 Coenzyme Q10
DM Diabetes mellitus
DM2 Diabetes mellitus type 2
GSH Reduced glutathione
HDL-c High density lipoprotein cholesterol
HOPE Heart Outcomes Prevention Evaluation
LDL-c Low-density lipoprotein cholesterol
NAD(P)H Nicotinamide adenine dinucleotide phosphate
NHANES National Health and Nutrition Examination Survey
PPARγ Peroxisome proliferator activated receptor γ
ROS Reactive oxygen species
SOD-Mn Manganese superoxide dismutase
TBARS Thiobarbituric acid reactive substances
VLDL Very low-density lipoproteins

INTRODUCTION

Diabetes mellitus (DM) is one of the major chronic diseases that affect mankind regardless of age, social condition and geographic location. Diabetes mellitus type 2 (DM2) is a heterogenous disorder characterized by impaired insulin action and secretion, which accounts for about 90% of the cases of diabetes. The age of onset of DM2 varies, although the disease is more frequent after 40 years of age, with a peak incidence at about 60 years. DM2 is typically a disease for which increased age is a risk factor [1].

According to recent data from the World Health Organization (WHO) [2], the mean prevalence of DM2 is 10%, although this rate can reach 33% in some regions such as the Pacific Islands. Factors such as growing urbanization, population aging, high-carbohydrate diets, reduced levels of physical activity, and obesity contribute to the high incidence of DM2 which, in turn, predisposes to cardiovascular diseases. Concomitantly, DM2 leads to depletion of the cellular antioxidant defense system, increasing the levels of free radicals and favoring a pro-oxidant state and consequent oxidative stress which causes tissue damage and cell death. The biological mechanisms whereby hyperglycemia acts on these processes are not fully understood, but evidence indicates that hyperglycemia, hyperinsulinemia and insulin resistance modify the lipid profile, predisposing to an increased production of free radicals and a possible reduction in plasma antioxidants such as vitamin E [3,4].

In the First National Health and Nutrition Examination Survey (NHANES I) Epidemiologic Follow-up Study, the use of vitamin supplements was found to be associated with a 24% lower risk of diabetes over 20 years of follow-up. However, only a few human trials have examined the association between antioxidant status, including vitamin E, in DM2, and the findings are contradictory.

VITAMIN E AND DIABETES

Vitamin E belongs to the group of liposoluble vitamins which are necessary for normal cell differentiation and function. The term vitamin E refers to a group of

Diabetes: Oxidative Stress and Dietary Antioxidants.
http://dx.doi.org/10.1016/B978-0-12-405885-9.00007-3

eight fat-soluble compounds with different biological activities, which are divided into two groups. The first group is derived from tocol (Figure 7.1) and includes four of the eight compounds: α-tocopherol (AT), β-tocopherol, γ-tocopherol, and δ-tocopherol. Tocopherols have a saturated side chain with 16 carbon atoms. There is an order of conversion among forms of tocopherol (Figure 7.2). Because of the efficiency of the transfer protein, AT is detected in the plasma at ten times the level of γ-tocopherol and its antioxidant potential in the biological environment varies, with $\alpha > \gamma > \delta > \beta$. The second group is derived from tocotrienol (Figure 7.3) and includes the remaining four forms of vitamin E with biological activity: α-tocotrienol, β-tocotrienol, γ-tocotrienol, and δ-tocotrienol [5].

All forms of vitamin E are absorbed by enterocytes and are released into the circulation inside chylomicrons.

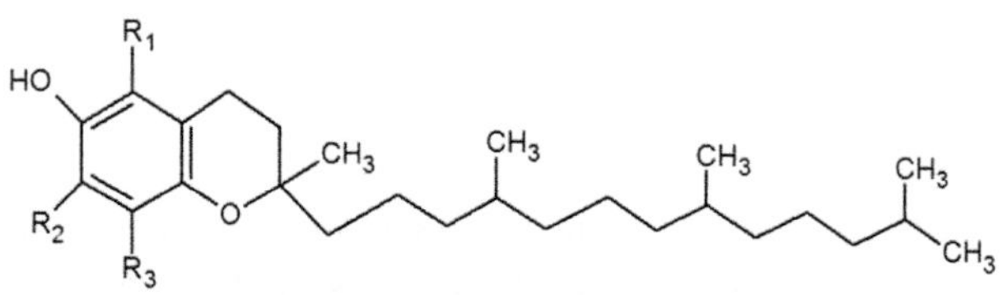

	R1	R2	R3
α-tocopherol	CH_3	CH_3	CH_3
β-tocopherol	CH_3	H	CH_3
γ-tocopherol	H	CH_3	CH_3
δ-tocopherol	H	H	CH_3

FIGURE 7.1 **Structural formula of the tocopherol isomers.**

In the liver, α-tocopherol transfer protein (α-TTP) incorporates vitamin E into very low-density lipoproteins (VLDL). Vitamin E is excreted mainly by secretion into bile and elimination in feces in the form of tocopheryl hydroquinone conjugated with glucuronic acid. About 1% is excreted in urine as glucuronic acid-conjugated tocopheronic acid. The other forms of vitamin E are much less retained and are generally excreted in urine or bile.

Of all vitamin E forms, AT, known as 2R,4R,8R-α-tocopherol or its abbreviated form RRR-α-tocopherol, is the natural compound with the highest biological activity. In plasma, AT accounts for 80% to 90% of all vitamin E forms and the remainder is mainly γ-tocopherol. Plasma levels of AT range from 5 to 16 μmol/L; plasma levels or serum concentrations of AT below 6.11 μmol/L usually indicate vitamin E deficiency, values between 11.6 and 16.2 μmol/L are considered low, and concentrations above 16.2 μmol/L refer to normalcy. The plasma levels of this vitamin are intimately related to the plasma levels of total lipids and cholesterol, hence it is recommended that concentrations of lipid which are AT-correlated values are usually expressed in the ratio AT/cholesterol. Levels below 2.2 μmol AT/μmol cholesterol indicate a risk of deficiency, while values above 5.2 are considered suitable for this reason (Table 7.1).

Decreased levels of vitamin E may indicate increased exposure to oxidative stress. AT has a strong antioxidant potential and is an important component of cell membranes, interrupting the lipid peroxidation chain reaction induced by free radicals *in vivo*, donating a hydrogen atom to a peroxyl radical and

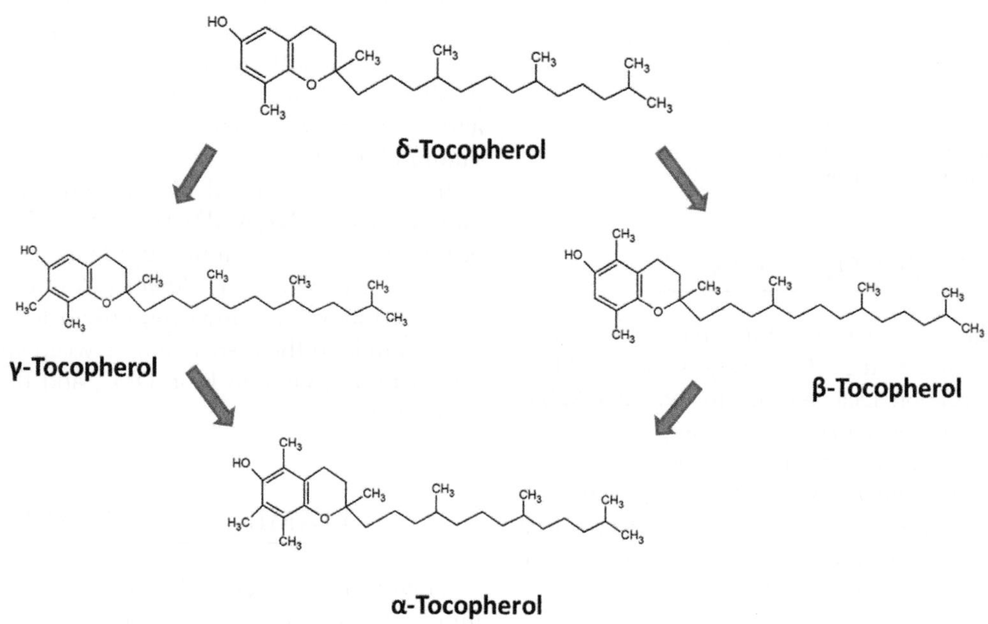

FIGURE 7.2 **Chemical structures of tocopherols and the order of conversions among forms.**

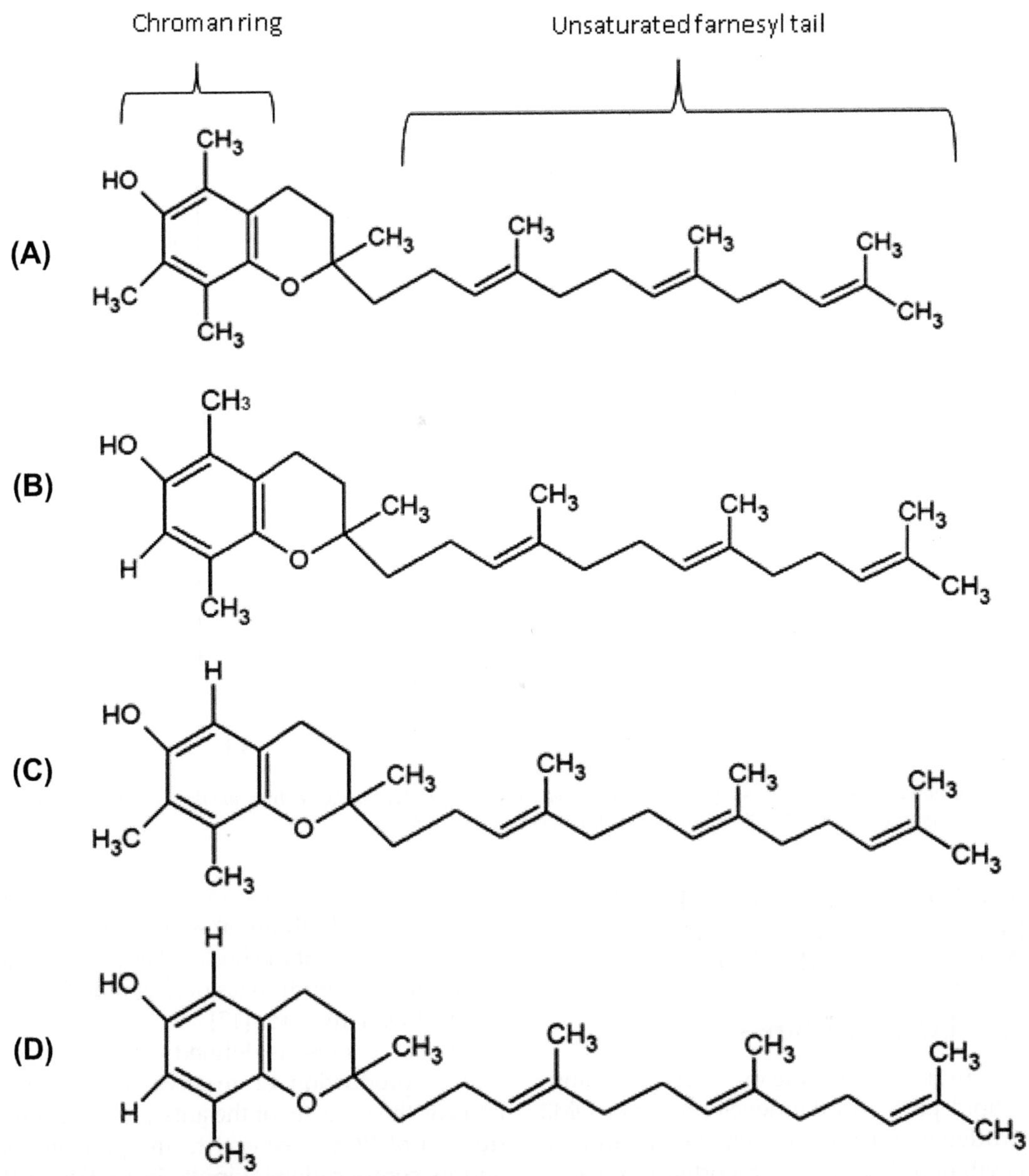

FIGURE 7.3 Tocotrienol structure. α-Tocotrienol (A) has three methyl groups on the chroman ring, β-tocotrienol (B) and γ-tocotrienol (C) have two methyl groups and δ-tocotrienol (D) has only one methyl group.

TABLE 7.1 Plasma Levels of α-Tocopherol

	α-Tocopherol Serum/Plasma		
Categories	**μmol/L**	**μg/mL**	**% Hemolysis in Erythrocyte (H_2O_2)**
Deficiency	<11.6	<5.0	> 20
Below	11.6–16.2	5.0–7.0	10–20
Normality	>16.2	>7.0	<10
α-tocopherol plasma / cholesterol (μg/mg) acceptable: >2.22 x 10^{-3}			

Sauberlich [6].

scavenging alkyl peroxy radicals (Figure 7.4). In addition to its antioxidant properties, vitamin E reduces cytotoxicity, minimizes the effect of oxidized lipoproteins, suppresses the proliferation of smooth muscle cells, reduces platelet adhesion and aggregation, and improves endothelial function [7]. There is strong evidence that oxidative stress plays a key role in the early stages of DM, and AT is a powerful chain-breaking antioxidant, which may be a protective factor against oxidative stress-related diseases [8–10]. Data from humans is controversial, and the most compelling evidence for the effect of vitamin E in diabetes is on protection against lipid peroxidation.

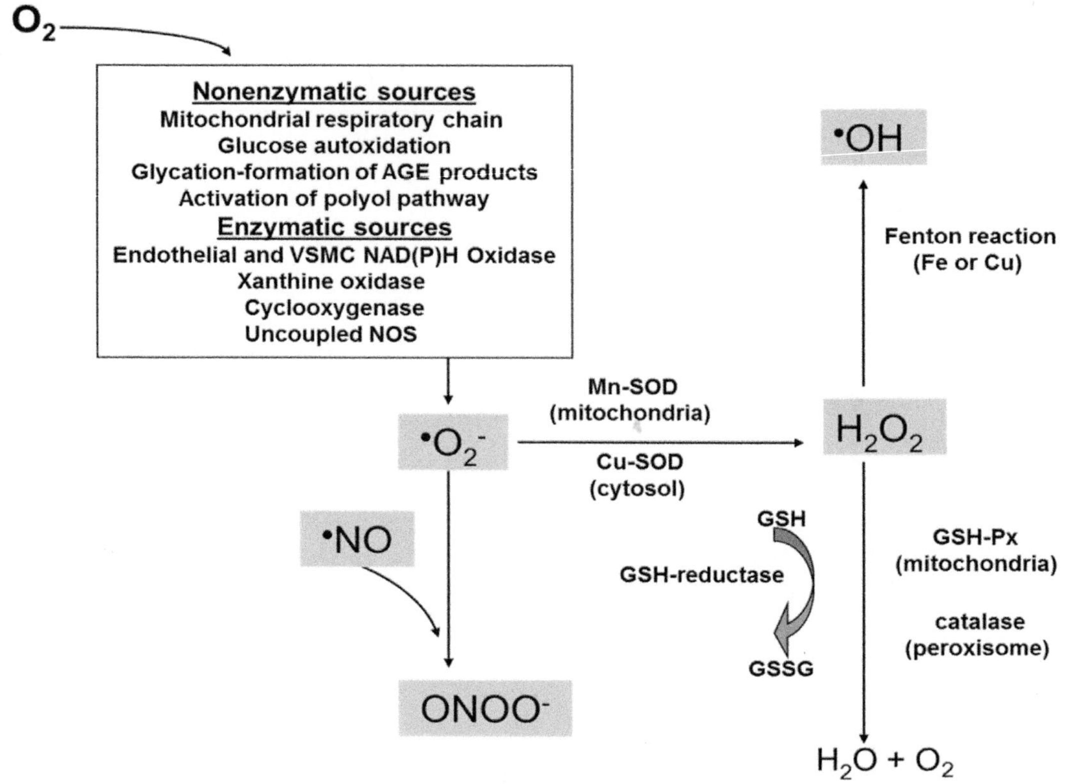

FIGURE 7.4 **Generation of reactive species.** *Figure reproduced from Johansen et al. [11]. Oxidative stress and the use of antioxidants in diabetes: Linking basic science to clinical practice. Published 2005 in Cardiovascular Diabetology 29;4(1):5.*

A POSSIBLE MECHANISM UNDERLYING THE EFFECTS OF α-TOCOPHEROL IN DIABETES MELLITUS

Lipid Profile and Oxidative Stress

A number of studies suggest the involvement of antioxidants and lipid profile in the development of DM2 [10–12], and different roles of non-enzymatic antioxidants such as vitamin E have been reported in reviews [13,14] and original papers [15].

Diabetic dyslipidemia, commonly observed in patients with DM2, is characterized by low plasma levels of high density lipoprotein cholesterol (HDL-c), increased levels of serum triglycerides and VLDL, and elevated plasma levels of small, dense, low-density, lipoprotein cholesterol (LDL-c) present as small, dense, atherogenic particles in the heterogeneous low-density lipoprotein sub fraction. These increase in people with hypertriglyceridemia, insulin resistance syndrome, metabolic syndrome, and DM2. Although plasma levels of LDL-c are either normal or only moderately elevated, the LDL-c particle is smaller, carries less cholesterol, and is more dense [16]. The strong correlation between AT and lipid profile is explained by the fact that, like lipids, this tocopherol is absorbed in the small intestine. The absorption of AT is impaired in the absence of bile acids or pancreatic secretions, and only minute quantities will be absorbed if both are absent. In addition, delivery of AT to the tissues of the body takes place through plasma lipoproteins by hydrolysis of chylomicrons and VLDL or via the LDL-c receptor [17].

Oxidative stress is defined as the state in which the rate of production of reactive oxygen species (ROS) exceeds the capacity of the antioxidant defense. The production of ROS is central to the pathogenesis of DM2 and its complications. Lipids, in particular the polyunsaturated fatty acid chains present in phospholipids, represent a main target of ROS attack [18]. However, there are multiple sources of oxidative stress in patients with DM2, including non-enzymatic, enzymatic, and mitochondrial pathways. The non-enzymatic sources of oxidative stress arise from the oxidative metabolism of glucose. In this respect, hyperglycemia can directly cause increased production of ROS, and glucose can undergo auto-oxidation and generate •OH radicals, among others [19]. Enzymatic sources of increased ROS generation in diabetic patients include NAD(P)H oxidase, xanthine oxidase, and nitric oxide synthase [20].

The respiratory mitochondrial chain is another non-enzymatic source of reactive free radicals. During the normal process of oxidative phosphorylation that culminates in the formation of adenosine triphosphate (ATP), the •OH radical is immediately eliminated by natural defense mechanisms. On the other hand, hyperglycemia has been shown to induce the generation of •OH radicals at the mitochondrial level, representing the initial trigger of the vicious cycle of oxidative stress in patients with DM [21,22].

Insulin Sensitivity

Important insights have been gained over the past decade in the biochemical pathways of insulin resistance, which is a key precursor of the development of DM2 [23]. Supplementation with high doses of vitamin E may improve insulin action and decrease plasma fasting insulin and glucose levels by decreasing cellular oxidative stress, altering membrane properties, and decreasing inflammatory activity. Administration of chronic doses of vitamin E (900 IU/day) ameliorates insulin action by improving the chemical-physical state of plasma membranes through a decrease in oxidative stress. This occurs because the resistance of peripheral tissues to glucose uptake is a consequence of permanently elevated lipid peroxidation due to low concentrations of liposoluble antioxidants such as vitamin E. Therefore, oxidative stress may compromise the action of insulin by altering the physical state of the plasma membrane of target cells. Although vitamin E may exert other effects that potentially modify the action of insulin, this vitamin inhibits the activity of protein kinase C, a fact that has been associated experimentally with insulin resistance.

According to Azzi et al. [5], vitamin E also regulates several genes; for example, it up-regulates the expression of peroxisome proliferator activated receptor γ (PPARγ), a nuclear receptor. Stimulation of PPARγ has been shown to improve glucose tolerance and insulin resistance in patients with DM2 and in an animal model [24]. Apparently, there are structural similarities between vitamin E and glucose-lowering agents such as thiazolidinediones, which are PPARγ agonists.

α-TOCOPHEROL SUPPLEMENTATION IN TYPE 2 DIABETES MELLITUS

Vitamin E exerts a protective effect mainly by suppressing lipid peroxidation. The Tolerable Upper Limit Intake (UL) for vitamin E is 1,000 mg. Deficiencies in vitamin E are rare, but this vitamin is depleted in DM. Dietary antioxidants have been suggested to attenuate oxidative stress, but the role of vitamin E supplementation in DM2 is less clear. Controversy exists in the literature as to whether antioxidant supplementation has an effect on dyslipidemia, hyperinsulinemia and hyperglycemia, particularly regarding the doses administered and time of intervention. Table 7.2 summarizes the results of relevant studies conducted over the last 10 years, which investigated the effects of AT intake or supplementation alone or in combination with other antioxidants on lipid profile and insulin resistance in DM2.

There are some studies showing that supplementation with individual nutrients such as vitamin E and C apparently does not reduce oxidative stress, cell adhesion molecule (CAM) expression, and insulin resistance and does not improve glucose disposal [37,38]. In fact, Skrha et al. [39] demonstrated enhanced oxidative stress and increased insulin resistance after supplementation with vitamin E alone. With respect to the vitamin E doses administered, experimental studies concluded that only megadoses of all-rac-α-tocopherol added to the diet or administered separately (25,000 mg/kg and 2,000 mg/kg body weight as supplement, respectively) are toxic [40,41]. In a double-blind study on patients with DM2, 2,000 mg of vitamin E was administered daily for six weeks. None of the participants presented adverse symptoms and levels of cholesterol, thyroid hormones and blood coagulation were normal. Elevated doses of vitamin E (e.g., 3,200 mg/day) used in human studies also showed no adverse effects [42].

In a meta-analysis conducted by Hamer and Chida [43], higher intakes of vitamin E and carotenoids, but not of vitamin C and flavonoids, were associated with a 25% reduction in DM2 risk, but the result for each antioxidant was based on two or three studies with dissimilar risks. On the other hand, in another meta-analysis, Miller et al. [44] reported that treatment with high doses of vitamin E may increase all-cause mortality. Some potential reasons for this fact were proposed by Steinberg et al. [45], such as a possible pro-oxidant effect on processes that occur in diseases characterized by high levels of oxidative stress. Concomitant with that study, Winterbone et al. [46], investigating the pro-oxidant effect of vitamin E, concluded that high dose supplementation of AT primes mononuclear cells from patients with DM2 for a potentially damaging response to acute hyperglycemia.

In the Alpha-Tocopherol, Beta-Carotene Cancer Prevention (ATBC) Study, Kataja et al. [15] randomized 29,133 male smokers aged 50–69 years to receive either AT (50 mg/day) or β-carotene (20 mg/day), both compounds, or placebo daily for 5–8 years (median: 6.1 years). The authors concluded that neither AT nor β-carotene supplementation prevented DM2 in male smokers. Serum levels of AT or β-carotene were not associated with DM2 risk.

The Effect of Vitamin E on Lipid Profile and Oxidative Stress

DM2 is known to be associated with dyslipidemia, LDL oxidation and consequently increased oxidative stress. In a study analyzing the effects of vitamin E on

TABLE 7.2 Studies Assessing α-Tocopherol Intake or α-Tocopherol Supplementation Alone or in Combination With Others Antioxidants on Lipid Profile and Insulin Resistance of Dm2 Patients (2002–2012)

References	Study Design	Age (Years)	Patients, n	Intervention (Groups)	Follow-Up	Results	Conclusions
Oliveira et al., 2011 [25]	Clinical trial	38–75	102 adults	AT (800 mg/day), LA (600mg/day), both, or placebo daily	4 months	Increased vitamin E/total cholesterol ratio in AT and AT+LA groups.	VitE alone or in combination with LA did not affect the lipid profile or insulin sensitivity
Lavie et al., 2011 [26]	Clinical trial	65 ± 10	236 male and 79 female	Two groups: antioxidant vitamins (AT 76% and vitamin C; AT 15%; vitamin C 9%) and placebo	3 months	There was no significant improvement in glycosylated hemoglobin. Both groups achieved statistically similar improvements in fasting blood glucose, body fat, and other CHD risk factors.	400 IU of vitamin E do not ameliorate the health benefits of exercise training, in CHD patients with manifest DM2
Palacka et al., 2010 [27]	Clinical trial	≥45	59 adults	AT (200IU), hydrosoluble CoQ10, (100 mg), ALA (60 mg) two daily doses	3 months	Supplementation with antioxidants decreased plasma lipid peroxides, increased concentration of CoQ10 and improved echocardiographic parameters.	Supportive therapy with PL along with the antioxidants hydrosoluble CoQ10, ALA and AT is an effective way of controlling the complications of DM2
Wang et al., 2010 [9]	Clinical trial	> 50	126 Chinese women	AT (100, 200 or 300 IU/day)	4 months	AT concentrations increased significantly after supplementation ($p < 0.01$). The protective decreases in plasma total cholesterol were significant in 200 IU/day and 300 IU/day VitE groups, but decreases in HDL-c were also significant in all the supplementation groups. Plasma TG was unaltered. The indicators of oxidative stress decreased substantially in all of the VitE supplementation groups. AT 300IU/day group showed the most significant effect.	VitE provided marked benefits in reducing oxidative stress levels and improving lipid status. AT 300 IU/day showed the optimal effect.
Song et al., 2009 [28]	Randomized clinical trial	≥40	8171 female	AT (600 IU every other day), vitamin C (500 mg every day), β-carotene (50 mg every other day), or their respective placebo.	10 years	The slight elevation in diabetes risk was observed in the AT group (RR: 1.13; 95% CI: 0.99, 1.29; $P = 0.07$).	No significant overall effects of AT, vitamin C, and β-carotene on risk of developing DM2.
Kataja-Tuomola et al., 2008 [15]	Double-blind, controlled trial	50–69	29133 male smokers	AT (50 mg/day), β-carotene (20 mg/day), both, or placebo daily	6.1 years	Baseline serum levels of AT and β-carotene were not associated with the risk of diabetes in the placebo group. Neither supplementation significantly affected the incidence of diabetes	Neither AT nor β-carotene supplementation prevented DM2 in male smokers.
Costacou et al 2008 [29]	Longitudinal, multicenter study	40–69	457 adults	1 year food frequency questionnaire	5 years	In multivariable regression analyses, no relationship was observed for AT intake and either IS or AIR. However, plasma AT concentration was positively associated with log-transformed IS, but not with log-transformed AIR.	Plasma concentration of AT may improve IS and pancreatic compensation for IS, although it does not seem to be related to acute IR

Devaraj S et al., 2008 [30]	Prospective clinical trials	56 ± 11	19 male and 61 female	AT (800 mg/day); GT (800 mg/day)), both, or placebo	6 weeks	There was a significant decrease in TNF-α with AT alone or in combination with GT. Plasma MDA/HNE and lipid peroxides were significantly decreased with AT, GT, or in combination. Nitrotyrosine levels were significantly decreased only with GT or GT+AT but not with AT compared to placebo.	The combination of AT and GT supplementation appears to be superior to either supplementation alone on biomarkers of oxidative stress
Wu et al., 2007 [31]	double-blind, placebo-controlled trial	43 ± 12	55 adults	AT (500 mg/day), mixed tocopherols rich in GT or placebo	6 weeks	Mixed Neutrophil AT and GT increased with mixed tocopherol supplementation, whereas AT increased and GT decreased after AT supplementation. Both AT and mixed tocopherol resulted in reduced plasma F2-isoprostanes	The ability of tocopherols to reduce systemic oxidative stress suggests potential benefits of vitE supplementation in DM2 patients.
Liu et al., 2006 [32]	Two-by-two factorial trial	> 45	38716 female	AT (600 IU) or placebo on alternate days	10 years	There was no evidence that DM2 risk factors including age, BMI, postmenopausal hormone use, multivitamin use, physical activity, alcohol intake, and smoking status modified the effect of vitamin E on the risk of DM2.	AT provided no significant benefit for DM2 in initially healthy women.
Sacco et al., 2003 [33]	Randomized, two-by-two factorial open trial	64.2 ± 7.5	1031 adults	AT (300 mg/day)	3.7 years	No significant reduction in any of the end points considered could be found among DM2 patients, whereas a marginal reduction in the risk of peripheral artery disease was documented in control individuals. Multivariate analyses confirmed no significant increase in those treated with AT.	No significant positive effect could be found with AT in either diabetic or nondiabetic subjects.
Ylönen et al 2003 [34]	Cross-sectional	> 53	81 male and 101female	3 days food records	Fasting and 2 hours	In women, dietary AT was inversely associated with fasting plasma glucose concentrations ($P < 0.05$). In both sexes, cholesterol-adjusted AT concentrations were directly associated with 2 hr plasma glucose concentrations ($P < 0.05$).	The available data do not show a consistent effect of carotenoids and tocopherols on glucose metabolism.
Mayer-Davis et al., 2002 [35]	Cohort IRAS study	55.8 ± 8.3	303 adults with IGT and 148 of whom developed DM2	food frequency interview	5 years	Among individuals who reported habitual use of vitamin E supplements (at least once per month in the year before baseline) no protective effect was observed for either reported intake of vitamin E or plasma concentration of AT.	A protective effect of vitamin E may exist within the range of intake available from food.
Park and Choi, 2002 [36]	Clinical trial	49 ± 10.1	88 adults	AT (200 IU/day)+CSII or placebo	2 months	Lipid peroxide concentrations in plasma and red blood cells decreased and AT concentrations in plasma and red blood cells increased after AT supplementation. However these changes were not affected significantly by CSII.	AT supplementation was beneficial in decreasing blood lipid peroxide concentrations without altering antioxidant enzyme activities.

DM2, diabetes mellitus type 2; AT, α-tocopherol; LA, lipoic acid; VitE, vitamin E; CHD, coronary heart disease; CoQ, coenzyme-Q; ALA, α-lipoic acid; PL, Polarized light; HDL-c, high density lipoprotein-cholesterol; TG, triglycerides; IS, insulin sensitivity; AIR, acute insulin response; TNF-α,tumor necrosia factor; GT, γ-tocopherol; MDA/HNE, malondialdehyde acid/ 4-hydroxy-2-nonenal; BMI, body mass index; TE, tocopherol equivalents; IRAS, The Insulin Resistance and Atherosclerosis Study; IGT, impaired glucose tolerance; CSII, continuous subcutaneous insulin Infusion.

lipid profile, glycated total serum protein, and serum glucose levels, 60 patients with DM2 were randomized to receive either 1,200 mg vitamin E/day or placebo for two months. The results showed no significant difference in glucose levels or lipid profile alterations between the supplemented and placebo groups [47]. However, using a similar dose administered over a period of three months, Hsu et al. [48] reported that AT supplementation significantly decreased titers of autoantibodies against oxidized-LDL in DM2 with and without macrovascular disease.

A study involving 30 patients with decompensated DM2 and 15 healthy controls evaluated the presence of oxidative stress based on the levels of thiobarbituric acid reactive substances (TBARS). After adjustment for diabetes, TBARS levels were significantly reduced ($p<0.001$), although levels continued to be higher when compared to the control group, indicating a partial reduction in lipid peroxidation. Analysis of post-supplementation results revealed no significant reduction of glucose levels ($p>0.05$), but TBARS levels were significantly lower ($p<0.001$). Vitamin E improved oxidative stress, demonstrating its effect on the reduction of cell and tissue damage induced by free radicals. Taken together, these results suggest that vitamin E, combined with conventional therapy, exerts a positive effect on the prevention of chronic complications of DM2 [49].

In a study designed to improve the complications of DM2, Palacka et al. [27] supplemented 59 patients with antioxidants (60 mg hydrosoluble CoQ10, 100 mg α-lipoic acid, and 200 mg vitamin E), administering two daily doses for three months. Supplementation with antioxidants decreased plasma lipid peroxides, and increased the concentration of hydrosoluble CoQ10. The authors concluded that supplementation is effective in controlling the complications of DM2.

Wang et al. [9] investigated the effects of supplementation with three different doses of AT (100, 200, and 300 IU/day) for four months in Chinese women with metabolic syndrome. The authors demonstrated that the protective decreases in plasma total cholesterol were significant in the 200 and 300 IU/day groups ($p<0.05$), but decreases in HDL-c were also significant in all supplemented groups ($p<0.05$), although plasma triglycerides were unchanged ($p>0.05$). Indicators of oxidative stress were substantially reduced in all of the vitamin E supplementation groups. Vitamin E provided marked benefits by reducing oxidative stress levels and improving lipid status in women with metabolic syndrome.

The Effect of Vitamin E on Insulin Sensitivity

Few studies have investigated the relationship of vitamin E with hyperinsulinemia and oxidative stress. Pharmacological doses of vitamin E have been shown to improve insulin-mediated glucose disposal. Almost two decades have passed since the classical study of Paolisso et al. [23], which investigated the effects of oral vitamin E administration on glucose metabolism in patients with DM2 and healthy subjects. Statistically significant reductions in glucose levels, and an increase in body glucose utilization and non-oxidative glucose metabolism were observed in the two groups supplemented with vitamin E at the end of the study. The authors concluded that in DM2 patients daily oral vitamin E supplements may reduce oxidative stress, thus improving membrane physical characteristics and related activities in glucose transport.

Manning et al. [50] examined the antioxidant capabilities of vitamin E in clinically healthy subjects, obese individuals, and patients with DM2, and found that vitamin E supplementation lowered plasma glucose, insulin and peroxide concentrations in the participants at three months. These results suggest that pharmacological doses of vitamin E can improve insulin action and may play a role in delaying the onset of diabetes in high risk individuals. Similarly, in a placebo-controlled clinical trial, Gokkusu et al. [38] investigated plasma oxidant and antioxidant status in patients with DM2, and the effect of vitamin E supplementation (800 IU/day) for 30 days on oxidative stress, antioxidant defense systems, and insulin action. At the end of the study, all lipid fractions were significantly reduced ($p<0.05$) in the DM2 group when compared to baseline values. Vitamin E also significantly reduced fasting glycemia, increased fasting insulin levels, and reduced TBARS levels ($p<0.01$, $p<0.001$ and $p<0.001$, respectively). In addition to this marker of oxidation, the authors evaluated superoxide dismutase and glutathione peroxidase, which were significantly elevated at baseline ($p<0.001$). The authors concluded that vitamin E supplementation in patients with DM2 improves beta-cell function, possibly by inducing the antioxidant capacity of the organism and/or reducing peripheral insulin resistance.

Although there is strong evidence of a positive correlation between vitamin E and increased insulin sensitivity, no positive effect was observed in obese patients with DM2 who received 600 IU vitamin E/day for 3 months, with supplementation even deteriorating the action of insulin [49]. Liu et al. [32], in a placebo-controlled supplementation trial following 38,716 initially healthy women for a period of 10 years, found no difference in the risk of developing DM2 between the group supplemented with AT (600 IU on alternate days) and the placebo group. Moreover, in a recent randomized, double-blind, placebo-controlled trial involving 102 patients with DM2, Oliveira et al. [25] suggested that vitamin E supplementation alone was associated with non-significant improvement in insulin resistance.

IS VITAMIN E SUPPLEMENTATION RECOMMENDED FOR DIABETIC COMPLICATIONS?

Despite strong evidence from experimental and observational studies on antioxidants indicating that vitamin E should confer beneficial effects in reducing complications in diabetes, there is insufficient clinical evidence for use of this vitamin. The Heart Outcomes Prevention Evaluation (HOPE) Study [51] is the largest trial on the use of antioxidants in diabetes conducted so far. In that study, daily administration of 400 IU vitamin E for an average of 4.5 years to 3,654 patients with diabetes had no effect on cardiovascular outcomes. On this ground, it is difficult to justify the recommendation of vitamin E supplementation in patients with DM2.

In addition to the fact that clinical trials administering vitamin E to patients with DM2 are limited, different variables can influence the objectives proposed and therefore should be monitored carefully. According to a review conducted by Robinson et al. [52], possible factors related to failure of vitamin E therapy are:

1) The inclusion of patients without biochemical evidence of increased oxidative stress,
2) A relatively short duration of supplementation,
3) The use of suboptimal dosages of vitamin E,
4) The suppression of γ-tocopherol by AT,
5) The administration of vitamin E supplementation without concurrent use of vitamin C,
6) The lack of inclusion of biochemical markers of oxidative stress,
7) The inappropriate administration of vitamins relative to meal ingestion, and
8) Poor patient compliance and the lack of monitoring of vitamin E levels.

In parallel, there are few studies examining the effects of antioxidants on cardiovascular events and mortality in DM2 [12], considering the strong association between DM2 and increased risk factors for cardiovascular disease.

Most clinical trials do not consider the interaction of AT with other tocopherol and tocotrienol stereoisomers, particularly γ-tocopherol. The metabolism of these two tocopherols is intimately related, with AT reducing the concentration of γ-tocopherol in plasma by the action of α-TTP, which preferentially incorporates AT into plasma, increasing the metabolism of γ-tocopherol. This mechanism may explain in part the lack of effect of vitamin E supplementation in patients with DM2.

Devaraj et al. [30] concluded that the effect of combined supplementation with AT and γ-tocopherol appears to be superior to either supplementation alone on biomarkers of oxidative stress in subjects with metabolic syndrome.

Furthermore, few studies have investigated the interactive effects between antioxidant vitamins [24,44–46]. Although not focusing on the lipid profile, Wu et al. [53] concluded that supplementation with antioxidants may help to attenuate the transient worsening of retinopathy in DM2 caused by acute intensive insulin therapy, showing that tocopherol can be regenerated from tocopheroxyl radical by ascorbic acid (vitamin C) or reduced glutathione (GSH). These findings confirm the interrelationship between micronutrients, in which water-soluble vitamin C regenerates liposoluble vitamin E. In contrast, Song et al. [28], in a randomized trial, found no significant overall effects of vitamin C, vitamin E, or β-carotene on the risk of developing DM2 in women at high risk of cardiovascular diseases.

When the objective was to correlate vitamin E supplementation with improvement in lipid profile, we found no studies investigating the size of LDL-c particles. Krayenbuehl et al. [17] observed that smaller LDL-c particle size reflects the impact of insulin resistance on lipoprotein metabolism more strictly than do the traditional lipid parameters. Another important factor that was not considered in many studies is the duration of diabetes and age of the patients. Oliveira et al. [25] explained part of their results by age and diabetes duration of the selected patients. According to the authors, the long-term complications of diabetes in these patients compromised the effects of vitamin E, which is more effective in patients with recent alterations. In addition to these variables, the difference in antioxidant metabolism between genders should be emphasized. In plasma, tocopherols are bound almost exclusively to HDL-c and LDL-c. However, a difference exists between genders, with most tocopherols being bound to HDL-c in women and to LDL-c in men.

Evidence in the literature indicates that the severity of DM2 alters the size and composition of LDL-c. In addition, the process of oxidation is complex. However, there are a wide variety of analytic methods to evaluate the degree of lipid peroxidation and antioxidant capacity. Although widely used, the TBARS method is not specific for the detection of lipid peroxidation products, since it quantifies the sum of different substances reactive to thiobarbituric acid. Therefore, TBARS values include substances that may interfere with the reaction of thiobarbituric acid with other compounds present in the sample. The measurement of urinary F2-isoprostanes provides a direct measure of lipid peroxidation and appears to be superior to indirect measures, such as LDL oxidative susceptibility.

The importance of the performance of antioxidants *in vivo* depends on the types of free radicals formed, where and how these radicals are generated, analysis and methods used for the identification of damage, and the ideal doses to achieve protection. It is therefore likely that one antioxidant acts as a protective agent in a certain system, but fails to protect or even increases the damage induced in other systems. Therefore, the method used to assess oxidative stress should be evaluated with caution, and techniques for this purpose need to be considered along with multiple factors, putting into question studies whose results are derived from a single assessment method.

Despite the growing evidence supporting a link between adiponectin and DM2 and the hypothesis that vitamin E modulates the expression of adiponectin in adipocytes, further clinical studies are needed to elucidate this interaction in patients with DM2. According to Landrier et al. [54], both AT and γ-tocopherol induce the expression of adiponectin, irrespective of their antioxidant capacity. The authors raised the hypothesis that this induction occurs through direct genetic regulation since the promoter of the human adiponectin gene contains a PPAR response element, and PPARγ plays an important role in the increased sensitivity to insulin.

FINAL CONSIDERATIONS

Studies designed to elucidate the mechanisms underlying the oxidative alterations in patients with DM2 are scarce. The evidence supporting the effect of AT on lipid profile and insulin sensitivity of DM2 patients is still not clear. Future studies should consider the potential of this vitamin, evaluating the benefit of this low-cost supplementation alone or in combination with other antioxidants. In this respect, the therapeutic window in which antioxidant supplementation would be effective needs to be identified.

SUMMARY POINTS

- α-tocopherol is a potential dietary antioxidant.
- Vitamin E is depleted in diabetes mellitus.
- In DM2, the requirement of antioxidants is increased.
- There are a high number of deaths from cardiovascular diseases in individuals with diabetes mellitus, probably a result of an increased production of ROS.
- The interactive effects between antioxidant vitamins have been investigated in human clinical trials.
- Apparently, intervention studies using vitamin E supplements do not have an impact on lipid profile and insulin resistance of DM2 individuals.

References

[1] Schwarz PE, Li J, Lindstrom J, Tuomilehto J. Tools for predicting the risk of type 2 diabetes in daily practice. Horm Metab Res 2009;41:86–97.
[2] World Health Organization – WHO Diabetes Program; 2012 Available from http://www.who.int/diabetes/en/ [accessed 12.09.12].
[3] Valko M, Dieter L, Moncol J, Cronin MTD, Mazura M, Telser J. Free radicals and antioxidants in normal physiological functions and human disease. Int J Biochem & Cell Biol 2007;39:44–84.
[4] Colas R, Pruneta-Deloche V, Guichardant M, Luquain-Costaz C, Cugnet-Anceau C, Moret M, et al. Increased Lipid Peroxidation in LDL from Type-2 Diabetic Patients. Lipids 2010;45:723–31.
[5] Azzi A, Gysin R, Kempna P, Munteanu A, Villacorta L, Visarius T, et al. Regulation of gene expression by alpha-tocopherol. Biol Chem 2004;385:585–91.
[6] Sauberlich HE. Laboratory tests for the assessment of nutritional status. CRC series in modern nutrition. 2nd ed. Boca Raton: CRC-Press; 1999. p. 486.
[7] Skyrme-Jones RA, O'Brien RC, Berry KL, Meredith IT. Vitamin E supplementation improves endothelial function in type I diabetes mellitus: a randomized, placebo-controlled study. J Am Coll Cardiol 2000;36:94–102.
[8] Mehta JL, Rasouli N, Sinha AK, Molavi B. Oxidative stress in diabetes: a mechanistic overview of its effects on atherogenesis and myocardial dysfunction. Int J Biochem Cell Biol 2006;38:794–803.
[9] Wang Q, Sun Y, Ma A, Li Y, Han X, Liang H. Effects of vitamin E on plasma lipid status and oxidative stress in Chinese women with metabolic syndrome. Int J Vitam Nutr Res 2010;80:178–87.
[10] Young IS, Woodside JV. Antioxidants in health and disease. J Clin Pathol 2001;54:176–86.
[11] Johansen JS, Harris AK, Rychly DJ, Ergul A. Oxidative stress and the use of antioxidants in diabetes: Linking basic science to clinical practice. Cardiovascular Diabetology 2005;4.
[12] Dembinska-Kiec A, Mykkänen O, Kiec-Wilk B, Mykkänen H. Antioxidant phytochemicals against type 2 diabetes. Br J Nutr 2008;99:109–17.
[13] Fardoun RZ. The use of vitamin E in type 2 diabetes mellitus. Clin Exp Hypert 2007;29:135–48.
[14] Pazdo R, Burgess JR. The role of vitamin E and oxidative stress in diabetes complications. Mechan Ageing and Develop 2010;131:276–86.
[15] Kataja-Tuomola M, Sundell JR, Männistö S, Virtanen MJ, Kontto J, Albanes D, et al. Effect of α-tocopherol and β-carotene supplementation on the incidence of type 2 diabetes. Diabetologia 2008;51:47–53.
[16] Shepherd J. Dyslipidaemia in diabetic patients: time for a rethink. Diabetes. Obesity and Metabolism 2007;9:609–16.
[17] Krayenbuehl PA, Wiesli P, Schmid C, Lehmann R, Giatgen A, Spinas GA, et al. Insulin sensitivity in type 2 diabetes is closely associated with LDL particle size. Swiss Med Wkly 2008;138:275–80.
[18] Spickett CM, Wiswedel I, Siems W, Zarkovic K, Zarkovic N. Advances in methods for the determination of biologically relevant lipid peroxidation products. Free Radic Res 2010;44:1172–202.
[19] Turko IV, Marcondes S, Murad F. Diabetes-associated nitration of tyrosine and inactivation of succinyl-CoA:3-oxoacid CoAtransferase. Am J Physiol Heart Circ Physiol 2001;281:H2289–94.
[20] Guzik TJ, Mussa S, Gastaldi D, Sadowski J, Ratnatunga C, Pillai R, et al. Mechanisms of increased vascular superoxide production in human diabetes mellitus: role of NAD(P)H oxidase and endothelial nitric oxide synthase. Circulation 2002;105:1656–62.
[21] Brownlee M. Biochemistry and molecular cell biology of diabetic complications. Nature 2001;414:813–20.
[22] Nishikawa T, Edelstein D, Du XL, Yamagishi S, Matsumura T, Kaneda Y, et al. Normalizing mitochondrial superoxide production blocks three pathways of hyperglycaemic damage. Nature 2000;404:787–90.

[23] Paolisso G, D'Amore A, Giugliano D, Ceriello A, Varricchio M, D'Onofrio F. Pharmacologic doses of vitamin E improve insulin action in healthy subjects and non-insulin-dependent diabetic patients. Am J Clin Nutr 2002;57:650–6.
[24] Picard F, Auwerx J. PPAR(gamma) and glucose homeostasis. Annu Rev Nutr 2002;22:167–97.
[25] Oliveira AM, Rondo PHC, Luzia LA, D'Abronzo FH, Illison VK. The effects of lipoic acid and α-tocopherol supplementation on the lipid profile and insulin sensitivity of patients with type 2 diabetes mellitus: A randomized, double-blind, placebo-controlled trial. Diabetes Res Clin Pract 2011;92:253–60.
[26] Lavie CJ, Jenna MD, Milani N. Do Antioxidant Vitamins Ameliorate the Beneficial Effects of Exercise Training on Insulin Sensitivity? J Cardiopul Rehab and Prev 2011;31:211–6.
[27] Palacka P, Kucharska J, Murin J, Dostalova K, Okkelova A, Cizova M, et al. Complementary therapy in diabetic patients with chronic complications: a pilot study. Bratisl Lek Listy 2010;111:205–11.
[28] Song Y, Cook NR, Albert CM, Denburgh M, Manson JE. Effects of vitamins C and E and β-carotene on the risk of type 2 diabetes in women at high risk of cardiovascular disease: a randomizedcontrolled trial. Am J Clin Nutr 2009;90:429–37.
[29] Costacou T, Ma B, King B, Mayer-Davis EJ. Plasma and dietary vitamin E in relation to insulin secretion and sensitivity. Diabetes. Obesity and Metabolism 2008;10:223–8.
[30] Devaraj S, Leonard S, Traber MG, Jialal I. Gamma-tocopherol supplementation alone and in combination with alpha-tocopherol alters biomarkers of oxidative stress and inflammation in subjects with metabolic syndrome. Free Rad Biol Med 2008;44:1203–8.
[31] Wu JHY, Ward NC, Indrawan AP. Effects of AT and mixed tocopherol supplementation on markers of oxidative stress and inflammation in type 2 diabetes. Clin Chem 2007;53:511–9.
[32] Liu S, Lee M, Song Y, Denburgh M, Cook NR, Manson JE, et al. Vitamin E and risk of Type 2 Diabetes in the women's health study randomized controlled trial Diabetes. 2006;55:2856–62.
[33] Sacco M, Pellegrini F, Roncaglioni MC, Avanzini F, Tognoni G, Nicolucci Aon behalf of the PPP Collaborative Group. Primary prevention of cardiovascular events with low-dose aspirin and vitamin e in type 2 diabetic patients -results of the primary prevention project (PPP) trial. Diabetes Care 2003;26:3264–72.
[34] Ylönen K, Alfthan G, Groop L, Saloranta C, Aro A, Virtanen SMand the Botnia Research Group. Dietary intakes and plasma concentrations of carotenoids and tocopherols in relation to glucose metabolism in subjects at high risk of type 2 diabetes: the Botnia Dietary Study. Am J Clin Nutr 2003;77:1434–41.
[35] Mayer-Davis EJ, Costacou T, King I, Zaccaro DJ, Bell RA. Plasma and dietary vitamin E in relation to incidence of type 2 diabetes – The Insulin Resistance and Atherosclerosis Study (IRAS). Diabetes Care 2002;25:2172–7.
[36] Park S, Choi SB. Effects of α tocopherol supplementation and continuous subcutaneous insulin infusion on oxidative stress in Korean patients with type 2 diabetes. Am J Clin Nutr 2002;75:728–33.
[37] Choi SW, Benzie IF, Collins AR, Hannigan BM, Strain JJ. Vitamins C and E: acute interactive effects on biomarkers of antioxidant defense and oxidative stress. Mutat Res 2004;551:109–17.
[38] Gökkusu C, Palanduz S, Ademoğlu E, Tamer S. Oxidant and antioxidant systems in NIDDM patients: influence of vitamin E supplementation. Endocr Res 2011;27:377–86.
[39] Skrha J, Sindelka G, Kvasnicka J, Hilgertova J. Insulin action and fibrinolysis influenced by vitamin E in obese Type 2 diabetes mellitus. Diab Res Clin Pract 1999;44:27–33.
[40] Igarashi O. Nutritional Requirement and Oral Safety. Vitamin E Its Usefulness in Health and in Curing Diseases. Tokio: Japan Scientific Societies Press and Karger; 1993. p. 131–42.
[41] Johnson LJ, Meacham SL, Kruskall LJ. The antioxidants, vitamin C, vitamin E, selenium, and carotenoids. J Agromedicine 2003;9:65–82.
[42] Garewal HS, Diplock AT. How 'safe' are antioxidant vitamins? Drug Safety 1995;13:8–14.
[43] Hamer M, Chida Y. Intake of fruit, vegetables and antioxidants and risk of type 2 diabetes: systematic review and metaanalysis. J Hypertens 2007;25:2361–9.
[44] Miller 3rd ER, Pastor-Barriuso R, Dalal D, Riemersma R, Appel L, Guallar E. Meta-analysis: high-dosage vitamin E supplementation may increase all-cause mortality. Ann Intern Med 2005;142: 37–46.
[45] Steinberg D, Witztum JL. Is the oxidative modification hypothesis relevant to human atherosclerosis: do the antioxidant trials conducted to date refute the hypothesis? Circulation 2002;105:2107–11.
[46] Winterbone MS, Sampson MJ, Saha S, Hughes JC, Hughes DA. Pro-oxidant effect of α-tocopherol in patients with Type 2 Diabetes after an oral glucose tolerance test– a randomised controlled trial. Cardiovascular Diabetology 2007;6:8.
[47] Gómez-Pérez FJ, Valles-Sanchez VE, López-Alvarenga JC, Choza-Romero R, Ibarra Pascuali JJ, González Orellana R, et al. Vitamin E modifies neither fructosamine nor HbA1c levels in poorly controlled diabetes. Rev Invest Clin 1996;48:421–4.
[48] Hsu RM, Devaraj S, Jialal I. Autoantibodies to oxidized low-density lipoprotein in patients with type 2 diabetes mellitus. Clin Chim Acta 2002;317:145–50.
[49] Sharma A, Kharb S, Chugh SN, Kakkar R, Singh GP. Evaluation of oxidative stress before and after control of glycemia and after vitamin E supplementation in diabetic patients. Metabolism 2000;49:160–2.
[50] Manning PJ, Sutherland WH, Walker RJ, Williams SM, De Jong SA, Ryalls AR, et al. Effect of high-dose vitamin E on insulin resistance and associated parameters in overweight subjects. Diabetes Care 2004;9:2166–71.
[51] Lonn E, Yusuf S, Hoogwerf B. Effects of vitamin E on cardiovascular and microvascular outcomes in high-risk patients with diabetes: results of the HOPE study and MICRO-HOPE sub study. Diabetes Care 2002;25:1919–27.
[52] Robinson I, de Serna DG, Gutierrez A, Schade DS. Vitamin E in humans: an explanation of clinical trial failure. Endocr Pract 2006;12:576–82.
[53] Wu H, Xu G, Liao Y, Ren H, Fan J, Sun Z, et al. Supplementation with antioxidants attenuates transient worsening of retinopathy in diabetes caused by acute intensive insulin therapy. Graefes Arch Clin Exp Ophthalmol 2012;250:1453–8.
[54] Landrier JF, Gouranton E, Yazidi C, Malezet C, Balaguer P, Borel P, et al. Adiponectin expression is induced by vitamin E via a peroxisome proliferator-activated receptor γ-dependent mechanism. Endocrinol 2009;150:5318–25.

CHAPTER

8

Effect of *Salvia miltiorrhiza* on Antioxidant Enzymes in Diabetic Patients

*Qingwen Qian**, *Shuhong Qian*†, *Vinood B. Patel***

*Department of Medicine, First Affiliated Hospital, Zhengzhou University, Zhengzhou, China, †Department of Clinical Laboratory, First Affiliated Hospital, Zhengzhou University, Zhengzhou, China, **Department of Biomedical Science, Faculty of Science & Technology, University of Westminster, London, UK

List of Abbreviations

AGE Advanced glycation end products
ApoE Apolipoprotein E
ATP Adenosine triphosphate
BUN Blood urea nitrogen
CDI Compound danshen injection
CDDP Compound danshen dripping pills
CDT Compound danshen tablet
ECG Electrocardiography
GSH Glutathione
GSH-Px Glutathione peroxidase
HUVEC Human umbilical vein endothelial cells
IL-6 Interleukin 6
IMA ischemia modified albumin
LDL Low density lipoprotein
MDA Malondialdehyde
NADPH Nicotinamide adenine dinucleotide phosphate
NO Nitric oxide
oxLDL Oxidative low density lipoprotein
PKC Protein kinase C
ROS Reactive oxygen species
S. miltiorrhiza *Salvia miltiorrhiza*
SalA Salvianolic acid A
SalB Salvianolic acid B
SOD Superoxide dismutase
STZ Streptozotocin
sVCAM-1 Soluble vascular cell adhesion molecule-1
TIIA Tanshinone IIA
T2DM Type 2 diabetes mellitus
UAER Urine albumin excretion rate
VSMC vascular smooth muscle cells
vWF von Willebrand factor

INTRODUCTION

The high prevalence of diabetes, especially among the older population, is increasing at an alarming rate. A report from Centers for Disease Control and Prevention, USA, showed that 25.8 million people in the United States had a diagnosis of diabetes mellitus, and 10.9 million or 26.9% of people aged 65 or older had diabetes in 2010 [1]. Moreover, according to a fact sheet from The World Health Organization, 346 million people worldwide were diagnosed as diabetic in 2011. Diabetes significantly increases the risk of chronic complications, including cardiovascular events, stroke, renal disease, blindness, and amputations in comparison with non-diabetic patients. Although the progress of diabetic chronic complications can be delayed with extensive tight control of hyperglycemia, hypertension and hyperlipidemia, the onset of diabetic chronic complications is still much higher than in non-diabetic patients.

Many studies have suggested that oxidative stress induced by hyperglycemia seems to be an activator of multiple signaling pathways involved in the pathogenesis of diabetic chronic complications. The signaling pathways include:

1) Intracellular advanced glycation end product (AGE) formation;
2) Polyol pathway;
3) Protein kinase C;
4) Hexoamine pathway (Figure 8.1) [2].

The studies demonstrate that all of these signaling pathways activate a single event – overproduction of reactive oxygen species (ROS) [3]. The evidence reveals that hyperglycemia is one of the major ways of inducing ROS formation and endothelial dysfunction in patients with diabetes [4]. The main sources of ROS include the oxidative phosphorylation of glucose, the mitochondrial electron transport chain, and uncoupling the NADPH oxidase and polyol pathways. Moreover,

Diabetes: Oxidative Stress and Dietary Antioxidants.
http://dx.doi.org/10.1016/B978-0-12-405885-9.00008-5

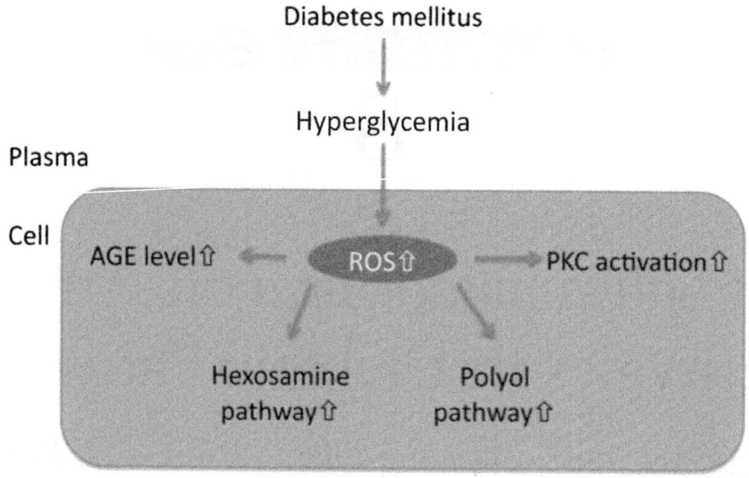

FIGURE 8.1 Hyperglycemia induced ROS formation activated major pathways related to hyperglycemic damage. The induction of oxidative stress by hyperglycemia resulted in the decrease of GSH, thereby reducing the activity of glyoxalase I. The inhibition of glyoxalase I stimulated the level of methylglyoxal – an important active reagent for the formation of AGE. High level of oxidative stress also increased UDP-GlcNac level (Hexosamine pathway), sorbitol level (Polyol pathway) and the flux of dihydroxyacetone phosphate to diacylglycerol, an activator of PKC (PKC pathway).

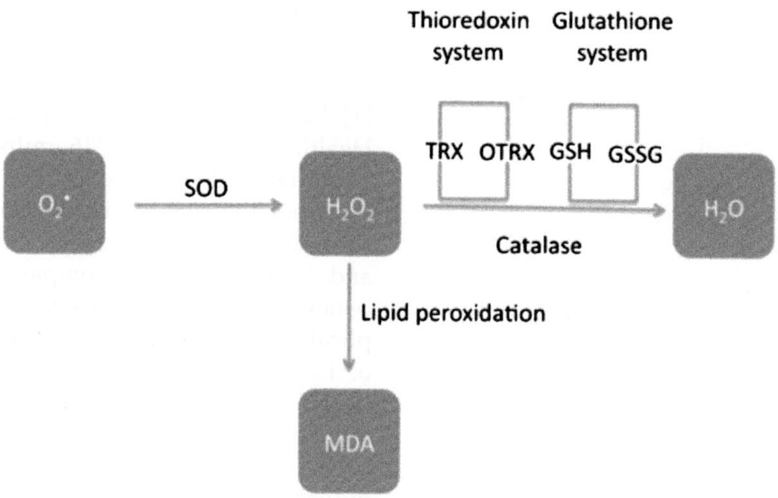

FIGURE 8.2 Cellular antioxidant defense system. Hydrogen peroxide (H_2O_2) is one of the major ROS generated during the process of dismutation of superoxide by the enzyme superoxide dismutase. H_2O_2 has the ability to trigger lipid peroxidation. In clinical studies, MDA reflected the degress of lipid peroxidation. H_2O_2 can be coverted into H_2O though the catalase, thioredoxin and glutathione systems. These systems and catalase play an important role in the amelioration of cellular oxidative stress.

the activities of antioxidative enzymes, such as superoxide dismutase (SOD), catalase, antioxidant enzymes of thioredoxin system and glutathione system, etc. (Figure 8.2) [5], decrease in diabetics and those with chronic vascular complications [2]. The increase of AGE product also stimulates cellular ROS formation [6]. Studies by Diamant et al. provided evidence that diabetic patients showed a reduction of diastolic function. This reduction was correlated to a decrease of phosphocreatine/ATP ratio in the heart [7]. Anderson's study showed that mitochondrial respiratory function was impaired, and hydrogen peroxide emission increased in the left atria appendage tissue of patients with type 2 diabetes mellitus (T2DM) undergoing coronary bypass surgery [8]. Studies of streptozotocin (STZ)-induced diabetes showed increased excretion of hydrogen peroxide, lipid peroxidation products, and nitric oxide products [9].

In summary, studies in diabetic animals and patients confirm that overproduction of ROS can be detected at every stage in diabetes, and also the increase of cellular ROS levels aggravates the development of chronic complications. Hence potential ways to alleviate oxidative stress have been explored; for example, vitamins C and E, alone or in combination have been tested in different clinical trials. Despite evidence from cohort studies showing an inverse relationship between dietary or supplemental vitamin E intake and the development of cardiovascular disease, conclusive findings on the beneficial effect of antioxidative supplements on diabetes and its related complications did not result [10–14]. It was concluded that most of these trials were performed in high-risk patients in whom vascular disease was presumably advanced. When antioxidant therapy was commenced, it was too late to have a substantial protective effect. The doses of antioxidant used also varied among trials. Therefore, it is important to explore new approaches to treating diabetic chronic complications early.

Danshen, the dried roots of *Salvia miltiorrhiza* (*S. miltiorrhiza*, red sage), is a popular herb in China, Japan, and Korea. It has been widely used in the treatment of cardiovascular disease, chronic hepatitis B infection, and ischemic stroke for more than 100 years. The compounds of *S. miltiorrhiza* are divided into two major groups, lipophilic diterpenoids and hydrophilic polyphenolic compounds. The lipophilic diterpenoids include tanshinone l, tanshinone llA (TIIA), tanshinone llB, tanshinone IV, cryptotanshinone, and 3a-hydroxytanshinone Il A. The hydrophilic extract contains danshensu, salvianolic acid A (SalA), salvianolic acid B (SalB), caffeic acid, rosmarinic acid, protocatechuic acid, salvianolic acid C, etc. [15]. In complimentary herbal medicine, *S. miltiorrhiza* has been used to prevent or delay the progress of diabetic chronic complications. It has been demonstrated that the treatment of herbal formulations containing *S. miltiorrhiza* has the ability to improve the symptoms and signs in diabetic patients with chronic heart disease [16]. In this review, our focus is on the antioxidative characterization of *S. miltiorrhiza* in diabetic patients with or without chronic complications.

COMBINATIONS CONTAINING S. MILTIORRHIZA

Combinations of *S. miltiorrhiza* and other herbs have been widely used in the treatment of diabetes or its chronic complications in Chinese clinics.

Compound Danshen

The most common combination of *S. miltiorrhiza* is called fufang danshen, or compound danshen. There are three different fufang danshens on the market (compound danshen tablet [CDT], compound danshen injection [CDI] and compound danshen dripping pills [CDDP]), containing different ingredients. CDT is made from *S. miltiorrhiza*, *radix notoginseng* and borneol; CDDP is made from the hydrophilic extract of *S. miltiorrhiza*, *radix notginseng* and borneol; CDI is made from equal amounts of the hydrophilic extracts of *S. miltiorrhiza* and *dalbergia*.

Compound Danshen Injection

In 1973, the first Chinese traditional patent medicine from *S. miltiorrhiza* – CDI – was announced in the *Chinese Journal of Pharmaceuticals* [17]. In 1990, Liu first used CDI to treat diabetic patients with neuropathy. In this study, the patients were treated for 20 days. After the treatment, amelioration of the symptoms of diabetic neuropathy was confirmed in 32 of the 37 patients [18]. This study extended the application of CDI to diabetes mellitus and its related chronic complications.

Since then, CDI has been widely used to treat diabetes mellitus and its related chronic complications. Jiang et al. investigated the therapeutic effect of CDI in patients with T2DM. Diabetes mellitus caused a significant decrease of SOD and an increase of malondialdehyde (MDA), compared with non-diabetic subjects. The treatment of CDI resulted in an improvement of SOD and MDA levels. Furthermore, there was no significant difference in MDA levels between the treatment group and non-diabetic subjects. These results indicated that treatment with CDI efficiently ameliorated the lipid peroxidation induced by diabetes [19]. Ren also observed the antioxidant effect of CDI in elderly patients with T2DM. The results of this randomized controlled clinical extended those of the previous study from Jang, as treatment with CDI for 30 days also alleviated hypertensive and proteinuria in diabetic patients. This was related to the increase in oxidative stress (SOD activity decreased) [20], which likely causes:

1) Decreased Na^+/K^+ ATP enzyme activity;
2) Stimulation of platelet activity, such as an increased ratio of thromboxane B2 to prostaglandin;
3) Glycation;
4) Increased flux along protein kinase C signaling pathway 21.

In summary, CDI ameliorated oxidative stress in patients with T2DM, and therefore, improved the microcirculation and delayed the development or progress of diabetic chronic vascular disease.

Compound Danshen Tablets

CDT was launched onto the market on September 2–3, 1976. Prior to launch, it was tested in multiple clinical centers in Southern China. 415 patients with coronary artery disease were recruited in this study. The results showed that the administration of CDT led to a 34.7% relief in the symptoms of unstable angina, and a 20.1% improvement in electrocardiography (ECG) results [22]. The patients in this study included diabetics.

According to the theory of Chinese herbal medicine, the therapeutic mechanism of CDT is to promote blood

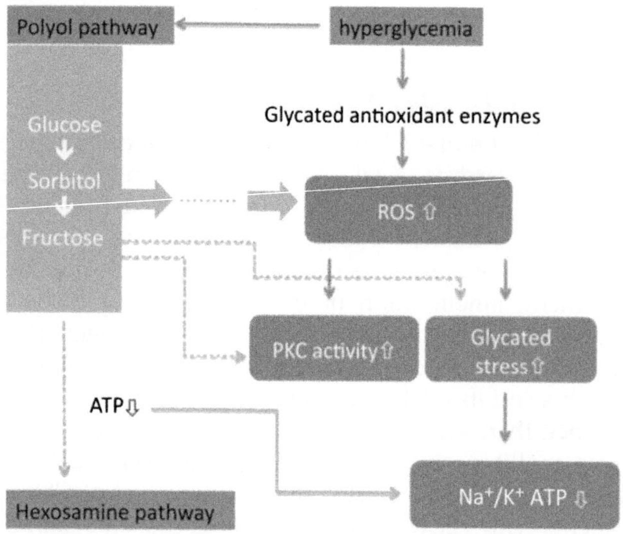

FIGURE 8.3 Polyol pathway in hyperglycemic condition has been associated with the pathogenesis of diabetic complications. Hyperglycemia resulted in an increase of glycated antioxidant enzymes and stimulation of the polyol pathway. The inactivated antioxidant enzymes and stimulation of polyol pathway led to high level of cellular ROS. At the same time, activation of the polyol pathway and increase in ROS deteriorated the increase of PKC activity and glycated stress. In addition to the above effect, the activation of the polyol pathway also caused low ATP levels, which inhibited cellular Na^+/K^+ ATP enzymes. All in all, hyperglycemia played a key role in the development of diabetic complications.

circulation, regulate Qi and activate blood analgesia. The studies of CDT in diabetic animals or patients focused on the improvement of microcirculation and the protection of endothelial function. The clinical study of Song et al. showed that the treatment with CDT for three months led to a significant improvement in blood viscosity, plasma viscosity, erythrocyte electrophoresis time and fibrinogen, and an increase of SOD activity, compared with the placebo group [23]. Studies using STZ-induced diabetic rats further revealed the role of oxidative stress in diabetes. Hyperglycemia activates the polyol pathway and increases the levels of its end products. Such activation mediates metabolic and osmotic alterations in many tissues (e.g., neurons, platelets). Increased glucose flux through the polyol pathway was associated with the pathogenesis of diabetic complications via several potential mechanisms, including sorbitol-osmotic effects, depletion of myoinositol [24], subsequent perturbations in Na^+/K^+ ATPase activity [25], activation of PKC [26], disturbances in cellular redox and free radical defenses, increased oxidative stress, and protein glycation (Figure 8.3). Although it had no effect on blood glucose, the administration of CDT reduced the level of sorbital in erythrocytes, neuron and cardiac myocytes. The inhibition of sorbital by CDT led to an increase in SOD activity and a decrease in MDA levels in diabetics [27]. This suggests that CDT treatment ameliorated the oxidative stress induced by hyperglycemia via the polyol pathway.

Compound Danshen Dripping Pills

Clinical studies revealed that the administration of CDDP increased coronary flow rate and SOD activity, expanded blood vessels, promoted blood circulation, relieved blood stasis, improved the microcycle, changed the blood's viscidity, and also decreased the oxygen consumption of the cardiac muscle [28]. In this section, we will focus mainly on diabetes and its related chronic complications.

DIABETIC CORONARY ARTERY DISEASE

Although most diabetic patients with coronary artery disease have severe atherosclerotic obstruction of the arteries, some such patients may have normal coronary arteries but develop spasm, which results in a variant of angina. Because administration of CDDP showed expansion of the blood vessels, it was effective in relieving angina due to coronary artery spasm. CDDP also improved the opening and formation of coronary collateral circulation, and thus protected the myocardium in patients with T2DM [29]. The cardioprotective effects of CDDP in reducing the infarct size and mortality in rats were impressive. These studies revealed that the protective effect occurred via sedative, antioxidant, and antiplatelet effects, and improvement of the coronary microcirculation [30]. CDDP improved cardiac function through multiple aspects, of which antioxidative protection is one of the most important for patients with T2DM.

Ischemia-modified albumin (IMA) is considered a biomarker for oxidative stress and ischemia. It has been shown that ischemic stress from hypoxic heart tissue induces modifications in circulating albumin, in which the binding capacity of the albumin's N-terminal to transitional metals, such as cobalt, copper and nickel. The level of IMA can be considered a biomarker of oxidative stress in patients with T2DM. Increasing levels of IMA were strongly associated with diabetic patients with ketosis. Therefore, our clinical retrospective study identified patients based on a diagnosis of T2DM and chronic artery disease (a detailed profile of these patients is shown in Table 8.1). As shown in Table 8.2, there was no significant difference in the levels of IMA and oxidative low density lipoprotein (oxLDL) between control and treatment groups at baseline. However, a three month treatment with CDDP caused a 4% decrease IMA levels and a 5% decrease in oxLDL levels compared to the control group. Those results indicated that treatment with CDDP ameliorated oxidative stress in diabetic patients with chronic artery disease.

TABLE 8.1 General Characteristics of Recruited Subjects in Control and Treatment Groups at Baseline (unpublished)

	Control		Treatment	
	N	%	N	%
number	122		74	
Age (yrs)	52–72		54–69	
Sex				
Male	74	60.7	42	56.8
Female	48	39.3	32	43.3
Smoking history	72	59	45	60.8
Blood pressure (mmHg)				
SBP	134.49±21.64		132.07±19.13	
DBP	82.95±14.08		80/91±14.24	
Medical history				
Cerebrovascular disease	51	41.8	40	54.1
Hypertension	110	90.2	65	87.8
Myocardial infarction	11	9	10	13.5

TABLE 8.2 The Effect of CDDP on the Levels of hsCRP, oxLDL and IMA in Diabetic Patients with Chronic Artery Disease (unpublished)

	Control		Treatment	
	Month 0	Month 3	Month	Month 3
hsCRP (mg/L)	2.80±0.73	2.79±0.71	2.76±0.70	2.51±0.74*
oxLDL(μg/dl)	0.55±0.08	0.57±0.08	0.54±0.09	0.52±0.08*
IMA (U/L)	56.85±3.64	26.29±3.80	55.83±4.13	52.14±3.64*

3-month treatment of CDDP resulted in a significant decrease of hsCRP, IMA, oxLDL level, compared with control group (*$p<0.05$).

DIABETIC NEPHROPATHY

T2DM is one of the leading causes of end-stage renal failure. The onset of diabetic nephropathy is related to oxidative stress [2]. This hypothesis is supported by a series of studies of antioxidants such as α-lipoic acid and vitamin C [31]. Based on regression analysis, plasma vitamin E was considered to be related to plasma creatinine levels in patients with T2DM [32]. Animal studies have shown that vitamin E supplementation reduced oxidative stress in the glomeruli of diabetic rats. Oxidative stress in the diabetic kidney is usually associated with tissue damage, which interferes with proper organ function, causing an increase in urinary protein excretion and blood urea nitrogen (BUN) [33]. Animal studies have shown that vitamin E supplementation reduced oxidative stress in the glomeruli of diabetic rats. To investigate whether CDDP confers similar protective properties to vitamin E, CDDP was supplemented for 40 weeks in a model of insulin resistance, and resulted in significant reductions in glomerulosclerosis compared to insulin resistant dogs [34]. Other studies confirmed that CDDP reduced BUN and serum creatinine in rats with T2DM, demonstrating a positive effect on kidney function [35]. At the cellular level, the mechanism of CDDP has been proposed to be the inhibition of oxidative stress-induced NF-κB activation and apoptosis in H_2O_2-treated HUVEC cells. These data indicate that the function of renal endothelial cells can be improved by CDDP. In a human clinical study involving supplementation with CDDP, the subjects in the treatment group showed the following:

1) A reduction of urine albumin excretion rate (UAER) in the danshen group after 12 weeks, and the same trend after treatment with irbesartan. However, there was no significant difference in UAER level between the irbesartan and danshen groups ($p>0.05$).
2) Stable levels of alanine aminotransferase, aspartate aminotransferase, BUN, creatine and serum potassium levels after 12 weeks of observation in two groups, compared with baseline [36].

These findings are important because elevated microalbumin in urine is an indicator of kidney disease.

DIABETIC RETINOPATHY

Diabetic retinopathy is the most common complication of the disease and threatens the sight of many people with diabetes. The condition involves microvascular damage, hemorrhage, and lipid accumulation affecting the retina, which may cause deterioration in the patient's vision [37]. Several studies have monitored the effect of intervention with vitamin E to prevent or slow outcomes of retinal degeneration by examining symptoms such as the formation of acellular capillaries and pericyte ghosts [38]. Clinical studies administering CDDP orally for six months showed a statistically significant improvement in diabetic retinopathy, such as in microaneurysms (39.5%), small bleeding point and bleeding spots (37.8%), compared with the groups treated with calcium dobesilate capsules. But there was no significant improvement in refractory macular edema between the CDDP and calcium dobesilate capsules treatments [39]. Results from diabetic rat studies revealed that characteristic retinal changes, including a decrease in pericytes, capillary microaneurysms, acellular capillaries and ghost pericytes, were detectable after six months of diabetes. The retinal parameters of the treatment group were better than those of the diabetic group. CDDP also protected retinal endothelial cells against high glucose levels, which showed as an induction of plasma nitric oxide (NO) levels, glutathione peroxidase (GSH-Px) activity and a reduction in MDA levels, tissue plasminogen activator and plasminogen activator inhibitor-1 activities by CDDP [40]. Clearly, CDDP showed protective effects in the diabetic retina in animal and clinical studies.

Besides retinal damage, diabetes mellitus also causes damage to the lids and conjunctiva, cornea, pupil, and optic nerve, leading to an increased risk of glaucoma and the formation of cataracts. In patients with diabetes mellitus, the cause of lens modified protein is oxidative stress [41]. Animal studies have demonstrated that treatment with CDDP significantly enhances the turbidity of the lens compared to the diabetic group, according to slit lamp microscopy results. The lens epithelial cells of the treatment group showed higher expression of SOD and lowers level of MDA than in the diabetic group [42]. All in all, animal studies have shown that treatment with DCCP benefited the eyes of diabetics, but there is insufficient evidence to confirm the effect of DCCP on cataracts in diabetic patients.

Hydrophilic Extracts

Hydrophilic Extract of **S. miltiorrhiza**

Our group recruited patients with the history of chronic heart disease and T2DM to investigate the therapeutic effect of hydrophilic extracts from *S. miltiorrhiza* in a 60 day study. The study measured serum levels of cell adhesion molecules, von Willebrand factor (vWF), and soluble vascular cell adhesion molecule-1 (sVCAM-1), as the accepted markers of vascular disease [43]. The results showed that there were no significant differences in the levels of vWF and sVCAM-1 between the treatment group and placebo. Linear regression analysis of sVCAM-1 and vWF in patients showed that the levels of sVCAM-1 ($r=0.42$, $p<0.05$) and vWF ($r=0.47$, $p<0.05$) were positively correlated with the level of oxLDL (Figure 8.4). However, the 60 day treatment of hydrophilic extract from *S. miltiorrhiza* resulted in a reduction of sVCAM-1 and vWF in the treatment group compared with the placebo group ($p<0.05$).

The antioxidative effect of the hydrophilic extract was investigated to further explore its protective mechanism in respect of diabetic chronic artery disease. Oxidative stress has been proposed as a causal factor in the onset of diabetic chronic complications [44]. A considerable number of studies have shown that oxidative stress was involved in many atherogenic changes in the vascular walls, such as expression of adhesion molecules, migration of macrophages and smooth muscle cells, release of chemokines, and impairment of endothelial nitric oxide production [45]. In this randomized, placebo-controlled trial, our findings demonstrated that supplementation with *S. miltiorrhiza* hydrophilic extract ameliorated oxidative stress. Subsequently, levels of oxLDL and MDA were attenuated, and serum GSH levels, and SOD, glutathione reductase and paraoxonase I activities increased [46]. Therefore, supplementation with *S. miltiorrhiza* induced an increase in antioxidant protection *in vivo*.

In summary, the results of our study confirmed that treatment with *S. miltiorrhiza* hydrophilic extract protected coronary arteries against the oxidative stress induced by hyperglycemia and hyperlipidemia. Moreover, the results also showed that the treatment did not give an improvement in glycemic control and dyslipidemia, which indicated that *S. miltiorrhiza* hydrophilic extract directly ameliorates reactive oxygen species and inhibits lipid peroxidation without regulating glycemic control or the lipid profile.

Salvianolate

Salvianolate is another common hydrophilic extract of *S. miltiorrhiza*. Its ingredients include salvianolic acid B, rosmarinic acid and lithospermic acid. A study by Xiong et al. showed that salvianolate inhibited the oxidation of low density lipoprotein (LDL) induced by $CuSO_4$ in endothelial cells. These results suggested that the administration of salvianolate had antioxidant activity in endothelial cells. Treatment with salvianolate might potentially improve the progress of atherosclerosis [47]. He et al. further demonstrated the antioxidative effect of salvianolate on high glucose cultured human umbilical vein endothelial cells (HUVEC). Their results revealed that such treatment at low, medium and high concentrations resulted in a significant increase in GSH-Px activity, and a decrease in MDA and endothelin-1 levels in comparison with the high glucose condition [48]. In conclusion, both of these studies confirmed that treatment with salvianolate could protect endothelial cells by scavenging reactive oxygen radicals, reducing lipid peroxidation and increasing the intracellular antioxidative enzymes' activities.

Based on results of these basic studies, Wu et al. administered salvianolate to patients with unstable angina, including non-diabetic subjects and those with T2DM. The results showed that giving salvianolate to unstable angina patients with or without T2DM for 10 days resulted in 96.67% relief from the symptoms of unstable angina, and 93.33% improvement in ECG results. In addition, the treatment significantly reduced levels of CRP and ET-1 [49]. In the meantime, Wang et al. also tested the protective effect of salvianolate in patients with T2DM. Their results showed that a reduction in prothrombin time, thrombin time and activated partial thromboplastin time in diabetic patients [50]. A further study by Feng et al. explored the ways in

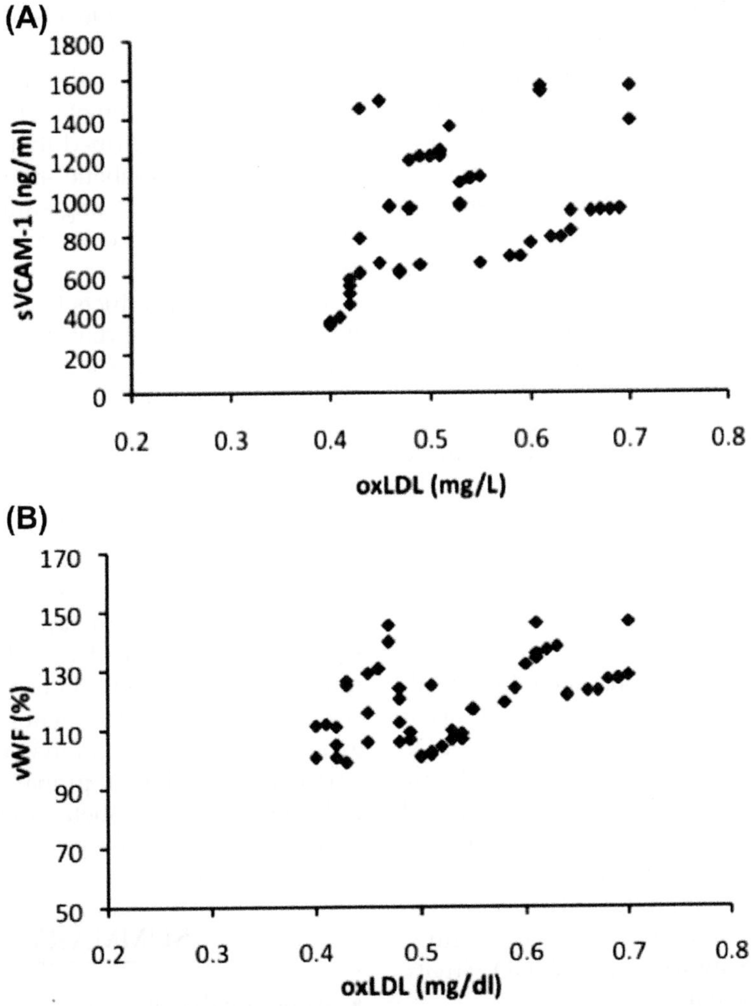

FIGURE 8.4 **The increase of VCAM-1 and vWF was correlated to the increase of oxLDL (unpublished).** Patients were recruited based on the diagnosis of diabetes mellitus and coronary artery disease. Serum levels of VCAM-1, vWF and oxLDL were measured at baseline. The levels of VCAM-1 and vWF were correlated to the level of oxLDL ($r=0.42$, $p<0.05$; $r=0.47$, $p<0.05$, respectively).

which this treatment could improve chronic artery disease and atherosclerosis. In this study, unstable angina patients with or without T2DM received salvianolate for 14 days. After treatment, the patients in the treatment group showed markedly improved symptoms, and the authors also found that the salvianolate treatment resulted in an increase of SOD activity and NO levels, and a decrease in MDA levels, compared with the placebo group [51]. All these studies indicate that salvianolate could be used as a treatment for coronary heart disease and atherosclerosis though amelioration of reactive oxygen species and inhibition of lipid peroxide.

In conclusion, these studies have demonstrated that treatment with salvianolate inhibited the progress of vascular disease and atherosclerosis, and potentially delayed the development of atherosclerosis in patients with T2DM. The protective mechanism of salvianolate was via the amelioration of oxidative stress.

ACTIVE COMPONENTS IN *S. MILTIORRHIZA*

Tanshinone IIA

TIIA is one of the major diterpenes found in *S. miltiorrhiza*. It has antioxidant properties and protects again lipid peroxidation *in vitro* and *in vivo*, making it a potential medicine for free radical-based disorders. In the clinic, it has been reported that TIIA is therapeutic in the treatment of diabetes and its chronic complications.

In their experimental model of diabetic vascular disease, Wang et al. demonstrated that supplementation of STZ-induced diabetic rats with TIIA for four weeks significantly reduced the formation of foam cells from macrophages, the aggregation of macrophages and the infiltration of T lymphocytes, monocytes, foam cells and other inflammatory cells in the area of atherosclerotic plaque without altering blood glucose levels or body weight. In the same study, further investigation revealed that treatment with TIIA also decreased the levels of H_2O_2 and MDA, and increased SOD activities in serum and thoracic aorta [52]. Another study by Lu et al. further confirmed the antioxidant effect of TIIA in high glucose cultured vascular smooth muscle cells (VSMC). The results from this study showed that the proliferation of VSMC induced by high glucose was inhibited by the administration of TIIA in a dose-dependent manner. Moreover, TIIA restored the activity of SOD and the level of MDA in the medium. These authors' results confirmed that the induction of cell proliferation by oxidative stress was the target of TIIA in high glucose cultured VSMC. High glucose levels cause oxidative stress by enhancing the activity of p38MAPK signaling pathway, and TIIA inhibits this pathway, resulting in an increase in mitogen-activated protein kinase phosphatase-1 mRNA levels, inducible nitric oxide synthase activity and NO levels, which initially led to the inhibition of VSMC proliferation in the diabetic condition [53].

Clinical studies have also demonstrated that treatment with TIIA for 14 days resulted in a significant decrease in serum total cholesterol, triglycerides, LDL cholesterol ($p<0.05$), whole blood viscosity and plasma viscosity ($p<0.05$) in patients with T2DM, compared with placebo. A further study by Li suggested that the 14-day TIIA treatment also led to a reduction in interleukin 6 (IL-6) in patients with T2DM. This reduction was correlated with an amelioration of oxidative stress, shown for example, by the improvement of SOD activity and MDA levels in diabetic patients.

All in all, the above studies confirmed that administration of TIIA inhibited the activity of signaling pathways related to cell proliferation and protein translation by relieving the oxidative stress induced by hyperglycemia. TIIA treatment has the ability to improve the progress of macro-vascular diseases in T2DM.

Potentially Active Components in *S. miltiorrhiza*

TIIA is the only component which has been approved by the State Food and Drug Administration, China. Recently, the other active components isolated from *S. miltiorrhiza*, such as SalB, have been tested in diabetic animal models.

A study using STZ-induced, apolipoprotein E gene knock-out (ApoE−/−) mice demonstrated that the administration of SalB significantly reduced the average optical density value of AGE and ratio of plaque area and vessel wall area, compared with a diabetic group [54]. The protective mechanism of SalB was further demonstrated in *in vitro* studies. The incubation of AGE and ox-LDL caused higher levels of LDH, MDA and apoptosis in HUVECs [55]. The treatment with SalB decreased the induction of LDL, alleviated lipid peroxidation and improved the secretion of NO from HUVECs [56]. These studies further confirmed that SalB has a strong capacity for reducing diabetic atherosclerosis and vascular complications. The strong antioxidative activity of SalB might relate to its protective regulation of the vascular endothelial system.

In summary, products from *S. miltiorrhiza* have been widely used to treat diabetes mellitus and its vascular complications. According to ancient traditional medicine, the administration of *S. miltiorrhiza* improved circulation and removed blood stasis. Basic and clinical studies have demonstrated that *S. miltiorrhiza* and its active components could protect endothelial cells, arterial smooth muscle cells, cardiomyocytes, etc., from free radical damage and peroxidation. In addition, *S. miltiorrhiza* attenuated cellular dysfunction by regulating intracellular signaling pathways. Taken together, the protective effect of *S. miltiorrhiza* is mediated by multiple molecular mechanisms that relate to oxidative stress, endothelial dysfunction, and inflammation. We expect that *S. miltiorrhiza* may be an ideal candidate for enriched, active herbal preparations to inhibit the multiple key events in diabetes and their chronic complications, with few adverse effects.

SUMMARY POINTS

- Although diabetes mellitus causes systemic dysfunction *in vivo*, oxidative stress is one of the key factors that is related to the development and progress of diabetic chronic complications.
- Combinations of *S. miltiorrhiza* and other herbs are commonly used in Chinese herbal medicine. Most combinations play an important role in the treatment of diabetes mellitus and its chronic complications.
- The combinations of *S. miltiorrhiza* and other herbs have demonstrable therapeutic effects in diabetic chronic complications. The therapeutic effect of those combinations is confirmed through multiple aspects. Of those aspects, amelioration of cellular oxidative stress has attracted intense interest.
- The crude extracts of *S. miltiorrhiza* have demonstrated antioxidative protection in diabetic patients with or without chronic complications.
- The study of active components of *S. miltiorrhiza* may potentially be an approach for protecting cellular function against the oxidative stress induced by hyperglycemia or hyperlipidemia in patients with diabetes mellitus.

References

[1] National diabetes fact sheet: national estimates and general information on diabetes and prediabetes in the United States. Atlanta, GA: Center for Disease Control and Prevention; 2011.

[2] Xue M, Qian Q, Adaikalakoteswari A, Rabbani N, Babaei-Jadidi R, Thornalley PJ. Activation of NF-E2-related factor-2 reverses biochemical dysfunction of endothelial cells induced by hyperglycemia linked to vascular disease. Diabetes 2008 Oct;57(10):2809–17.

[3] Giacco F, Brownlee M. Oxidative stress and diabetic complications. Circ Res 2010 Oct 29;107(9):1058–70.

[4] Busik JV, Mohr S, Grant MB. Hyperglycemia-induced reactive oxygen species toxicity to endothelial cells is dependent on paracrine mediators. Diabetes 2008 Jul;57(7):1952–65.

[5] Bellinger FP, Raman AV, Reeves MA, Berry MJ. Regulation and function of selenoproteins in human disease. Biochem J 2009 Aug 15;422(1):11–22.

[6] Cai W, He JC, Zhu L, Chen X, Striker GE, Vlassara H. AGE-receptor-1 counteracts cellular oxidant stress induced by AGEs via negative regulation of p66shc-dependent FKHRL1 phosphorylation. Am J Physiol Cell Physiol 2008 Jan;294(1):C145–52.

[7] Diamant M, Lamb HJ, Groeneveld Y, Endert EL, Smit JW, Bax JJ, et al. Diastolic dysfunction is associated with altered myocardial metabolism in asymptomatic normotensive patients with well-controlled type 2 diabetes mellitus. J Am Coll Cardiol 2003 Jul 16;42(2):328–35.

[8] Anderson EJ, Kypson AP, Rodriguez E, Anderson CA, Lehr EJ, Neufer PD. Substrate-specific derangements in mitochondrial metabolism and redox balance in the atrium of the type 2 diabetic human heart. J Am Coll Cardiol 2009 Nov 10;54(20):1891–8.

[9] Jang YY, Song JH, Shin YK, Han ES, Lee CS. Protective effect of boldine on oxidative mitochondrial damage in streptozotocin-induced diabetic rats. Pharmacol Res 2000 Oct;42(4):361–71.

[10] Hamdy NM, Suwailem SM, El-Mesallamy HO. Influence of vitamin E supplementation on endothelial complications in type 2 diabetes mellitus patients who underwent coronary artery bypass graft. J Diabetes Complications 2009 May–Jun;23(3):167–73.

[11] Tousoulis D, Antoniades C, Vasiliadou C, Kourtellaris P, Koniari K, Marinou K, et al. Effects of atorvastatin and vitamin C on forearm hyperaemic blood flow, asymmentrical dimethylarginine levels and the inflammatory process in patients with type 2 diabetes mellitus. Heart 2007 Feb;93(2):244–6.

[12] Chen H, Karne RJ, Hall G, Campia U, Panza JA, Cannon 3rd RO, et al. High-dose oral vitamin C partially replenishes vitamin C levels in patients with Type 2 diabetes and low vitamin C levels but does not improve endothelial dysfunction or insulin resistance. Am J Physiol Heart Circ Physiol 2006 Jan;290(1):H137–45.

[13] Manuel Y, Keenoy B, Shen H, Engelen W, Vertommen J, Van Dessel G, et al. Long-term pharmacologic doses of vitamin E only moderately affect the erythrocytes of patients with type 1 diabetes mellitus. J Nutr 2001 Jun;131(6):1723–30.

[14] Bursell SE, Clermont AC, Aiello LP, Aiello LM, Schlossman DK, Feener EP, et al. High-dose vitamin E supplementation normalizes retinal blood flow and creatinine clearance in patients with type 1 diabetes. Diabetes Care 1999 Aug;22(8):1245–51.

[15] Qu FN, Qi LW, Wei YJ, Wen XD, Yi L, Luo HW, et al. Multiple target cell extraction and LC-MS analysis for predicting bioactive components in Radix Salviae miltiorrhizae. Biol Pharm Bull 2008 Mar;31(3):501–6.

[16] Cheng TO. Cardiovascular effects of danshen. Int J Cardiol 2007 Sep 14;121(1):9–22.

[17] Factory StP. The new drug for coronary heart disease – danshen and compound danshen injection (Chinese). Pharm Industry 1973;1:14–20.

[18] Li YL. The new application for compound danshen injection (Chinese). Clinical Focus 1990;5:236.

[19] Jiang ZY, Zhang SL, Cai XJ, Xing WJ, Wang SX. Effect of *Salvia miltiorrhiza composita* on superoxide dismutase and malonyldialdehyde in treating patients with non-insulin dependent diabetes mellitus (NIDDM) (Chinese). Chinese Journal of Integrated Traditional and Western Medicine 1997;01:236.

[20] Ren ZL. The effect of compound danshen injection on activity of superoxide dismutase and blood flow deformation in elderly patients with type 2 diabetes mellitus (Chinese). Proc Clin Med 2002;4:907–8.

[21] Brownlee M. The pathobiology of diabetic complications: a unifying mechanism. Diabetes 2005 Jun;54(6):1615–25.

[22] Report of compound danshen tablets appraisal meeting (Chinese). Pharm Industry 1976;10:38.

[23] Song HF, Lin LH. The Effect of *Miltiorrhizae composita* tablets on superoxide dismutase and hemorrheology of diabetics. Prog Pharma Sci 2000;3:170–2.

[24] Kinoshita JH, Merola LO, Satoh K, Dikmak E. Osmotic changes caused by the accumulation of dulcitol in the lenses of rats fed with galactose. Nature 1962 Jun 16;194:1085–7.

[25] Hotta N, Kawamori R, Atsumi Y, Baba M, Kishikawa H, Nakamura J, et al. Stratified analyses for selecting appropriate target patients with diabetic peripheral neuropathy for long-term treatment with an aldose reductase inhibitor, epalrestat. Diabet Med 2008 Jul;25(7):818–25.

[26] Hamada Y, Nakamura J. Clinical potential of aldose reductase inhibitors in diabetic neuropathy. Treat Endocrinol 2004;3(4):245–55.

[27] Wu L, Yang GZ, Huang KJ, Chen JM. Effects of compound Red-rooted Salvia tablets on the oxidative stress in diabetic rats (Chinese). Ningxia Med J 2008;30(5):396–8.

[28] Chu Y, Zhang L, Wang XY, Guo JH, Guo ZX, Ma XH. The effect of compound danshen dripping pills, a Chinese herbal medicine, on the pharmacokinetics and pharmacodynamics of warfarin in rats. J Ethnopharmacol 2011 Oct 11;137(3):1457–61.

[29] Liu D, Tang JY, Yan L. Effect of compound danshen dripping pill on arterial intima-media thickness in patients with newly diagnosed type 2 diabetes mellitus. Zhongguo Zhong Xi Yi Jie He Za Zhi 2010 Dec;30(12):1265–68.

[30] Ng CS, Wang SP, Cheong JL, Wu YD, Jia YL, Leung SW. Systematic review and meta-analysis of randomized controlled trials comparing Chinese patent medicines Compound danshen Dripping Pills and Di'ao Xinxuekang in treating angina pectoris. Zhong Xi Yi Jie He Xue Bao 2012 Jan;10(1):25–34.

[31] Davis RL, Lavine CL, Arredondo MA, McMahon P, Tenner Jr TE. Differential indicators of diabetes-induced oxidative stress in New Zealand White rabbits: role of dietary vitamin E supplementation. Int J Exp Diabetes Res 2002 Jul-Sep;3(3):185–92.

[32] Zitouni K, Harry DD, Nourooz-Zadeh J, Betteridge DJ, Earle KA. Circulating vitamin E, transforming growth factor beta1, and the association with renal disease susceptibility in two racial groups with type 2 diabetes. Kidney Int 2005 May;67(5):1993–8.

[33] Zhu B, Shen H, Zhou J, Lin F, Hu Y. Effects of simvastatin on oxidative stress in streptozotocin-induced diabetic rats: a role for glomeruli protection. Nephron Exp Nephrol 2005;101(1):e1–8.

[34] Guo XL, Zhang L, Jia HX, He EH, Che YZ. The role of hyperlipidemia in insulin resistant beagle dog multi-organ injury. Chinese Journal of Cardiovascular Review 2006;4(4):292–4.

[35] Chen P, Zhang QL, Chen WY, Wang YQ, Xu XJ. The effects of danshen dripping pills on the expressions of HIF-1α and VEGF in renal tissues of type 2 diabetic rats (Chinese). Chin J Health Care Med 2011;13(3):200–3.

[36] Lu WH, Shi BY, Li SL, Wei DG, Liu WD. Effect of compound danshen dropping pills on type 2 diabetes mellitus with microalbuminuria. J Shanxi Med Univ 2010;41(4).

[37] Negre-Salvayre A, Salvayre R, Auge N, Pamplona R, Portero-Otin M. Hyperglycemia and glycation in diabetic complications. Antioxid Redox Signal 2009 Dec;11(12):3071–109.
[38] Kowluru RA, Tang J, Kern TS. Abnormalities of retinal metabolism in diabetes and experimental galactosemia. VII. Effect of long-term administration of antioxidants on the development of retinopathy. Diabetes 2001 Aug;50(8):1938–42.
[39] Li X. Clinical study on treatment of diabetic retinology by compound danshen dripping pills. Chi J Modern Drug Appl 2011;5(10):108–9.
[40] Zhou YP, Guo ZY, Tong XL, Pan L, Zhao JB. Effect of composite salvia pellets on diabetic retinopathy in streptozotocin induced diabetic rats. Chin J Integrated Tradit West Med 2002;30(S1):174–8.
[41] Pazdro R, Burgess JR. The role of vitamin E and oxidative stress in diabetes complications. Mech Ageing Dev 2010 Apr;131(4):276–86.
[42] Zhou SP, Guo ZX, Tong XL, Pan L, Zhao JB. Effect of composite salvia pellets on diabetic retinopathy in streptozotocin induced diabetic rats. Chin J Integrated Tradit West Med 2002;22(S1): 174–8.
[43] Qian S, Wang S, Fan P, Huo D, Dai L, Qian Q. Effect of Salvia miltiorrhiza hydrophilic extract on the endothelial biomarkers in diabetic patients with chronic artery disease. Phytother Res 2012 Oct;26(10):1575–8.
[44] Galle J, Hansen-Hagge T, Wanner C, Seibold S. Impact of oxidized low density lipoprotein on vascular cells. Atherosclerosis 2006 Apr;185(2):219–26.
[45] Ishigaki Y, Katagiri H, Gao J, Yamada T, Imai J, Uno K, et al. Impact of plasma oxidized low-density lipoprotein removal on atherosclerosis. Circulation 2008 Jul 1;118(1):75–83.
[46] Qian Q, Qian S, Fan P, Huo D, Wang S. Effect of Salvia miltiorrhiza hydrophilic extract on antioxidant enzymes in diabetic patients with chronic heart disease: a randomized controlled trial. Phytother Res 2012 Jan;26(1):60–6.
[47] Tao X, Wu XJ, Wang YP. Inhibition of salvianolate on LDL oxidation (Chinese). Pharmacol Clin Chin Mater Medica 2004;20(4): 7–10.
[48] He SH, Yan JF, Yuan B, Yan FD, Zhang J, Chen S. Protective effect of salvianolate on human umbilical vein endothelial cells induced by high glucose. Chin J Arteriosclerosis 2008;24(12):948–52.
[49] Wu ZM, Luo XY, Wang SH. Effect of salvianolate on the level of CRP, NO, ET-1 in patients with unstable angina. Henan Tradit Med 2012;32(7):864–5.
[50] Wang L, Jia HY, Bai Y. Effect of salvianolate on hemostatic changes in elderly patients with type 2 diabetes mellitus (Chinese). Chin J Basic Med Tradit Chin Med 2011;17 (889+893):889.
[51] Feng ZH, Ji XW. Clinical study of salvianolate in early admission period in patients with unstable angina. J Liaoning University Tradit Chin Med 2010;12(4):54–6.
[52] Wang L, Li XR, Deng XL, Lu L. The effect of ganshinone II A on oxygen free radicals in type II diabetes (Chinese). J Clin Exp Med 2007;6(7):8–10.
[53] Lu L, Li XY, Deng XL. Effect of tanshinone II A on p38MAPK signal transduction pathway of rats' vascular smooth muscle cells under high glucose concentration (Chinese). J Southeast University (Medical Science Edition) 2008;27(2):130–3.
[54] Fang Z, Jiang XJ, Wang YC, Fan YC. Effects of salvianolic acid b on atherosclerotic plaque area and expressions of AGEs/RAGE in ApoE-Gene knock-out mice treated with stz and high fat diet (Chinese). Tianjin Med J 2010;38(9):777–80.
[55] Pau LY, Zhang J, Jiang XJ, Fan YC. Effect of salvianolic acid b on apoptosis of high-fat HUVECs induced by AGEs (Chinese). J Liaoning University of Tradit Chin Med 2010;10:23–4.
[56] Wang XB, Yu F, Liu F. The protective effect of salvianolic acid a on endothelial damage (Chinese). J Southeast Univ 2008;27(1): 42–6.

CHAPTER

9

Antioxidant Spices and Herbs Used in Diabetes

Roberta Cazzola, Benvenuto Cestaro

Department of Biomedical and Clinical Sciences 'L. Sacco', University of Milan, Milan, Italy

List of Abbreviations

ACSOs S-alk(en)yl-l-cysteine sulfoxides
AGEs Advanced glycation end-products
MCSO S-methyl-l-cysteine sulfoxide
1-PeCSO S-1-propenyl-l-cysteine sulfoxide
2-PeCSO S-2-Propenyl-l-cysteine sulfoxide
SGLT-1 Na^+/glucose cotransporter-1

INTRODUCTION

Diabetes mellitus is a metabolic disorder characterized by chronic hyperglycemia associated with complete or partial deficiencies in insulin secretion or function and is one of the most common chronic diseases affecting millions of people globally [1]. Type 1 diabetes is an autoimmune disease caused by the destruction of pancreatic beta cells, and characterized by a deficiency in the secretion of insulin, while type 2 diabetes is due to abnormal secretion and/or action of insulin, or both. Hyperglycemia and insulin resistance promote an oxidative stress and a pro-inflammatory state, two factors that increase the risk of developing type 2 diabetes and diabetic co-morbidities, such as ischemic heart disease, stroke, neuropathy, nephropathy, and retinopathy. Type 2 diabetes (the most common form of this disease) is one of the world's fastest growing metabolic diseases. It is often, but not always, associated with obesity, which itself can cause insulin resistance and lead to elevated blood sugar levels. Type 2 diabetes has evolved in association with cultural and social changes, aging populations, increasing urbanization, dietary changes, reduced physical activity, and other unhealthy lifestyle factors. In industrialized countries, along with the aging of the population and the increasing prevalence of obesity, the incidence of diabetes has increased steadily in the last decades.

Diet has been recognized as a cornerstone in the management of diabetes mellitus. Before the introduction of the therapeutic use of insulin, diet was the main form of treatment of the disease, and dietary measures included the use of culinary herbs and spices. From the terminological point of view, culinary herbs are considered to be the leaves of a plant used to flavor foods, and spices are any other part of the plant used in cooking, often in the dry state. Generally, while spices have an aromatic and pungent taste which restricts their use, culinary herbs have a more delicate and pleasant taste that makes it possible to use them in larger quantities and in a greater number of food preparations. For thousands of years, spices and herbs have been used not only to flavor and preserve foods, but also as medicaments. In ancient civilizations, the choice of herbs or spices to be used for therapeutic purposes depended on their local availability; for example, in ancient Greece and Rome the herbs were more commonly used, while spices were prevalent in the Middle East, North Africa, and India. In Europe, the new geographical discoveries of the fifteenth and sixteenth centuries allowed a large availability of spices, but the great abundance of scents and flavors that invested the tables of that epoch, later provoked a tiredness towards them and, consequently, a gradual reduction in their use, especially in France and in Italy, where the spices were largely replaced with aromatic herbs, such as garlic, rosemary, sage, laurel, thyme, oregano, and marjoram. These herbs are also used in significant amounts in the Mediterranean diet, a diet associated with a reduced incidence of diabetes and other chronic pathologies, such as heart disease and cancer.

Even nowadays some spices and culinary herbs play an important role in primary health care and in the treatment of diabetes, especially in developing countries [2]. Recently, they have been recognized as sources of

Diabetes: Oxidative Stress and Dietary Antioxidants.
http://dx.doi.org/10.1016/B978-0-12-405885-9.00009-7

various phytochemicals, many of which possess a high antioxidant activity, which, however, can be affected by various factors such as variety, and growing and storage conditions. In particular, almost all spices and the majority of culinary herbs are rich in polyphenols, plant secondary metabolites having high antioxidant activity [3–5] arising from their ability to scavenge a wide spectrum of free radicals, chelate redox-active metals, and/or quench singlet oxygen [4]. They are also known to play an important role in stabilizing lipid peroxidation and in inhibiting various types of oxidizing enzymes [6]. In addition, most of these phenolic compounds have antimicrobial properties that together with their antioxidant capacity are a valuable aid in food preservation. Spices and culinary herbs also possess a high anti-glycant potential arising mainly from their polyphenol content [7]. The non-enzymatic glycation of proteins (Maillard reaction) is a process closely linked to oxidative stress and is associated with increased production of hydrogen peroxide and other highly reactive oxidants that in turn leads to the formation of complex compounds, the advanced glycation end-products (AGEs), which alter the structure and functions of proteins. AGEs are involved in the pathogenesis of diabetes, and contribute to several pathophysiologies associated with aging and diabetes mellitus, such as chronic renal insufficiency, Alzheimer's disease, nephropathy, neuropathy, and cataract [7]. Hyperglycemia accelerates the formation of AGEs and the degree of accumulation of AGEs is correlated to the severity of diabetic complications [7].

Most polyphenols maintain the main features of their structure even after ingestion and metabolism; however, the stability and bioavailability of these secondary plant metabolites could be affected by several factors [8]. Moreover, most polyphenols are poorly absorbed by humans and the real concentrations that can be reached in plasma of individuals subjected to a reasonable polyphenol consumption are transient, because of the rapid metabolism of these compounds, and are more modest (nanomolar range) than those of other plasma antioxidants (micromolar range) [8]. However, as a consequence of this low bioavailability, these compounds can be present in the gastrointestinal tract at much greater concentrations. The gastrointestinal tract is an important site of reactive species production because is much more exposed than other tissues to pro-oxidants, such as hydroxyl radicals generated in the stomach by the interaction of copper and iron contained in foods and ascorbic acid from diet and/or gastric juice, oxidized lipids derived from foods or from lipid peroxidation in the gastrointestinal tract, nitrous acid and nitrosamines originated by nitrites, and reactive species produced by immune system [9]. Therefore, the seasoning of foods with spices and/or culinary herbs, by increasing antioxidant contents of meals, can reduce the production of pro-oxidants not only during storage and cooking, but also in the course of digestion. Moreover, in the gastrointestinal tract, spices and culinary herbs can also have another anti-diabetic effect because of their ability to decrease the activity of digestive enzymes, including α-amylase and disaccharidases [3,10,11], and, as a result, post-prandial hyperglycemia.

The aim of this chapter is to discuss the antioxidant activity and the potential anti-diabetic role of some herbs and spices used to flavor foods, such as sage, marjoram, oregano, peppermint, thyme, garlic, laurel, ginger, turmeric, cumin, coriander, mustard, and pepper.

CULINARY HERBS

Lamiaceae

The family of Lamiaceae or Labiatae includes several widely used culinary herbs, such as sage, oregano, peppermint, marjoram, thyme, and basil. These herbs are particularly rich in phenolic compounds (Table 9.1) which possess a high antioxidant capacity [5,12], anti-glycant action (Table 9.2) and other beneficial properties, such as anti-inflammatory and anticancer activities [13]. In addition, they can affect glycemia by acting on several factors which influence glucose homeostasis (Table 9.3). Along with basic plant antioxidants, culinary herbs of Lamiaceae contain specific characteristic antioxidants (Table 9.1), such as lamiatic acid, carnosic acid, carvacrol, and various methyl and ethyl esters of these substances and derivatives of phenolic acids, such as rosmarinic acid, one of the most effective antioxidant compounds in these plants [4,14]. Both extracts and isolated antioxidant compounds from these herbs have been shown to possess potential anti-diabetic properties.

Sage (*Salvia officinalis L*) is a member of *Salvia*, the largest genus of the Lamiaceae's family which includes about 900 species, spread throughout the world. Many species of *Salvia* have been used as traditional herbal medicines against several diseases, but sage has been one of the most commonly used plants in folk medicine since antiquity, as indicated by its Latin genus name *Salvia*, meaning 'to cure' and species name *officinalis*, meaning 'medicinal'. The plant is reported to have a wide range of biological activities, including anti-oxidative properties [15], hypoglycemic [16] and anti-inflammatory effects [11]. The beneficial effects of sage are the result of numerous compounds from diverse chemical groups acting together, including many phenolic compounds of which the main is rosmarinic acid [14]. Several studies have demonstrated that sage has high *in vitro* antioxidant activity [3,6,11,14,15,17,18], mainly due to its phenolic compounds. Moreover, sage tea has been shown to improve liver glutathione levels in mice and rats [19]. In addition, Lima et al.

TABLE 9.1 Major Antioxidant and Active Compounds of Culinary Herbs

	Major Antioxidants and Active Compounds
Sage (*Salvia officinalis*) Family Lamiaceae	Ascorbic acid, beta carotene, beta-sitosterol, camphene, carnosic acid, carnosol, gamma-terpinene, hispidulin, labiatic acid, oleanolic acid, terpinen-4-ol, ursolic acid, selenium [4], salvigenin, nevadensin, apigenin, cirsileol, cirsimaritin
Oregano (*Origanum vulgaris*) Family Lamiaceae	Camphene, carvacol, gamma-terpinene, thymol, terpinen-4-ol, myricene, linalyl-acetate [4]
Marjoram (*Origanum majorana*) Family Lamiaceae	Ascorbic acid, beta carotene, caffeic acid, rosmarinic acid, tannin, eugenol, hydroquinone, myrcene, phenol, terpinen-4-ol, trans-anethole, ursolic acid, beta-sitosterol, oleanolic acid [4]
Peppermint (*Mentha* x *piperita*) Family Lamiaceae	Ascorbic acid, beta carotene, narirutin, eriodictyol, eriodictyol 7-O-β-glucoside, eriocitrin, hesperidin, isorhoifolin, luteolin 7-O-β-glucoside, luteolin 7-O-rutinoside, diosmin, rosmarinic acid, caffeic acid, piperitoside, menthoside, lithospermic acid [26]
Thyme (*Thymus vulgaris*) Family Lamiaceae	Ascorbic acid, beta carotene, isochlorogenic acid, labiatic acid, p-coumaric acid, rosmarinic acid [4]
Garlic (*Allium sativum*) Family Liliaceae	caffeic, vanillic, p-hydroxybenzoic, and p-coumaric acids [37], allicin [33]
Onion (*Allium cepa*) Family Liliaceae	Quercetin, kaempferol, cyanidin glucosides, peonidin glucosides, taxifolin [36], allicin [33]
Laurel or bay leaf (*Laurus nobilis L.*) Family Lauraceae	Ascorbic acid, beta carotene, tocopherols, eugenol, methyl eugenol, eudesmol [48] kaempferol, kaempferol-3-rhamnopyranoside, kaempferol-3,7-dirhamnopyranoside, 8-cineole, α-terpinyl acetate, terpinen-4-ol, catechin, cinnamtannin B1[47]

For more details see the text and the bibliographic references.

TABLE 9.2 Anti-Glycant Activity of Culinary Herbs

	Experimental Model	Material
Sage	*In vitro*	Water extracts [3]
	In vitro	Methanol extracts [3]
	In vitro	Ethanol extracts [31]
Oregano	*In vitro*	Water extracts [22]
	In vitro	Methanol extracts [22]
Marjoram	*In vitro*	Water extracts [3]
	In vitro	Methanol extracts [3, 23]
	In vitro	Ethanol extracts [31]
	Animal, type 1 diabetes	Methanol extracts [23]
Garlic	*In vitro*	Water extracts [44]
Onion	*In vitro*	Water extracts [44]

For more details see the text and the bibliographic references.

[20] demonstrated dose-dependent anti-diabetic activity of sage tea comparable to the standard anti-diabetic drug glibenclamide (metformin) in rats [20]. This study demonstrated that sage significantly reduced fasting plasma glucose by increasing hepatocyte glucose consumption, decreasing fasting gluconeogenesis and inhibiting the stimulation of hepatic glucose production by glucagon. Greek sage (*Salvia fruticosa*) tea has been demonstrated to prevent the deterioration of glucose homeostasis in streptozotocin diabetic rats (one of the most employed animal models for type 1 diabetes), by abrogating the streptozotocin-induced increase in the intestinal Na^+/glucose cotransporter-1 (SGLT-1). This anti-diabetic effect of Greek sage appears to be due to the modulation of SGLT-1 trafficking caused by rosmarinic acid [21].

Oregano (*Origanum vulgare*) and marjoram (*Oregano majorana*) are plants traditionally used in diabetes control and treatment in North Africa and the Middle East; however their anti-diabetic effects have not yet definitively been proven. *In vitro* studies suggest a potential anti-diabetic effect of oregano due to its antioxidant content [6,10,15,22], anti-glycant capacity [22,23], and inhibition

TABLE 9.3 Hypoglycemic Effects of Culinary Herbs

	Experimental Model	Proposed Mechanism of Action
Sage	Healthy rats Type 1 diabetic rats *In vitro*	Decreased liver gluconeogenesis [20] Intestinal glucose absorption [21] Inhibition of α-amylase and α-glucosidase [3]
Oregano	*In vitro*	Inhibition of amylase enzymes [24]
Laurel	Type 2 diabetic patients	Not investigated [49]
Garlic	Type 1 diabetic animal models	Insulin secretagogues and sensitizing [40]
Onion	Type 1 and 2 diabetic patients	Glucogenic [46]

For more details see the text and the bibliographic references.

of carbohydrate digesting enzymes [10,24]. An aqueous extract of marjoram has been shown to have anti-hyperglycemic activity similar to that of the hypoglycemic drug sodium-vanadate in streptozotocin diabetic rats [25].

The genus *Mentha L* includes 18 species and about 11 hybrids, of which the most used and cultivated are *Mentha spicata* (spearmint) and the hybrid *Mentha* x *piperita* (peppermint). Mints are available in all five continents, are used in traditional medicine for the prevention and therapy of several diseases, and are a well-known herbal remedy used for their aromatic, stomachic, choleretic, carminative, and stimulant properties. The most active compounds in mints are the essential oil and polyphenols. The main phenolic compounds are phenolic acids and flavonoids [6,26,27]. Studies on the anti-diabetic effects of mint are scarce, despite their appreciable total phenolic content. Water extracts of peppermint have been shown to improve glycemia and lipidemia in offspring of streptozotocin-induced diabetic rats [28]. Nevertheless, Narendhirakannan et al. [29] have shown that peppermint ethanolic extracts have no effect on insulin, C-peptide levels, and glucose tolerance in the same animal model.

Studies on the anti-diabetic effects of Lamiaceae's extracts have shown that basil, sage, marjoram, oregano, and thyme significantly inhibit the activity of α-amylase and α-glucosidase, two key enzymes of carbohydrate digestion, *in vitro* [3,10,30] and *in vivo* [30]. Lamiaceae's extracts have also been demonstrated to possess significant anti-glycant capacity *in vitro* [3,22,23,31] and *in vivo* [23]. Büyükbalci et al. [18], have investigated *in vitro* the antioxidant and anti-diabetic effects of herbal teas traditionally used in the treatment of diabetes in Turkey, and found that peppermint and thyme have high antioxidant activity and inhibitory effects on glucose absorption, whereas sage was less effective.

Garlic

Garlic (*Allium sativum*) and onion (*Allium cepa*) are two species widely used for flavoring foods and in folk medicine. Onion, though not strictly an herb, is presented for comparison as it is used in flavoring food, albeit in large amounts. Both these species of *Allium* are rich in sulfur-containing compounds that are products of the transformation of S-alk(en)yl-l-cysteine sulfoxides (ACSOs) by the enzyme alliinase and subsequent reactions. The ACSOs detected in intact onion are S-1-propenyl-l-cysteine sulfoxide (1-PeCSO), S-methyl-l-cysteine sulfoxide (MCSO), and S-propyl-l-cysteine sulfoxide. S-2-Propenyl-l-cysteine sulfoxide (2-PeCSO) is the predominant ACSO in garlic, with smaller amounts of MCSO, 1-PeCSO and S-Ethyl-l-cysteine sulfoxide [32]. In intact *Allium* tissues, ACSOs are located in the cytosol, where they are protected from lysis by alliinase stored in vacuoles. Enzyme and substrates react rapidly upon disruption of the tissue, and the sulfoxides are converted into thiosulfinates, such as allicin [33]. These thiosulfinates and their derivatives were found experimentally to have a wide variety of potential therapeutic effects [32,34,35], including antioxidant and anti-inflammatory activities. Onion and garlic are rich also in phenolic compounds (Table 9.1), and onions are among the most important dietary sources of flavonoids. The main flavonoids in onions are quercetin, kaempferol, myricetin, cyanidin, peonidin, and taxifolin and their derivatives [36]. The main phenolic compounds of garlic are phenolic acids, in particular, caffeic, vanillic, p-hydroxybenzoic, and p-coumaric acids [37]. Moreover, garlic and onion are able to uptake and accumulate selenium from the soil readily, and use it for the biosynthesis of selenocysteine, an amino acid required for the synthesis of seleno-proteins, including the antioxidant enzymes glutathione peroxidase, thioredoxin reductase and iodothyronine deiodinases. Many studies have reported the role of *Allium* species in the prevention and treatment of several human pathologies, including diabetes [38–41], metabolic syndrome [42], and cardiovascular disease [35,43]. An *in vitro* anti-glycant activity has been found both in garlic and onion [44]. Moreover, both garlic and onion have been shown to have hypoglycemic effects in different animal models and in limited human trials [13,40,45,46]. However, recently, a meta-analysis of their anti-diabetic effect in experimental diabetic rats has shown that onion

TABLE 9.4 Major Antioxidant and Active Compounds of Spices

	Major Antioxidants and Active Compounds
Ginger (*Zingiber officinalis*) Family Zingiberaceae	6-Gingerol, 6-shogaol, ascorbic acid, beta carotene, caffeic acid, camphene, gamma-terpinene, p-coumaric-acid, terpinen-4-ol [4]
Turmeric (*Curcuma domestica*) Family Zingiberaceae	Ascorbic acid, carotenes, caffeic acid, curcumin, p-cumaric-acid [4]
Cumin (*Cuminum cyminum*) Family Apiaceae	Apigenin, luteolin, cuminaldehyde, cuminic alcohol, p-cymene, β-pinene, cuminal, cumin alcohol, γ-terpinene [55]
Coriander (*Coriandrum sativum*) Family Apiaceae	beta carotene, beta-sitosterol, caffeic acid, camphene, gamma-terpinene, isoquercitrin, myrcene, myristicin, p-hydroxy-benzoic-acid, protocatechuic-acid, quercetin, rhamnetin, rutin, scopoletin, tannin, terpinen-4-ol, trans-anethole, vanillic-acid [4]
Mustards (*Brassica nigra, alba, juncea*) Family Brassicaceae	Carotenes, glucosinolates [58]
Black Pepper (*Piper nigrum*) Family Piperaceae	Ascorbic acid, beta carotene, ubiquinone, camphen, carvacrol, eugenol, gamma-terpinene, methyl eugenol, piperine [4]

For more details see the text and the bibliographic references.

extracts and single components of both species (S-allyl-cysteine sulfoxide, S-methylcysteine sulfoxide, and diallyl trisulfide) have significant positive effects on blood glucose concentration and body weight, while garlic has no significant anti-diabetic effects [39].

Laurel (Bay Leaves)

Laurel (*Laurus nobilis*, Family Lauraceae) is used as a valuable flavoring agent in the culinary and food industry. This plant is used in folk medicine, in stomachic and carminative remedies, and for the treatment of digestive disease. Laurel contains several compounds with antioxidant activity (Table 9.1). Both the water extract and the non-polar fraction of leaves have been shown to possess high antioxidant activity, the former mainly because of its polyphenol content [47], and the latter for its high levels of terpenes [48]. A clinical trial showing that laurel improves glycemia and lipid profiles in type 2 diabetes patients [49] makes this culinary herb a promising anti-diabetic agent.

SPICES

Spices are an excellent source of antioxidants [12], and some of them even outperform synthetic antioxidants with the advantage of being more secure from the point of view of health. Generally, they contain large amounts of phenolic substances (Table 9.4), many of which have received great attention with regard to their antioxidant and anti-inflammatory properties. Among the spices, ginger, turmeric, cumin, coriander, and mustard have been reported to have anti-diabetic potential due to their anti-glycant activity (Table 9.5) and possible blood sugar lowering effects (Table 9.6).

TABLE 9.5 Anti-Glycant Activity of Spices

	Experimental Model	Material
Ginger	*In vitro* *In vitro*	Ethanol extracts [31] Water extracts [44]
Turmeric	*In vitro*	Water extracts [44]
Cumin	*In vitro*	Water extracts [44]
Mustard	*In vitro*	Water extracts [44]
Black Pepper	*In vitro*	Water extracts [44]

For more details see the text and the bibliographic references.

TABLE 9.6 Hypoglycemic Effects of Spices

	Experimental Model	Proposed Mechanism of Action
Ginger	Type 2 diabetic patients and diabetic animal models	Improvement of insulin action [51]
Turmeric	Type 2 diabetic animal models	Improvement in insulin action [53]
Cumin	Type 1 diabetic rat	Delay of diabetic cataract [56]
Mustards	Type 1 diabetic rats	Increased serum insulin [58]

For more details see the text and the bibliographic references.

Ginger and Turmeric

Ginger (*Zingiber officinalis*) and turmeric (*Curcuma longa*) are members of the botanical family of the Zingiberaceae (ginger family), whose rhizome is used as a spice. Both these spices are among the most commonly used worldwide and are also widely employed in traditional medicines. Ginger contains several antioxidant compounds (Table 9.4) [15,50], comprising different phenolic substances among which are the gingerols (in particular, 6-gingerol), the compounds responsible for the pungency of the fresh rhizome. Cooking ginger transforms gingerols into zingerones, which are less pungent and have a spicy-sweet aroma, while drying and thermal treatment of the rhizome leads to an increase in the concentration of shogaols, the dehydrated form of gingerols, in particular 6-shogaol. The pungent constituents of the rhizome are responsible for ginger's anti-nausea action, and its antimicrobial and antiviral activities. Along with antioxidant properties, ginger has even been shown to possess antiglycant activity [31,44] and other potential anti-diabetic effects. In fact, recent data from *in vitro*, *in vivo*, and clinical trials showed an anti-hyperglycemic effect of ginger due to improved insulin signaling and metabolism of carbohydrates and lipids [51]. In addition, ginger has shown potential protective effects on diabetic complications of the liver, kidney, eye, and neural system [44,51].

Turmeric is widely used in cooking and gives the flavor and yellow color to the Indian curry, a mixture of spices in which turmeric is the major component (about 40–50%). It is also used in mustard sauces and for coloring butter and cheese. Turmeric has been used in traditional medicines as an anti-inflammatory agent, to treat digestive and liver problems, skin diseases, and wounds. Turmeric is valued mainly for its principal pigment, curcumin, which, along with few other related pigments, gives the yellow color to the rhizome of the plant. Chemically, these pigments are polyphenols and all together they are called curcuminoids. Turmeric and, in particular, curcumin have been extensively investigated in the last decades for their antioxidant and anti-inflammatory properties [52]. The results of these investigations have demonstrated that curcumin is a powerful antioxidant and immuno-modulant. These activities of curcumin come from its ability to modulate numerous signaling molecules in humans, such as pro-inflammatory cytokines, apoptotic proteins, transcription factors (in particular, NF-κB), cyclooxygenases, lipoxigenases and adhesion molecules [52]. Some promising effects have been observed in patients with various pro-inflammatory diseases, including diabetes, diabetic nephropathy and diabetic microangiopathy [52]. Curcumin has also been shown to have an anti-hyperglycemic effect and the ability to improve insulin sensitivity, and this last action has been attributed, at least in part, to its anti-inflammatory properties [52,53]. These anti-inflammatory properties are also responsible of the beneficial effects of turmeric and curcumin on diabetic complications, such as diabetic nephropathy and microangiopathy [52].

Cumin and Coriander

Cumin (*Cuminum cyminum*) and coriander (*Coriandrum sativum*) are two plants of the Apiaceae family (parsley family), whose dried seeds are used as a spice. Cumin, like turmeric, is a component of curries and is also used as a condiment and flavoring in many oriental dishes. These two spices are also widely used in traditional medicines and contain high concentrations of antioxidant compounds, including phenolic acids and flavonoids [50,54] (Table 9.4), whose antioxidant activity has been demonstrated in several *in vitro* and animal models of oxidative stress [15,50,55]. Cumin and coriander have been demonstrated to exert anti-glycant activity *in vitro* [44,56,57] and a hypoglycemic action [38,56] in animal models of diabetes.

Mustards

Mustards are several plant species in the genera *Brassica* and *Sinapis* belonging to the Brassicaceae family whose seeds are used as spices. The most cultivated are black mustard (*Brassica nigra*), white mustard (*Brassica* or *Sinapis alba*), and oriental or Indian mustard (*Brassica juncea*). Mustards are used as food flavoring and in traditional medicine as emetics and diuretics, as well as a topical treatment for inflammatory conditions such as arthritis and rheumatism. Mustard seeds contain numerous chemical constituents, including carotenes and phenolic compounds, but the most investigated are glucosinolates, the thiocyanate glycosides from which derive the spice flavor. These glucosinolates, when hydrolyzed by the enzyme myrosinase to flavor-active isothiocyanates, are responsible of the pungency of the spice. Glucosinolates are typical constituents of Brassica species, which also include broccoli, cabbage, cauliflower, Brussels sprouts, caper, etc. They have been extensively investigated for their potential beneficial effects, especially as potential anticancer agents, because of their detoxification activity that derives primarily from their ability to affect the metabolism of carcinogenic substances, including several pro-oxidants, through the modulation of drug-metabolizing enzymes, i.e., the induction of phase II enzymes and the inhibition of phase I enzymes [58]. The mechanisms of action of glucosinolates and related isothiocyanates are multiple, and include also antioxidant, anti-inflammatory, and immuno-modulatory activities [58]. The anti-diabetic potential of mustard is suggested by a few animal studies that have shown a hypoglycemic effect in rats of black and oriental mustard [13,59].

Pepper

Before concluding this section, we would like to mention also black pepper (*Piper nigrum*, Family Piperaceae), among the most widespread and most used spice in the world, although it has not yet been shown that it possesses significant anti-diabetic effects, except an anti-glycant activity *in vitro* [44]. However, pepper has, in addition to a high antioxidant activity, other properties that might enhance the anti-diabetic and antioxidant properties of the other spices. The antioxidant activity of pepper is mainly due to piperine, the alkaloid contributing to the pungency of this spice. Black pepper or piperine treatment has been demonstrated to inhibit or quench free radicals and reactive oxygen species, and to positively influence cellular thiol status, antioxidant molecules and antioxidant enzymes *in vitro*, and reduce lipid peroxidation *in vivo* [60]. In addition, piperine strongly inhibits hepatic and intestinal aryl hydrocarbon hydroxylase and UDP-glucuronyl transferase, two enzymes involved in both the bio-transforming reactions of drugs and phytochemicals, including phenolic substances, and the modulation of the bioavailability of these compounds. In addition, piperine enhances the bioavailability of a number of therapeutic drugs and phytochemicals, also through an interaction with the ultra-structure of intestinal brush border that causes an increase in intestinal absorption of these substances [60]. The effect of piperine on the bioavailability of phytochemicals deserves to be investigated more thoroughly, in order to clarify potential synergistic effects on the anti-diabetic and antioxidant activities of other spices.

CONCLUSIONS

Spices and culinary herbs are rich in compounds with different and often very high antioxidant activities, and potential pharmacological effects on diabetes and its complications. Considering the well-established role of oxidative stress as a trigger factor for type 2 diabetes and diabetic complications, the antioxidant activities of spices and culinary herbs may act synergistically with their hypoglycemic properties in exerting an overall anti-diabetic action. However, the real effectiveness of these spices and herbs and/or of compounds isolated from them must be tested more thoroughly because of the lack of scientific evidence from human studies and inconsistent data from animal studies. Considering the wealth of bioactive compounds in these plants, and the encouraging results of *in vitro* and pilot clinical studies, further studies on their preventive and therapeutic effects against diabetes, especially of type 2, are desirable in the future. Bearing in mind that diabetic subjects generally use different drugs, and that these foods also contain substances that may interfere with the metabolism of drugs, extensive basic and clinical research to evaluate the effects of these interactions would also be desirable.

SUMMARY POINTS

- Oxidative stress increases the risk for developing type 2 diabetes and diabetic co-morbidities.
- Spices and culinary herbs contain high concentrations of antioxidant compounds, including phenolic substances.
- The seasoning of foods with spices and/or culinary herbs increases the daily intake of antioxidants and protects foods during storage, cooking, and digestion.
- Spice and culinary herb antioxidants also have other potential anti-diabetic effects, such as anti-glycant, anti-inflammatory and hypoglycemic activities.
- Further clinical researches are needed to confirm the real effectiveness of spices and herbs and/or of compounds isolated from them in diabetes prevention and treatment.

References

[1] Shaw JE, Sicree RA, Zimmet PZ. Global estimates of the prevalence of diabetes for 2010 and 2030. Diabetes Res Clin Pract 2010;87:4–14.

[2] Dham S, Shah V, Hirsch S, Banerji MA. The role of complementary and alternative medicine in diabetes. Curr Diab Rep 2006;6:251–8.

[3] Cazzola R, Camerotto C, Cestaro B. Anti-oxidant, anti-glycant, and inhibitory activity against alpha-amylase and alpha-glucosidase of selected spices and culinary herbs. Int J Food Sci Nutr 2011;62:175–84.

[4] Suhaj M. Spice antioxidants isolation and their antiradical activity: a review. J Food Composit Anal 2006;19:531–7.

[5] Yi W, Wetzstein HY. Biochemical, biological and histological evaluation of some culinary and medicinal herbs grown under greenhouse and field conditions. J Sci Food Agric 2010;90:1063–70.

[6] Shan B, Cai YZ, Sun M, Corke H. Antioxidant capacity of 26 spice extracts and characterization of their phenolic constituents. J Agric Food Chem. 2005;53:7749–59.

[7] Elosta A, Ghous T, Ahmed N. Natural products as anti-glycation agents: possible therapeutic potential for diabetic complications. Curr Diabetes Rev. 2012;8:92–108.

[8] Manach C, Scalbert A, Morand C, Remesy C, Jimenez L. Polyphenols: food sources and bioavailability. Am J Clin Nutr 2004;79:727–47.

[9] Halliwell B, Zhao K, Whiteman M. The gastrointestinal tract: a major site of antioxidant action? Free Radic Res. 2000;33:819–30.

[10] Kwon YI, Vattem DA, Shetty K. Evaluation of clonal herbs of Lamiaceae species for management of diabetes and hypertension. Asia Pac J Clin Nutr 2006;15:107–18.

[11] Chohan M, Naughton DP, Jones L, Opara EI. An investigation of the relationship between the anti-inflammatory activity, polyphenolic content, and antioxidant activities of cooked and *in vitro* digested culinary herbs. Oxid Med Cell Longev 2012;2012:627843.

[12] Carlsen MH, Halvorsen BL, Holte K, Bohn SK, Dragland S, Sampson L, et al. The total antioxidant content of more than 3100 foods, beverages, spices, herbs and supplements used worldwide. Nutr J 2010;9:3.

[13] Srinivasan K. Plant foods in the management of diabetes mellitus: Spices as beneficial antidiabetic food adjuncts. Int J Food Sci Nutr 2005;56:399–414.

[14] Generalic I, Skroza D, Surjak J, Mozina SS, Ljubenkov I, Katalinic A, et al. Seasonal variations of phenolic compounds and biological properties in sage (Salvia officinalis L.). Chem Biodivers 2012; 9:441–57.

[15] Skrovankova S, Misurcova L, Machu L. Antioxidant activity and protecting health effects of common medicinal plants. Adv Food Nutr Res 2012;67:75–139.

[16] Alarcon-Aguilar FJ, Roman-Ramos R, Flores-Saenz JL, Aguirre-Garcia F. Investigation on the hypoglycaemic effects of extracts of four Mexican medicinal plants in normal and alloxan-diabetic mice. Phytother Res. 2002;16:383–6.

[17] Bozin B, Mimica-Dukic N, Samojlik I, Jovin E. Antimicrobial and antioxidant properties of rosemary and sage (*Rosmarinus officinalis L.* and *Salvia officinalis L.*, Lamiaceae) essential oils. J Agric Food Chem 2007;55:7879–85.

[18] Buyukbalci A, El SN. Determination of *in vitro* antidiabetic effects, antioxidant activities and phenol contents of some herbal teas. Plant Foods Hum Nutr 2008;63:27–33.

[19] Lima CF, Andrade PB, Seabra RM, Fernandes-Ferreira M, Pereira-Wilson C. The drinking of a *Salvia officinalis* infusion improves liver antioxidant status in mice and rats. J Ethnopharmacol 2005;97:383–9.

[20] Lima CF, Azevedo MF, Araujo R, Fernandes-Ferreira M, Pereira-Wilson C. Metformin-like effect of *Salvia officinalis* (common sage): is it useful in diabetes prevention? Br J Nutr 2006;96:326–33.

[21] Azevedo MF, Lima CF, Fernandes-Ferreira M, Almeida MJ, Wilson JM, Pereira-Wilson C. Rosmarinic acid, major phenolic constituent of Greek sage herbal tea, modulates rat intestinal SGLT1 levels with effects on blood glucose. Mol Nutr Food Res 2011;55(Suppl. 1):S15–25.

[22] Cervato G, Carabelli M, Gervasio S, Cittera A, Cazzola R, Cestaro B. Antioxidant properties of oregano (*Origanum vulgare*) leaf extracts. J Food Biochem 2000;24:453–65.

[23] Perez Gutierrez RM. Inhibition of advanced glycation end-product formation by *Origanum majorana* L. *In vitro* and in streptozotocin-induced diabetic rats. Evid Based Complement Alternat Med 2012;2012:598638.

[24] McCue P, Vattem D, Shetty K. Inhibitory effect of clonal oregano extracts against porcine pancreatic amylase *in vitro*. Asia Pac J Clin Nutr 2004;13:401–8.

[25] Lemhadri A, Zeggwagh NA, Maghrani M, Jouad H, Eddouks M. Anti-hyperglycaemic activity of the aqueous extract of *Origanum vulgare* growing wild in the Tafilalet region. J Ethnopharmacol 2004;92:251–6.

[26] Fecka I, Turek S. Determination of water-soluble polyphenolic compounds in commercial herbal teas from Lamiaceae: peppermint, melissa, and sage. J Agric Food Chem 2007;55:10908–17.

[27] Guedon DJ, Pasquier BP. Analysis and distribution of flavonoid glycosides and rosmarinic acid in 40 *Mentha* x *piperita* clones. J Agric Food Chem 1994;42:679–84.

[28] Barbalho SM, Damasceno DC, Spada AP, da Silva VS, Martuchi KA, et al. Metabolic profile of offspring from diabetic Wistar rats treated with *Mentha piperita* (Peppermint). Evid Based Complement Alternat Med 2011:430237; 2011.

[29] Narendhirakannan RT, Subramanian S, Kandaswamy M. Biochemical evaluation of antidiabetogenic properties of some commonly used Indian plants on streptozotocin-induced diabetes in experimental rats. Clin Exp Pharmacol Physiol 2006;33:1150–7.

[30] Koga K, Shibata H, Yoshino K, Nomoto K. Effects of 50% ethanol extract from rosemary (*Rosmarinus officinalis*) on α-glucosidase inhibitory activity and the elevation of plasma glucose level in rats, and its active compound. J Food Sci. 2006;71:S507–12.

[31] Dearlove RP, Greenspan P, Hartle DK, Swanson RB, Hargrove JL. Inhibition of protein glycation by extracts of culinary herbs and spices. J Med Food 2008;11:275–81.

[32] Chan JY, Yuen AC, Chan RY, Chan SW. A review of the cardiovascular benefits and antioxidant properties of allicin. Phytother Res 2013;27:637–46.

[33] Briggs WH, Xiao H, Parkin KL, Shen C, Goldman IL. Differential inhibition of human platelet aggregation by selected Allium thiosulfinates. J Agric Food Chem 2000;48:5731–5.

[34] Butt MS, Sultan MT, Iqbal J. Garlic: nature's protection against physiological threats. Crit Rev Food Sci Nutr 2009;49:538–51.

[35] Ali M, Thomson M, Afzal M. Garlic and onions: their effect on eicosanoid metabolism and its clinical relevance. Prostaglandins Leukot Essent Fatty Acids 2000;62:55–73.

[36] Slimestad R, Fossen T, Vagen IM. Onions: a source of unique dietary flavonoids. J Agric Food Chem 2007;55:10067–80.

[37] Beato VM, Orgaz F, Mansilla F, Montano A. Changes in phenolic compounds in garlic (*Allium sativum* L.) owing to the cultivar and location of growth. Plant Foods Hum Nutr 2011;66:218–23.

[38] Srinivasan K. Plant foods in the management of diabetes mellitus: spices as beneficial antidiabetic food adjuncts. Int J Food Sci Nutr 2005;56:399–414.

[39] Kook S, Kim GH, Choi K. The antidiabetic effect of onion and garlic in experimental diabetic rats: meta-analysis. J Med Food 2009;12:552–60.

[40] Liu CT, Sheen LY, Lii CK. Does garlic have a role as an antidiabetic agent? Mol Nutr Food Res. 2007;51:1353–64.

[41] Padiya R, Banerjee SK. Garlic as an anti-diabetic agent: recent progress and patent reviews. Recent Pat Food Nutr Agric 2012.

[42] Vazquez-Prieto MA, Rodriguez Lanzi C, Lembo C, Galmarini CR, Miatello RM. Garlic and onion attenuates vascular inflammation and oxidative stress in fructose-fed rats. J Nutr Metab 2011;2011:475216.

[43] Kendler BS. Garlic (*Allium sativum*) and onion (*Allium cepa*): A review of their relationship to cardiovascular disease. Preventive Medicine 1987;16:670–85.

[44] Saraswat M, Reddy PY, Muthenna P, Reddy GB. Prevention of non-enzymic glycation of proteins by dietary agents: prospects for alleviating diabetic complications. Br J Nutr 2009;101:1714–21.

[45] Kumar R, Chhatwal S, Arora S, Sharma S, Singh J, Singh N, et al. Antihyperglycemic, antihyperlipidemic, anti-inflammatory and adenosine deaminase- lowering effects of garlic in patients with type 2 diabetes mellitus with obesity. Diabetes Metab Syndr Obes 2013;6:49–56.

[46] Taj Eldin IM, Ahmed EM, Elwahab HMA. preliminary study of the clinical hypoglycemic effects of *Allium cepa* (Red Onion) in Type 1 and Type 2 diabetic patients. Environ Health Insights 2010;4:71–7.

[47] Dall'Acqua S, Cervellati R, Speroni E, Costa S, Guerra MC, Stella L, et al. Phytochemical composition and antioxidant activity of *Laurus nobilis L.* leaf infusion. J Med Food 2009;12:869–76.

[48] Conforti F, Statti G, Uzunov D, Menichini F. Comparative chemical composition and antioxidant activities of wild and cultivated *Laurus nobilis L.* leaves and *Foeniculum vulgare* subsp. *piperitum* (Ucria) coutinho seeds. Biol Pharm Bull 2006;29:2056–64.

[49] Khan A, Zaman G, Anderson RA. Bay leaves improve glucose and lipid profile of people with type 2 diabetes. J Clin Biochem Nutr 2009;44:52–6.

[50] El-Ghorab AH, Nauman M, Anjum FM, Hussain S, Nadeem M. A comparative study on chemical composition and antioxidant activity of ginger (*Zingiber officinale*) and cumin (*Cuminum cyminum*). J Agric Food Chem. 2010;58:8231–7.

[51] Li Y, Tran VH, Duke CC, Roufogalis BD. preventive and protective properties of *Zingiber officinale* (ginger) in diabetes mellitus, diabetic complications, and associated lipid and other metabolic disorders: a brief review. Evid Based Complement Alternat Med 2012;2012:516870.

[52] Gupta SC, Patchva S, Aggarwal BB. Therapeutic roles of curcumin: lessons learned from clinical trials. AAPS J 2013; 15:195–218.

[53] El-Moselhy MA, Taye A, Sharkawi SS, El-Sisi SF, Ahmed AF. The antihyperglycemic effect of curcumin in high fat diet fed rats. Role of TNF-alpha and free fatty acids. Food Chem Toxicol 2011;49:1129–40.
[54] de Almeida Melo E, Mancini Filho J, Barbosa Guerra N. Characterization of antioxidant compounds in aqueous coriander extract (*Coriandrum sativum L.*). LWT-Food Sci Technol 2005;38: 15–9.
[55] Sowbhagya HB. Chemistry, technology, and nutraceutical functions of cumin (*Cuminum cyminum L*): an overview. Crit Rev Food Sci Nutr 2013;53:1–0.
[56] Jagtap AG, Patil PB. Antihyperglycemic activity and inhibition of advanced glycation end product formation by *Cuminum cyminum* in streptozotocin induced diabetic rats. Food Chem Toxicol 2010;48:2030–6.
[57] Kumar PA, Reddy PY, Srinivas PN, Reddy GB. Delay of diabetic cataract in rats by the antiglycating potential of cumin through modulation of alpha-crystallin chaperone activity. J Nutr Biochem 2009;20:553–62.
[58] Steinkellner H, Rabot S, Freywald C, Nobis E, Scharf G, Chabicovsky M, et al. Effects of cruciferous vegetables and their constituents on drug metabolizing enzymes involved in the bioactivation of DNA-reactive dietary carcinogens. Mutat Res. 2001;480–481:285–97.
[59] Thirumalai T, Therasa SV, Elumalai EK, David E. Hypoglycemic effect of *Brassica juncea* (seeds) on streptozotocin induced diabetic male albino rat. Asian Pacific J Tropical Biomed 2011;1:323–5.
[60] Srinivasan K. Black pepper and its pungent principle-piperine: a review of diverse physiological effects. Crit Rev Food Sci Nutr 2007;47:735–48.

CHAPTER

10

Resveratrol and Oxidative Stress in Diabetes Mellitus

Pál Brasnyó, Balázs Sümegi†, Gábor Winkler**, István Wittmann**

*Second Department of Medicine and Nephrological Center, Faculty of Medicine, University of Pécs, Pécs, Hungary, †Department of Biochemistry and Medical Chemistry, Faculty of Medicine, University of Pécs, Pécs, Hungary, **Second Department of Internal Medicine-Diabetology, St. John's Hospital, Budapest, Hungary

List of Abbreviations

Akt(PKB) Protein kinase B
AMPK Adenosine monophosphate-activated protein kinase
ATP Adenosine triphosphate
CCR 6 Chemokine receptor 6
CGMS Continuous glucose monitoring system
eNOS Endothelial nitric oxide synthase
ERK Extracellular signal regulated kinase
FOXO Forkhead box O
GLUT4 Glucose transporter type 4
HbA_{1C} Hemoglobin A_{1C}
HOMAβ homeostatic model assessment of β cell
$HOMA_{IR}$ Homeostasis model assessment insulin resistance
IL-1β Interleukin-1 beta
IL-6 Interleukin-6 iNOS inducible nitric oxide synthase
IRS Insulin receptor substrat
JNK c-Jun-N-terminal kinase
MAPK Mitogen-activated protein kinase
NADH Nicotinamide adenine dinucleotide reduced form
NADPH Nicotinamide adenine dinucleotide phosphate reduced form
NF-κB Nuclear factor-κB
NO Nitric oxide
Nrf2 Nuclear factor erythroid 2-related factor 2
PARP Poly(ADP-ribose) polymerase
PGC Peroxisome proliferator-activated receptor-γ coactivator
PI3-K Phosphatidylinositol 3-kinase
SirT Silent information regulator / sirtuin
STZ Streptozotocin
TNF-α Tumor necrosis factor-alpha
UCP2 Uncoupling protein 2

INTRODUCTION

It was estimated in the fifth edition of The International Diabetes Federation Diabetes Atlas that the global prevalence of diabetes mellitus continues to increase, and the number of diabetic patients will have risen from 366.2 million people in 2011 to 551.8 million by 2030. As a result of our modern way of life, diabetes mellitus has become a public healthcare problem of considerable magnitude in several countries. Whilst there is an increasing number of type 1 diabetic patients, mostly in Europe, the escalating prevalence of type 2 diabetes mellitus is responsible for the major health burden world-wide. This manifests in adulthood, largely due to unfavorable lifestyle factors and it accounts for 90% of all diabetes cases, as well as their associated cardiovascular co-morbidities [1,2].

In type 1 diabetes mellitus, increased levels of reactive oxygen species released from white blood cells during immune-mediated responses could induce the destruction of β-cells, which already possess a relatively low antioxidant capacity [3]. Oxidative stress induced by various factors (e.g., obesity, food intake) plays a pivotal role in the pathogenesis of type 2 diabetes by provoking insulin resistance and thus leading to development of the disease; in addition, the augmented oxidative stress resulting from adverse metabolic alterations also largely contributes to its progression [4,5].

Several mechanisms have been implicated in the increased oxidative stress in overt diabetes mellitus [4,6–9]. The levels of ortho-tyrosine and meta-tyrosine, both of which are exclusively generated from phenylalanine in response to hydroxyl free radical damage, have been found to closely correlate with the level of malondialdehyde products and oxidized fatty acids, and the activity of the pro-oxidant NADPH oxidase enzyme [10].

Insulin-mediated signaling cascades (e.g., phosphorylation of insulin receptor substrates [IRS], activation

Diabetes: Oxidative Stress and Dietary Antioxidants.
http://dx.doi.org/10.1016/B978-0-12-405885-9.00010-3

of the phosphatidylinositol 3-kinase [PI3-K], pathway, activation of Akt [protein kinase B] and other regulating proteins, translocation of the glucose transporter 4 [GLUT4] to the plasma membrane) are responsible for physiological, insulin-dependent, glucose uptake. Insulin is capable of increasing the availability of nitric oxide (NO), and this has an important role in the recruitment of precapillary nutritive arterioles via the IRS-1 – PI3K – Akt pathway [11–13].

In diabetes mellitus, the inactivation of Akt and the loss of GLUT4 translocation can be observed [14]. In response to oxidative stress, these aforementioned critical signaling pathways could be inhibited at several points, increasing the degree of insulin resistance, and thus contributing to the development of metabolic syndrome and type 2 diabetes, or further aggravating the metabolic disturbance associated with manifest diabetes mellitus [11,12,15].

Administration of antioxidants could represent a valuable strategy in both the prevention and management of diabetes mellitus. Ford et al. have fully discussed the possible links between metabolic syndrome and antioxidants [16].

The preventive effects of polyphenols, specifically of resveratrol, were first noticed in the analysis of the results of the so-called 'French Paradox' study, which recognized that, in France, regular consumption of small amounts of red wine resulted in decreased cardiovascular morbidity and mortality, in spite of the high fat food intake. The disease rates were low even with respect to other countries with comparable economic development and risk factors [19]. Following this observation, several animal and human studies have shown that moderate wine consumption decreases the risk of metabolic syndrome and its cardiovascular co-morbidities. Of more than 500 chemical compounds found in red wine, the beneficial effect has been primarily linked to the polyphenol resveratrol [20].

A number of studies have also investigated the beneficial effects of resveratrol in the prevention and treatment of diabetes, these findings will be discussed in more detail in the following sections.

THE ROLE OF RESVERATROL IN THE PREVENTION OF DIABETES MELLITUS

The Relationship of Resveratrol with Endothelial Nitric Oxide Synthase and Metabolic Syndrome

A number of beneficial effects have been put forward to explain the possible role of the antioxidant resveratrol [21] in the prevention/treatment of type 2 diabetes mellitus (Figure 10.1).

eNOS (endothelial nitric oxide synthase) plays a fundamental role in endothelially-dependent vasodilation via the synthesis of NO. A lack of eNOS activation and consequent abnormalities in the recruitment of nutritive precapillary arterioles could contribute to enhanced insulin resistance [12]. This hypothesis is supported by findings showing that features of metabolic syndrome were present in eNOS-depleted mice [20]. Human studies investigating the consequences of eNOS gene polymorphisms have demonstrated identical findings [20].

On the other hand, the polyphenols in red wine have been reported to improve endothelial dysfunction by

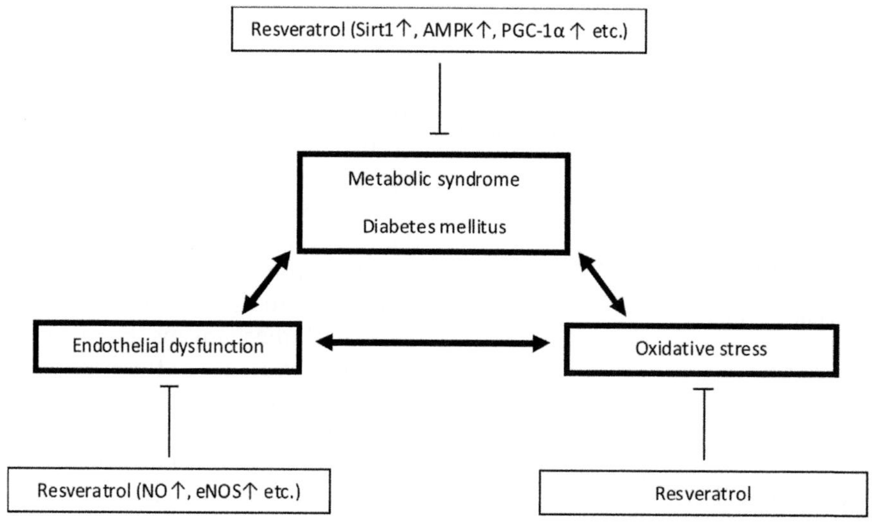

FIGURE 10.1 **The putative role of resveratrol in the prevention and treatment of diabetes mellitus.** Oxidative stress increases in insulin resistant conditions (e.g., metabolic syndrome, pre-diabetes, type 2 diabetes mellitus) and decreases eNOS activation, leading to endothelial dysfunction and decreased recruitment of nutritive precapillary arterioles, and as a vicious circle it could contribute to the enhanced insulin resistance. Resveratrol, via its direct and indirect antioxidant effects may decrease endothelial dysfunction by activating the eNOS-NO pathway, and this may play a role in the prevention of insulin resistance. *Unpublished figure.*

increasing NO production in *in vitro* cell studies. The polyphenols improved NO bioavailability due to their direct antioxidative action [22]. Alternatively, addition of polyphenols led to the activation of eNOS by increasing its activating phosphorylation [23]. Expression of the eNOS gene was also increased in endothelial cells treated with red wine polyphenols [24]. All the mechanisms leading to activation of the NO-eNOS pathway by resveratrol were found consistently in a wide array of *in vitro* cell studies (in endothelial cells, in aortic smooth muscle cells, in the aorta of mice), therefore it is conceivable that this is the pathway by which resveratrol contributes to the prevention of metabolic syndrome [9,25].

The Relationship between Resveratrol, Caloric Restriction and Metabolic Syndrome

Metabolic syndrome and caloric restriction could be considered as two opposite arms of a single metabolic spectrum. Liu et al. summarized the advantageous effects of caloric restriction: by counteracting components of metabolic syndrome, it defends against associated disorders, including cardiovascular disease, cancer, diabetes mellitus, and neurodegenerative disease [20]. Therefore, regulators which offer similar effects may have an important role in the prevention of metabolic syndrome and the other related diseases mentioned above. Accumulating evidence suggests that resveratrol could have a significant impact in modulating these mechanisms [20].

Recent studies have focused intensively on the molecule sirtuin1 (SirT1), a member of the sirtuins (SirTs) family [26]. Several reviews have acknowledged SirTs as important regulators of the biogenesis of mitochondria in the liver and muscle, as they increase oxidative phosphorylation via the deacetylation of peroxisome proliferator-activated receptor-γ coactivator (PGC)-1α. The SirTs could induce the mobilization of lipids in adipose tissue by inhibiting adipogenesis and activating lipolysis, and could protect pancreatic β-cells against hyperglycemia-induced oxidative stress via the deacetylation of Forkhead Box O (FOXO) transcription factors [20,27]. In addition, sirtuins in the pancreas could also stimulate the glucose-induced secretion of insulin by β-cells [28]. Furthermore, activation of SirT1 via FOXO increases the synthesis of adiponectin, which is known to improve sensitivity to insulin [29,30]. In the background, suppression of the oxidative stress regulated nuclear factor-κB (NF-κB) pathway seems to be involved through the neutralization of the toxic effects of tumor necrosis factor-α (TNF-α), suggesting that resveratrol could be important in decreasing oxidative stress [31]. The SirT1-induced activation of PGC-1α, and activation of the adenosine monophosphate-activated protein kinase (AMPK) pathway have been also shown to mediate the beneficial metabolic effects of resveratrol in experiments using mice [32,33].

In obese patients, treatment with resveratrol resulted in the activation of AMPK in muscles, while it also increased SirT1 and PGC-1α levels. In this study, decreased systolic blood pressure values and improved insulin resistance (HOMA index, Homeostasis model assessment) were also found after resveratrol treatment [34].

Activation of c-Jun-N-terminal kinase (JNK) in response to increased oxidative stress due to a high-calorie diet augmented insulin resistance in obese rats by blocking insulin signaling, an effect which could be prevented by antioxidants [35]. Augmentation of the insulin resistant state due to glucotoxicity- and lipotoxicity-induced oxidative stress has been shown to be associated with decreased SirT1 gene and protein expression levels, which could be prevented with resveratrol treatment, since the latter acts as a SirT1 activator. In addition, resveratrol markedly reduced p53 protein and JNK activity, and these are known to be important pathogenic factors in atherosclerosis, obesity, and insulin resistance [26]. Thus, the antioxidant effects of resveratrol could be also mediated via these putative mechanisms.

The responses seen with AMPK and SirT1 activation were analogous, which could be explained by noting that AMPK can be activated via SirT1, although this occurs in a dose-dependent manner with resveratrol (independent SirT1 activation takes place only with higher doses of resveratrol) [36].

The effects of resveratrol have been examined in prenatal hypoxia-induced intrauterine growth-restricted rats, an animal model of increased postnatal susceptibility to metabolic syndrome. Continued postnatal administration of resveratrol in rats fed a high-calorie diet decreased abdominal fat tissue, improved the lipid profile, and reduced the triglyceride accumulation compared to control littermates, even though they were kept on the same high-calorie diet. Administration of resveratrol also improved insulin sensitivity and glucose tolerance, indicating that it could prevent components of metabolic syndrome in these animals [37].

In endothelial cells, activation of AMPK was shown to activate eNOS by increasing its activating phosphorylation; thus, it is likely that activation of SirT1 via this mechanism could also contribute to reduced insulin resistance [20].

Resveratrol and the Prevention of Type 1 Diabetes Mellitus

Recent evidence indicates that oxidative stress plays an important role in the pathogenesis of type 1 diabetes mellitus [3]. T-cells in particular have been implicated in the destruction of pancreatic β-cells. One major consequence of activated T-cells is the release of inflammatory cytokines (e.g., TNF-α) which together with other factors increase the level of oxidative stress (e.g., iNOS activation) in β-cells, contributing to their decline [38]. The effects of resveratrol treatment in non-obese, diabetic mice showed that it inhibited the formation of chemokine receptor 6 (CCR6), by which it also suppressed the cellular infiltration of the pancreas islets [39]. This protective effect of resveratrol has also been confirmed in other reports. It has been documented that the signaling pathways of the c-Jun transcription factor, after its deacetylation by SirT1, are involved in T-cell mediated immune responses. In addition, administration of resveratrol increases the activity of SirT1 [39a,39b]. Moreover, involvement of CCR6 was found to be essential in activating T-helper 17 cells, and this has been linked to the development of type 1 diabetes in human studies [39c,39d,39e,39f]. Furthermore, inhibiting CCR6 formation with resveratrol resulted in suppressed cellular infiltration of the pancreas islets, with a concomitant decrease in oxidative stress, and thereby reduced β-cell injury [39]. Previous studies of isolated islet cells demonstrated that resveratrol prevented the inflammatory cytokines (i.e., interleukine-1β, interferone-γ) inducing β-cell injury by inhibiting the NF-κB pathway via SirT1 [40].

Ku et al. have studied potential mechanisms of β-cell injury and the effect of resveratrol pre-treatments in streptozotocin (STZ) induced diabetes, the most widely employed animal model of type 1 diabetes [41a]. A highly toxic and β-cell specific substance, STZ is known to induce the apoptosis of β-cells. It acts by inducing the increased production of reactive oxygen species and activating poly(ADP-ribose) polymerase (PARP). Treatment of rats with resveratrol inhibited the STZ-induced activation of PARP in the pancreas, while it had no effect on the synthesis of PARP. In addition, resveratrol treatment also inhibited the pro-apoptotic caspase-3 enzyme [41a]. Another workgroup studied human chondrocytes, and found that resveratrol was able to decrease PARP activation by inhibiting the caspase pathway, thus the abrogated PARP activation seen in the former study may also be mediated via the inhibition of caspase-3 [41b].

THE ROLE OF RESVERATROL IN THE TREATMENT OF DIABETES MELLITUS

The Effect of Resveratrol on Insulin Secretion

To date, only a small number of polyphenols have been shown to be beneficial to diabetes, but accumulating evidence suggests that resveratrol does indeed exert anti-diabetogenic effects. In 2004, electrophysiological studies using an INS-1 (beta) cell-line revealed that resveratrol caused the closure of pancreatic adenosine triphosphate (ATP) sensitive potassium channels by binding to sulfanylurea receptors, and this effect – similar to that seen with sulfanylureas – resulted in increased insulin secretion [42].

Moreover, resveratrol also enhanced ATP synthesis in β-cells by activating sirT1 and by inhibiting uncoupling protein 2 (UCP2) leading to increased insulin secretion. These effects could be verified in both the INS-1E (beta) cell-line and human pancreas islet cells [28].

The glucose-lowering effect of the incretin type glucagon-like peptide 1 (GLP-1) has been attributed, at least in part, to increases in glucose-dependent insulin secretion. In diabetic rats, GLP-1 secretion and the resultant insulin secretion were both increased after resveratrol treatment. Moreover, improved glucose tolerance due to other mechanisms could be also observed [43].

In other studies, treatment of diabetic rats with resveratrol was shown not only to improve blood sugar levels, but also to decrease the level of reactive oxygen species in the plasma and pancreatic tissue in conjunction with increased activity of antioxidant enzymes (superoxide dismutase, catalase, glutathione peroxidase, glutathione-S-transferase). Based on these findings, resveratrol could have broad application in contributing to decreasing oxidative stress in pancreatic β-cells, and thus improving insulin secretion [44].

Recently, a growing body of data supporting the beneficial effects of resveratrol has been reported. Resveratrol treatment was shown to alleviate higher levels of insulin secretion both in hyperinsulinemic rats and in the rat pancreas [44a,44b]. This could have an important role in preventing the β-cell depletion that results from sustained increases in insulin secretion, the major hallmark of type 2 diabetes mellitus. It is well known that intracellular glucose transport, oxidative glucose metabolism, hyperpolarization of the mitochondrial membrane, increased ATP synthesis, and a higher ratio of ATP/ADP are all important regulatory determinants of glucose-dependent insulin secretion [44c,44d]. Based on recent findings demonstrating that pre-treatment with resveratrol decreased the oxidation of glucose in pancreatic islet cells, and resulted in reduced activity of the mitochondrial respiratory chain, it is likely that reduced ATP levels in pancreatic islets could elicit transient and reversible reductions in insulin secretion [44].

In our previous human studies, we found that administration of resveratrol had no effect on insulin secretion, since HOMA values ($HOMA_\beta$) did not show a statistically significant change after resveratrol treatment (95.91 ± 19.32 vs. 74.68 ± 11.00) [45]. On the other hand, no resveratrol-induced significant changes were found in incretin levels (glucagon-like peptide 1, glucose-dependent insulinotropic peptide, amylin) [45].

Resveratrol, Oxidative Stress and the Treatment of Diabetes Mellitus

A promising therapeutic approach for the treatment of diabetes is provided by the fact that resveratrol is capable of decreasing oxidative stress via a number of different mechanisms (Figure 10.2).

Accordingly, resveratrol decreased the hyperglycemia-induced oxidative stress in human leukemia K562 cells as indicated by reduced levels of reactive oxygen species and suppressed activation of JNK and caspase-3, with concomitant decreases in apoptosis [46]. The impact of activating the SirT1-FOXO pathway on decreasing hyperglycemia-induced oxidative stress could be also present in manifest diabetes, since resveratrol was shown to enhance the production of superoxide dismutase 1 and 2 via the FOXO3 in diabetic mice [47]. Resveratrol treatment also decreased oxidative stress in STZ- and nicotinamide-induced diabetic rats, as indicated by reduced levels of lipid peroxide products, hydroperoxide, and protein carbonyl compounds in both the plasma and pancreas, while it led to the increased activity of superoxide dismutase, catalase, glutathione peroxidase, and glutathione-S-transferase enzymes in the pancreas. These changes were clearly associated with simultaneous reductions in the level of various pro-inflammatroy cytokines (i.e., TNF-α, IL-1β, IL-6). In addition, reduced blood glucose and glycated hemoglobin levels of rats could be also observed [44]. Consistent findings were demonstrated

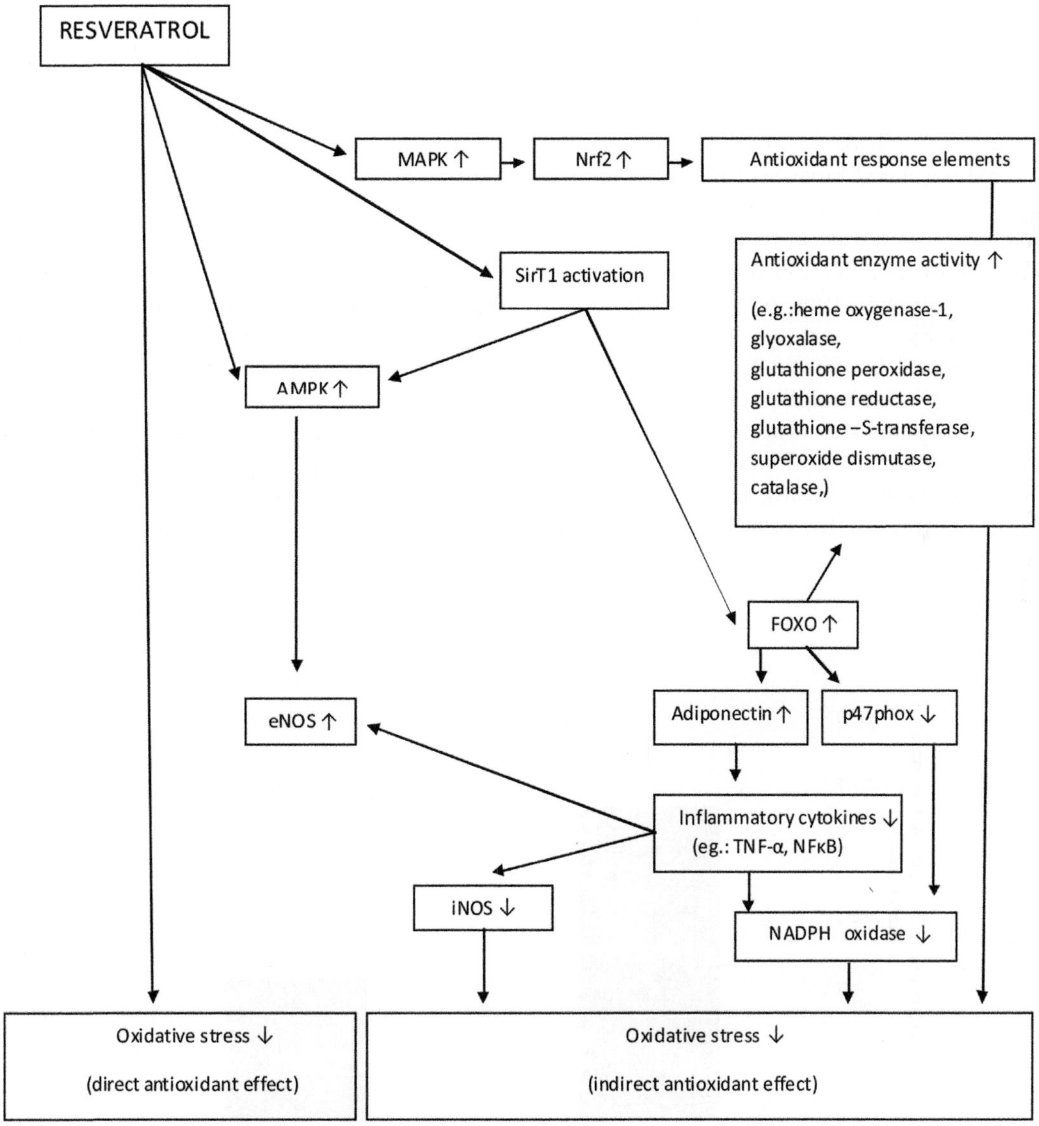

FIGURE 10.2 The direct and indirect antioxidant effects of resveratrol. The direct antioxidant properties of resveratrol could ensue from its activity as a free radical scavenger. It has the ability to indirectly activate antioxidant enzymes and other mechanisms. These indirect effects could be conferred either via increased expression/activation of SirT1, Nrf2, antioxidant enzymes or the suppression of iNOS and p47phox translocation/expression with the resultant inhibition of NAD(P)H oxidase. *Unpublished figure.*

in other experiments, which showed that resveratrol treatment of diabetic rats ameliorated glycated hemoglobin levels and reduced oxidative stress by increasing the level of reduced glutathione and antioxidant enzymes (i.e., superoxide dismutase, glutathione peroxidase, and catalase) [48].

The nuclear factor erythroid 2-related factor 2 (Nrf2) is known to be a key transcription factor in mediating the activation of antioxidant enzymes. Typically, binding of Nrf2 to the antioxidant-response elements induces and promotes the transcription of catalase, glutathione peroxidase, glutathione reductase, glutathione-S-transferase, superoxide dismutase, and heme oxygenase-1 [49]. It has been suggested that activation of Nrf2 by phosphorylation is regulated by MAPK, a pathway which could be activated by resveratrol [9]. In HepG2 cells exposed to methylglyoxal – which is a highly reactive dicarbonyl compound formed via the metabolism of glucose – resveratrol treatment augmented the activation of Nrf2 and elevated the levels of glyoxalase and heme oxygenase-1. In this study, resveratrol was found to activate the extracellular signal regulated kinase (ERK) by which the effect of resveratrol on activating Nrf2 could be mediated. Additional findings of this study included increases in intracellular glucose uptake, and a decrease in insulin resistance. However, activation of the JNK pathway could not be verified [8].

In monocytes isolated from type 1 diabetic patients, addition of resveratrol attenuated increases in hyperglycemia-induced superoxide anion production by eliciting the up-regulation of SirT1 and the induction of FOXOa3, as well as suppressing the expression of p47phox, an important regulator of monocyte NADPH oxidase localized in the cytosol [50].

The pro-oxidant enzyme iNOS is known to have a central role in mediating many oxidative-stress-induced deleterious effects, including ischemia/reperfusion-induced oxidative injury. Due to an additive effect, treatment of diabetic rats with resveratrol and insulin significantly improved blood glucose levels and insulin signaling (Akt/GLUT4), whereas it reduced the expression of iNOS/nitrotyrosine and superoxide anion production. In addition, resveratrol treatment alone resulted in enhanced survival rates [9]. In type 2 diabetic mice, administration of resveratrol increased eNOS expression in the myocardium, and decreased NAD(P)H oxidase activity, iNOS activation, mRNA synthesis of TNF-α, and NF-κB activation. These findings indicate that resveratrol reduces oxidative stress by inhibiting NAD(P)H oxidase and iNOS by suppressing TNF-α-mediated NF-κB. Alternatively, resveratrol could decrease endothelial dysfunction by up-regulating eNOS expression, which is crucial for preventing the recruitment of precapillary nutritive arterioles [51].

Resveratrol is able to substantially reduce the level of reactive oxygen species both *in vitro* and in a number of animal models of diabetes *in vivo*, either as a consequence of its direct antioxidant effects, or by increasing the activity/level of antioxidant enzymes, and/or inhibiting pro-oxidants. Administration of resveratrol in patients with type 2 diabetes mellitus resulted in decreased urinary ortho-tyrosine excretion rates, possibly due to the antioxidant actions of resveratrol (Figure 10.3) [45].

The Effect of Resveratrol on Insulin Resistance by Reducing Oxidative Stress

Insulin resistance could be enhanced by oxidative stress through activation of the JNK pathway. This

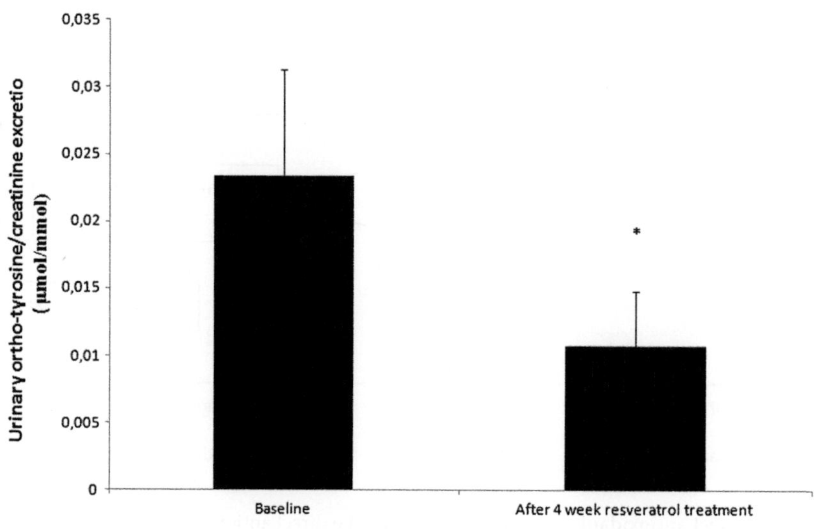

FIGURE 10.3 Urinary excretion rates of ortho-tyrosine/creatinine upon resveratrol treatment. Urinary excretion rates of ortho-tyrosine/creatinine, a marker of oxidative stress were significantly decreased (*$p < 0.05$) after resveratrol treatment for four weeks in type 2 diabetic patients. Values are means ± SEM. *Unpublished figure.*

could lead to, among other effects, inactivating the phosphorylation of IRS-1 which would inhibit insulin signaling at this point [35]. By interfering with multiple mechanisms, resveratrol is capable of reducing oxidative stress, and as shown earlier, it efficiently decreased JNK activity in human cell studies [26]. Resveratrol treatment improved blood sugar levels in diabetic rats, and this was associated with significant increases in the activating phosphorylation of Akt, which is considered as one of the key elements of the insulin signaling cascade. There were subsequent increases in the activating phosphorylation of eNOS, and the activation of the antioxidant thioredoxin and heme oxygenase-1 [52]. Our earlier studies found that treatment of diabetic patients with resveratrol reduced oxidative stress and improved the glycemic state, and these effects were also associated with increases in the activating phosphorylation of Akt (Figure 10.4) [45].

It has been demonstrated *in vitro* (e.g., in endothelial cells, aortic smooth muscle cells, aortas of mice) that resveratrol activates eNOS by increasing its PI3K/Akt-mediated activating phosphorylation and/or eNOS gene expression. Given that resveratrol is chemically analogous to estrogen, by binding to its receptor, resveratrol most likely induces the activation of the mitogen-activated protein kinase (MAPK) pathway. it has been shown in human umbilical cells that activation of MAPK could also lead to increased eNOS activation [9,25].

The loss of eNOS activation and consequent recruitment of nutritive pre-capillary arterioles could make important contributions to the augmentation of the insulin resistant state [12]. Taken together, the effect of resveratrol on reducing the insulin resistance can be attributed to increased eNOS activation resulting from the decreased oxidative stress and hence improved signaling responses to insulin.

Resveratrol treatment of diabetic rats has been found to increase the expression of GLUT4 transporter, thus this mechanism could also contribute to the observed decrease in insulin resistance [44]. The pro-inflammatory cytokines (e.g., TNF-α, IL-6) are the major mediating factors responsible for enhancing insulin resistance [53,54], and their levels were found to show a reciprocal relationship with adiponectin levels [55]. It has been demonstrated that resveratrol suppressed NF-κB activation in a TNF-α-mediated manner in cells isolated from human umbilical veins [56], and that it increased adiponectin levels mediated via the protein kinase B (Akt)/FOXO1 and AMPK signaling pathways in L3T3-L1 adipocytes; this appeared to be independent of SirT1 activation [57]. In diabetic rats, administration of resveratrol improved the glycemic state and was also associated with reduced levels of inflammatory mediators (i.e., TNF-α, IL-1β, IL-6) and the activation of the p65 subunit of NF-κB transcription factor. Using the linoleinic acid-induced model of insulin resistance, addition of resveratrol to human adipocytes reduced the inflammatory cytokine levels by suppressing the inflammatory prostaglandin pathway, as well as enhancing PPAR-γ activity, leading to increases in insulin-dependent glucose uptake [44]. Resveratrol in diabetic rats blocked the effect of TNF-α and the subsequent activation of NAD(P)H oxidase, which is known to increase oxidative stress. These changes were also associated with increased eNOS phosphorylation at the serine residue [15]. Moreover, resveratrol treatment in bovine aortic

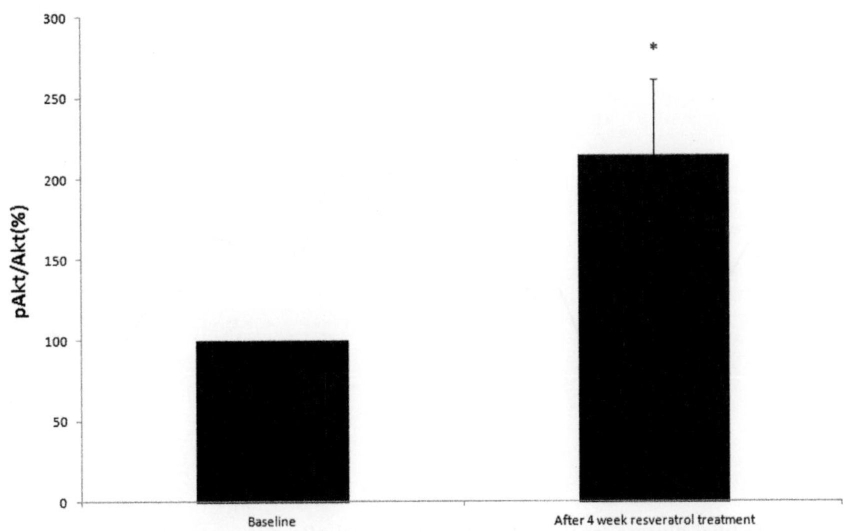

FIGURE 10.4 Changes of activating phosphorylation of Akt in platelets upon resveratrol treatment. The activating phosphorylation of Akt, a key regulating factor of the insulin signaling pathway showed a significant increase (*P < 0.05) in platelets isolated from type 2 diabetic patients treated with resveratrol for four weeks. Values after resveratrol treatment are means ± SEM. *Unpublished figure.*

endothelial cells also increased the activating phosphorylations of Akt, eNOS, and ERK. In addition, resveratrol blunted the activation of NADP(H) oxidase in cells subjected to exogenously given TNF-α in a dose-dependent manner [58]. Intraperitoneal administration of resveratrol to rats resulted in enhanced blood flow in the muscle microvasculature via an eNOS-dependent mechanism, which could be blunted with TNF-α infusions applied prior to resveratrol treatment [58].

These findings indicate that resveratrol could significantly reduce the effects of inflammatory cytokines and oxidative stress in diabetes. As noted above, its effect on eNOS activation could decrease the recruitment of precapillary nutritive arterioles, and thus also decrease insulin resistance.

In addition to the notion that resveratrol improves insulin-mediated signaling responses, there is an alternative mechanism by which resveratrol could decrease the insulin resistance and increase eNOS activation, and this is via the activation of the SirT1 – PGC-1α – AMPK pathway [26,32,33,47,57].

We found that resveratrol treatment of type 2 diabetic patients consistently attenuated insulin resistance, as assessed by decreased HOMA indices. This was possibly due to reduced levels of oxidative stress (Figure 10.5) [45].

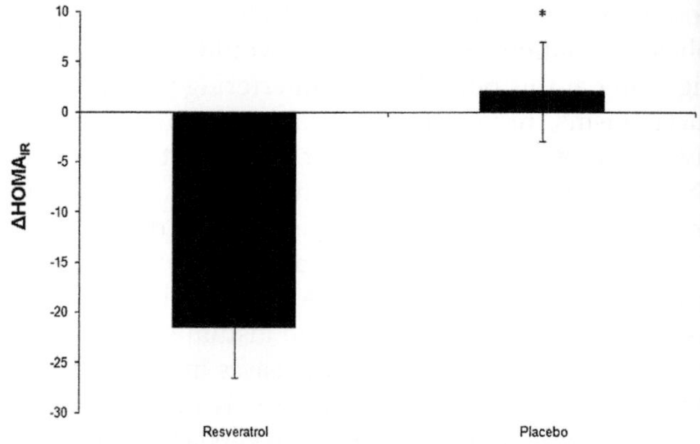

FIGURE 10.5 Percentile changes of insulin resistance upon resveratrol treatment. Insulin resistance was significantly decreased ($^*P<0.05$) in type 2 diabetic patients following resveratrol treatment for four weeks, as indicated by significant reductions in $HOMA_{IR}$ values (homeostasis model assessment insulin resistance). Values between baseline and week 4 for the placebo and resveratrol groups are means ± SEM. *Unpublished figure.*

Resveratrol Affects Serum Glucose Levels by Reducing Oxidative Stress

Resveratrol treatment of diabetic animals reduces oxidative stress, increases sensitivity to insulin, and restores critical events downstream to the insulin signaling pathway, all of which result in improvements in glucose metabolism [44,48]. Our findings also indicated that by reducing oxidative stress, improving the insulin signaling pathway, and increasing insulin sensitivity, resveratrol could ameliorate blood glucose levels and the glycemic state of patients with type 2 diabetes, which we demonstrated by measurements using a continuous glucose monitoring system (CGMS) [45] (Figure 10.6). We found that the time intervals before the appearance of maximal interstitial glucose levels following test meals were significantly increased in resveratrol-treated patients [45] (Figure 10.7), however, possible involvement of an incretin-induced effect (glucagon-like peptide 1,

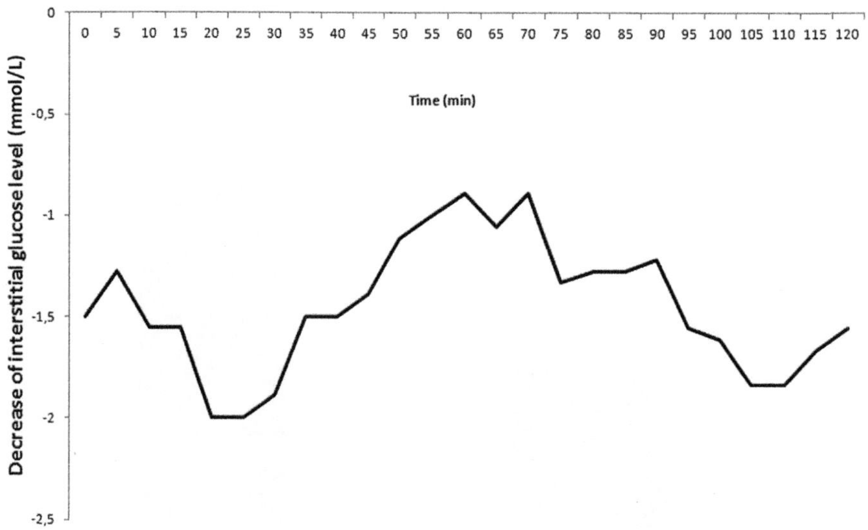

FIGURE 10.6 Postprandial interstitial glucose levels following a test meal after resveratrol treatment. Postprandial interstitial glucose levels following a test meal were decreased in type 2 diabetic patients after four weeks of resveratrol treatment. This figure demonstrates a calculated representative differential curve of two records of interstitial glucose levels registered at baseline and week 4 using CGMS (continuous glucose monitoring system). In resveratrol-treated patients, the mean value of interstitial glucose levels at the 25th, 30th, and 35th minutes were significantly reduced ($p<0.05$) compared to the baseline values, and also suggested a decreasing tendency at all measured time-points. *Unpublished figure.*

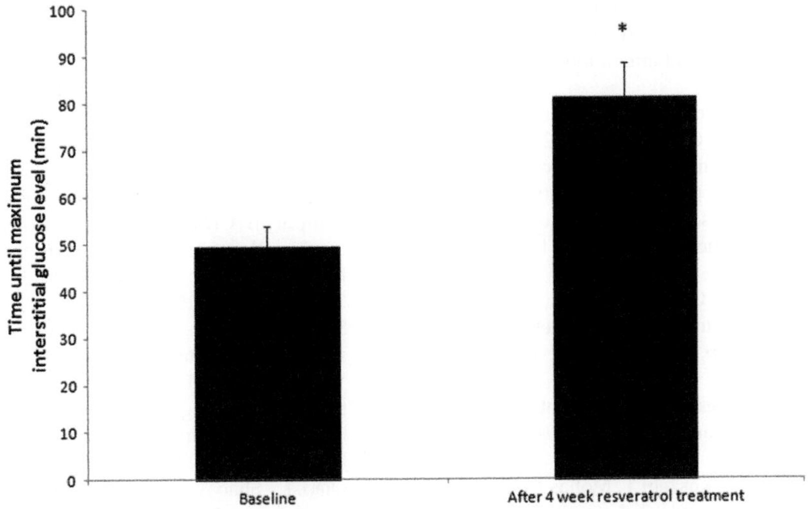

FIGURE 10.7 **Time until maximum interstitial glucose level after resveratrol treatment.** Lag time between test meal intake and the appearance of maximal interstitial glucose concentrations, as measured by CGMS (continuous glucose monitoring system) in type 2 diabetic patients, was significantly lengthened (*$p < 0.05$) after resveratrol treatment for four weeks. Values are means ± SEM. *Unpublished figure.*

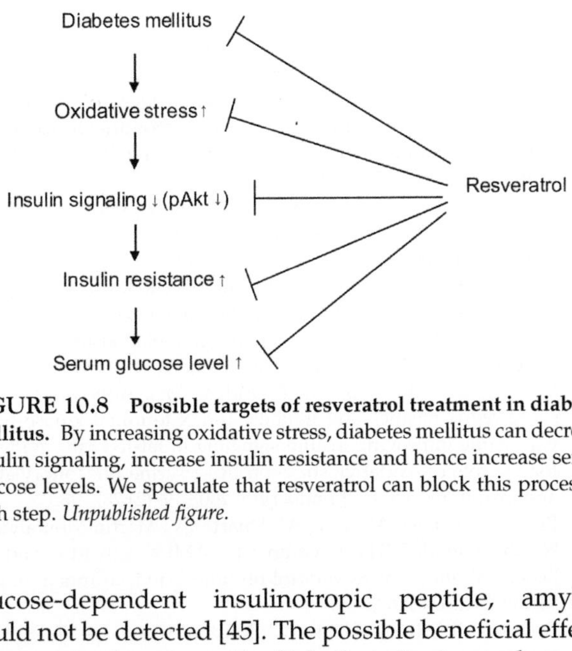

FIGURE 10.8 **Possible targets of resveratrol treatment in diabetes mellitus.** By increasing oxidative stress, diabetes mellitus can decrease insulin signaling, increase insulin resistance and hence increase serum glucose levels. We speculate that resveratrol can block this process at each step. *Unpublished figure.*

glucose-dependent insulinotropic peptide, amylin) could not be detected [45]. The possible beneficial effects of resveratrol treatment in diabetic patients are shown in Figure 10.8.

Reports by other groups have also demonstrated the beneficial effects of resveratrol in type 2 diabetes mellitus. Accordingly, diabetic patients taking supplementation by resveratrol in addition to regular oral hypoglycemic agents showed significantly reduced HbA_{1c} values, systolic blood pressure, and total cholesterol levels [59].

SUMMARY POINTS

- The global prevalence of diabetes mellitus is increasing.
- Diabetes mellitus and related micro- and macrovascular complications are major causes of morbidity and mortality.
- Oxidative stress plays a key role in the pathogenesis of type 1 and 2 diabetes mellitus and their related complications.
- Resveratrol has advantageous effects in insulin resistant conditions by decreasing oxidative injury via direct and indirect antioxidant effects.
- In diabetics, antioxidant resveratrol treatment could markedly decrease insulin resistance and serum glucose levels via an increase in insulin signaling.
- Resveratrol could also improve carbohydrate metabolism by promoting similar beneficial metabolic processes to those found in caloric restriction via the activation of SirT1.
- Administration of resveratrol in combination with healthier dietary food intake and regular physical activity (i.e., healthier lifestyle) may be an effective strategy for the prevention of diabetes mellitus, and together with oral anti-diabetic agents an effective strategy for its treatment.

References

[1] Shaw JE, Sicree RA, Zimmet PZ. Global estimates of the prevalence of diabetes for 2010 and 2030. Diabetes Res Clin Pract 2010;87(1):4–14.
[2] International Diabetes Federation: IDF Diabetes Atlas. 5th ed. Brussels: Belgium; 2011. www.idf.org/diabetesatlas.
[3] Oberley LW. Free radicals and diabetes. Free Radic Biol Med 1988:113–24.
[4] Ceriello A, Motz E. Is oxidative stress the pathogenic mechanism underlying insulin resistance, diabetes, and cardiovascular disease? The common soil hypothesis revisited. Arterioscler Thromb Vasc Biol 2004;24(5):816–23.

[5] Garcia-Bailo B, El-Sohemy A, Haddad PS, Arora P, Benzaied F, Karmali M, et al. Vitamins D, C, and E in the prevention of type 2 diabetes mellitus: modulation of inflammation and oxidative stress. Biologics 2011;5:7–19.

[6] King GL, Loeken MR. Hyperglycemia-induced oxidative stress in diabetic complications. Histochem Cell Biol 2004;122(4):333–8.

[7] Folli F, Corradi D, Fanti P, Davalli A, Paez A, Giaccari A, et al. The role of oxidative stress in the pathogenesis of type 2 diabetes mellitus micro- and macrovascular complications: avenues for a mechanistic-based therapeutic approach. Curr Diabetes Rev 2011;7(5):313–24.

[8] Cheng AS, Cheng YH, Chiou CH, Chang TL. Resveratrol up-regulates nrf2 expression to attenuate methylglyoxal-induced insulin resistance in hep g2 cells. J Agric Food Chem 2012;60(36):9180–7.

[9] Turan B, Tuncay E, Vassort G. Resveratrol and diabetic cardiac function: focus on recent *in vitro* and *in vivo* studies. J Bioenerg Biomembr 2012;44(2):281–96.

[10] Molnár GA, Wagner Z, Markó L, Kőszegi T, Mohás M, Kocsis B, et al. Urinary ortho-tyrosine excretion in diabetes mellitus and renal failure: evidence for hydroxyl radical production. Kidney Int 2005;68(5):2281–7.

[11] Mlinar B, Marc J, Janez A, Pfeifer M. Molecular mechanisms of insulin resistance and associated diseases. Clin Chim Acta 2007;375(1–2):20–35.

[12] Jonk AM, Houben AJ, de Jongh RT, Serné EH, Schaper NC, Stehouwer CD. Microvascular dysfunction in obesity: a potential mechanism in the pathogenesis of obesity-associated insulin resistance and hypertension. Physiology (Bethesda) 2007;22:252–60.

[13] Chakraborty C, Roy SS, Hsu MJ, Agoramoorthy G. Landscape mapping of functional proteins in insulin signal transduction and insulin resistance: a network-based protein-protein interaction analysis. PLoS One 2011;6(1):e16388.

[14] Tirosh A, Potashnik R, Bashan N, Rudich A. Oxidative stress disrupts insulin-induced cellular redistribution of insulin receptor substrate-1 and phosphatidylinositol 3-kinase in 3T3-L1 adipocytes. A putative cellular mechanism for impaired protein kinase B activation and GLUT4 translocation. J Biol Chem 1999;274(15):10595–602.

[15] Zhang H, Zhang J, Ungvari Z, Zhang C. Resveratrol improves endothelial function: role of TNF{alpha} and vascular oxidative stress. Arterioscler Thromb Vasc Biol 2009;29(8):1164–71.

[16] Ford ES, Mokdad AH, Giles WH, Brown DW. The metabolic syndrome and antioxidant concentrations: findings from the Third National Health and Nutrition Examination Survey. Diabetes 2003;52(9):2346–52.

[17] Halliwell B, Gutteridge JMC. Free radicals in biology and medicine. Oxford: Clarendon Press; 1989.

[18] Flechner I, Maruta K, Burkart V, Kawai K, Kolb H, Kiesel U. Effects of radical scavengers on the development of experimental diabetes. Diabetes Res 1990;13(2):67–73.

[19] Renaud S, de Lorgeril M. Wine, alcohol, platelets, and the French paradox for coronary heart disease. Lancet 1992;339(8808):1523–6.

[20] Liu L, Wang Y, Lam KS, Xu A. Moderate wine consumption in the prevention of metabolic syndrome and its related medical complications. Endocr Metab Immune Disord Drug Targets 2008;8(2):89–98.

[21] Frombaum M, Le Clanche S, Bonnefont-Rousselot D, Borderie D. Antioxidant effects of resveratrol and other stilbene derivatives on oxidative stress and *NO bioavailability: Potential benefits to cardiovascular diseases. Biochimie 2012;94(2):269–76.

[22] Soleas GJ, Diamandis EP, Goldberg DM. Wine as a biological fluid: history, production, and role in disease prevention. J Clin Lab Anal 1997;11(5):287–313.

[23] Ndiaye M, Chataigneau T, Chataigneau M, Schini-Kerth VB. Red wine polyphenols induce EDHF-mediated relaxations in porcine coronary arteries through the redox-sensitive activation of the PI3-kinase/Akt pathway. Br J Pharmacol 2004;142(7):1131–6.

[24] Leikert JF, Räthel TR, Wohlfart P, Cheynier V, Vollmar AM, Dirsch VM. Red wine polyphenols enhance endothelial nitric oxide synthase expression and subsequent nitric oxide release from endothelial cells. Circulation 2002;106(13):1614–7.

[25] Takahashi S, Nakashima Y. Repeated and long-term treatment with physiological concentrations of resveratrol promotes NO production in vascular endothelial cells. Br J Nutr 2012;107(6):774–80.

[26] de Kreutzenberg SV, Ceolotto G, Papparella I, Bortoluzzi A, Semplicini A, Dalla Man C, et al. Downregulation of the longevity-associated protein sirtuin 1 in insulin resistance and metabolic syndrome: potential biochemical mechanisms. Diabetes 2010;59(4):1006–15.

[27] Schwer B, Verdin E. Conserved metabolic regulatory functions of sirtuins. Cell Metab 2008;7(2):104–12.

[28] Vetterli L, Brun T, Giovannoni L, Bosco D, Maechler P. Resveratrol potentiates glucose-stimulated insulin secretion in INS-1E beta-cells and human islets through a SIRT1-dependent mechanism. J Biol Chem 2011;286(8):6049–60.

[29] Qiao L, Shao J. SIRT1 regulates adiponectin gene expression through Foxo1-C/enhancer-binding protein alpha transcriptional complex. J Biol Chem 2006;281(52):39915–24.

[30] Banks AS, Kon N, Knight C, Matsumoto M, Gutiérrez-Juárez R, Rossetti L, et al. SirT1 gain of function increases energy efficiency and prevents diabetes in mice. Cell Metab 2008;8(4):333–41.

[31] Nakanishi S, Yamane K, Kamei N, Nojima H, Okubo M, Kohno N. A protective effect of adiponectin against oxidative stress in Japanese Americans: the association between adiponectin or leptin and urinary isoprostane. Metabolism 2005;54(2):194–9.

[32] Lagouge M, Argmann C, Gerhart-Hines Z, Meziane H, Lerin C, Daussin F, et al. Resveratrol improves mitochondrial function and protects against metabolic disease by activating SIRT1 and PGC-1alpha. Cell 2006;127(6):1109–22.

[33] Baur JA, Pearson KJ, Price NL, Jamieson HA, Lerin C, Kalra A, et al. Resveratrol improves health and survival of mice on a high-calorie diet. Nature 2006;444(7117):337–42.

[34] Timmers S, Konings E, Bilet L, Houtkooper RH, van de Weijer T, Goossens GH, et al. Calorie restriction-like effects of 30 days of resveratrol supplementation on energy metabolism and metabolic profile in obese humans. Cell Metab 2011;14(5):612–22.

[35] Vinayagamoorthi R, Bobby Z, Sridhar MG. Antioxidants preserve redox balance and inhibit c-Jun-N-terminal kinase pathway while improving insulin signaling in fat-fed rats: evidence for the role of oxidative stress on IRS-1 serine phosphorylation and insulin resistance. J Endocrinol 2008;197(2):287–96.

[36] Price NL, Gomes AP, Ling AJ, Duarte FV, Martin-Montalvo A, North BJ, et al. SIRT1 is required for AMPK activation and the beneficial effects of resveratrol on mitochondrial function. Cell Metab 2012;15(5):675–90.

[37] Dolinsky VW, Rueda-Clausen CF, Morton JS, Davidge ST, Dyck JR. Continued postnatal administration of resveratrol prevents diet-induced metabolic syndrome in rat offspring born growth restricted. Diabetes 2011;60(9):2274–84.

[38] Atkinson MA, Bluestone JA, Eisenbarth GS, Hebrok M, Herold KC, Accili D, et al. How does type 1 diabetes develop? The notion of homicide or β-cell suicide revisited. Diabetes 2011;60(5):1370–9.

[39] Lee SM, Yang H, Tartar DM, Gao B, Luo X, Ye SQ, et al. Prevention and treatment of diabetes with resveratrol in a non-obese mouse model of type 1 diabetes. Diabetologia 2011;54(5):1136–46.

[39a] Borra MT, Smith BC, Denu JM. Mechanism of human SIRT1 activation by resveratrol. J Biol Chem 2005;280(17):17187–95.

[39b] Zhang J, Lee SM, Shannon S, Gao B, Chen W, Chen A, et al. The type III histone deacetylase Sirt1 is essential for maintenance of T cell tolerance in mice. J Clin Invest 2009;119(10):3048–58.

[39c] Reboldi A, Coisne C, Baumjohann D, Benvenuto F, Bottinelli D, Lira S, et al. C-C chemokine receptor 6-regulated entry of TH-17 cells into the CNS through the choroid plexus is required for the initiation of EAE. Nat Immunol 2009;10(5):514–23.

[39d] Emamaullee JA, Davis J, Merani S, Toso C, Elliott JF, Thiesen A, et al. Inhibition of Th17 cells regulates autoimmune diabetes in NOD mice. Diabetes 2009;58(6):1302–11.
[39e] Marwaha AK, Crome SQ, Panagiotopoulos C, Berg KB, Qin H, Ouyang Q, et al. Cutting edge: Increased IL-17-secreting T cells in children with new-onset type 1 diabetes. J Immunol 2010;185(7):3814–8.
[39f] Honkanen J, Nieminen JK, Gao R, Luopajarvi K, Salo HM, Ilonen J, et al. IL-17 immunity in human type 1 diabetes. J Immunol 2010;185(3):1959–67.
[40] Lee JH, Song MY, Song EK, Kim EK, Moon WS, Han MK, et al. Overexpression of SIRT1 protects pancreatic beta-cells against cytokine toxicity by suppressing the nuclear factor-kappaB signaling pathway. Diabetes 2009;58(2):344–51.
[41a] Ku CR, Lee HJ, Kim SK, Lee EY, Lee MK, Lee EJ. Resveratrol prevents streptozotocin-induced diabetes by inhibiting the apoptosis of pancreatic β-cell and the cleavage of poly (ADP-ribose) polymerase. Endocr J 2012;59(2):103–9.
[41b] Shakibaei M, John T, Seifarth C, Mobasheri A. Resveratrol inhibits IL-1 beta-induced stimulation of caspase-3 and cleavage of PARP in human articular chondrocytes *in vitro*. Ann N Y Acad Sci 2007;1095:554–63.
[42] Zhang Y, Jayaprakasam B, Seeram NP, Olson LK, DeWitt D, Nair MG. Insulin secretion and cyclooxygenase enzyme inhibition by cabernet sauvignon grape skin compounds. J Agric Food Chem 2004;52(2):228–33.
[43] Dao TM, Waget A, Klopp P, Serino M, Vachoux C, Pechere L, et al. Resveratrol increases glucose induced GLP-1 secretion in mice: a mechanism which contributes to the glycemic control. PLoS One 2011;6(6):e20700.
[44] Szkudelski T, Szkudelska K. Anti-diabetic effects of resveratrol. Ann N Y Acad Sci 2011;1215:34–9.
[44a] Rivera L, Morón R, Zarzuelo A, Galisteo M. Long-term resveratrol administration reduces metabolic disturbances and lowers blood pressure in obese Zucker rats. Biochem Pharmacol 2009;77(6):1053–63.
[44b] Szkudelski T. Resveratrol inhibits insulin secretion from rat pancreatic islets. Eur J Pharmacol 2006;552(1–3):176–81.
[44c] Henquin JC. Triggering and amplifying pathways of regulation of insulin secretion by glucose. Diabetes 2000;49(11):1751–60.
[44d] Maechler P. Mitochondria as the conductor of metabolic signals for insulin exocytosis in pancreatic beta-cells. Cell Mol Life Sci 2002;59(11):1803–18.
[45] Brasnyó P, Molnár GA, Mohás M, Markó L, Laczy B, Cseh J, et al. Resveratrol improves insulin sensitivity, reduces oxidative stress and activates the Akt pathway in type 2 diabetic patients. Br J Nutr 2011;106(3):383–9.
[46] Chan WH. Effect of resveratrol on high glucose-induced stress in human leukemia K562 cells. J Cell Biochem 2005;94(6):1267–79.
[47] Kim MY, Lim JH, Youn HH, Hong YA, Yang KS, Park HS, et al. Resveratrol prevents renal lipotoxicity and inhibits mesangial cell glucotoxicity in a manner dependent on the AMPK-SIRT1-PGC1α axis in db/db mice. Diabetologia 2013;56(1):204–17.
[48] Soufi FG, Sheervalilou R, Vardiani M, Khalili M, Alipour MR. Chronic resveratrol administration has beneficial effects in experimental model of type 2 diabetic rats. Endocr Regul 2012;46(2):83–90.
[49] Kobayashi M, Yamamoto M. Nrf2-Keap1 regulation of cellular defense mechanisms against electrophiles and reactive oxygen species. Adv Enzyme Regul 2006;46:113–40.
[50] Yun JM, Chien A, Jialal I, Devaraj S. Resveratrol up-regulates SIRT1 and inhibits cellular oxidative stress in the diabetic milieu: mechanistic insights. J Nutr Biochem 2012;23(7):699–705.
[51] Zhang H, Morgan B, Potter BJ, Ma L, Dellsperger KC, Ungvari Z, et al. Resveratrol improves left ventricular diastolic relaxation in type 2 diabetes by inhibiting oxidative/nitrative stress: *in vivo* demonstration with magnetic resonance imaging. Am J Physiol Heart Circ Physiol 2010;299(4):H985–94.
[52] Thirunavukkarasu M, Penumathsa SV, Koneru S, Juhasz B, Zhan L, Otani H, et al. Resveratrol alleviates cardiac dysfunction in streptozotocin-induced diabetes: Role of nitric oxide, thioredoxin, and heme oxygenase. Free Radic Biol Med 2007;43(5):720–9.
[53] Winkler G, Lakatos P, Salamon F, Nagy Z, Speer G, Kovács M, et al. Elevated serum TNF-alpha level as a link between endothelial dysfunction and insulin resistance in normotensive obese patients. Diabet Med 1999;16(3):207–11.
[54] Cseh K, Baranyi E, Melczer Z, Csákány GM, Speer G, Kovács M, et al. The pathophysiological influence of leptin and the tumor necrosis factor system on maternal insulin resistance: negative correlation with anthropometric parameters of neonates in gestational diabetes. Gynecol Endocrinol 2002;16(6):453–60.
[55] Hays NP, Galassetti PR, Coker RH. Prevention and treatment of type 2 diabetes: current role of lifestyle, natural product, and pharmacological interventions. Pharmacol Ther 2008;118(2):181–91.
[56] Labinskyy N, Csiszar A, Veress G, Stef G, Pacher P, Oroszi G, et al. Vascular dysfunction in aging: potential effects of resveratrol, an anti-inflammatory phytoestrogen. Curr Med Chem 2006;13(9):989–96.
[57] Wang A, Liu M, Liu X, Dong LQ, Glickman RD, Slaga TJ, et al. Up-regulation of adiponectin by resveratrol: the essential roles of the Akt/FOXO1 and AMP-activated protein kinase signaling pathways and DsbA-L. J Biol Chem 2011;286(1):60–6.
[58] Wang N, Ko SH, Chai W, Li G, Barrett EJ, Tao L, et al. Resveratrol recruits rat muscle microvasculature via a nitric oxide-dependent mechanism that is blocked by TNFα. Am J Physiol Endocrinol Metab 2011;300(1):E195–201.
[59] Bhatt JK, Thomas S, Nanjan MJ. Resveratrol supplementation improves glycemic control in type 2 diabetes mellitus. Nutr Res 2012;32(7):537–41.

CHAPTER

11

Vitamin D, Oxidative Stress and Diabetes: Is There A Link?

Tirang R. Neyestani

National Nutrition and Food Technology Research Institute (NNFTRI) and Faculty of Nutrition Science and Food Technology, Shahid Beheshti University of Medical Sciences, Tehran, Iran

List of Abbreviations

AGEs Advanced glycation end products
AOPPs Advanced oxidation protein products
ATP adenosine triphosphate
CGD Chronic granulomatous disease
CVD Cardiovascular disease
DBP Vitamin D binding protein
DR-3 Direct repeat-3
FGF Fibroblast growth factor
GGT γ-glutamyl transpeptidase
GSH Glutathione
GSH-Px Glutathione peroxidase
G6PD Glucose-6-phosphate dehydrogenase
hsCRP Highly sensitive C-reactive protein
IFG Impaired fasting glucose
IL Interleukin
LDL Low density lipoprotein
MDA Malondialdehyde
MPO Myeloperoxidase
OS Oxidative stress
ox-LDL Oxidized low density lipoprotein
PCO Protein carbonyl
QUICKI Quantitative insulin sensitivity check index
RAGE Advanced glycation end products receptor
ROS Reactive oxygen species
SOD Superoxide dismutase
T2D Type 2 diabetes
VCAM-1 Vascular cell adhesion molecule-1
VDR Vitamin D receptor

INTRODUCTION

From the phylogenic and ontogenic points of view, the formation of reactive oxygen species (ROS) is among the earliest innate defense mechanisms against pathogenic invaders. A plant cell produces superoxide or hydrogen peroxide in response to an invading pathogen. By this, it reinforces its cell wall and makes a lattice-work around the pathogen to restrict its further movement and reproduction. In higher animals, including humans, immune cells, notably macrophages, play their role in ROS production when they encounter intruding pathogens. Following binding of microbial molecules to macrophage cell surface receptors, a myriad of reactions are triggered, resulting in engulfment and internalization of the pathogen by the macrophage. To complete its job, the macrophage generates ROS to kill the pathogen through a series of reactions called 'respiratory burst'. Impairment of the respiratory burst often seen in chronic granulomatous disease (CGD) is accompanied by high occurrence of opportunistic infections [1].

Generation of ROS, though crucial, is not confined just to the immune reactions. In aerobic organisms, ROS are formed as normal products of cellular metabolism. Conversion of the cellular energy to the usable form adenosine triphosphate (ATP) in mitochondria is accompanied by the generation of ample amounts of free radicals, which leak out to the cytosol where they form ROS molecules such as superoxide anion and hydroxyl radicals. Because they have unpaired electrons, free radicals may attack other molecules and make them into new free radicals – so a chain reaction may occur. Since the attacked molecule is oxidized by losing electrons, free radicals may also be called 'pro-oxidants' (or proxidants, in short). It is believed that the excess amounts of these proxidants are deactivated by endogenous and exogenous antioxidants so there is a 'balance' between free radicals and antioxidants. However, under certain circumstances, such as impairment of endogenous antioxidant systems, low intake of dietary antioxidant-rich foods (notably fruits and vegetables) and/or overproduction of free radicals, this balance would be disturbed with a shift towards proxidants, a condition known as

Diabetes: Oxidative Stress and Dietary Antioxidants.
http://dx.doi.org/10.1016/B978-0-12-405885-9.00011-5

'oxidative stress' (OS). A great deal of evidence has associated OS with many human pathologies including cancers, atherosclerosis and diabetes [2]. Though augmented OS has been shown in most, if not all, of these conditions, the causality is still unclear. Indeed, exacerbation of OS in these conditions is like finding a man with a smoking gun in hand at the murder scene!

Nevertheless, the link between OS and development of diabetes and its long-term complications has been documented [3], raising the hope of combating the morbidities with antioxidants. However, although short-term interventions have provided evidence on attenuation of OS following antioxidant supplementation, most long-term studies failed to show any significant clinical improvement in diabetic patients due to antioxidant supplementation [4].

Vitamin D can be endogenously synthesized in the body under the influence of the ultraviolet component of sunlight. However, many people are not sufficiently exposed to the sun due to environmental, cultural, and geographical factors, or fear of skin cancer. On the other hand, there are very limited dietary sources of the vitamin. In many countries, including Iran, most, if not all, dietary sources of vitamin D are not part of the household food basket in appreciable amounts. Consequently, vitamin D deficiency has become pandemic.

The relation of vitamin D with several chronic diseases, including cardiovascular disease (CVD), cancers and both types of diabetes, has become a hot topic especially during the last decade [5]. Poor vitamin D status has been associated with insulin resistance, diabetes and its advanced complications. The link between OS and the development of diabetes and its complications has also been documented. It is therefore likely that vitamin D, OS and insulin resistance are interrelated.

VITAMIN D

Vitamin D is a generic term for a group of compounds with similar functions in the body. There are primarily two forms of the vitamin; ergocalciferol or D2, mostly found in plants, and cholecalciferol or D3, which has an animal origin. Cholecalciferol is a steroid molecule which is synthesized in skin layers from 7-dehydrocholesterol under the influence of solar ultra violet (UV) light in the wavelength range 280–320 nm. The vitamin D thus produced is biologically inactive unless it is transformed to its daughter steroid hormone, 1,25-dihydroxycholecalciferol (1,25(OH)2D3) (Figure 11.1). This complicated process is accomplished via two major hydroxylation steps in the liver and kidney to yield 25(OH)D3 and 1,25(OH)2D3/or 24R,25(OH)2D3, respectively. The physiological importance of 24,25(OH)2D3 is controversial. This metabolite is produced by 24R-hydroxylase which is expressed in the kidney and in the vast majority of 1,25(OH)2 D3 target cells. It is believed that the enzyme has a regulatory role by inactivating 1,25(OH)2D3 to 1α,24R,25(OH)3D3 in the target cells. About 37 vitamin D3 metabolites have been isolated and chemically characterized thus far. Regulation of 1,25(OH)2D biosynthesis is under the influence of many factors including circulating calcium, phosphate, parathyroid hormone (PTH), caclcitriol, and fibroblast growth factor (FGF)23, which suppresses renal 1,α-hydroxylase and stimulates 24-hydroxylase. To do its job, FGF23 needs a signaling cofactor, named klotho, a multifactorial protein. Klotho may have a regulatory role via suppression of 1,25(OH)2D synthesis. Calcitriol is an inducer of klotho gene expression, while in the absence of klotho, 1-α-hydroxylase is induced [6].

As a fat-soluble molecule, vitamin D is immiscible with the aqueous environment of blood. Nature has overcome the problem by evolving a specific protein carrier, vitamin D binding protein (DBP), which conveys all vitamin D metabolites to their sites of metabolism and target organs. The biologically active form of the vitamin, 1,25(OH)2D3, like many other steroid hormones (e.g., estradiol, testosterone and cortisol) exerts its effects via its action on gene transcription. This pathway is referred to as the classic genomic response, and it involves an interaction of 1,25(OH)D3 and a specific nuclear receptor, vitamin D receptor (VDR). On binding of calcitriol, VDR undergoes heterodimerization with retinoid receptor, RXR. It is believed that 9-cis retinoic acid at very high concentrations may sequester RXR as homodimer thereby antagonizing the nuclear functions of vitamin D [6]. VDR has been found on a variety of cells including adipocytes, suggesting a role for vitamin D in inhibiting adipogenesis [7].

The genomic response to vitamin D takes at least a few hours to be accomplished. However, there are several known functions of the vitamin (such as the effect on gut calcium absorption) that occur in a matter of seconds to minutes. These 'rapid' non-genomic responses are mediated through membrane VDRs which are present on the plasma membrane caveolae of a variety of cells. Vitamin D has at least two non-genomic actions [8]:

1. Recruitment of membrane calcium transport proteins from intracellular vesicles to the cell surface and thus a rapid increase in calcium absorption. This is accomplished before induction of calcium-binding protein (calbindin) expression.
2. Opening of intracellular calcium channels and activation of protein kinase C and mitogen-activated protein kinases (MAP kinases), resulting in the inhibition of cellular proliferation and the induction of cellular differentiation.

Vitamin D influences cellular proliferation and differentiation as well as immune function. Activated macrophages express 25(OH)D 1-α-hydroxylase to convert calidiol to calcitriol, indicating a paracrine role for

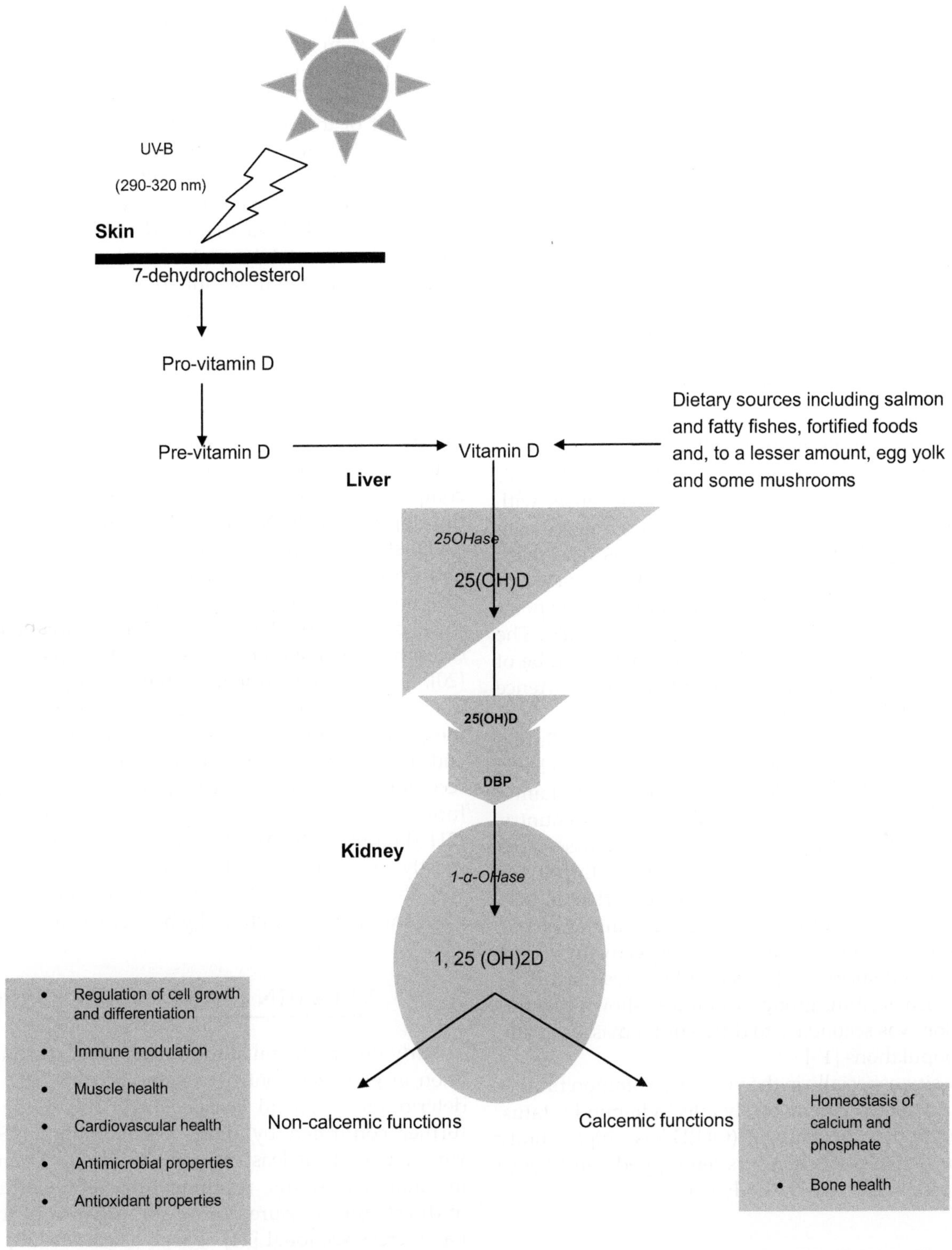

FIGURE 11.1 **Vitamin D biosynthesis and functions.**

vitamin D in the immune system [9]. Cholecalciferol can therefore be considered a 'hormone' with endocrine and paracrine functions. The vitamin D endocrine system comprises the following components [10]:

(a) Photoconversion of 7-dehydrocholesterol to pre-pro-vitamin D3 and/or dietary intake of calciferol.

(b) Hydroxylation of pre-pro-vitamin D to pro-vitamin D, i.e., 25(OH)D, in the liver. 25(OH)D is the most abundant circulating and storage form of the vitamin.

(c) Hydroxylation of 25(OH)D to produce 1α,25(OH)2D (the active form of the vitamin) and 24R,25(OH)2D in the kidney, the endocrine organ.

(d) Transportation of calcitriol to the target organs by DBP.
(e) Interaction of the vitamin with its receptor, VDR, to generate biological responses.

As long as humans and animals have enough direct sunlight exposure, there is no need for dietary calciferol. However, many geographical, social, cultural and environmental factors disrupt this natural relationship of humans with the sun, thus making calciferol a real 'vitamin' with a dietary requirement.

FACTORS AFFECTING VITAMIN D STATUS

When one considers the main source of vitamin D, it is not surprising that its status is influenced by many biosocial factors. In the areas above 33° in latitude, the sun's emission angle may be less effective than areas with lower latitude. Type of clothing is another issue of concern. According to Islamic regulations, girls who reach puberty must cover their bodies, except for the face and the hands from the wrists down. From the Islamic point of view, the age of pubescence is 9 years for girls. The problem of poor vitamin D status in females will be of more concern when several reports of higher occurrence of vitamin D deficiency in females in non-Islamic communities are taken into consideration [11]. Air pollution and sunscreen use also markedly decreases the efficiency of sun exposure in the endogenous synthesis of vitamin D. In a recent study from Australia, a sunny country, higher incidence of poor vitamin D status was associated with age, female gender, high latitude and adiposity. In this study, vitamin D deficiency was reported in 42% of women and 27% of men during the summer or fall, and this increased to 58% and 35%, respectively, during the winter and spring [12]. Vitamin D status may differ among various ethnic groups, but it was shown that this association was secondary to different fat masses in ethnic subpopulations [13].

Adiposity, especially in the viscera, a common finding in type 2 diabetes, can inversely affect vitamin D status. It is thought that circulating 25(OH)D has a high affinity for adipose tissue wherein it is 'entrapped', and hence will be less available to the body [14].

OXIDATIVE STRESS IN DIABETES: DEVELOPMENT AND COMPLICATIONS

A growing body of evidence has pointed to OS as a promoting factor for diabetic complications. Both acute and chronic variations in blood glucose may exacerbate OS, which is linked to the systemic inflammation often seen in both obesity and T2D [15]. It has recently been shown that the severity of OS is correlated with arterial stiffness in subjects with newly diagnosed T2D [16]. A link between OS and diabetic neuropathy has also been reported [17]. Whether OS is a causative agent or the result of the pathologic process of chronic disease, including diabetes, is still controversial [18].

Type 2 diabetes (T2D) is a multifactorial disease with an accelerating rate of occurrence worldwide. Although genetic factors do their share in development of the disease, environmental determinants of diabetes, including diet, have attracted more attention since, unlike genetic makeup, they are modifiable, presenting a means whereby the risk of disease could be reduced dramatically [19]. Diabetic complications are another issue of concern. Uncontrolled diabetes is often accompanied by early and late complications. While short-term complications are usually symptomatic early enough to be detected and (most of the time) managed, long-term complications are commonly insidious, unless they develop noxiously. Micro- and macro-vascular injuries, CVD, stroke, kidney involvement, immune-depression and purulent oozing wounds especially in limb terminals are among these complications. CVD is the main cause of death in T2D subjects. Many, if not all, of these comorbidities have been linked to the augmented OS [20]. To date, the present evidence suggests that ROS may contribute to diabetic long-term complications via the polyol pathway, generation of advanced glycation end products (AGEs) and over-expression of the related receptors, i.e., RAGE, activation of protein kinase C isoforms and increased activity of hexosamine pathway [21] (Figure 11.2). As the exacerbated OS in diabetes mostly originates from high circulating blood glucose [15], those antioxidants lacking ameliorating effects on glycemic status may clinically be inefficient.

VITAMIN D AND DIABETES

Early observational studies revealed a seasonal variation in glycemic control in subjects with T2D, with a deterioration in cold seasons [22]. This finding was further confirmed by more recent studies [23]. This variation may, at least in part, be due to fluctuations in vitamin D status, resulting from shorter durations of direct sun exposure during cold seasons of the year. Later, cross-sectional [24] as well as cohort [25] studies showed that vitamin D may be a modulator of diabetes risk. From these observational data, the need emerged for randomized trials to investigate the actual effects of vitamin D intake on both the glycemic status of diabetic subjects and the occurrence of T2D. In a clinical trial conducted by our research group, the effect of daily intake of vitamin D, either alone or together with calcium, on glycemic status of 90 T2D subjects aged 30–60 yrs of

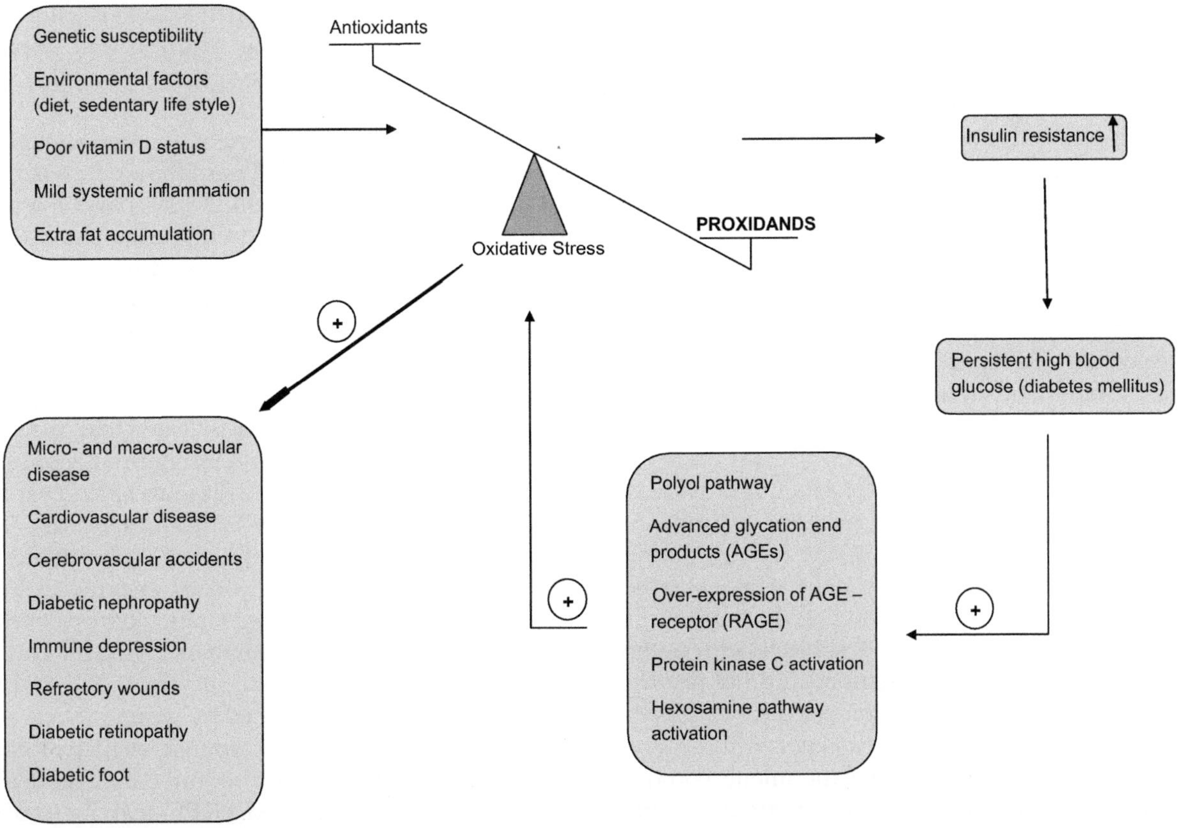

FIGURE 11.2 Inter-relationship among life style, vitamin D status, oxidative stress and development/complications of diabetes. Some links are not depicted here. For instance, while obesity may result in undesirable concentrations of circulating 25(OH)D, poor vitamin D status may also have some role in adipogenesis.

both sexes was investigated. In this study, the Persian yogurt drink (*doogh*) was fortified with either vitamin D (500 IU/250 mL) or vitamin D and calcium (500 IU and 250 mg/250 mL, respectively). After 12 weeks intervention, fasting serum glucose, insulin, insulin resistance, waist circumference and body fat improved. However, additional calcium did not confer further benefit [26]. A glycemic optimizing effect of vitamin D intake was further demonstrated in another trial [27].

One of the major issues of concern in T2D is the late complications, notably CVD, often seen in the course of the disease. Though CVD is known as the major cause of death in subjects with diabetes, vascular complications cause considerable morbidity and disability [28]. Involvement of blood vessels leading to micro- and macro-angiopathy is predisposed by both hyperinsulinemia and OS, both commonly found in T2D [29].

Despite some evidence provided by a few clinical trials of the beneficial effect of vitamin D on blood glucose, the issue is still controversial [30]. Even if the glycemic optimizing effect of vitamin D is accepted, an axial question would be whether vitamin D-induced decrement of blood glucose would be accompanied by appropriate amelioration of systemic inflammation and OS. Anti-inflammatory effects of vitamin D intake were reported in a few clinical trials [27, 31–32]. Although some animal studies provided evidence for an antioxidative effect of vitamin D [33], this issue needs to be addressed in further clinical studies.

VITAMIN D AS AN ANTIOXIDANT

Among non-calcemic functions of vitamin D, antioxidative action has only recently been investigated (Table 11.1). About two decades ago, the antioxidant properties of vitamin D isoforms, i.e., 7-dehydrocholesterol (pro-vitamin D3), cholecalciferol, ergocalciferol (vitamin D2) and calcitriol, were demonstrated by inhibiting lipid peroxidation in an experimental model. This antioxidant function of vitamin D compounds, structurally related to the cholesterol core, was comparable with that of an anticancer drug, tamoxifen, and its 4-hydroxy metabolite [34]. In an *in vitro* study, the antioxidative effect of vitamin D3, as judged by inhibition of MDA formation in brain homogenates, was even more than that of Trolox (a water-soluble analog of vitamin E), β-estradiol and melatonin [35]. In accordance with these findings, vitamin D protected keratinocytes against caspase-independent cell death induced by OS *in vitro* [36].

These findings were further supported by animal studies (Table 11.2). Vitamin D deficiency-induced vascular OS was shown in a rat model [37]. In a murine colon, oxidative damage to DNA, as judged by expression of 8-hydroxy-2'-deoxyguanosine (8-OHdG), was significantly augmented with complete loss of VDR, suggesting the necessity of calcitriol genomic action to protect DNA from oxidative damage [38]. Later, upregulation of the antioxidant enzymes, superoxide dismutase (SOD), catalase and glutathione peroxidase (GSH-Px), by 207, 52 and 72%, respectively, following administration of calcitriol was reported in diabetic rat model [33]. However, vitamin D supplementation did not convey additional benefit over insulin injection alone in suppressing OS [39].

Exploration of the association of vitamin D with OS has ignited the eagerness of investigators to find possible links in the clinical setting. Contrary to the findings of *in vitro* and animal studies, daily intake of either vitamin D (800 IU/d) or calcium (2g/d), alone or in combination, for six months by 92 subjects with pathologically confirmed colorectal adenoma did not result in significant decrease in 8-OHG in biopsied cancerous tissues [40]. Part of the discrepancies between these findings and the evidence from animal experiments could be due to the evaluation of localized versus circulating biomarkers of OS in different pathological or physiological settings. In support of this notion, the antioxidant effect of intravenous calcitriol in hemodialysis patients was demonstrated by measuring oxidized and unoxidized albumin [41], suggesting the systemic antioxidant effect of vitamin D.

Several studies have reported an inverse relationship between circulating 25(OH)D and the amount of fat mass (FM). An undesirable vitamin D status in obese subjects may, therefore, be associated with augmented OS. This assumption was further encouraged by a recent report of increased levels of malondialdehyde (MDA), myeloperoxidase (MPO), 3-nitrotyrosine, interleukin (IL)-6, and soluble vascular cell adhesion molecule (VCAM)-1 in obese children with vitamin D insufficiency [42].

An interesting *in vitro* study revealed that calcitriol has a selective antioxidative effect in non-malignant human prostate epithelial cell lines (BPH-1 and RWPE-1) but not in malignant cell lines (CWR22R and DU 145). Further investigation showed that glucose-6-phosphate dehydrogenase (G6PD), an antioxidant enzyme in the glucose metabolism pathway, was induced by calcitriol in a dose- and time-dependent manner. Using the chromatin immunoprecipitation method, it was found that G6PD gene expression was regulated by vitamin D via a direct repeat-3 (DR3) vitamin D response element located in the first intron which can be bounded by liganded VDR. Therefore, calcitriol-induced G6PD activity and glutathione (GSH) can scavenge ROS [43]. The antioxidative action of vitamin D deserves further study.

TABLE 11.1 *In Vitro* Studies Evaluating the Antioxidative Effects of Vitamin D

Study	Cell Type/line	Primary Outcome
Wiseman, 1993 [34]	Brain liposomes	Inhibition of iron-induced MDA formation
Lin et al., 2005 [35]	Cortical brain homogenate	Reduced zinc-induced MDA and its dihydropyridine polymers
Diker-Cohen et al., 200 [36]	HaCaT keratinocytes	Reduced oxidative stress-induced cell death
Bao et al., 2008 [43]	BPH-1 and RWPE-1	Calcitriol dose- and time-dependent activation of G6PD and increased glutathione

TABLE 11.2 Animal Studies Evaluating the Antioxidative Properties of Vitamin D

Study	Animal	Induction of Oxidative Stress	Primary Outcome
Lin et al., 2005 [35]	Adult rat	Infusion of zinc chloride into substantia nigra	Reduced MDA and its dihydropyridine polymers
Argacha et al., 201 [37]	Growing rat	Vitamin D deficiency	Increased superoxide anion production in the aortic wall
Kallay et al., 2002 [38]	Mouse	Complete loss of VDR in colon	Over-expression of 8-hydroxy-2'-deoxyguanosine (8-OHdG)
Hamden et al., 2009 [33]	Diabetic rat	Diabetes	Increased plasma SOD, catalase and GSH-Px by 207, 52 and 72%, respectively
Noyan et al., 2005 [39]	Diabetic rat	Diabetes	Increased kidney MDA in insulin+vitamin D compared to insulin alone, increased heart SOD and catalase due to insulin injection alone compared to insulin+vitamin D; unaltered GSH-Px

ANTIOXIDANT EFFECT OF VITAMIN D IN DIABETES: DIRECT VS. INDIRECT EFFECT

Data on a possible antioxidant function of vitamin D in diabetes is scarce. Persistent hyperglycemia may induce OS through several ways, including the polyol pathway. In a recent cross-sectional study on elder subjects with impaired fasting glucose (IFG) or T2D, a significant inverse association was found between serum 25(OH)D and circulating OS biomarkers including AGEs, advanced oxidation protein products (AOPPs), low density lipoprotein (LDL) susceptibility to oxidation and nitric oxide metabolites [44]. Therefore, one may expect that vitamin D can potentially attenuate OS in diabetic subjects, at least through glycemic normalization (Figure 11.3).

To examine this idea, we conducted two separate clinical trials on the effect of daily vitamin D intake on different aspects of diabetic host responses including glycemic, lipidemic, immunologic, inflammatory, and OS. In both studies, a vitamin D-fortified Persian yogurt drink (*doogh*) was employed to improve the vitamin D status of the subjects. In the first experiment, the efficacy of a daily intake of *doogh* fortified either with vitamin D (DD; 500 IU/d) alone or a combination of vitamin D and calcium (CDD; 500 IU and 250 mg/d, respectively) was evaluated. Participants were instructed to drink two 250 mL bottles of *doogh* a day preferably with their meals, i.e., one with lunch and the other with dinner. Compared to plain *doogh* (PD), both fortified products resulted in a significant amelioration of glycemic [26] and inflammatory biomarkers [31]. In this study, serum concentrations of MDA, oxidized low density lipoprotein (ox-LDL), protein carbonyl (PCO), cardiac myeloperoxidase (MPO) and AGEs were measured as markers of OS. Although serum MDA and ox-LDL did not differ significantly among the groups, final values of PCO and MPO, compared to initial ones, decreased significantly in both groups whichreceived fortified *doogh*, and there was no significant difference between DD and CDD groups [45]. Interestingly, serum AGEs also decreased in the DD and CDD groups compared to the PD group [46].

Another clinical trial investigated the effect of vitamin D intake on OS biomarkers. One hundred subjects with T2D were randomly assigned to receive two 250 mL bottles of *doogh*/d which was either plain (PD, n_1=50) or fortified with 500IU/250mL vitamin D (FD, n_2=50). After 12 weeks intervention, MDA decreased by 15.6% (p=0.004), only in the FD group, and this was accompanied by a significant rise in both total antioxidant capacity (TAC) (21%; $p<0.001$) and GSH (12.6%; p=0.007). The significant differences in TAC and GSH between PD and FD disappeared after controlling for changes of serum 25(OH)D (p=0.39 and p=0.13, respectively). However, after controlling for changes of quantitative insulin sensitivity check index (QUICKI), an indicator of insulin sensitivity, while the difference of TAC was still insignificant (p=0.31), GSH changes remained significant (p=0.001), suggesting the glycemic status-independent upregulating effect of vitamin D on GSH (unpublished data). The direct upregulating effect of calcitriol on endogenous antioxidant effectors, γ-glutamyl transpeptidase (GGT) and

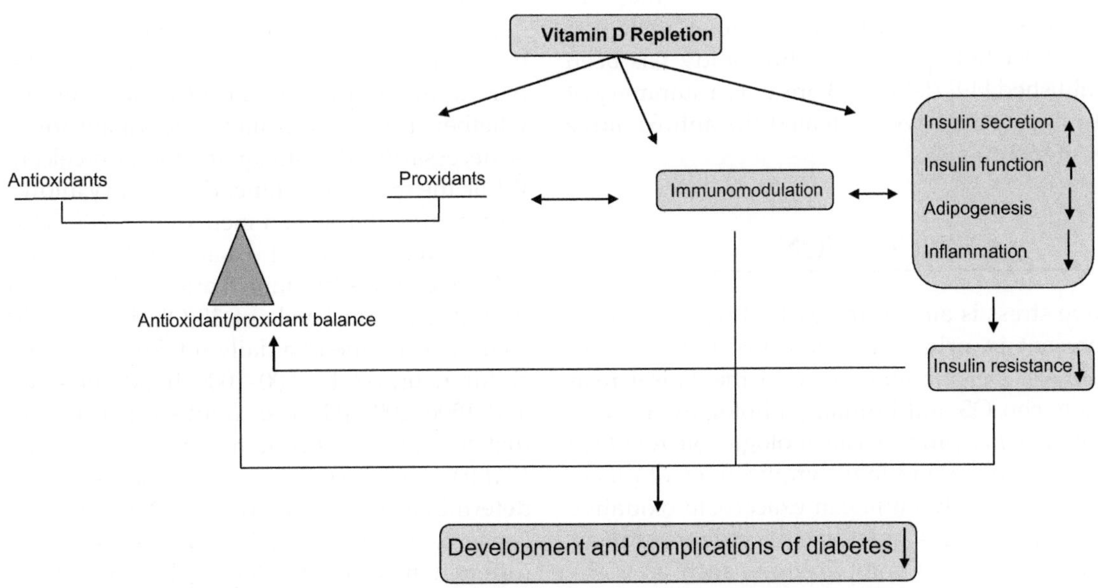

FIGURE 11.3 **Vitamin D may have both direct and indirect effects on antioxidant/proxidant balance in diabetes.** While vitamin D may act as a membrane antioxidant, some endogenous antioxidant effectors like glutathione can be upregulated by calcitriol. Decreased production of reactive oxygen species due to amelioration of glycemic and inflammatory status can mediate calcitriol indirect effects on antioxidant defense system.

TABLE 11.3 Human Studies Evaluating Antioxidative Effects of Vitamin D

Study	Type of Study	Intervention	Duration	Population	Primary Outcome
Fedirko et al., 2010 [40]	RCT	800 IU/d vitamin D or calcium 2g/d, alone or in combination	6 months	92 subjects with at least one pathologically confirmed colorectal adenoma	No significant decrease in 8(OH)G in biopsied cancerous tissues
Tanaka et al., 2011 [41]	Pre- post trial	Weekly intravenous injection of 1.5 microgram calcitriol	4 weeks	11 hemodialysis patients with secondary hyperparathyroidism	Reduced oxidized/unoxidized albumin; increased serum thiol content; increased radical scavenging activity of albumin
Tayebinejad et al., 2012 [46]	RCT	1,000 IU/d vitamin D with or without 500 mg calcium in the form of fortified yogurt drink	12 weeks	90 T2D subjects randomly divided in three groups to receive plain, vitamin D-fortified or vitamin D-calcium-fortified yogurt drink	No significant change in serum MDA and ox-LDL; significant decrease in circulating AGEs; no additional benefit of extra calcium
Nikooyeh et al., 2012 [45]	RCT	1,000 IU/d vitamin D in the form of fortified yogurt drink	12 weeks	100 T2D subjects randomly divided in two groups to receive either plain or vitamin D-fortified yogurt drink	Significant 15.6% decrease in MDA but 21% and 12.6% increase in TAC and GSH, respectively

glutathione, has been shown in rat primary astrocytes [47]. The way that vitamin D increases TAC needs further investigation.

In an attempt to evaluate the role of genetic factors in various aspects of the diabetic host response to vitamin D intake, we analyzed the Vitamin D receptor *FokI* polymorphisms for 140 subjects with T2D, who received FD for 12 weeks. We found that VDR *FokI* ff were 'low-responders' to vitamin D in terms of rise in circulating 25(OH)D and amelioration of some inflammatory markers, including highly sensitive C-reactive protein (hsCRP) and IL-6 [48]. However, further analyses revealed no between-group difference in changes of TAC, MDA, GSH, SOD and GSH-Px among VDR *FokI* genotypes. The whole protocol of this study has been already published [49]. Table 11.3 presents a summary of human studies which have evaluated the antioxidative properties of vitamin D.

CONCLUSION

Oxidative stress is among the earliest defense mechanisms, present in primitive organisms as well as in higher animals. Despite ambiguity in the causal relationship between OS and human pathologies, a growing body of evidence proposes an etiologic role for OS in both the development and late complications of diabetes. Persistent hyperglycemia can exacerbate oxidative conditions in many ways, including the polyol pathway, leading to very noxious complications such as CVD, nephropathy and stroke. Vitamin D, a secosterol, has a well-known function in the maintenance of bone health. However, there is an increasing understanding of the non-calcemic actions of the vitamin, one of the less studied of which is its antioxidative function. Evidence from observational studies as well as recent clinical trials support the beneficial effect of vitamin D on glycemic control [26] and subsiding systemic/vascular inflammation in T2D [27, 31–32]. Glycemic normalization can lead to the attenuation of OS. Moreover, some experimental and clinical findings noted a direct genomic action of calcitriol on upregulated of endogenous antioxidants, notably glutathione.

Despite these promising effects, there are still many questions to be answered. One of the most controversial issues in vitamin D has been, and continues to be, 'adequate intake'. Most recommendations have been made based on its calcemic actions (calcium absorption or parathyroid hormone concentrations), and it is not clear whether a vitamin D intake adequate for bone health is necessarily also adequate for non-calcemic actions. While the recent recommended dietary allowance (RDA) for vitamin D has been increased to 600 IU (from a previously recommended dosage of 400 IU), most experts still believe this amount would be insufficient to make desirable serum levels of 25(OH)D of 75–100 nmol/L, so they recommend a daily intake of 400–1000 IU/d for children under 1y, 600–1000 IU/d for children 1–18y, and 1500–2000 IU/d for adults [5]. The requirement in diabetic carriers of certain genotypic variants (like VDR *FokI* ff) may prove to be even higher [48]. The method of determination of circulating 25(OH)D is another issue of concern. As there may be some disagreement between different methods (including high-performance liquid chromatography, competitive protein binding assay and radioimmunoassay) [50], cutoffs of 25(OH)D should be based on a specific method. In addition, it is needless to say that vitamin D repletion of diabetic subjects, despite countless beneficial effects, would still be regarded as an adjunct to conventional therapy. Healthy life style, including weight management and a healthy diet, still comprises the core of the treatment.

SUMMARY POINTS

- Formation of reactive oxygen species (ROS) is among the earliest innate defense mechanisms against pathogens.
- Excess amounts of the ROS (proxidants) are deactivated by endogenous and exogenous antioxidants so there is a 'balance' between free radicals and antioxidants. However, under certain circumstances, this balance is disturbed, with a shift towards proxidants; a condition known as 'oxidative stress' (OS).
- There is a link between OS and development of diabetes and its long-term complications.
- Hyperglycemia exacerbates OS.
- Vitamin D, a hormone synthesized in the skin under the influence of ultraviolet light, is involved in insulin secretion and function.
- Vitamin D has antioxidant properties. It also upregulates certain endogenous antioxidants like superoxide dismutase, catalase, glutathione and glutathione peroxidase.
- Vitamin D-induced glycemic amelioration can also attenuate diabetic OS.

References

[1] Falcone EL, Holland SM. Invasive fungal infection in chronic granulomatous disease: insights into pathogenesis and management. Curr Opin Infect Dis 2012 Dec;25(6):658–69.

[2] Giustarini D, Dalle-Donne I, Tsikas D, Rossi R. Oxidative stress and human diseases: Origin, link, measurement, mechanisms, and biomarkers. Crit Rev Clin Lab Sci 2009;46(5–6):241–81.

[3] Sasaki S, Inoguchi T. The role of oxidative stress in the pathogenesis of diabetic vascular complications. Diabetes Metab J 2012 Aug;36(4):255–61.

[4] Johansen JS, Harris AK, Rychly DJ, Ergul A. Oxidative stress and the use of antioxidants in diabetes: linking basic science to clinical practice. Cardiovasc Diabetol 2005;4(1):5.

[5] Holick MF. Evidence-based D-bate on health benefits of vitamin D revisited. Dermatoendocrinol 2012 Apr 1;4(2):183–90.

[6] Haussler MR, Whitfield GK, Kaneko I, Haussler CA, Hsieh D, Hsieh JC, et al. Molecular Mechanisms of Vitamin D Action. Calcif Tissue Int 2012 Jul 11.

[7] Wood RJ. Vitamin D and adipogenesis: new molecular insights. Nutr Rev 2008 Jan;66(1):40–6.

[8] Haussler MR, Jurutka PW, Mizwicki M, Norman AW. Vitamin D receptor (VDR)-mediated actions of 1alpha,25(OH)(2)vitamin D(3): genomic and non-genomic mechanisms. Best Pract Res Clin Endocrinol Metab 2011 Aug;25(4):543–59.

[9] Adams JS, Hewison M. Extrarenal expression of the 25-hydroxyvitamin D-1-hydroxylase. Arch Biochem Biophys 2012 Jul 1;523(1): 95–102.

[10] Adorini L, Penna G. Control of autoimmune diseases by the vitamin D endocrine system. Nat Clin Pract Rheumatol 2008 Aug;4(8):404–12.

[11] Lu HK, Zhang Z, Ke YH, He JW, Fu WZ, Zhang CQ, et al. High prevalence of vitamin d insufficiency in china: relationship with the levels of parathyroid hormone and markers of bone turnover. PLoS One 2012;7(11):e47264.

[12] Daly RM, Gagnon C, Lu ZX, Magliano DJ, Dunstan DW, Sikaris KA, et al. Prevalence of vitamin D deficiency and its determinants in Australian adults aged 25 years and older: a national, population-based study. Clin Endocrinol (Oxf) 2012 Jul;77(1):26–35.

[13] Sulistyoningrum DC, Green TJ, Lear SA, Devlin AM. Ethnic-specific differences in vitamin D status is associated with adiposity. PLoS One 2012;7(8):e43159.

[14] Cheng S, Massaro JM, Fox CS, Larson MG, Keyes MJ, McCabe EL, et al. Adiposity, cardiometabolic risk, and vitamin D status: the Framingham Heart Study. Diabetes 2010 Jan;59(1):242–8.

[15] Chang CM, Hsieh CJ, Huang JC, Huang IC. Acute and chronic fluctuations in blood glucose levels can increase oxidative stress in type 2 diabetes mellitus. Acta Diabetol 2012 Dec;49(Suppl. 1): S171–7.

[16] Ha CY, Kim JY, Paik JK, Kim OY, Paik YH, Lee EJ, et al. The association of specific metabolites of lipid metabolism with markers of oxidative stress, inflammation and arterial stiffness in men with newly diagnosed type 2 diabetes. Clin Endocrinol (Oxf) 2012 May;76(5):674–82.

[17] Kasznicki J, Kosmalski M, Sliwinska A, Mrowicka M, Stanczyk M, Majsterek I, et al. Evaluation of oxidative stress markers in pathogenesis of diabetic neuropathy. Mol Biol Rep 2012 Sep;39(9): 8669–78.

[18] Naviaux RK. Oxidative shielding or oxidative stress? J Pharmacol Exp Ther 2012 Sep;342(3):608–18.

[19] Lazarou C, Panagiotakos D, Matalas AL. The role of diet in prevention and management of type 2 diabetes: implications for public health. Crit Rev Food Sci Nutr 2012;52(5):382–9.

[20] Giacco F, Brownlee M. Oxidative stress and diabetic complications. Circ Res 2010 Oct 29;107(9):1058–70.

[21] Folli F, Corradi D, Fanti P, Davalli A, Paez A, Giaccari A, et al. The role of oxidative stress in the pathogenesis of type 2 diabetes mellitus micro- and macrovascular complications: avenues for a mechanistic-based therapeutic approach. Curr Diabetes Rev 2011 Sep;7(5):313–24.

[22] Asplund J. Seasonal variation of HbA1c in adult diabetic patients. Diabetes Care 1997 Feb;20(2):234.

[23] Gikas A, Sotiropoulos A, Pastromas V, Papazafiropoulou A, Apostolou O, Pappas S. Seasonal variation in fasting glucose and HbA1c in patients with type 2 diabetes. Prim Care Diabetes 2009 May;3(2):111–4.

[24] Nsiah-Kumi PA, Erickson JM, Beals JL, Ogle EA, Whiting M, Brushbreaker C, et al. Vitamin D insufficiency is associated with diabetes risk in Native American children. Clin Pediatr (Phila) 2012 Feb;51(2):146–53.

[25] Kirii K, Mizoue T, Iso H, Takahashi Y, Kato M, Inoue M, et al. Calcium, vitamin D and dairy intake in relation to type 2 diabetes risk in a Japanese cohort. Diabetologia 2009 Dec;52(12): 2542–50.

[26] Nikooyeh B, Neyestani TR, Farvid M, Alavi-Majd H, Houshiarrad A, Kalayi A, et al. Daily consumption of vitamin D- or vitamin D + calcium-fortified yogurt drink improved glycemic control in patients with type 2 diabetes: a randomized clinical trial. Am J Clin Nutr 2011 Apr;93(4):764–71.

[27] Shab-Bidar S, Neyestani TR, Djazayery A, Eshraghian MR, Houshiarrad A, Gharavi A, et al. Regular consumption of vitamin D-fortified yogurt drink (*Doogh*) improved endothelial biomarkers in subjects with type 2 diabetes: a randomized double-blind clinical trial. BMC Med 2011;9:125.

[28] Avitabile NA, Banka A, Fonseca VA. Glucose control and cardiovascular outcomes in individuals with diabetes mellitus: lessons learned from the megatrials. Heart Fail Clin 2012 Oct;8(4):513–22.
[29] Sobel BE, Schneider DJ. Cardiovascular complications in diabetes mellitus. Curr Opin Pharmacol 2005 Apr;5(2):143–8.
[30] Mitri J, Muraru MD, Pittas AG. Vitamin D and type 2 diabetes: a systematic review. Eur J Clin Nutr 2011 Sep;65(9):1005–15.
[31] Neyestani TR, Nikooyeh B, Alavi-Majd H, Shariatzadeh N, Kalayi A, Tayebinejad N, et al. Improvement of vitamin D status via daily intake of fortified yogurt drink either with or without extra calcium ameliorates systemic inflammatory biomarkers, including adipokines, in the subjects with type 2 diabetes. J Clin Endocrinol Metab 2012 Jun;97(6):2005–11.
[32] Shab-Bidar S, Neyestani TR, Djazayery A, Eshraghian MR, Houshiarrad A, Kalayi A, et al. Improvement of vitamin D status resulted in amelioration of biomarkers of systemic inflammation in the subjects with type 2 diabetes. Diabetes Metab Res Rev 2012 Jul;28(5):424–30.
[33] Hamden K, Carreau S, Jamoussi K, Miladi S, Lajmi S, Aloulou D, et al. 1Alpha,25 dihydroxyvitamin D3: therapeutic and preventive effects against oxidative stress, hepatic, pancreatic and renal injury in alloxan-induced diabetes in rats. J Nutr Sci Vitaminol (Tokyo) 2009 Jun;55(3):215–22.
[34] Wiseman H. Vitamin D is a membrane antioxidant. Ability to inhibit iron-dependent lipid peroxidation in liposomes compared to cholesterol, ergosterol and tamoxifen and relevance to anticancer action. FEBS Lett 1993 Jul 12;326(1–3):285–8.
[35] Lin AM, Chen KB, Chao PL. Antioxidative effect of vitamin D3 on zinc-induced oxidative stress in CNS. Ann N Y Acad Sci 2005 Aug;1053:319–29.
[36] Diker-Cohen T, Koren R, Liberman UA, Ravid A. Vitamin D protects keratinocytes from apoptosis induced by osmotic shock, oxidative stress, and tumor necrosis factor. Ann N Y Acad Sci 2003 Dec;1010:350–3.
[37] Argacha JF, Egrise D, Pochet S, Fontaine D, Lefort A, Libert F, et al. Vitamin D deficiency-induced hypertension is associated with vascular oxidative stress and altered heart gene expression. J Cardiovasc Pharmacol 2011 Jul;58(1):65–71.
[38] Kallay E, Bareis P, Bajna E, Kriwanek S, Bonner E, Toyokuni S, et al. Vitamin D receptor activity and prevention of colonic hyperproliferation and oxidative stress. Food Chem Toxicol 2002 Aug;40(8):1191–6.
[39] Noyan T, Balaharoglu R, Komuroglu U. The oxidant and antioxidant effects of 25-hydroxyvitamin D3 in liver, kidney and heart tissues of diabetic rats. Clin Exp Med 2005 May;5(1):31–6.
[40] Fedirko V, Bostick RM, Long Q, Flanders WD, McCullough ML, Sidelnikov E, et al. Effects of supplemental vitamin D and calcium on oxidative DNA damage marker in normal colorectal mucosa: a randomized clinical trial. Cancer Epidemiol Biomarkers Prev 2010 Jan;19(1):280–91.
[41] Tanaka M, Tokunaga K, Komaba H, Itoh K, Matsushita K, Watanabe H, et al. Vitamin D receptor activator reduces oxidative stress in hemodialysis patients with secondary hyperparathyroidism. Ther Apher Dial 2011 Apr;15(2):161–8.
[42] Codoner-Franch P, Tavarez-Alonso S, Simo-Jorda R, Laporta-Martin P, Carratala-Calvo A, Alonso-Iglesias E. Vitamin D status is linked to biomarkers of oxidative stress, inflammation, and endothelial activation in obese children. J Pediatr 2012 Nov;161(5):848–54.
[43] Bao BY, Ting HJ, Hsu JW, Lee YF. Protective role of 1 alpha, 25-dihydroxyvitamin D3 against oxidative stress in nonmalignant human prostate epithelial cells. Int J Cancer 2008 Jun 15;122(12):2699–706.
[44] Gradinaru D, Borsa C, Ionescu C, Margina D, Prada GI, Jansen E. Vitamin d status and oxidative stress markers in elderly with impaired fasting glucose and type 2 diabetes mellitus. Aging Clin Exp Res 2012 Dec;24(6):595–602.
[45] Nikooyeh B, Neyestani TR, Tayebinejad N, Alavi-Majd H, Shariatzadeh N, Kalayi A, et al. Daily intake of vitamin D- or calcium-vitamin D-fortified Persian yogurt drink (doogh) attenuates diabetes-induced oxidative stress: evidence for antioxidative properties of vitamin D. J Hum Nutr Diet. 2013 Jul 5.
[46] Tayebinejad N, Neyestani TR, Rashidkhani B, Nikooyeh B, Kalayi A, Shariatzadeh N, et al. The effect of daily consumption of Iranian yogurt drink *doogh* fortified with vitamin D or vitamin D plus calcium on the serum advanced glycation end products (AGEs) and oxidized LDL concentrations in type 2 diabetes patients: a randomized clinical trial. Iranian J Nutr Sci Food Tech 2012;7(3):1–9.
[47] Garcion E, Sindji L, Leblondel G, Brachet P, Darcy F. 1,25-dihydroxyvitamin D3 regulates the synthesis of gamma-glutamyl transpeptidase and glutathione levels in rat primary astrocytes. J Neurochem 1999 Aug;73(2):859–66.
[48] Neyestani TR, Djazayery A, Shab-Bidar S, Eshraghian MR, Kalayi A, Shariatzadeh N, et al. Vitamin D Receptor Fok-I Polymorphism Modulates Diabetic Host Response to Vitamin D Intake: Need for a nutrigenetic approach. Diabetes Care 2013 Mar;36(3):550–6.
[49] Shab-Bidar S, Neyestani TR, Djazayery A. Efficacy of vitamin D3-fortified-yogurt drink on anthropometric, metabolic, inflammatory and oxidative stress biomarkers according to vitamin D receptor gene polymorphisms in type 2 diabetic patients: a study protocol for a randomized controlled clinical trial. BMC Endocr Disord 2011;11:12.
[50] Neyestani TR, Gharavi A, Kalayi A. Determination of serum 25-hydroxy cholecalciferol using high-performance liquid chromatography: a reliable tool for assessment of vitamin D status. Int J Vitam Nutr Res 2007 Sep;77(5):341–6.

CHAPTER

12

Glutamine and Antioxidant Potential in Diabetes

Sung-Ling Yeh, Yu-Chen Hou

School of Nutrition and Health Sciences, Taipei Medical University, Taipei, Taiwan

List of Abbreviations

AGE Advanced glycation end product
AR Aldose reductase
DM Diabetes mellitus
GFAT 1 Glutamine fructose-6-phosphate transaminase
GLN Glutamine
GLP-1 Glucagon-like peptide 1
GPx Glutathione peroxidase
GRd Glutathione reductase
GSH Glutathione
GSSG Glutathione disulfide
HSP Heat shock protein
IL Interleukin
NADPH Nicotinamide adenine dinucleotide phosphate
NF-κB Nuclear factor-κB
NO Nitric oxide
PAI-1 Plasminogen activator inhibitor
PKC Protein kinase C
PPAR Peroxisome proliferator-activated receptor
RAGE Receptor of AGEs
ROS Reactive oxygen species
SOD Superoxide dismutase
Txnip Thioredoxin-interacting protein

INTRODUCTION TO GLUTAMINE

Glutamine (GLN) is the most abundant amino acid in mammalian plasma and intracellular pools. The physiological level of GLN is 500~600 μM [1]. Because GLN can be synthesized *de novo* in virtually all tissues of the body, it was historically designated a 'non-essential' amino acid. GLN is present in nearly all dietary proteins. In most food proteins, GLN makes up 4–8% of the amino acid residues, so approximately 10 g of dietary GLN is consumed daily by the average person. Additional supplementation is not necessary for healthy adults, but this amount of GLN might not be sufficient to meet requirements during the course of a catabolic condition such as when a person experiences surgery, trauma, or infection. Studies in patients undergoing major operations showed that plasma GLN concentrations diminished by 50% during the acute postoperative period [2]. Profound GLN depletion and poor outcomes develop, indicating that the ability of GLN production to meet requirements during a catabolic disease is impaired. A study on stressed patients suggested that considerably larger amounts of GLN are necessary to maintain GLN homeostasis [3]. Thus it is considered a 'conditionally essential' amino acid in catabolic conditions.

GLN has a high turnover rate in the body because there is a wide array of metabolic functions that directly or indirectly depend on it. Its functions within cells can generally be classified as follows:

1) GLN works as a vehicle for the shuttling of nitrogen transport. Approximately one-third of all nitrogen derived from protein metabolism is transported in the blood in the form of GLN. It is also the major source of nitrogen in hepatic ureagenesis.
2) GLN is important in maintaining the cellular redox state. As a source of intracellular glutamate, GLN provides one of the constituents of glutathione (GSH) that may protect cells against oxidative injury [3].
3) GLN is an important source of carbon and nitrogen for metabolic intermediates and macromolecular synthesis, such as purine and pyrimidine nucleotide production, fatty acid synthesis, and gluconeogenesis.
4) GLN is an energy source for rapidly proliferating cells such as enterocytes and immune cells. The oxidation of GLN can generate adenosine triphosphate (ATP) for cellular respiration [3] (Figure 12.1).

Diabetes: Oxidative Stress and Dietary Antioxidants.
http://dx.doi.org/10.1016/B978-0-12-405885-9.00012-7

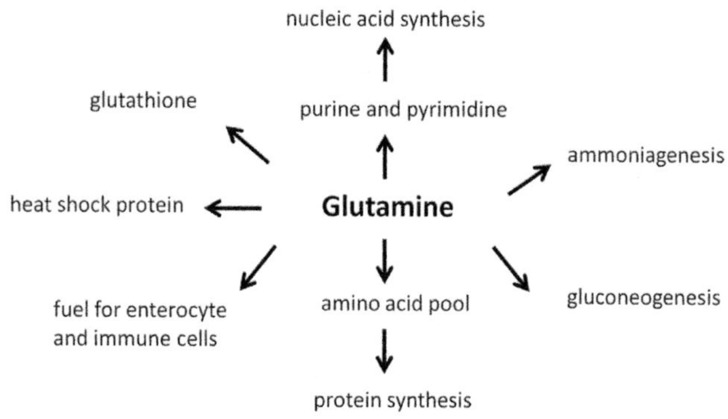

FIGURE 12.1 **Important functions of glutamine in the body.**

IMMUNOMODULATORY EFFECTS OF GLN

In addition to the important role of GLN in human metabolism, special emphasis should be given to its non-nutritive function, since it is a potent immune regulator. Numerous studies have shown that GLN has immunomodulatory properties, and suppresses inflammatory responses in critical illness [4,5]. It has been shown to regulate the expression of many genes related to cell defense and repair, and to activate intracellular signal pathways [6]. A previous study showed that GLN supplementation attenuated proinflammatory cytokine release, protected against organ damage, and decreased mortality in a lipopolysaccharide-treated animal model [7]. Kozar et al. [8] showed that GLN maintains small-bowel barrier function after gut ischemia/reperfusion injury in rats. We recently completed a study of intravenous GLN therapy in a cecal ligation and puncture model of sepsis in mice, and found that GLN administration prevented apoptosis of intestinal intraepithelial lymphocyte γδT-cells, and down-regulated γδT-cell-expressed inflammatory mediators that may consequently ameliorate the severity of sepsis-induced intestinal epithelial injury [9]. Also, GLN reduced the expressions of high-mobility group box-1 related mediators and thus ameliorated acute kidney injury induced by sepsis [10]. A meta-analysis of clinical trials found that GLN administration improves gut permeability in burn patients, and in patients undergoing abdominal surgery [11]. It was suggested that therapeutic intervention with GLN can protect tissues against injury, mitigate inflammation, and preserve metabolic function that may be beneficial in preventing or treating multiple organ dysfunction syndromes resulting from sepsis or other injuries [5]. Enteral GLN-containing formulas are commonly used in nutrition regimens for critically ill patients. Because free GLN is unstable in solution and rapidly degrades to ammonia, many studies used alanyl-glutamine as a substitute. The alanyl-glutamine dipeptide is stable in aqueous solution, and is widely used for critically ill patients on total parenteral nutrition [12,13], where it serves as a source of free GLN [14]. According to former investigations, acute administration of GLN in a dose of up to 30~40g/70 kg body weight is safe in critically ill patients [15,16].

GLN AND DIABETES

Diabetes mellitus (DM) is a metabolic disorder characterized by chronic hyperglycemia and the development of various micro- and macrovascular diseases. There are close links among hyperglycemia, oxidative stress, and diabetic complications [17,18]. A previous study showed that in rats with short- and long-term diabetes, there was a marked decrease in GLN with a concomitant increase in ketone bodies in arterial concentrations. These results indicated that diabetic rats exhibit decreased rates of GLN metabolism, and such decreases were partially compensated for by enhanced ketone body utilization [19]. A previous report showed that patients with type 2 diabetes exhibited significant reductions in GLN levels, which can lead to disturbances in insulin secretion and its actions [20]. GLN plays an essential role in promoting and maintaining the functionality of various organs and cells, including pancreatic β-cells. Rat islets consume high rates of GLN [21]. Previous studies found that parenteral supplementation with the alanyl-glutamine dipeptide was associated with better insulin sensitivity in multiple-trauma patients, which also proved that GLN plays a critical role as a signal molecule in insulin secretion [22,23]. Those results suggest that GLN supplementation may be needed in diabetic conditions. A study performed by Opara et al. [24] investigated the effects of dietary GLN on the development of hyperglycemia and excessive weight gain. They used a genetically overweight and hyperglycemically-predisposed B/6J mouse model, and found that GLN supplementation of a high-fat diet reduced body weight and attenuated hyperglycemia and hyperinsulinemia. The authors suggested that the possible mechanism of GLN's action on body weight reduction could involve its attenuation of insulin resistance induced by fat. Greenfield et al. [25] investigated whether GLN increases circulating glucagon-like peptide (GLP)-1 and glucose-dependent insulinotropic polypeptide concentrations, thus increasing plasma insulin levels. The authors recruited three groups of subjects with eight persons in each group. One group consisted of healthy, normal-weight volunteers, while the other group contained obese individuals with type 2 DM or impaired glucose tolerance. The third group comprised obese non-diabetic subjects. Oral glucose, GLN, and water were administered on three separate days in random order to the three groups. The authors found that GLN effectively increased circulating incretin

TABLE 12.1 Studies Demonstrating Benefits of Glutamine in Diabetes

Study	Ref	Subject	Effects of Glutamine
Greenfield et al.	25	Obese or obese with type 2 DM subjects	Increased circulating incretin and insulin concentrations
Samacha-Bonet et al.	26	Type 2 DM patients	Enhanced circulating GLP-1 and decreased postprandial glycemia
Opera et al.	24	Overweight and hyperglycemic mice	Reduced body weight and improved hyperglycemia and hyperinsulinemia
Tsai et al.	27	Type 1 DM mice	Decreased leukocyte adhesion molecule expression and reduced oxidative damage to organs
Tsai et al.	35	Type 2 DM rats	Decreased oxidative-related gene expressions and attenuated renal oxidative damage
Tsai et al.	28	Type 2 DM rats	Downregulated inflammatory mediator expression
Tashima et al.	29	Diabetic rats	Improved neuronal density in the proximal colon
Pereira et al.	30	Diabetic rats	Prevented neuron loss and had gliatrophic effects in the ileum
Ugurlucan et al.	54	Diabetic rats	Enhanced heat shock protein expression and had a cardioprotective effect
Jang et al.	53	Islet cells	Attenuated interleukin-1β-induced islet injury and apoptosis

hormones and insulin concentrations in all study groups. This result may represent a novel therapeutic approach to stimulating insulin secretion and possibly improving glycemic control in obese subjects and those with type 2 DM. Samacha-Bonet et al. [26] designed a randomized, crossover study to evaluate the effect of a single oral dose of 30 g GLN on postprandial glycemia and increased total and active GLP-1 concentrations in type 2 DM patients. They found that GLN treatment enhanced the postprandial insulin response, stimulated GLP-1 concentrations, and limited postprandial glycemia in type 2 DM patients. Because there was no corresponding increase in C-peptides, the authors suggested that GLN may affect insulin clearance rather than secretion, and the effect of GLN on glycemia may possibly be mediated through a slowing of gastric emptying. A recent animal study performed by our laboratory showed that supplemental dietary GLN did not affect plasma glucose. However, leukocyte adhesion molecule expression, organ nitrotyrosine concentrations, and liver neutrophil infiltration were lower in diabetic animals when GLN was administered [27]. We also investigated the effects of GLN supplementation on gene expressions of inflammatory mediators and cytokines in diabetic rats. We found that messenger RNA expressions of interleukin (IL)-6, IL-23, monocyte chemotactic protein-1, and the receptor of the advanced glycated end products (RAGE) were lower in the GLN-diabetic group. Those results suggest that supplemental dietary GLN down-regulated inflammatory mediator expression in a diabetic condition [28]. Tashima et al. [29] studied the neuronal density and size of myenteric neurons and epithelial cell proliferation and crypt depth in the proximal colon of diabetic rats after GLN supplementation. They found that there were no changes in crypt depth or metaphasic index among the experimental groups. However, dietary 1% GLN supplementation resulted in an improvement in neuronal density compared to that of the untreated diabetic group. Consistent with that report, a recent study also found that GLN supplementation prevented myenteric neuron loss and had gliatrophic effects in the ileum of diabetic rats [30] (Table 12.1).

GLN AND HYPERGLYCEMIA-INDUCED COMPLICATIONS

There are five main hypotheses about the way in which hyperglycemia causes diabetic complications:

1) Increased polyol pathway flux;
2) Increased AGE formation;
3) Increased RAGE expression;
4) Activation of protein kinase C (PKC) isoforms;
5) Increased hexosamine pathway flux [31].

These metabolic pathways are major contributors to the overproduction of reactive oxygen species (ROS) and high oxidative stress during hyperglycemia [18,32] (Table 12.2). We analyzed the gene expression of key enzymes which regulate the above-mentioned pathways, including aldose reductase (AR), glutamine fructose-6-phosphate transaminase 1 (GFAT), and PKC in blood mononuclear cells of rodents. AR is the first enzyme in the polyol pathway. It catalyzes the Nicotinamide

TABLE 12.2 Major Pathways Involved in the Pathogenesis of Diabetic Complications

- Increased polyol pathway flux: This may result in sorbitol-induced osmotic stress, decreased ATPase activity, an increase in cytosolic NADH/NAD+, and a decrease in cytosolic NADPH.
- Increased advanced glycated end product (AGE) formation: AGEs are a group of compounds formed via non-enzymatic reactions between reducing sugars and amine residues on proteins, lipids, and nucleic acids. AGEs can act directly to induce cross-linking of long-lived proteins, thus altering the vascular structure and function.
- Increased receptor of AGE (RAGE) expression: RAGE is a multi-ligand receptor. Interactions of AGEs with the RAGE result in oxidative stress and elicit inflammation.
- Activation of protein kinase C (PKC): Hyperglycemia increases *de novo* synthesis of diacylglycerol which activates PKC. PKC activation inhibits endothelial nitric oxide synthase which enhances endothelin-1 and vascular endothelial growth factor expressions that may result in abnormalities of blood flow and permeability.
- Increased hexosamine pathway: The rate limiting enzyme is glutamine fructose-6-phosphate transaminase 1 (GFAT) which converts glucose to glucosamine. This pathway is associated with activation of plasminogen activator inhibitor (PAI)-1 and plays important roles in hyperglycemia-induced insulin resistance.

adenine dinucleotide phosphate (NADPH)-dependent reduction of various carbonyl compounds. GFAT is the rate limiting enzyme in the hexosamine pathway, which converts glucose to glucosamine [31,32]. RAGE and thioredoxin-interacting protein (Txnip) gene expressions were also measured. Binding of AGEs to RAGE activates a number of pathways implicated in chronic inflammation and the development of diabetic complications [33]. Hyperglycemia induces Txnip expression and thus inhibits thioredoxin's ROS-scavenging function [34]. Our results showed that diabetic rats had higher Txnip gene expression than the normal controls. Compared to the diabetic group without GLN, GLN supplementation resulted in lower GFAT, RAGE, and Txnip gene expressions by blood mononuclear cells [35] (Figure 12.2).

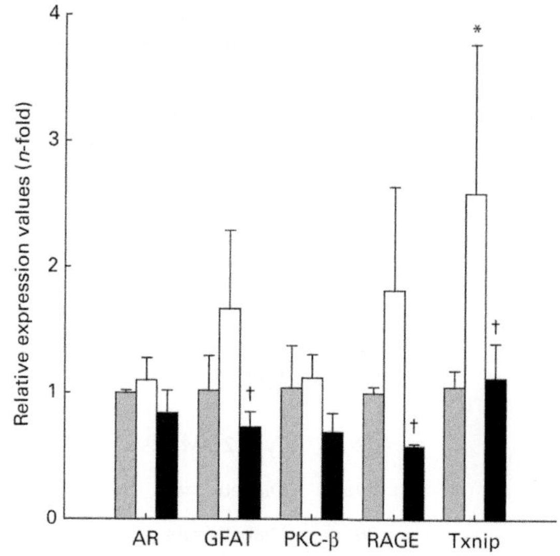

FIGURE 12.2 Relative mRNA expressions of aldose reductase (AR), glutamine fructose-6-phosphate transaminase 1 (GFAT), protein kinase C (PKC)-β, receptor of advanced glycation end products (RAGE), and thioredoxin-interacting protein (Txnip) by blood mononuclear cells. Values are the means of duplicate measurements, with standard deviations represented by vertical bars (n=4). Differences among groups were analyzed by a one-way ANOVA followed by Duncan's post-hoc test. *Mean values significantly differed from those of the normal control group (NC,■; $p<0.05$). †Mean values significantly differed from those of the diabetes mellitus group (DM,□; $p<0.05$). DM-GLN (■), diabetes with glutamine. *Reprinted from Tsai et al. [34] with permission from Cambridge University Press.*

MECHANISMS OF GLN IN ATTENUATING OXIDATIVE STRESS

Oxidative stress occurs as a consequence of an imbalance between the production of ROS and the body's ability to detoxify the reactive intermediates. This imbalance can result from the overproduction of ROS or a decrease in the capacity of antioxidant enzymes. Since oxidative stress plays a major role in the mechanisms of diabetic complications, it is likely that any therapy that successfully reduces oxidative stress will have a significant impact in treating the disease. The GSH system is one of the major mechanisms for reducing oxidative stress. A previous study found alterations in GSH metabolism in patients with diabetes [36]. An abnormal cellular GSH redox status decreases insulin sensitivity and affects the β-cell response to glucose in type 2 DM patients [37]. In addition, antioxidant enzyme activities were found to have changed in response to high levels of free radicals [35].

GSH

GSH (γ-glutamyl-cysteinyl-glycine) is a ubiquitous thiol (-SH)-containing tripeptide in mammalian cells, which plays a central role in modulating the cellular redox status. GSH is found in millimolar concentrations (0.5–10 mmol/L) intracellularly, and most (85%–90%) of the cellular GSH is localized in the cytosol [38]. GSH is composed of glutamate, cysteine, and glycine, and the thiol of the cysteine residue is responsible for its reducing ability. As a major component of the cellular antioxidant, GSH protects cells from free-radical damage by the following mechanisms:

1) GSH directly reacts with electrophilic substances, and is an important non-enzymatic free-radical scavenger; and
2) GSH participates in the reaction catalyzed by glutathione peroxidase (GPx) to eliminate hydrogen peroxide and is oxidized to glutathione disulfide (GSSG) which is recycled to GSH by glutathione reductase (GRd) in an NADPH-dependent reaction [39–41].

The ratio of GSH to GSSG is an indicator of the cellular redox status. In physiological conditions, GRd activity and NADPH availability are sufficient to maintain the GSH/GSSG ratio at >100 [42]. GSH plays a key role in detoxifying xenobiotics via the catalytic reaction of glutathione-S-transferase, and its metabolites are ultimately excreted in the urine and feces [43]. The GSH concentration was found to decrease in most organs of animals with chemically induced diabetes. However, there is also some contradictory evidence of increased GSH concentrations in diabetic rat kidneys and lenses [44].

Antioxidant Enzymes and Reactive Nitrogen Species

GPx and GRd are two enzymes that are found in the cytoplasm, mitochondria, and nuclei. GPx metabolizes H_2O_2 to water using reduced GSH as a hydrogen donor. Glutathione disulfide is recycled back to GSH by GRd. Catalase, located in peroxisomes, decomposes H_2O_2 to water and oxygen. Superoxide dismutase (SOD) converts superoxide anion radicals produced in the body to H_2O_2, thereby reducing the likelihood of superoxide anions interacting with nitric oxide (NO) to form reactive peroxynitrite. Animals with diabetes were found to have higher nitrotyrosine levels in their organs. Nitrotyrosine is the major product of a peroxynitrite attack on proteins, and is considered a good marker of oxidative damage to proteins and of oxidative stress. Higher nitrotyrosine levels indicate the extent of NO oxidation, which is increased in diabetes [45] (Figure 12.3). There is no total agreement about the effects of diabetes on antioxidant enzymes. Antioxidant enzyme activities are erratic and depend on the species of animal, and the duration and type of diabetes. Different species originating from different tissues also causes antioxidant enzyme activities to vary [44].

Heat Shock Proteins (HSPs)

HSPs comprise a highly conserved, ubiquitously expressed family of stress-response proteins. They can function as molecular chaperones, facilitating protein folding, preventing protein aggregation, or targeting improperly folded proteins to degradative pathways. HSPs are classified into subfamilies according to their molecular weight. Under normal physiological conditions, expressions of HSPs are at low levels; however, in response to cellular stress, their expressions dramatically increase. HSPs participate in a number of cellular processes that occur during and after exposure to oxidative stress. Activation of inflammatory pathways is one of the events that occur following oxidative stress. Prolonged oxidative stress can lead to cell death via activation of the apoptotic cell death pathway. Mechanisms of

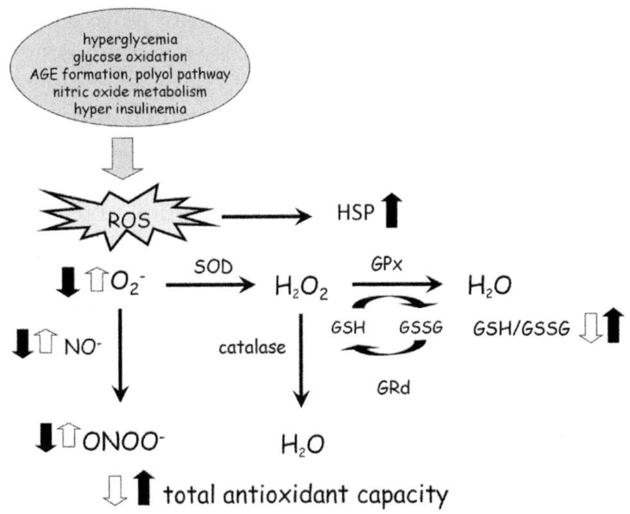

FIGURE 12.3 General catalytic reaction of antioxidant enzymes and the possible role of glutamine in reducing oxidative stress induced by hyperglycemia and related pathways. Glutamine supplementation reduces the production of peroxynitrite, increases the total antioxidant capacity, and reverses changes in antioxidant enzyme activities. Hollow arrows indicate the prooxidant substance and redox ratio in a diabetic condition; black arrows indicate the intervention of glutamine in diabetes. SOD, superoxide dismutase; GPx, glutathione peroxidase; GRd, glutathione reductase; GSH/GSSG, glutathione redox ratio; ROS, reactive oxygen species; O_2^-, superoxide; NO^-, nitric oxide; $ONOO^-$, peroxynitrite.

the protective action of HSPs following oxidative stress include:

1) Recognizing redox changes within the intracellular environment;
2) Repairing and eliminating damaged proteins;
3) Possessing antiapoptotic effects under stressed conditions; and
4) Binding to nuclear factor NF-κB and thus inhibiting transcriptional expressions of downstream inflammatory mediators [46].

GLN and Redox Capacity

GLN provides a source of glutamate and is considered to be a precursor in the synthesis of GSH. GLN was found to be rate limiting for GSH synthesis, and the availability of GLN is critical for generating GSH stores [47]. A previous *in vitro* study found that GLN prevented oxidative damage to hepatocytes induced by H_2O_2 and NO, and this was possibly mediated by GSH synthesis [48]. An animal study also showed that GLN-supplemented nutrition preserved GSH stores after treatment with an antineoplastic agent [49]. Studies performed by our laboratory revealed that GLN supplementation significantly increased the GSH/GSSG ratio in kidneys of diabetic mice and normalized the changes in the antioxidant enzyme system. Also, peroxynitrite production was reduced when GLN was administered under a diabetic condition [27,35]. Since activation of NF-κB relies on the cellular redox potential and intracellular GSH/GSSG ratio [50], a higher antioxidant capacity may thus prevent NF-κB activation and reduce subsequent diabetes-induced inflammation and organ injury (Figure 12.3).

HSP expression is vital to cellular and tissue protection after stress or injury. The HSP 70 family is the most conserved and best investigated class of all HSPs. GLN supplementation was found to enhance HSP70 and protect animals against various catabolic-stress conditions [51,52]. In an *in vitro* study, Jang et al. [53] divided rats into two groups after islet isolation. Isolated rat islets were cultured with IL-1β to induce tissue injury. One group of islet cells did not receive GLN in its culture medium. In the other group, islet cells were cultured with 10 mM GLN for 24 h. Results showed that the GLN-treated group had higher HSP70 expression and higher GSH levels. Also, expression of the antiapoptotic Bcl-2 markedly increased. Those results suggest that GLN administration can attenuate IL-1β-induced islet cell injury and apoptosis, possibly by enhancing HSP70 and GSH expressions, implying that it may be a potential nutrient for mitigating ischemic damage and inflammation to islet cells through a self-protective mechanism. A study performed by Ugurlucan et al. [54] also found that parenteral administration of GLN enhanced serum and tissue HSP70 expressions that may protect left atrial and ventricular tissues in hearts of diabetic rats (Table 12.1).

PROPOSED MOLECULAR MECHANISMS OTHER THAN ANTIOXIDANT EFFECTS

The action of GLN on attenuating diabetes or other disease-induced tissue injury may involve a complex mechanism. Generating an HSP response and enhancing GSH synthesis that leads to lower oxidative stress may be part of several contributory mechanisms. NF-κB is a protein complex that controls the transcription of DNA. It is retained in the cytoplasm in an inactive state by being bound to IκBα. Upon stimulation, IκB kinase is activated and subsequently phosphorylates the IκBα protein, which promotes degradation of IκBα and leads to nuclear translocation of NF-κB. A recent study found that GLN inhibited NF-κB activation through the PI3K/Akt/mTOR pathway and suppressed NF-κB-DNA binding activity, which led to repression of the expression of NF-κB target genes [55]. This study also showed that GLN inhibits the activation of the stress kinase pathway, reduces inflammatory cytokine release, and prevents acute respiratory distress syndrome following sepsis [56].

In addition, GLN can activate peroxisome proliferator activated receptor (PPAR) expression. There are three distinct PPARs: α, β, and γ, each encoded by a separate gene and distributed in different tissues. PPAR-α and PPAR-γ have been shown to control the expression of genes implicated in the inflammatory response via negative interference with proinflammatory pathways. PPAR-γ is expressed primarily in adipose tissue and the intestine and is activated by several ligands, suggesting their potential role in inflammation. Once activated by a ligand, PPAR heterodimerizes with the retinoid X receptor and binds to specific PPAR-responsive elements of DNA to promote transcription of a wide variety of genes. GLN is a ligand for PPAR-γ. A previous study revealed that luminal GLN induced the expression of PPAR-γ following mesenteric ischemia/reperfusion. This result represents a novel protective mechanism for GLN against intestinal inflammation [57].

GLN was also found to decrease cellular apoptosis after stress or injury (Table 12.3). An *in vitro* study showed that L-GLN deprivation of hybridoma cells rapidly triggers intracellular events, leading to the cytosolic release of apoptogenic factors, the activation of caspases-9 and -3, and commitment to the cell death program [58]. GLN limitation, even in the presence of an adequate glucose supply, impacts stress-related gene expression, differentially modulates receptor-mediated apoptosis, and directly elicits apoptosis through signaling mechanisms and caspase cascades [59]. Apoptotic destruction of the insulin-producing pancreatic β-cell is involved in the etiology of both type 1 and type 2 DM. The loss of pancreatic β-cells in type 1 DM occurs as a result of apoptotic signals from high concentrations of inflammatory cytokines or T-cells in the islet microenvironment. Similar to type 1, type 2 DM is also characterized by progressive loss of β-cells. The inflammatory cytokine IL-1β represents a common mediator of β-cell death in both types of DM. Hyperglycemia has been reported to induce β-cell apoptosis via the induction of autocrine production of IL-1β by β-cells [60]. Determining whether GLN decreases inflammatory cytokine secretion that may consequently inhibit apoptosis of β-cells and mitigate the severity of diabetes requires further investigation.

TABLE 12.3 Proposed Mechanisms by Which Glutamine Can Improve Outcomes in Diabetes

- Antioxidant potential
- Enhanced glutathione synthesis
- Promotion of heat shock protein expression
- Mitigation of inflammatory reaction
- Attenuated proinflammatory cytokine production
- Attenuated NF-κB/stress kinase activation
- Enhanced PPAR-γ expression
- Decreased cellular apoptosis
- Enhanced insulin secretion and attenuated insulin resistance

CONCLUSIONS

Numerous studies have found that GLN enhances the insulin response, reduces inflammatory mediator production, and decreases expression of genes associated with the main pathways that cause diabetic complications. GLN is a precursor of GSH. Also, GLN enhances HSP expression. GLN supplementation increases the antioxidant potential, which may play an important role in mitigating the tissue injury induced by diabetes. Other factors, including attenuating inflammatory reactions, decreasing cellular apoptosis, and enhancing insulin secretion, may also contribute to the benefits of GLN in diabetes.

SUMMARY POINTS

- GLN is a non-essential amino acid with many physiological functions. Currently, it is considered conditionally essential for patients with catabolic diseases.
- Profound GLN depletion was found during major injury, indicating that additional supplementation is needed to maintain GLN homeostasis in such situations.
- Many studies have demonstrated the benefits of GLN administration to immune function in various disease conditions.
- Plasma GLN levels decrease in diabetic patients, and this may lead to disturbances of insulin secretion and its actions.
- GLN is a precursor of GSH and promotes HSP expression.
- GLN has antioxidant potential in attenuating diabetes-induced oxidative stress.
- The influences of GLN on improving outcomes of diabetes may involve other mechanisms, including attenuating inflammatory reactions, decreasing cellular apoptosis, and enhancing insulin secretion.

References

[1] Parry-Billings M, Evans J, Calder PC, Newsholme EA. Does glutamine contribute to immunosuppression after major burns? Lancet 1990;336:523–5.
[2] Greig JE, Keast D, Garcia-Webb P, Crawford P. Inter-relationships between glutamine and other biochemical and immunological changes after major vascular surgery. Br J Biomed Sci 1996;53: 116–21.
[3] Labow BI, Souba WW. Glutamine. World J Surg 2000;24:1503–13.
[4] Coeffier M, Dechelotte P. The role of glutamine in intensive care unit patients: mechanisms of action and clinical outcome. Nutr Rev 2005;63:65–9.
[5] Wischmeyer PE. Glutamine: mode of action in critical illness. Crit Care Med 2007;35:S541–4.
[6] Curi R, Lagranha CJ, Doi SQ, Sellitti DF, Procopio J, Pithon-Curi TC, et al. Molecular mechanisms of glutamine action. J Cell Physiol 2005;204:392–401.
[7] Wischmeyer PE, Kahana M, Wolfson R, Ren H, Musch MM, Chang EB. Glutamine reduces cytokine release, organ damage, and mortality in a rat model of endotoxemia. Shock 2001; 16:398–402.
[8] Kozar RA, Schultz SG, Bick RJ, Poindexter BJ, DeSoignie R, Moore FA. Enteral glutamine but not alanine maintains small bowel barrier function after ischemia/reperfusion injury in rats. Shock 2004;21:433–7.
[9] Lee WY, Hu YM, Ko TL, Yeh SL, Yeh CL. glutamine modulates sepsis-induced changes to intestinal intraepithelial gammadeltat lymphocyte expression in mice. Shock 2012;38:288–93.
[10] Hu YM, Pai MH, Yeh CL, Hou YC, Yeh SL. Glutamine administration ameliorates sepsis-induced kidney injury by downregulating the high-mobility group box protein-1-mediated pathway in mice. Am J Physiol Renal Physiol 2012;302:F150–8.
[11] De-Souza DA, Greene LJ. Intestinal permeability and systemic infections in critically ill patients: effect of glutamine. Crit Care Med 2005;33:1125–35.
[12] Fuentes-Orozco C, Anaya-Prado R, Gonzalez-Ojeda A, Arenas-Marquez H, Cabrera-Pivaral C, Cervantes-Guevara G, et al. L-alanyl-L-glutamine-supplemented parenteral nutrition improves infectious morbidity in secondary peritonitis. Clin Nutr 2004;23:13–21.
[13] Goeters C, Wenn A, Mertes N, Wempe C, Van Aken H, Stehle P, et al. Parenteral L-alanyl-L-glutamine improves six month outcomes in critically ill patients. Crit Care Med 2002;30:2032–7.
[14] Furst P, Albers S, Stehle P. Glutamine-containing dipeptides in parenteral nutrition. JPEN J Parenter Enteral Nutr 1990;14:118S–24S.
[15] Soeters PB, van de Poll MC, van Gemert WG, Dejong CH. Amino acid adequacy in pathophysiological states. J Nutr 2004;134: 1575S–82S.
[16] Garlick PJ. Assessment of the safety of glutamine and other amino acids. J Nutr 2001;131:2556S–61S.
[17] Wei W, Liu Q, Tan Y, Liu L, Li X, Cai L. Oxidative stress, diabetes, and diabetic complications. Hemoglobin 2009;33:370–7.
[18] Giacco F, Brownlee M. Oxidative stress and diabetic complications. Circ Res 2010;107:1058–70.
[19] Ardawi MS. Glutamine and ketone-body metabolism in the gut of streptozotocin-diabetic rats. Biochem J 1988;249:565–72.
[20] Menge BA, Schrader H, Ritter PR, Ellrichmann M, Uhl W, Schmidt WE, et al. Selective amino acid deficiency in patients with impaired glucose tolerance and type 2 diabetes. Regul Pept 2010;160:75–80.
[21] Curi R, Lagranha CJ, Doi SQ, Sellitti DF, Procopio J, Pithon-Curi TC, et al. Molecular mechanisms of glutamine action. J Cell Physiol 2005;204:392–401.
[22] Li C, Buettger C, Kwagh J, Matter A, Daikhin Y, Nissim IB, et al. A signaling role of glutamine in insulin secretion. J Biol Chem 2004;279:13393–401.
[23] Bakalar B, Duska F, Pachl J, Fric M, Otahal M, Pazout J, et al. Parenterally administered dipeptide alanyl-glutamine prevents worsening of insulin sensitivity in multiple-trauma patients. Crit Care Med 2006;34:381–6.
[24] Opara EC, Petro A, Tevrizian A, Feinglos MN, Surwit RS. L-glutamine supplementation of a high fat diet reduces body weight and attenuates hyperglycemia and hyperinsulinemia in C57BL/6J mice. J Nutr 1996;126:273–9.
[25] Greenfield JR, Farooqi IS, Keogh JM, Henning E, Habib AM, Blackwood A, et al. Oral glutamine increases circulating glucagon-like peptide 1, glucagon, and insulin concentrations in lean, obese, and type 2 diabetic subjects. Am J Clin Nutr 2009;89:106–13.
[26] Samocha-Bonet D, Wong O, Synnott EL, Piyaratna N, Douglas A, Gribble FM, et al. Glutamine reduces postprandial glycemia and augments the glucagon-like peptide-1 response in type 2 diabetes patients. J Nutr 2011;141:1233–8.

[27] Tsai PH, Liu JJ, Chiu WC, Pai MH, Yeh SL. Effects of dietary glutamine on adhesion molecule expression and oxidative stress in mice with streptozotocin-induced type 1 diabetes. Clin Nutr 2011;30:124–9.
[28] Tsai PH, Yeh CL, Liu JJ, Chiu WC, Yeh SL. Effects of dietary glutamine on inflammatory mediator gene expressions in rats with streptozotocin-induced diabetes. Nutrition 2012;28:288–93.
[29] Tashima CM, Tronchini EA, Pereira RV, Bazotte RB, Zanoni JN. Diabetic rats supplemented with L-glutamine: a study of immunoreactive myosin-V myenteric neurons and the proximal colonic mucosa. Dig Dis Sci 2007;52:1233–41.
[30] Pereira RV, Tronchini EA, Tashima CM, Alves EP, Lima MM, Zanoni JN. L-glutamine supplementation prevents myenteric neuron loss and has gliatrophic effects in the ileum of diabetic rats. Dig Dis Sci 2011;56:3507–16.
[31] Brownlee M. Biochemistry and molecular cell biology of diabetic complications. Nature 2001;414:813–20.
[32] Johansen JS, Harris AK, Rychly DJ, Ergul A. Oxidative stress and the use of antioxidants in diabetes: linking basic science to clinical practice. Cardiovasc Diabetol 2005;4:5.
[33] Bierhaus A, Humpert PM, Morcos M, Wendt T, Chavakis T, Arnold B, et al. Understanding RAGE, the receptor for advanced glycation end products. J Mol Med (Berl) 2005;83:876–86.
[34] Nishiyama A, Matsui M, Iwata S, Hirota K, Masutani H, Nakamura H, et al. Identification of thioredoxin-binding protein-2/vitamin D(3) up-regulated protein 1 as a negative regulator of thioredoxin function and expression. J Biol Chem 1999;274:21645–50.
[35] Tsai PH, Liu JJ, Yeh CL, Chiu WC, Yeh SL. Effects of glutamine supplementation on oxidative stress-related gene expression and antioxidant properties in rats with streptozotocin-induced type 2 diabetes. Br J Nutr 2012;107:1112–8.
[36] Roth E, Oehler R, Manhart N, Exner R, Wessner B, Strasser E, et al. Regulative potential of glutamine – relation to glutathione metabolism. Nutrition 2002;18:217–21.
[37] De Mattia G, Bravi MC, Laurenti O, Cassone-Faldetta M, Armiento A, Ferri C, et al. Influence of reduced glutathione infusion on glucose metabolism in patients with non-insulin-dependent diabetes mellitus. Metabolism 1998;47:993–7.
[38] Lu SC. Regulation of glutathione synthesis. Curr Top Cell Regul 2000;36:95–116.
[39] Wu G, Fang YZ, Yang S, Lupton JR, Turner ND. Glutathione metabolism and its implications for health. J Nutr 2004;134:489–92.
[40] Fang YZ, Yang S, Wu G. Free radicals, antioxidants, and nutrition. Nutrition 2002;18:872–9.
[41] Kehrer JP, Lund LG. Cellular reducing equivalents and oxidative stress. Free Radic Biol Med 1994;17:65–75.
[42] Akerboom TP, Bilzer M, Sies H. The relationship of biliary glutathione disulfide efflux and intracellular glutathione disulfide content in perfused rat liver. J Biol Chem 1982;257:4248–52.
[43] Hayes JD, McLellan LI. Glutathione and glutathione-dependent enzymes represent a co-ordinately regulated defense against oxidative stress. Free Radic Res 1999;31:273–300.
[44] Maritim AC, Sanders RA, Watkins III JB. Diabetes, Oxidative Stress, and Antioxidants: A Review. J Biochem Mol Toxicol 2003;17:24–38.
[45] Piconi L, Quagliaro L, Ceriello A. Oxidative stress in diabetes. Clin Chem Lab Med 2003;41:1144–9.
[46] Kalmar B, Greensmith L. Induction of heat shock proteins for protection against oxidative stress. Adv Drug Deliv Rev 2009;61:310–8.
[47] Welbourne TC. Ammonia production and glutamine incorporation into glutathione in the functioning rat kidney. Can J Biochem 1979;57:233–7.
[48] Babu R, Eaton S, Drake DP, Spitz L, Pierro A. Glutamine and glutathione counteract the inhibitory effects of mediators of sepsis in neonatal hepatocytes. J Pediatr Surg 2001;36:282–6.
[49] Yu JC, Jiang ZM, Li DM, Yang NF, M-X B. Alanyl-glutamine preserves hepatic glutathione stores after 5-FU treatment. Clin Nutr 1996;15:261–5.
[50] Sen CK, Khanna S, Reznick AZ, Roy S, Packer L. Glutathione regulation of tumor necrosis factor-alpha-induced NF-kappa B activation in skeletal muscle-derived L6 cells. Biochem Biophys Res Commun 1997;237:645–9.
[51] Singleton KD, Wischmeyer PE. Glutamine's protection against sepsis and lung injury is dependent on heat shock protein 70 expression. Am J Physiol Regul Integr Comp Physiol 2007;292:R1839–45.
[52] Morrison AL, Dinges M, Singleton KD, Odoms K, Wong HR, Wischmeyer PE. Glutamine's protection against cellular injury is dependent on heat shock factor-1. Am J Physiol Cell Physiol 2006;290:C1625–32.
[53] Jang HJ, Kwak JH, Cho EY, We YM, Lee YH, Kim SC, et al. Glutamine induces heat-shock protein-70 and glutathione expression and attenuates ischemic damage in rat islets. Transplant Proc 2008;40:2581–4.
[54] Ugurlucan M, Erer D, Karatepe O, Ziyade S, Haholu A, Gungor Ugurlucan F, et al. Glutamine enhances the heat shock protein 70 expression as a cardioprotective mechanism in left heart tissues in the presence of diabetes mellitus. Expert Opin Ther Targets 2010;14:1143–56.
[55] Hou YC, Chiu WC, Yeh CL, Yeh SL. Glutamine modulates lipopolysaccharide-induced activation of NF-κB via the Akt/mTOR pathway in lung epithelial cells. Am J Physiol Lung Cell Mol Physiol 2012;302:L174–83.
[56] Singleton KD, Beckey VE, Wischmeyer PE. Glutamine prevents activation of NF-kappaB and stress kinase pathways, attenuates inflammatory cytokine release, and prevents acute respiratory distress syndrome (ards) following sepsis. Shock 2005;24:583–9.
[57] Sato N, Moore FA, Kone BC, Zou L, Smith MA, Childs MA, et al. Differential induction of PPAR-gamma by luminal glutamine and iNOS by luminal arginine in the rodent postischemic small bowel. Am J Physiol Gastrointest Liver Physiol 2006;290:G616–23.
[58] Paquette JC, Guerin PJ, Gauthier ER. Rapid induction of the intrinsic apoptotic pathway by L-glutamine starvation. J Cell Physiol 2005;202:912–21.
[59] Fuchs BC, Bode BP. Stressing out over survival: glutamine as an apoptotic modulator. J Surg Res 2006;131:26–40.
[60] Ryan A, Murphy M, Godson C, Hickey FB. Diabetes mellitus and apoptosis: inflammatory cells. Apoptosis 2009;14:1435–50.

CHAPTER

13

The Anti-Oxidative Component of Docosahexaenoic Acid (DHA) in the Brain in Diabetes

*Emma Arnal**, *María Miranda***, *Siv Johnsen-Soriano**, *Francisco J. Romero**, †

*Fundación Oftalmológica del Mediterráneo, Valencia, Spain, **Universidad CEU Cardenal Herrera, Moncada, Spain, †Facultad de Medicina, Universidad Católica de Valencia 'San Vicente Mártir', Valencia, Spain

List of Abbreviations

AA Arachidonic acid
ALA Alfa-linolenic acid
ARPE-19 Human retinal pigment epithelial cell line
CNS Central nervous system
COX Cyclooxygenase
DHA Docosahexaenoic acid
EPA Eicosapentanoic acid
GSH Glutathione
IL Interleukin
LOX Lipoxygenase
MCI Mild cognitive impairment
NPD1 Neuroprotectin D1
PUFA Polyunsaturated fatty acid
ROS Reactive oxygen species
RPE Retinal pigment epithelium
SOD Superoxide dismutase

INTRODUCTION: OXIDATIVE STRESS IN DIABETES

Neuronal cells are particularly sensitive to oxidative insults, and reactive oxygen species (ROS) are involved in many neurodegenerative processes such as diabetes [1–3]. In these pathological conditions, cellular stress triggers mitochondrial oxidative damage, which may result in apoptosis and/or necrosis [4], and apoptosis induced by oxidative stress has been related to neurogenesis inhibition [5].

ROS generated by high glucose levels causes metabolic abnormalities which are involved in the development of diabetes [6]. Previous studies have shown that oxidative stress is closely linked to apoptosis in a variety of cell types under hyperglycemic conditions [7]; furthermore apoptosis mediated by caspase-3 is activated in the brain of diabetic rats, and antioxidants are able to inhibit these activations [8–10] (Figure 13.1). Chronic degenerative brain disease in diabetes, known as 'diabetic encephalopathy', is a recognized complication that can occur in patients whose diabetes is long-standing. The mechanisms underlying diabetic encephalopathy are only partially understood, and can involve impairments in learning, memory, problem solving, and mental and motor speed (Figure 13.2) which are more common in type 1 diabetic patients than in the general population [11]. Neuronal cells are particularly sensitive to oxidative insults and ROS are involved in many neurodegenerative processes (not only diabetes but also Alzheimer's, Parkinson's, and Huntington's diseases, acute brain ischemia, and excitotoxicity) [1–3].

The possible source of oxidative stress in brain injury includes auto-oxidation of glucose, lipid peroxidation, decreased tissue concentrations of low molecular weight antioxidants such as reduced glutathione (GSH) (Figure 13.3) and impaired activities of antioxidant defense enzymes such as superoxide dismutase (SOD) and catalase [6,12,13]. Convincing evidence is now available from previous studies to prove the role of oxidative stress in the development of neuronal injury in the diabetic brain and the beneficial effects of antioxidants.

Diabetes: Oxidative Stress and Dietary Antioxidants.
http://dx.doi.org/10.1016/B978-0-12-405885-9.00013-9

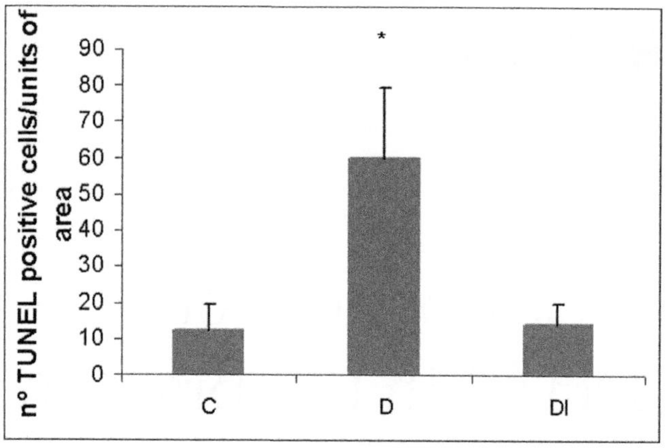

FIGURE 13.1 Number of TUNEL-positive cells in the dentate gyrus of the hippocampus of diabetic and control rats. (*$p<0.05$ vs. all groups). C, control; D, untreated diabetic rats; DI, diabetic rats treated with insulin.

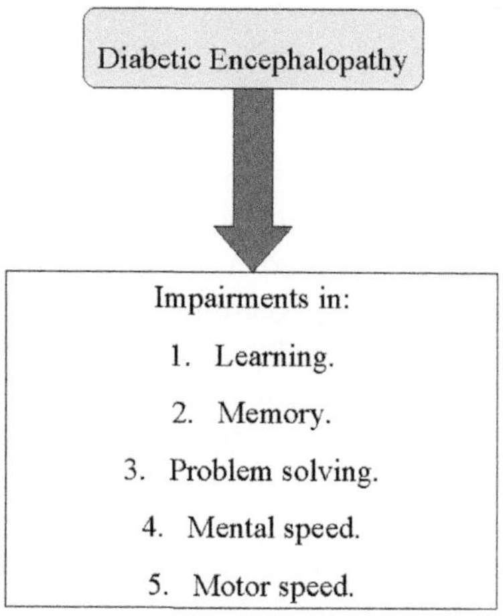

FIGURE 13.2 Schematic representation of the potential impairments in diabetic encephalopathy.

However clinical trials testing the efficacy of antioxidants in the treatment of different diseases, including diabetes, have produced contradictory findings. This could be because most studies have focused on the use of antioxidants to block the production of ROS and other compounds, and perhaps it is too late to observe any beneficial effect and focus should be placed on blocking changes in intracellular signaling produced by oxidative stress. In this sense, many studies demonstrate the ability of antioxidant administration to revert the perjudicial effects of diabetes. The beneficial effect of lutein and DHA in diabetic animals and the way that these substances were able to ameliorate the oxidative stress present in diabetes have been studied [14].

DOCOSAHEXAENOIC ACID (DHA)

DHA;4 22:6(n-3) (Figure 13.4); is a dietary essential (n-3) PUFA highly enriched in fish oils and concentrated up the food chain from photosynthetic and heterotrophic microalgae. In addition to these essential marine sources, DHA is also synthesized via the elongation and desaturation of the 20-carbon eicosapentanoic acid (EPA 20:5(n-3)), or by elongation of the 18-carbon (n-3) fatty acid, a-linolenic acid (ALA; 18:3(n-3)) enriched in flax (Linaceae), walnut (Juglandaceae), chia (*Salvia hispanica*), and other photosynthesizing terrestrial plants (Figure 13.5) [15–17]. In the brain, the glial and endothelial cells of the microvasculature, but not neurons, have some capacity to synthesize DHA from ALA and other (n-3) precursor fatty acids, but whether or not this contributes significantly to total brain DHA is not clear. The high concentration of DHA in the capillary endothelium suggests that DHA is taken up from the diet via

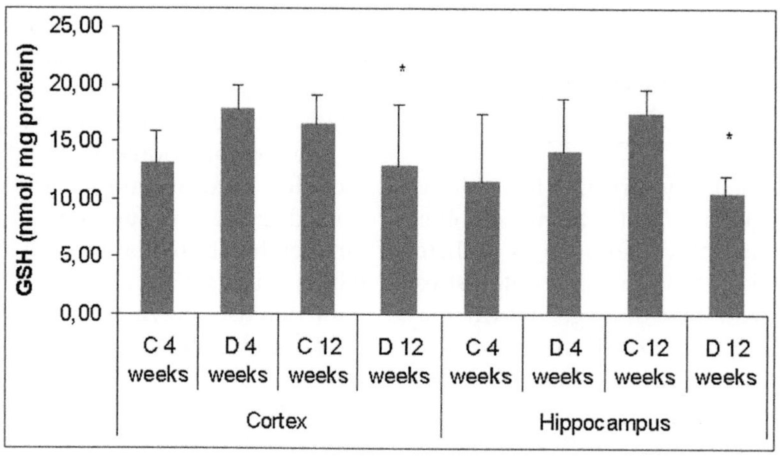

FIGURE 13.3 GSH concentration in the cortex and hippocampus of control and 4 or 12 weeks diabetic rats (*$p<0.05$ vs. control 12 weeks groups). C, control; D, untreated diabetic rats.

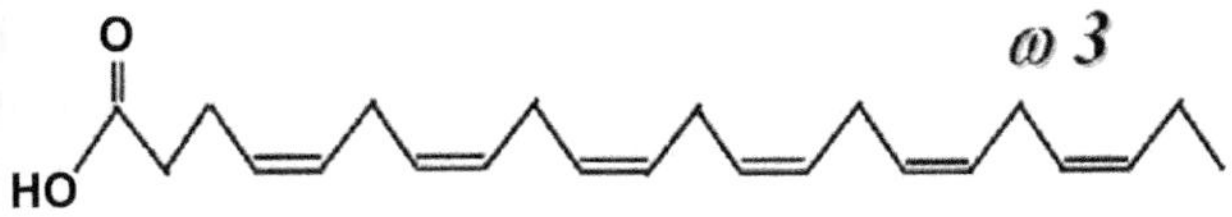

FIGURE 13.4 DHA structure.

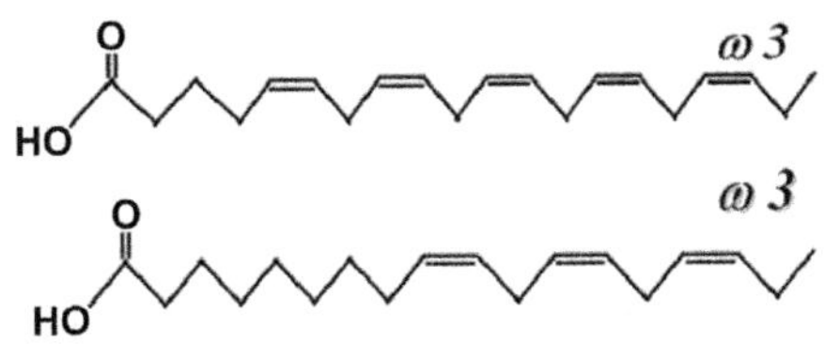

FIGURE 13.5 Eicosapentanoic acid and α-linolenic acid structures.

blood plasma DHA transporters including specific fatty-acid-binding lipoprotein carriers [17–19].

DHA is an absolute requirement for the development of the human central nervous system (CNS), and the continuous maintenance of brain cell function, illustrating the strong mechanistic link between an adequate supply of essential PUFA in the diet and the sustenance of cognitive health. During postnatal development, rapid accretion of DHA in the brain and retina takes place [16–18]. DHA attains its highest concentration in CNS synapses and in retinal photoreceptors; in fact, up to 60% of all fatty acids esterified in neuronal plasma membrane phospholipid consist of DHA. By means of a postnatal mouse development experimental model, it has been determined that dietary ALA is first taken up by the liver, where elongation and desaturation to DHA occurs, followed by its supply through the bloodstream to brain and retina, coinciding with photoreceptor development and synaptogenesis [17,19]. Brain and retinal cells therefore have a convenient and readily accessible supply of DHA that, through highly regulated, phospholipase-mediated exoprotease activities, liberates membrane-bound DHA to serve in neuroprotective and cell fate-signaling roles [20–26]. The beneficial neurophysiological actions of DHA occur in part through its direct maintenance of neuronal plasma membrane fluidity and functional integrity, and in part through the generation of docosanoids. The first identified DHA-derived mediator, neuroprotectin D1 (NPD1; MW 359), is formed through tandem phospholipase A2 (PLA2)-lipoxygenase (LOX) action on free DHA, via a 16,17S-DHA epoxide intermediate [20,24,27,28].

DHA AND OXIDATIVE STRESS

DHA is most highly concentrated in photoreceptors, the nervous system, and testes, in descending order of concentration [26]. Both neurons and glia are richly endowed with this fatty acid. The outer segments of photoreceptors display the highest content of DHA in the human body. Moreover, DHA is present in much smaller quantities in non-nervous system cells. DHA is esterified at C2 of the glycerol backbone of phospholipids. In contrast the other major polyunsaturated fatty acyl group of cell phospholipids, the omega-6 family member arachidonic acid (AA), is distributed throughout the human body. Arachidonoyl chains of phospholipids are the reservoir of biologically active eicosanoids, and docosahexaenoyl chains of phospholipids are a reservoir for biologically active docosanoids. Both polyunsaturated fatty acids are also a target for free radical-mediated lipid peroxidation.

Free (unesterified) AA and DHA are released from membrane phospholipids through the action of phospholipases in response to stimulation (e.g., neurotransmitters, cytokines, seizures, ischemia, neurotrauma, etc.) [26,29]. This response tells us that phospholipases are a regulatory gatekeeper in the initiation of the eicosanoid and docosanoid pathways under both physiological and pathological conditions. It remains to be determined whether any of the docosanoids are esterified back into phospholipids, which might, in turn, serve as reservoirs for readily-made bioactive mediators. In connection with this, there are examples of AA-derived lipoxygenation products incorporated into phospholipids of the nervous tissue [30]. During basal cell function, active ATP-dependent reacylation of AA and DHA takes place in membrane phospholipids [31,32].

Oxidative stress in the brain generates neuroprostanes from DHA through enzyme-independent reactions [33]. It has recently been shown that electrophilic cyclopentenone neuroprostanes elicit anti-inflammatory activity [34]. These compounds are formed from the peroxidation of DHA; therefore, it remains to be determined how the production of these compounds might be regulated and how they might exert specific actions such as anti-inflammatory activity.

DHA is required for brain and retina development [35] and has been implicated in several functions, including those of excitable membranes [36,37], memory [37], photoreceptor biogenesis and function [38], and neuroprotection [39]. One property the retina and brain share (insofar as omega-3 fatty acids are concerned) is their unusual ability to retain DHA even during prolonged dietary deprivation of essential fatty acids of the omega-3 family. To effectively reduce the DHA content in retinas and brains of rodents and non-human primates, dietary deprivation for more than one generation has been required [40,41]. This in turn produces impairments of retinal and brain function. Studies on DHA-mediated neuroprotection have prompted the following questions: Is the prosurvival action of DHA the result of replenishing the fatty acid into membrane phospholipids? Is it due to a more selective signaling by a DHA-derived mediator? Or is there a combination of mechanisms?

This review highlights the elucidation of a specific DHA mediator that promotes the homeostatic regulation of cell integrity and retina and brain protection.

NEUROPROTECTIN D1

The retina forms mono-, di- and trihydroxy derivatives of DHA. Since lipoxygenase inhibitors block the formation of these derivatives, it was suggested that a lipoxygenase enzyme catalyzes their synthesis, and the name 'docosanoids' was introduced for the family of enzyme-derived products of DHA [42]. At the time of that study, the stereochemistry and bioactivity of these DHA-oxygenated derivatives were not defined. It was suggested, however, that these lipoxygenase-reaction products might be neuroprotective [42]. Upon the advent of mediator lipidomic analysis based on liquid chromatography, photodiode array, electrospray ionization, and tandem mass spectrometry (LC-MS/MS), Bazan and colleagues [43] identified oxygenation pathways for the synthesis of the stereospecific docosanoid NPD1 during brain ischemia-reperfusion [44], in human RPE cells [45–47], in human brain cells [20], and in the human brain. NPD1 synthesis occurs through DHA oxygenation by 15-lipoxygenase-1 (15-LOX-1). NPD1 then works through a stereospecific site, implying that this mediator acts in an autocrine fashion, and/or diffuses through the intercellular space (e.g., interphotoreceptor matrix to act in paracrine mode on nearby cells). One paracrine target in the retina could be photoreceptor cells and/or Müller cells. In addition, this group described the way that interleukin (IL)-1β, oxidative stress, or the Ca^{2+} ionophore A23187 activates the synthesis of NPD1 in ARPE-19 cells (spontaneously transformed human RPE cells) [45]. NPD1 in turn is a potent inhibitor of oxidative stress-induced apoptosis and of cytokine-mediated pro inflammatory induction of cyclooxygenase 2 (COX-2). The name 'neuroprotectin D1' [47] was proposed, based on its neuroprotective bioactivity in oxidatively stressed RPE cells or brain and its potent ability to inactivate pro-apoptotic and pro-inflammatory signaling. 'D1' refers to this being the first identified neuroprotective mediator derived from DHA.

DHA AND OXIDATIVE STRESS IN THE BRAIN

Oxidative stress results from an imbalance between the formation and the degradation of pro-oxidants or impaired cellular antioxidant mechanisms, and excessive oxidative stress leads to cell damage and apoptosis [48].

The brain is particularly susceptible to oxidative stress, because it has a high content of easily peroxidizable long-chain PUFAs such as DHA and AA. Mitochondrial consumption of a large quantity of glucose to fuel the brain's normal energy requirements also results in relatively high production of free radicals [49]. In diabetes, the oxidative stress situation increases the production of free radicals, resulting in increased lipid peroxidation in the brain [50]. Crucial oxidative damage has also been observed in subjects with mild cognitive impairment (MCI), suggesting an early role of oxidative stress [51]. Lipid peroxide levels are significantly lower in DHA-administered rats and reciprocally correlate with the DHA/AA ratio [52], indicating that dietary DHA contributes to the antioxidant defense, decreases oxidative stress, and protects against memory loss. This inference is consistent with the fact that DHA also increases the levels of antioxidant enzymes such as

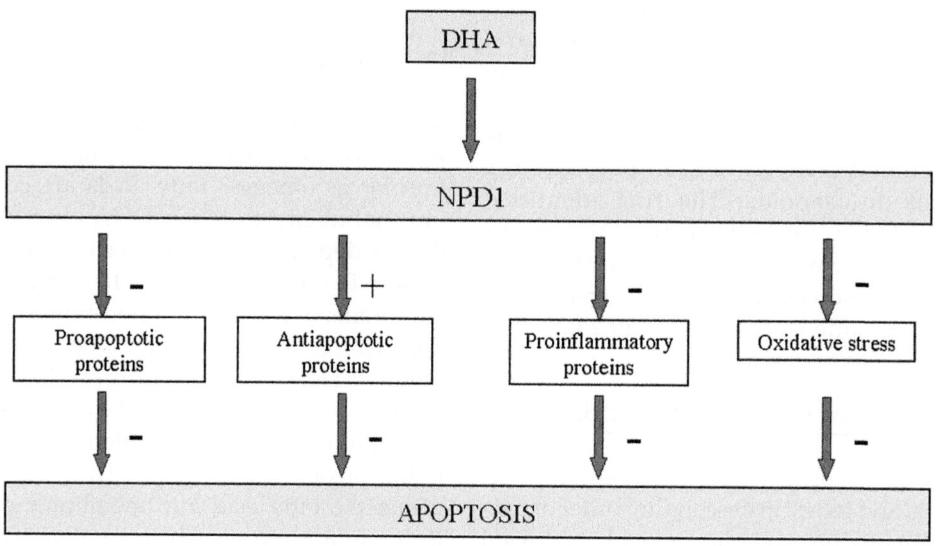

FIGURE 13.6 **Schematic representation of the potential DHA and NPD1 actions that may lead to apoptosis inhibition.**

catalase and glutathione peroxidase, and reduces glutathione levels with a concomitant decrease in the levels of ROS in the cortex and hippocampus of diabetes rat models [53]. Further, DHA has free radical-scavenging properties such as protection against lipid and protein peroxidation in developing and adult brains and attenuation of neuronal loss and cognitive and locomotor deficits in animal models of ischemia-reperfusion brain injury [54]. The antioxidant action of DHA in the brain has been underscored [55], despite the fact that its molecular structure contains six double bonds, which theoretically makes it a molecular target for peroxidation and sensitizes cells to ROS. Moreover, DHA can produce docosatrienes and resolvins, collectively known as docosanoids. In particular, NPD1 is formed through tandem phospholipase A2-lipoxygenase action on free DHA; it is a docosatriene that appears to be a major bioactive effector in neuronal tissues. Even a minute amount of NPD1 can promote anti-inflammatory and neuroprotective activity and inhibit oxidative stress-induced apoptosis [20] (Figure 13.6). These results suggest the notable role of DHA and/or DHA-derived mediators in the inhibition of oxidative stress.

References

[1] Jackson GR, Werrbach-Perez K, Pan Z, Sampath D, Perez-Polo JR. Neurotrophin regulation of energy homeostasis in the central nervous system. Dev Neurosci 1994;16:285–90.

[2] Dugan LL, Sensi SL, Canzoniero LM, Handran SD, Rothman SM, Lin TS, et al. Mitochondrial production of reactive oxygen species in cortical neurons following exposure to N-methyl-D-aspartate. J Neurosci 1995;15:6377–88.

[3] Yuan J, Yankner BA. Apoptosis in the nervous system. Nature 2000;407:802–9.

[4] Merad-Boudia M, Nicole A, Santiard-Baron D, Saillé C, Ceballos-Picot I. Mitochondrial impairment as an early event in the process of apoptosis induced by glutathione depletion in neuronal cells: relevance to Parkinson's disease. Biochem Pharmacol 1998;56:645–55.

[5] Cui X, Zuo P, Zhang Q, Li X, Hu Y, Long J, et al. Chronic systemic D-galactose exposure induces memory loss, neurodegeneration, and oxidative damage in mice: protective effects of R-alpha-lipoic acid. J Neurosci Res 2006;84(3):647–54.

[6] Brownlee M. Biochemistry and molecular cell biology of diabetic complications. Nature 2001;414:813–20.

[7] Cui Y, Xu X, Bi H, Zhu Q, Wu J, Xia X, et al. Expression modification of uncoupling proteins and MnSOD in retinal endothelial cells and pericytes induced by high glucose: the role of reactive oxygen species in diabetic retinopathy. Exp Eye Res 2006;83:807–16.

[8] Kowluru RA, Tang J, Kern TS. Abnormalities of retinal metabolism in diabetes and experimental galactosemia. VII. Effect of long-term administration of antioxidants on the development of retinopathy. Diabetes 2001;50:1938–42.

[9] Kowluru RA. Effect of reinstitution of good glycemic control on retinal oxidative stress and nitrative stress in diabetic rats. Diabetes 2003;52:818–23.

[10] Arnal E, Miranda M, Johnsen-Soriano S, Alvarez-Nölting R, Díaz-Llopis M, Araiz J, et al. Beneficial effect of docosahexanoic acid and lutein on retinal structural, metabolic, and functional abnormalities in diabetic rats. Curr Eye Res 2009;34:928–38.

[11] Li ZG, Zhang W, Grunberger G, Sima AA. Hippocampal neuronal apoptosis in type 1 diabetes. Brain Res 2002;946:221–31.

[12] Kowluru RA, Kern TS, Engerman RL, Armstrong D. Abnormalities of retinal metabolism in diabetes or experimental galactosemia. III. Effects of antioxidants. Diabetes 1996;45:1233–7.

[13] Haskins K, Bradley B, Powers K, Fadok V, Flores S, Ling X, et al. Oxidative stress in type 1 diabetes. Ann N Y Acad Sci 2003;1005:43–54.

[14] Arnal E, Miranda M, Johnsen-Soriano S, Alvarez-Nölting R, Díaz-Llopis M, Araiz J, et al. Beneficial effect of docosahexanoic acid and lutein on retinal structural, metabolic, and functional abnormalities in diabetic rats. Curr Eye Res 2009;34: 928–38.

[15] Marszalek JR, Lodish HF. Docosahexaenoic acid, fatty acid-interacting proteins, and neuronal function: breastmilk and fish are good for you. Annu Rev Cell Dev Biol 2005;21:633–57.

[16] Rapoport SI, Rao JS, Igarashi M. Brain metabolism of nutritionally essential polyunsaturated fatty acids depends on both the diet and the liver. Prostaglandins Leukot Essent Fatty Acids 2007;77:251–61.

[17] Innis SM. Dietary (n-3) fatty acids and brain development. J Nutr 2007;137:855–9.

[18] Spector AA. Plasma free fatty acid and lipoproteins as sources of polyunsaturated fatty acid for the brain. J Mol Neurosci 2001;16:159–65; discussion 215–221.

[19] Scott BL, Bazan NG. Membrane docosahexaenoate is supplied to the developing brain and retina by the liver. Proc Natl Acad Sci U S A 1989;86:2903–7.

[20] Lukiw WJ, Cui JG, Marcheselli VL, Bodker M, Botkjaer A, Gotlinger K, et al. A role for docosahexaenoic acid-derived neuroprotectin D1 in neural cell survival and Alzheimer disease. J Clin Invest 2005;115:2774–83.

[21] Mancuso M, Coppede F, Migliore L, Siciliano G, Murri L. Mitochondrial dysfunction, oxidative stress and neurodegeneration. J Alzheimers Dis 2006;10:59–73.

[22] Kazantsev AG. Cellular pathways leading to neuronal dysfunction and degeneration. Drug News Perspect 2007;20:501–9.

[23] Smith DG, Cappai R, Barnham KJ. The redox chemistry of the Alzheimer's disease amyloid beta peptide. Biochim Biophys Acta 2007;1768:1976–90.

[24] Mukherjee PK, Chawla A, Loayza MS, Bazan NG. Docosanoids are multifunctional regulators of neural cell integrity and fate: significance in aging and disease. Prostaglandins Leukot Essent Fatty Acids 2007;77:233–8.

[25] Lukiw WJ, Bazan NG. Survival signaling in Alzheimer's disease. Biochem Soc Trans 2006;34:1277–82.

[26] Bazan NG. Synaptic lipid signaling: significance of polyunsaturated fatty acids and platelet-activating factor. J Lipid Res 2003;44:2221–33.

[27] Brand A, Schonfeld E, Isharel I, Yavin E. Docosahexaenoic acid-dependent iron accumulation in oligodendroglia cells protects from hydrogen peroxide-induced damage. J Neurochem 2008;105:1325–35.

[28] Uauy R, Dangour AD. Nutrition in brain development and aging: role of essential fatty acids. Nutr Rev 2006;64:S24–33; discussion S72–91.

[29] Sun GY, Xu J, Jensen MD, Simonyi A. Phospholipase A2 in the central nervous system: implications for neurodegenerative diseases. J Lipid Res 2004;45:205–13.

[30] Birkle DL, Bazan NG. (19849. Effect of K+ depolarization on the synthesis of prostaglandins and hydroxyeicosatetra(5,8,11,14) enoic acids (HETE) in the rat retina. Evidence for esterification of 12-HETE in lipids. Biochim Biophys Acta 795, 564–573.

[31] Reddy TS, Bazan NG. Long-chain acyl CoA synthetase in microsomes from rat brain gray matter and white matter. Neurochem Res 1985;10:377–86.

[32] Reddy TS, Bazan NG. Synthesis of arachidonoyl coenzyme A and docosahexaenoyl coenzyme A in synaptic plasma membranes of cerebrum and microsomes of cerebrum, cerebellum, and brain stem of rat brain. J Neurosci Res 1985;13:381–90.
[33] Roberts LJ, Montine TJ, Markesbery WR, Tapper AR, Hardy P, Chemtob S, et al. Formation of isoprostane-like compounds (neuroprostanes) *in vivo* from docosahexaenoic acid. J Biol Chem 1998;273:13605–12.
[34] Musiek ES, Brooks JD, Joo M, Brunoldi E, Porta A, Zanoni G, et al. Electrophilic cyclopentenone neuroprostanes are anti-inflammatory mediators formed from the peroxidation of the omega-3 polyunsaturated fatty acid docosahexaenoic acid. J Biol Chem 2008;283:19927–35.
[35] Diau GY, Hsieh AT, Sarkadi-Nagy EA, Wijendran V, Nathanielsz PW, Brenna JT. The influence of long chain polyunsaturate supplementation on docosahexaenoic acid and arachidonic acid in baboon neonate central nervous system. BMC Med 2005;3:11.
[36] Litman BJ, Niu SL, Polozova A, Mitchell DC. The role of docosahexaenoic acid containing phospholipids in modulating G protein-coupled signaling pathways: visual transduction. J Mol Neurosci 2001;16:237–42; discussion 79–84.
[37] Salem N, Litman B, Kim HY, Gawrisch K. Mechanisms of action of docosahexaenoic acid in the nervous system. Lipids 2001;36:945–59.
[38] Organisciak DT, Darrow RM, Jiang YL, Blanks JC. Retinal light damage in rats with altered levels of rod outer segment docosahexaenoate. Invest Ophthalmol Vis Sci 1996;37:2243–57.
[39] Kim HY, Akbar M, Lau A, Edsall L. Inhibition of neuronal apoptosis by docosahexaenoic acid (22:6n-3). Role of phosphatidylserine in antiapoptotic effect. J Biol Chem 2000;275:35215–23.
[40] Neuringer M, Connor WE, Lin DS, Barstad L, Luck S. Biochemical and functional effects of prenatal and postnatal omega 3 fatty acid deficiency on retina and brain in rhesus monkeys. Proc Natl Acad Sci U S A 1986;83:4021–5.
[41] Weisinger HS, Armitage JA, Jeffrey BG, Mitchell DC, Moriguchi T, Sinclair AJ, et al. Retinal sensitivity loss in third-generation n-3 PUFA-deficient rats. Lipids 2002;37:759–65.
[42] Bazan NG, Birkle DL, Reddy TS. Docosahexaenoic acid (22:6, n-3) is metabolized to lipoxygenase reaction products in the retina. Biochem Biophys Res Commun 1984;125:741–7.
[43] Bazan NG. Cellular and molecular events mediated by docosahexaenoic acid-derived neuroprotectin D1 signaling in photoreceptor cell survival and brain protection. Prostaglandins Leukot Essent Fatty Acids 2009;81:205–11.
[44] Marcheselli VL, Hong S, Lukiw WJ, Tian XH, Gronert K, Musto A, et al. Novel docosanoids inhibit brain ischemia-reperfusion mediated leukocyte infiltration and pro-inflammatory gene expression. J Biol Chem 2003;278:43807–17.
[45] Mukherjee PK, Marcheselli VL, de Rivero Vaccari JC, Gordon WC, Jackson FE, Bazan NG. Photoreceptor outer segment phagocytosis attenuates oxidative stress-induced apoptosis with concomitant neuroprotectin D1 synthesis. Proc Natl Acad Sci U S A 2007;104:13158–63.
[46] Mukherjee PK, Marcheselli VL, Barreiro S, Hu J, Bok D, Bazan NG. Neurotrophins enhance retinal pigment epithelial cell survival through neuroprotectin D1 signaling. Proc Natl Acad Sci U S A 2007;104:13152–7.
[47] Mukherjee PK, Marcheselli VL, Serhan CN, Bazan NG. Neuroprotectin D1: a docosahexaenoic acid-derived docosatriene protects human retinal pigment epithelial cells from oxidative stress. Proc Natl Acad Sci U S A 2004;101:8491–6.
[48] Steele M, Stuchbury G, Münch G. The molecular basis of the prevention of Alzheimer's disease through healthy nutrition. Exp Gerontol 2007;42:28–36.
[49] Floyd RA, Hensley K. Oxidative stress in brain aging. Implications for therapeutics of neurodegenerative diseases. Neurobiol Aging 2002;23:795–807.
[50] Alvarez-Nölting R, Arnal E, Barcia JM, Miranda M, Romero FJ. Protection by DHA of early hippocampal changes in diabetes: possible role of CREB and NF-κB. Neurochem Res 2012;37:105–15.
[51] Migliore L, Fontana I, Trippi F, Colognato R, Coppedè F, Tognoni G, et al. Oxidative DNA damage in peripheral leukocytes of mild cognitive impairment and AD patients. Neurobiol Aging 2005;26:567–73.
[52] Hossain MS, Hashimoto M, Gamoh S, Masumura S. Antioxidative effects of docosahexaenoic acid in the cerebrum versus cerebellum and brainstem of aged hypercholesterolemic rats. J Neurochem 1999;72:1133–8.
[53] Arnal E, Miranda M, Barcia J, Bosch-Morell F, Romero FJ. Lutein and docosahexaenoic acid prevent cortex lipid peroxidation in streptozotocin-induced diabetic rat cerebral cortex. Neuroscience 2010;166(1):271–8.
[54] Cao DH, Xu JF, Xue RH, Zheng WF, Liu ZL. Protective effect of chronic ethyl docosahexaenoate administration on brain injury in ischemic gerbils. Pharmacol Biochem Behav 2004;79:651–9.
[55] Yavin E, Brand A, Green P. Docosahexaenoic acid abundance in the brain: a biodevice to combat oxidative stress. Nutr Neurosci 2002;5:149–57.

CHAPTER

14

Diabetic Nephropathy and Tocotrienol

Kanwaljit Chopra, Vipin Arora, Anurag Kuhad

Pharmacology Research Laboratory, University Institute of Pharmaceutical Sciences, UGC Center of Advanced Study, Panjab University, Chandigarh, India

List of Abbreviations

DN Diabetic nephropathy
ESRD End stage renal disease
ICAM-1 Intercellular adhesion molecule-1
NF-κB Nuclear Factor kappa-light-chain-enhancer of activated B cells
PPAR Peroxisome proliferator-activated receptors
STZ Streptozotocin
TNF-α Tumor necrosis factor-alpha
TGF-β1 Transforming growth factor beta
TBARS Thiobarbituric acid reactive substance

INTRODUCTION

Diabetic nephropathy (DN) is a leading cause of end stage renal disease (ESRD), and the incidence of diabetes mellitus had already reached epidemic proportions by the beginning of this millennium [1]. According to the World Health Organization, it is expected that the number of patients with diabetes worldwide will rise to 370 million by 2030 [2], but in recent reports, these figures are further augmented to 439 million in 2030 [3]. This steep increase will be sharpest in developing countries, particularly in India and China (69%) compared to developed countries (20%) [4]. India has the largest number of diabetic patients in the world, estimated to be 40.9 million in the year 2007 and expected to increase to 69.9 million by the year 2025 [5], this gives India the title of 'Diabetic Capital of the World' [6]. Over 90% of people with diabetes will have type 2 diabetes, and it has also been reported that about 25–40% of diabetic patients develop DN within 20–25 years of the onset of diabetes [7]. Appreciating the growing global threat of DN, the renal community declared 11th March, 2010 as 'World Kidney Day' in numerous countries, focusing on DN with the slogan *'Protect Your Kidneys, Control Diabetes'* [8].

In 1959, Gellman et al. first reported an overview and clinical correlation of findings on renal biopsies from patients with DN [9]. DN is defined as an increase in urinary albumin excretion, accompanied by rising blood pressure and a decline in glomerular filtration rate. Early DN may be identified by persistent microalbuminuria, defined as an albumin excretion rate of 20–200 μg/min, or urine albumin to creatinine ratio of 30–300 mg/g in males and 20–200 mg/g in females. Overt DN is marked by proteinuria >500 mg/24 h or albuminuria >300 mg/24 h. Decreased estimated glomerular filtration rate <60 ml/min/1.73 m^2 may be another manifestation of overt DN [4].

BIOLOGICAL MARKERS INVOLVED IN THE PATHOPHYSIOLOGY OF DIABETIC NEPHROPATHY

In recent years, our knowledge of the pathophysiological processes that lead to diabetic nephropathy has notably improved, both on a genetic and a molecular level. Thus, the classic view of metabolic and hemodynamic alterations as the main causes of renal injury in diabetes has been transformed significantly, with clear evidence indicating that these traditional factors are only part of a much more complex picture [10]. It is likely that the pathophysiology of diabetic nephropathy involves a multifactorial interaction between metabolic and hemodynamic factors. Metabolic factors involve glucose-dependent pathways, such as advanced glycation end-products and their receptors. Hemodynamic factors include various vasoactive hormones, such as components of the renin-angiotensin system. It is likely that these metabolic and hemodynamic factors interact through shared molecular and signaling pathways, such

Diabetes: Oxidative Stress and Dietary Antioxidants.
http://dx.doi.org/10.1016/B978-0-12-405885-9.00014-0

as chemokines (monocyte chemoattractant protein-1), adhesion molecules (intercellular adhesion molecule-1 (ICAM-1) [11,12], enzymes (cyclooxygenase-2, nitric oxide synthase) [13,14], growth factors (vascular endothelial growth factor, growth hormone, IGF, TGF-β1) [15–17], and nuclear factors (NF-κB) [18,19], with associated reactive oxygen species generation [20,21] implicated in processes related to diabetic nephropathy.

In terms of renoprotective strategies in patients with DN, large clinical trials such as the United Kingdom Prospective Diabetes Study [22] and the Diabetes Control and Complications Trial [23] revealed that strict control of blood glucose or use of agents blocking the renin-angiotensin system significantly reduced the development and progression of diabetic nephropathy in both type 1 and type 2 diabetes. Although these therapeutic options slow the progression of diabetic nephropathy, the burden and mortality rate of the disease remains very high, and the majority of patients with diabetic nephropathy continue to progress to end stage renal disease. This imperfection points to the need for newer therapeutic agents that have the potential to affect primary mechanisms contributing to the pathogenesis of diabetic nephropathy [24]. Increasing evidence in both experimental and clinical studies suggests that there is a close link between hyperglycemia, oxidative stress induced inflammatory cascade, and diabetic complications [25,26]. Activation of the oxidative stress induced inflammatory pathway in diabetes likely contributes to the pathogenesis of diabetic nephropathy and its progression to end stage renal disease [27,28,29]. Therefore investigations into antioxidant and anti-inflammatory strategies may offer new approaches of further effect.

TOCOTRIENOLS

Tocochromanols encompass a group of compounds with vitamin E activity which are essential for human nutrition. Structurally, natural vitamin E includes eight chemically distinct molecules: α-, β-, γ- and δ-tocopherol; and α-, β-, γ- and δ-tocotrienol. Thus, tocotrienols may be viewed as being members of the natural vitamin E family not only structurally but also functionally. Palm oil and rice bran oil represent two major nutritional sources of natural tocotrienol. Taken orally, tocotrienols are bioavailable to all vital organs. Tocotrienols are thought to have more potent antioxidant properties than α-tocopherol [30,31]. The unsaturated side chain of tocotrienol allows for more efficient penetration into tissues that have saturated fatty layers, such as the brain and liver [32]. Experimental research examining the antioxidant, free radical scavenging effects of tocopherol and tocotrienols have revealed that tocotrienols appear to be superior due to their better distribution in the fatty layers of the cell membrane [32,33]. The present chapter will deal with the renoprotective effects of tocotrienols in a rat model of diabetic nephropathy.

EXPERIMENTAL STUDY STATING THE USE OF TOCOTRIENOL IN DIABETIC NEPHROPATHY

Diabetes was induced by injecting the β-cytotoxin, streptozotocin, dissolved in citrate buffer, into rats (Figure 14.1). A total of 100 rats were employed for the study, divided into nine groups of 10–12 animals each. Group 1 was the non-diabetic control, and these animals received a single vehicle injection of citrate buffer and oral gavage of Tween 80 vehicle. Group 2 was the diabetic control, and these animals received a single intraperitoneal injection of streptozotocin (45 mg/kg) and oral gavage of Tween 80 vehicle. Group 3 comprised the diabetic animals, which received subcutaneous injections of insulin (10 IU/kg, s.c.). Groups 4, 5 and 6 consisted of diabetic animals which received oral gavage of tocotrienol at 25, 50 and 100 mg/kg/day respectively. Group 7 consisted of diabetic animals treated with insulin (10 IU/kg, s.c.) + tocotrienol (100 mg/kg/day, oral gavage). Group 8 consisted of control animals which received tocotrienol (100 mg/kg, oral gavage). Group 9 consisted of diabetic animals treated with α-tocopherol [34].

The drug treatment was started from the fifth week after STZ injection and continued until the eighth week (Figure 14.2). Drug solutions were freshly prepared and administered in a constant volume of 10 mL/kg body weight. Tocotrienol was freshly prepared by dissolving in double distilled water after triturating with 5% Tween 80. At the end of eighth week, the animals were sacrificed under deep anesthesia, blood was collected by carotid bleeding and plasma separated. Kidneys were rapidly removed and weighed. A 10% (w/v) tissue homogenate was prepared in 0.1 M phosphate buffer (pH 7.4).

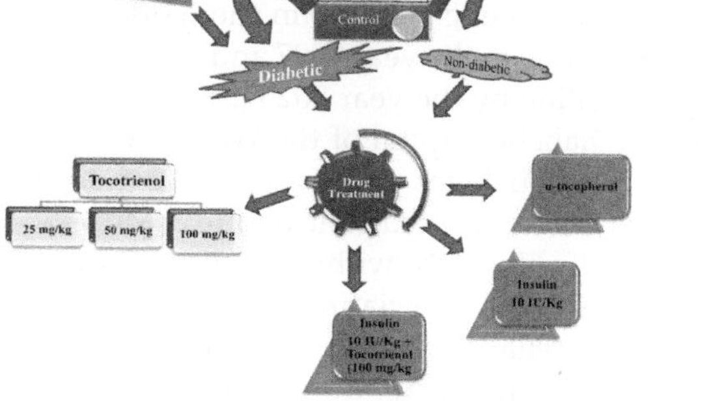

FIGURE 14.1 Study design. This figure is reproduced in color in the color section.

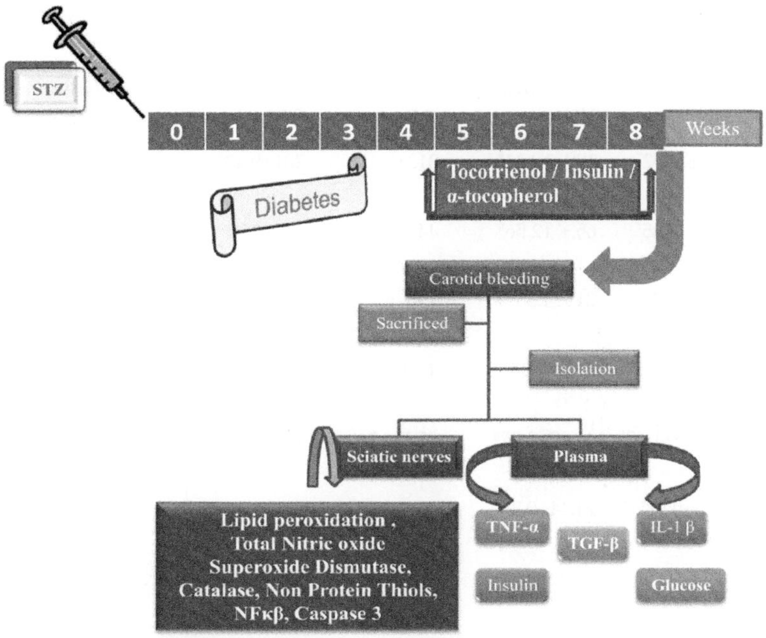

FIGURE 14.2 **Experimental protocol.** This figure is reproduced in color in the color section.

Homogenates were centrifuged at 200 g for 10 min, at 4°C and supernatant was used for estimation of lipid peroxidation, total nitric oxide, superoxide dismutase, catalase and non-protein thiols. Cytoplasmic and nuclear fractions were prepared for the quantification of caspase-3 and p65 subunit of NF-κB. Plasma was used for the estimation of TNF-α, TGF-β1 and IL-1 β. The samples were stored at −80°C until processed for biochemical estimations [34].

TOCOTRIENOL AND DIABETIC NEPHROPATHY: POSSIBLE MECHANISM OF ACTION

DN is one of the major chronic complications of type 2 diabetes. It finally progresses to end stage renal disease, requiring dialysis therapy. Glomerular changes, such as capillary basement membrane thickening, mesangial proliferation, and nodular glomerulosclerosis, are pathogenomic for DN [35]. Tubulointerstitial fibrosis is a predictor of progressive renal failure [36]. Traditionally, DN has been considered a non-immune, degenerative disease. However, in 1991, Bohle et al. described the presence of monocytes, macrophages, T-cells, and fibroblasts associated with the tubulointerstitial changes seen in DN [37]. Reports have suggested that inflammation may underlie disease progression in DN [38,39]. The activation of NF-κB-linked regulatory pathways generally underlies inflammatory processes, and an increase in the nuclear translocation of NF-κB has been demonstrated in human DN [40,41].

EFFECT ON GLYCEMIC INDEX AND RENAL PHYSIOLOGY

STZ-injected rats demonstrate typical characteristics of diabetes mellitus, such as hyperglycemia, polyuria, growth retardation, and an increase in urinary albumin excretion. With the onset of diabetes mellitus, there is a subsequent decrease in creatinine and urea clearance. Four weeks after STZ injection, diabetic animals exhibited increased blood glucose levels (111±7.94 and 402±10.52 mg/dl; for control and diabetic rats, respectively; $p > 0.01$) and decreased body weight (232±2.15 and 171±1.32g for control and diabetic rats, respectively; $p < 0.05$) compared with controls. Chronic treatment with tocotrienol in diabetic rats between the fifth and eighth weeks ameliorated plasma glucose levels as well as the decreased body weight, compared with vehicle-treated diabetic rats. These results are also in accordance with the study done by Budin et al., who showed that tocotrienol-rich fractions reduced serum glucose and glycated hemoglobin concentrations of streptozotocin-induced diabetic rats [42]. Treatment with a higher dose of tocotrienol attenuated the decrease in body weight in diabetic rats but this effect was not significant compared with vehicle-treated diabetic rats (Table 14.1). Further, a significant increase in food intake, water intake and systolic blood pressure in STZ-injected rats were attenuated with tocotrienol treatment. Diabetic rats exhibited marked polyuria, increased urinary albumin excretion, high serum creatinine as well as blood urea nitrogen. Chronic treatment with tocotrienol (25, 50 and 100 mg/kg/day) significantly and dose dependently reduced diabetic proteinuria, polyuria and

TABLE 14.1 Effect of Tocotrienol on Plasma Glucose, Plasma Insulin Levels and Renal Functions in Diabetic Rats (Mean±SEM)

Groups	Control	STZ	STZ+ Insulin (10)	STZ+ Toco (25)	STZ+ Toco (50)	STZ+ Toco (100)	STZ + Insulin (10) +Toco (100)	STZ + α-Tocopherol (100)
Plasma Glucose (mg/dL)	111±7.94	402±10.52*	199±10.34#	313±7.18#	281±9.43#	211±7.89#	145±9.83#	279±4.28#
Plasma Insulin (pmol/L)	102 ± 5.51	25 ± 18.45*	65 ± 12.56#	44 ± 23.48	41 ± 25.89	23 ± 11.47	52 ± 9.04#	29 ± 24.87
Body Weights (g)	232±2.15	171±1.32*	215±4.35#	156±8.22	187±4.54#	209±1.89#	221±2.11#	176±3.84#
Food Intake (g)	28.25±1.652	58.75±2.689*	32.6±1.33#	49.42±1.08#	43.32±1.11#	37.1±1.12#	30.09±1.06#	44.49±1.02#
Water Intake (mL)	35.26±1.23	108.25±1.65*	44.47±3.02#	95.51±3.96#	70.58±2.05#	51.51±1.11#	39.16±1.00#	72.41±3.37#
Urine Output (mL)	9.37±0.63	42.5±0.81*	24.44±0.36#	38.42±1.21#	26.27±1.98#	19.13±1.26#	15.01±0.89#	28.11±2.21#
Urine Albumin (mg/dL)	3.83±0.49	11.25±0.54*	7.76±0.57#	10.98±0.50#	8.93±0.41#	6.87±0.37#	4.76±0.10#	9.56±0.68#
Serum Creatinine (mg/dL)	0.31±0.02	1.42±0.11*	0.73±0.03#	1.29±0.27#	0.96±0.09#	0.65±0.05#	0.46±0.03#	0.92±0.12#
Blood Urea Nitrogen (mg/dL)	24.5±0.64	58.25±1.75*	45.02±1.00#	52.78±2.08#	46.59±2.01#	37.81±1.10#	29.76±1.09#	47.86±3.04#
Creatinine Clearance (mL/24 h)	0.71±0.01	0.25±0.02*	0.50±0.01#	0.32±0.03#	0.49±0.03#	0.60±0.02#	0.68±0.03#	0.43±0.10#
Urea Clearance (mL/24 h)	0.8±0.06	0.31±0.06*	0.57±0.05#	0.37±0.06#	0.55±0.04#	0.64±0.03#	0.76±0.07#	0.48±0.07#
BP (mm Hg)	112±3.27	205±11.18*	132±11.33#	182±9.12	145±9.58#	131±10.20#	119±8.39#	151±11.08#

**P<0.05 as compared to control group.*
#P<0.05 as compared to streptozotocin (STZ) treated group.
Toco (25) = Tocotrienol 25mg/kg, Toco (50) = Tocotrienol 50mg/kg, Toco (100) = Tocotrienol 100mg/kg, α-Tocopherol 100 = α-Tocopherol 100 mg/kg. Adapted from Kuhad and Chopra (2009) [34].

increased serum creatinine and blood urea nitrogen. Creatinine and urea clearance were also significantly improved following the administration of tocotrienol (25, 50 and 100 mg/kg/day) to diabetic rats compared with untreated diabetic rats (Table 14.1). However, insulin levels were not significantly altered in tocotrienol-treated diabetic rats.

Tocotrienol produced more pronounced effects than α-tocopherol. Moreover, diabetic rats treated with an insulin-tocotrienol combination significantly prevented this alteration in renal function compared to their respective control groups (diabetic rats treated with insulin and tocotrienol alone). It has also been observed that increased blood urea nitrogen and serum creatinine in diabetic rats indicates progressive renal damage, which is taken as an index of altered GFR in diabetic nephropathy [43]. Hence the results are indicative of the protective action of tocotrienol, if we see them in terms of blood glucose levels, blood urea nitrogen and serum creatinine levels. This protective action of tocotrienol may also be attributed to its action on the peroxisome proliferator-activated receptors that play essential roles in energy metabolism. Importantly, synthetic PPARα and PPARγ ligands are currently used for treating hyperlipidemia and diabetes, as the study carried out by Fang and coworkers showed that tocotrienols enhanced the interaction between the purified ligand-binding domain of PPARα with the receptor-interacting motif of coactivator PPARγ coactivator-1α. In addition, the tocotrienol-rich fraction of palm oil improved whole body glucose utilization and insulin sensitivity of diabetic db/db mice by selectively regulating PPAR target genes [44].

TABLE 14.2 Effect of Tocotrienol on Lipid Peroxide, Non-Protein Thiols, Superoxide Dismutase, Catalase and Nitric Oxide Levels (Mean±SEM)

Treatment	LPO (nmol/mg protein)	Non-Protein Thiols (moles)	SOD (units/mg protein)	Catalase (k/min)	Total NO (μmol/liter)
Control	1.01 ± 0.06	32.53 ± 3.21	8.89 ± 0.38	3.94 ± 0.31	99± 0.50
STZ	2.10 ± 0.07[a]	12.87 ± 2.19[a]	4.02 ± 0.28[a]	0.91 ± 0.08[a]	267 ± 2.16[a]
STZ + Insulin (10)	1.79 ± 0.10[b]	18.52 ± 1.21[b]	6.10 ± 0.10[b]	1.57 ± 0.11[b]	244 ± 1.33[b]
STZ + Toco (25)	1.74 ± 0.07[b,c]	19.42 ± 1.14[b,c]	5.73 ± 0.11[b,c]	1.78 ± 0.16[b,c]	191 ± 1.38[b,c]
STZ + Toco (50)	1.49 ± 0.11[b,c]	25.02 ± 1.07[b,c]	6.95 ± 0.08[b,c]	2.48 ± 0.07[b,c]	169 ± 1.29[b,c]
STZ + Toco (100)	1.18 ± 0.08[b,c]	29.72 ± 1.00[b,c]	8.28 ± 0.10[b,c]	3.02 ± 0.10[b,c]	134 ± 0.82[b,c]
STZ + Insulin (10) + Toco (100)	1.07 ± 0.05[b,d]	31.35 ± 1.02[b,d]	8.64 ± 0.11 [b,d]	3.46 ± 0.11 [b,d]	106 ± 1.76 [b,d]

[a]*different from control.*
[b]*different from diabetic.*
[c]*different from one another.*
[d]*different from their per se group ($p<0.05$).*
Toco (25) = Tocotrienol 25mg/kg, Toco (50) = Tocotrienol 50mg/kg, Toco (100) = Tocotrienol 100mg/kg, α-Tocopherol 100 = α-Tocopherol 100 mg/kg. Adapted from Kuhad and Chopra (2009) [34].

PREVENTION OF RENAL OXIDATIVE STRESS

A number of *in vitro* and *in vivo* studies demonstrate a marked oxidative stress in diabetic nephropathy patients as well as in animal models of diabetes [25,45,46]. Excess intracellular glucose increases superoxide radical formation in the mitochondria at the electron transport chain and directly increases H_2O_2 generation in mesangial cells, leading to lipid peroxidation of glomeruli and mesangial cells in a dose dependent manner, which is highly supportive of the presence of increased oxidative stress in diabetic glomeruli [47,48]. Lack of effects of either L-glucose or mannitol on H_2O_2 generation and lipid peroxidation of mesangial cells suggest that high glucose-induced lipid peroxidation in this tissue is related to the metabolism of glucose [49,50]. It is thus suggested that there is a high correlation between oxidative stress in diabetes and the development of complications including diabetic nephropathy. We observed a marked increase in thiobarbituric acid reactive substance (TBARS) levels in the kidneys of diabetic rats as compared to the control group (Table 14.2). Chronic treatment with tocotrienol produced a significant and dose dependent reduction in thiobarbituric acid reactive substance levels in STZ-treated rats. Tocotrienol was more potent in inhibiting TBARS than α-tocopherol. However, diabetic rats treated with an insulin-tocotrienol combination significantly prevented this rise in lipid peroxidation as compared to their respective control groups (diabetic rats treated with insulin and tocotrienol alone) [$F(7,67)=39.76$ ($p<0.05$)]. The non-protein thiols [$F(7,67)=28.67$ ($p<0.05$)], enzyme activity of superoxide dismutase [$F(7,67)=18.59$ ($p<0.05$)], and catalase [$F(7,67)=34.28$ ($p<0.05$)] significantly decreased in the kidneys of diabetic rats compared to the control group (Table 14.2). This reduction was significantly and dose dependently improved by the treatment with tocotrienol in the kidneys of STZ-treated rats. Tocotrienol produced more pronounced effects than α-tocopherol. However, diabetic rats treated with insulin-tocotrienol combination significantly restored the endogenous antioxidant profile as compared to their respective control groups (diabetic rats treated with insulin and tocotrienol alone). The restoration of the antioxidant enzyme levels and lipid levels to the control values confirms its antioxidant potential, and that of tocotrienol is also corroborated by recent studies done by other research groups [40,51]. Budin and coworkers recently demonstrated that a tocotrienol-rich fraction lowers the blood glucose level and levels of oxidative stress markers in streptozotocin-induced diabetic rats. Siddiqui and colleagues showed that the tocotrienol-rich fraction from palm oil significantly improved the glycemic status and renal function in type 1 diabetic rats [42,51].

INHIBITORY EFFECT ON PROINFLAMMATORY AND PROFIBROTIC CYTOKINES

Tubulointerstitial fibrosis is the final manifestation of end stage renal disease [52], and renal injury is correlated to the degree of renal interstitial fibrosis. Transforming growth factor-β1 (TGF-β1) is known to be one of the major mediators that leads to fibrosis. GW788388, a new TGF-beta type I receptor inhibitor, significantly reduced renal fibrosis and decreased the mRNA levels of key mediators of extracellular matrix deposition in the kidneys of the db/db mouse [53]. Further, experimental studies have consistently reported that mRNA encoding TNF-α

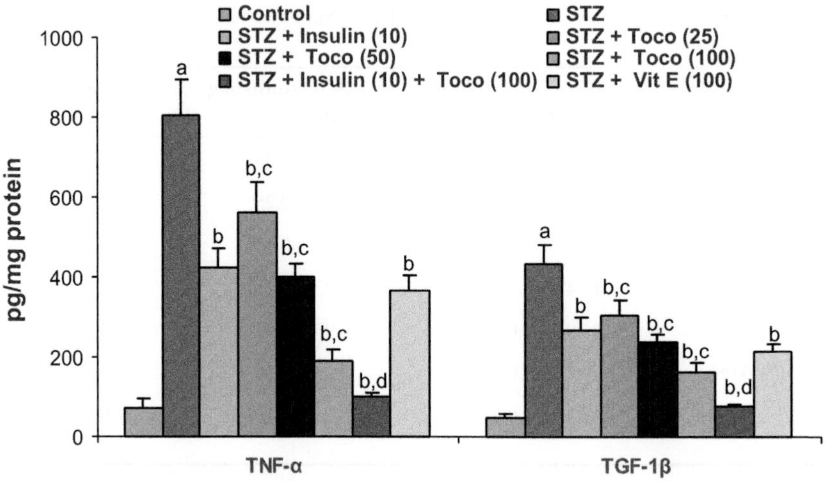

FIGURE 14.3 Effect of tocotrienol (Toco) and its combination with insulin on TNF-α and TGF-β1 levels in the kidneys of diabetic rats. Data are expressed as mean ± S.E.M. a different from control; b different from diabetic group; c different from one another; d different from tocotrienol and insulin per se groups. Toco (25) = Tocotrienol 25mg/kg, Toco (50) = Tocotrienol 50mg/kg, Toco (100) = Tocotrienol 100mg/kg, Vit E (100) = α-Tocopherol 100 mg/kg. *Adapted from Kuhad and Chopra (2009) [34].* This figure is reproduced in color in the color section.

and protein levels increase in glomerular and proximal tubule cells of diabetic rats [43,54-56]. These investigations demonstrated a significant role of TNF-α in the development of renal hypertrophy and hyperfunction, two main alterations observed during the initial stage of diabetic nephropathy [54,56]. TNF-α has a stimulatory effect on sodium-dependent solute uptake in cultured mouse proximal tubular cells [57] and in these studies, diabetic rats exhibited enhanced urinary TNF-α excretion, sodium retention, and renal hypertrophy, which were prevented by administration of the anti-TNF-α agent TNFR:Fc, a soluble TNF-α receptor fusion protein [54,57]. Uncontrolled diabetes significantly enhanced TNF-α and TGF-β1 levels in diabetic rat kidneys [58]. In our study, tocotrienol treatment significantly and dose dependently inhibited TNF-α and TGF-β1 levels in the STZ-treated rats (Figure 14.3). Tocotrienol produced more pronounced effects than α-tocopherol. Moreover, diabetic rats treated with insulin-tocotrienol combination more significantly inhibited TNF-α [$F(7,67)=62.84$ ($p<0.01$)] and TGF-β1 [$F(7,67)=157.53$ ($p<0.01$)] levels compared to their respective control groups (diabetic rats treated with insulin and tocotrienol alone). This significant inhibition of TNF-α and TFG-β1 levels by tocotrienol observed in our study is indicative of the fact that tocotrienol contributes to beneficial effects seen in diabetic nephropathy.

EFFECT ON NF-κB SIGNALING AND RENAL APOPTOSIS

The final common pathway for progressive renal diseases such as DN is the development of tubular atrophy and chronic interstitial fibrosis, which is generally preceded by or associated with an inflammatory infiltrate. Increased steady-state mRNA levels of inflammatory genes are shown to be associated with interstitial fibrosis and progressive human DN [18]. The transcription factor NF-κB helps to control the expression of numerous genes activated during inflammation. NF-κB is induced by various cell stress-associated stimuli including growth factors, vasoactive agents, cytokines, and oxidative stress [59,60]. NF-κB in turn controls the regulation of genes encoding proteins involved in immune and inflammatory responses (i.e., cytokines, chemokines, growth factors, immune receptors, cellular ligands, and adhesion molecules). The activation and nuclear translocation of NF-κB in human DN has been demonstrated in intrinsic cells of the kidney [38,39]. Further activation of the NF-κB signaling pathway leads to renal dysfunction in diabetic animals which is positively correlated with increased oxidative-nitrosative stress and inflammation. In the present study, NF-κB p65 subunit was significantly elevated in the kidneys of diabetic animals (Figure 14.4). Tocotrienol treatment significantly and dose dependently prevented reactive oxygen species induced NF-κB p65 subunit expression in the nuclear fraction of STZ-treated rats. Tocotrienol produced more pronounced effects in comparison to α-tocopherol. The levels of NF-κB p65 subunit were further significantly reduced by insulin-tocotrienol combination as compared to their respective groups (diabetic rats treated with insulin and tocotrienol alone) [$F(7,67)=171.38$ ($p<0.05$)]. These results are in line with the previous study done by Ahn et al. who demonstrated that γ-tocotrienol inhibited the NF-κB activation pathway [61].

To better understand the pathway leading to apoptosis in diabetes, we investigated the expression of apoptosis-related proteins such as caspase-3 in the

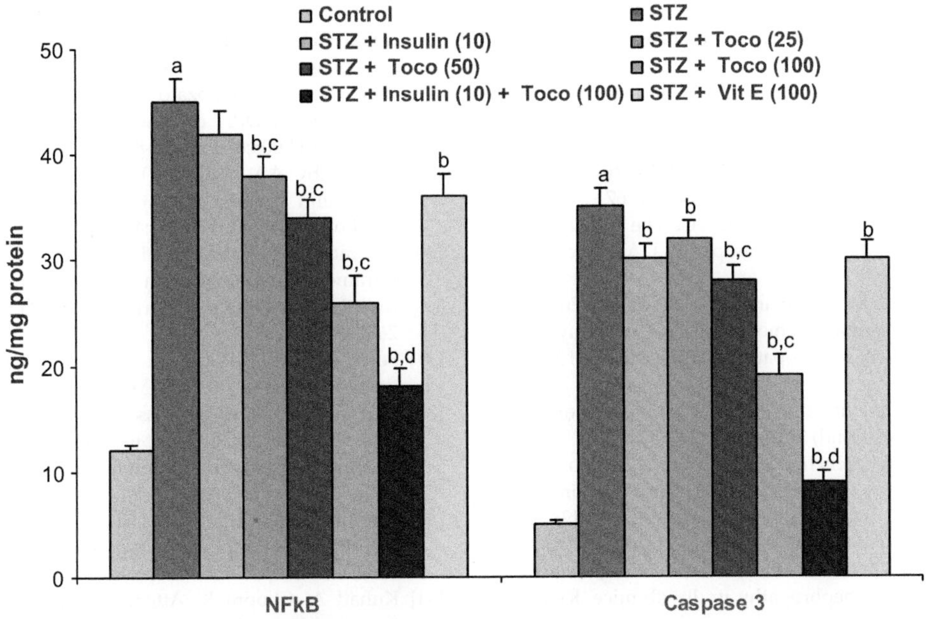

FIGURE 14.4 Effect of tocotrienol (Toco) and its combination with insulin on p65 subunit of NFκβ and caspase-3 levels in the kidneys of diabetic rats. Data are expressed as mean ± S.E.M. a different from control; b different from diabetic group; c different from one another; d different from tocotrienol and insulin per se groups. Toco (25) = Tocotrienol 25mg/kg, Toco (50) = Tocotrienol 50mg/kg, Toco (100) = Tocotrienol 100mg/kg, Vit E (100) = α-Tocopherol 100 mg/kg. *Adapted from Kuhad and Chopra (2009) [34].* This figure is reproduced in color in the color section.

diabetic rat's kidneys. It has been demonstrated that high glucose levels cause the generation of peroxynitrite, leading to caspase-mediated apoptosis. Ebselen and a caspase-3 inhibitor provided significant protection against high glucose-mediated apoptosis, implicating peroxynitrite as a proapoptotic ROS in early diabetic nephropathy [62]. In the present study, caspase-3 levels were significantly elevated in the diabetic rat kidney (Figure 14.4). Tocotrienol treatment significantly and dose dependently inhibited apoptosis in the STZ-injected rats. Tocotrienol again displayed more marked inhibition of caspase 3 compared to α-tocopherol. However, diabetic rats treated with an insulin-tocotrienol combination produced a more pronounced attenuation of caspase 3 expression compared to their respective control groups (diabetic rats treated with insulin and tocotrienol alone) [$F(7,67)=94.37$ ($p<0.05$)]. This amenable effect of tocotrienol on caspase 3 is in concurrence with the study done by Osakada et al., who showed that the tocotrienol-rich fraction of the edible oil derived from palm oil (Tocomin 50%), which contains α-tocopherol, and α-, γ- and δ-tocotrienols, significantly inhibited hydrogen peroxide (H_2O_2)-induced neuronal death, Moreover, tocotrienols have been shown to block oxidative stress-mediated cell death with apoptotic DNA fragmentation caused by an inhibitor of glutathione synthesis, L-buthionine-[S,R]-sulfoximine [63]. In an another study done by Mazlan and coworkers, it was demonstrated that primary astrocyte cultures pretreated with either α-tocopherol or γ-tocotrienol reduced apoptosis to the same degree but α-tocopherol was less effective in maintaining the viable cell number [64].

CONCLUSION

The major finding of the study is that tocotrienol alone as well as in combination with insulin not only attenuated the diabetic condition but also reversed renal dysfunction through modulation of oxidative stress, release of profibrotic and proinflammatory cytokines and renal apoptosis in diabetic rats. However, insulin alone corrected the hyperglycemia and partially reversed the renal dysfunction in diabetic rats. Thus, these findings indicate the strong renoprotective potential of tocotrienol in diabetic patients.

References

[1] Zimmet P, Alberti KG, Shaw J. Global and societal implications of the diabetes epidemic. Nature 2001;414(6865):782–7.

[2] Wild S, Roglic G, Green A, Sicree R, King H. Global prevalence of diabetes: estimates for the year 2000 and projections for 2030. Diabetes Care 2004;27(5):1047–53.

[3] Shaw JE, Sicree RA, Zimmet PZ. Global estimates of the prevalence of diabetes for 2010 and 2030. Diabetes Res Clin Pract 2010;87(1):4–14.

[4] Reutens AT, Atkins RC. Epidemiology of diabetic nephropathy. Contrib Nephrol 2011;170:1–7.

[5] Unnikrishnan RI, Rema M, Pradeepa R, Deepa M, Shanthirani CS, Deepa R, et al. Prevalence and risk factors of diabetic nephropathy in an urban South Indian population: the Chennai Urban Rural Epidemiology Study (CURES 45). Diabetes Care 2007;30(8):2019–24.

[6] Mohan V, Sandeep S, Deepa R, Shah B, Varghese C. Epidemiology of type 2 diabetes: Indian scenario. Indian J Med Res 2007;125(3):217–30.

[7] Remuzzi G, Schieppati A, Ruggenenti P. Clinical practice. Nephropathy in patients with type 2 diabetes. N Engl J Med 2002;346(15):1145–51.
[8] Tang SC. Diabetic nephropathy: a global and growing threat. Hong Kong Med J 2010;16(4):244–5.
[9] Gellman DD, Pirani CL, Soothill JF, Muehrcke RC, Kark RM. Diabetic nephropathy: a clinical and pathologic study based on renal biopsies. Medicine (Baltimore) 1959;38:321–67.
[10] Navarro-Gonzalez JF, Mora-Fernandez C. The role of inflammatory cytokines in diabetic nephropathy. J Am Soc Nephrol 2008;19(3):433–42.
[11] Navarro-Gonzalez JF, Mora-Fernandez C, Muros de Fuentes M, Garcia-Perez J. Inflammatory molecules and pathways in the pathogenesis of diabetic nephropathy. Nat Rev Nephrol 2011;7(6): 327–40.
[12] Wada J, Makino H. Inflammation and the pathogenesis of diabetic nephropathy. Clin Sci (Lond) 2013;124(3):139–52.
[13] Green T, Gonzalez AA, Mitchell KD, Navar LG. The complex interplay between cyclooxygenase-2 and angiotensin II in regulating kidney function. Curr Opin Nephrol Hypertens 2012;21(1):7.
[14] Cheng H, Wang H, Fan X, Paueksakon P, Harris RC. Improvement of endothelial nitric oxide synthase activity retards the progression of diabetic nephropathy in db/db mice. Kidney Int 2012;82(11):1176–83.
[15] Oh Y. The insulin-like growth factor (IGF) system in chronic kidney disease: Pathophysiology and therapeutic opportunities. Kidney Research and Clinical Practice. Volume 2012;31(1):26–37.
[16] Brennan EP, Morine MJ, Walsh DW, Roxburgh SA, Lindenmeyer MT, Brazil DP, et al. Next-generation sequencing identifies TGF-beta1-associated gene expression profiles in renal epithelial cells reiterated in human diabetic nephropathy. Biochim Biophys Acta 2012;1822(4):589–99.
[17] Kanwar YS, Sun L, Xie P, Liu FY, Chen S. A glimpse of various pathogenetic mechanisms of diabetic nephropathy. Annu Rev Pathol 2011;6:395–423.
[18] Schmid H, Boucherot A, Yasuda Y, Henger A, Brunner B, Eichinger F, et al. Modular activation of nuclear factor-kappaB transcriptional programs in human diabetic nephropathy. Diabetes 2006;55(11):2993–3003.
[19] Xie X, Peng J, Chang X, Huang K, Huang J, Wang S, et al. Activation of RhoA/ROCK regulates NF-kappaB signaling pathway in experimental diabetic nephropathy. Mol Cell Endocrinol 2013; 369(1–2):86–97.
[20] Singh DK, Winocour P, Farrington K. Oxidative stress in early diabetic nephropathy: fueling the fire. Nat Rev Endocrinol 2011;7(3):176–84.
[21] Kafle D, Singh N, Singh S, Singh N, Bhargav V, Singh A. Persistent hyperglycemia generating reactive oxygen species in renal cells, a probable cause of inflammation in type2 diabetic nephropathy subjects. Biomed Res 2012;23(4):501.
[22] UK Prospective Diabetes Study (UKPDS) Group. Intensive blood-glucose control with sulphonylureas or insulin compared with conventional treatment and risk of complications in patients with type 2 diabetes (UKPDS 33). Lancet 1998;352(9131):837–53.
[23] The Diabetes Control and Complications Trial Research Group. The effect of intensive treatment of diabetes on the development and progression of long-term complications in insulin-dependent diabetes mellitus. N Engl J Med 1993;329(14):977–86.
[24] Williams MD, Nadler JL. Inflammatory mechanisms of diabetic complications. Curr Diab Rep 2007;7(3):242–8.
[25] Giacco F, Brownlee M. Oxidative stress and diabetic complications. Circ Res 2010;107(9):1058–70.
[26] Pan HZ, Zhang L, Guo MY, Sui H, Li H, Wu WH, et al. The oxidative stress status in diabetes mellitus and diabetic nephropathy. Acta Diabetol 2010;47(Suppl. 1):71–6.
[27] Wolf G. New insights into the pathophysiology of diabeti nephropathy: from haemodynamics to molecular pathology. Eur Clin Invest 2004;34(12):785–96.
[28] Asaba K, Tojo A, Onozato ML, Goto A, Quinn MT, Fujita T, et al Effects of NADPH oxidase inhibitor in diabetic nephropathy Kidney Int 2005;67(5):1890–8.
[29] Elmarakby AA, Sullivan JC. Relationship between Oxidative Stress and Inflammatory Cytokines in Diabetic Nephropathy Cardiovasc Ther 2012;30(1):49–59.
[30] Serbinova E, Kagan V, Han D, Packer L. Free radical recycling and intramembrane mobility in the antioxidant properties of alpha-tocopherol and alpha-tocotrienol. Free Radic Biol Med 1991;10(5): 263–75.
[31] Serbinova EA, Packer L. Antioxidant properties of alpha-tocopherol and alpha-tocotrienol. Methods Enzymol 1994;234:354–66.
[32] Suzuki YJ, Tsuchiya M, Wassall SR, Choo YM, Govil G, Kagan VE, et al. Structural and dynamic membrane properties of alpha-tocopherol and alpha-tocotrienol: implication to the molecular mechanism of their antioxidant potency. Biochemistry 1993;32(40):10692–9.
[33] Sen CK, Khanna S, Roy S. Tocotrienols in health and disease: the other half of the natural vitamin E family. Mol Aspects Med 2007;28(5–6):692–728.
[34] Kuhad A, Chopra K. Attenuation of diabetic nephropathy by tocotrienol: involvement of NFkB signaling pathway. Life Sci 2009;84(9–10):296–301.
[35] O'Connor AS, Schelling JR. Diabetes and the kidney. Am J Kidney Dis 2005;46(4):766–73.
[36] Gilbert RE, Cooper ME. The tubulointerstitium in progressive diabetic kidney disease: more than an aftermath of glomerular injury? Kidney Int 1999;56(5):1627–37.
[37] Bohle A, Wehrmann M, Bogenschutz O, Batz C, Muller CA, Muller GA. The pathogenesis of chronic renal failure in diabetic nephropathy. Investigation of 488 cases of diabetic glomerulosclerosis. Pathol Res Pract 1991;187(2–3):251–9.
[38] Navarro JF, Mora C. Role of inflammation in diabetic complications. Nephrol Dial Transplant 2005;20(12):2601–4.
[39] Galkina E, Ley K. Leukocyte recruitment and vascular injury in diabetic nephropathy. J Am Soc Nephrol 2006;17(2):368–77.
[40] Mezzano S, Aros C, Droguett A, Burgos ME, Ardiles L, Flores C, et al. NF-kappaB activation and overexpression of regulated genes in human diabetic nephropathy. Nephrol Dial Transplant 2004;19(10):2505–12.
[41] Sakai N, Wada T, Furuichi K, Iwata Y, Yoshimoto K, Kitagawa K, et al. Involvement of extracellular signal-regulated kinase and p38 in human diabetic nephropathy. Am J Kidney Dis 2005;45(1): 54–65.
[42] Budin SB, Othman F, Louis SR, Bakar MA, Das S, Mohamed J. The effects of palm oil tocotrienol-rich fraction supplementation on biochemical parameters, oxidative stress and the vascular wall of streptozotocin-induced diabetic rats. Clinics (Sao Paulo) 2009;64(3):235–44.
[43] Sugimoto H, Shikata K, Wada J, Horiuchi S, Makino H. Advanced glycation end products-cytokine-nitric oxide sequence pathway in the development of diabetic nephropathy: aminoguanidine ameliorates the overexpression of tumor necrosis factor-alpha and inducible nitric oxide synthase in diabetic rat glomeruli. Diabetologia 1999;42(7):878–86.
[44] Fang F, Kang ZF, Wong CW. Vitamin E tocotrienols improve insulin sensitivity through activating peroxisome proliferator-activated receptors. Mol Nutr Food Res 2010;54(3):345–52.
[45] Calabrese V, Mancuso C, Sapienza M, Puleo E, Calafato S, Cornelius C, et al. Oxidative stress and cellular stress response in diabetic nephropathy. Cell Stress Chaperones 2007;12(4):299–306.
[46] Pazdro R, Burgess JR. The role of vitamin E and oxidative stress in diabetes complications. Mech Ageing Dev 2010;131(4):276–86.

[47] Ruiz-Munoz LM, Vidal-Vanaclocha F, Lampreabe I. Enalaprilat inhibits hydrogen peroxide production by murine mesangial cells exposed to high glucose concentrations. Nephrol Dial Transplant 1997;12(3):456–64.
[48] Trachtman H, Futterweit S, Bienkowski RS. Taurine prevents glucose-induced lipid peroxidation and increased collagen production in cultured rat mesangial cells. Biochem Biophys Res Commun 1993;191(2):759–65.
[49] Ha H, Lee SH, Kim KH. Effects of rebamipide in a model of experimental diabetes and on the synthesis of transforming growth factor-beta and fibronectin, and lipid peroxidation induced by high glucose in cultured mesangial cells. J Pharmacol Exp Ther 1997;281(3):1457–62.
[50] Steffes MW, Osterby R, Chavers B, Mauer SM. Mesangial expansion as a central mechanism for loss of kidney function in diabetic patients. Diabetes 1989;38(9):1077–81.
[51] Siddiqui S, Rashid Khan M, Siddiqui WA. Comparative hypoglycemic and nephroprotective effects of tocotrienol rich fraction (TRF) from palm oil and rice bran oil against hyperglycemia induced nephropathy in type 1 diabetic rats. Chem Biol Interact 2010;188(3):651–8.
[52] Zeisberg M, Strutz F, Muller GA. Role of fibroblast activation in inducing interstitial fibrosis. J Nephrol 2000;13(Suppl. 3):S111–20.
[53] Petersen M, Thorikay M, Deckers M, van Dinther M, Grygielko ET, Gellibert F, et al. Oral administration of GW788388, an inhibitor of TGF-beta type I and II receptor kinases, decreases renal fibrosis. Kidney Int 2008;73(6):705–15.
[54] DiPetrillo K, Coutermarsh B, Gesek FA. Urinary tumor necrosis factor contributes to sodium retention and renal hypertrophy during diabetes. Am J Physiol Renal Physiol 2003;284(1):F113–21.
[55] Navarro JF, Milena FJ, Mora C, Leon C, Garcia J. Renal proinflammatory cytokine gene expression in diabetic nephropathy: effect of angiotensin-converting enzyme inhibition and pentoxifylline administration. Am J Nephrol 2006;26(6):562–70.
[56] DiPetrillo K, Gesek FA. Pentoxifylline ameliorates renal tumor necrosis factor expression, sodium retention, and renal hypertrophy in diabetic rats. Am J Nephrol 2004;24(3):352–9.
[57] Schreiner GF, Kohan DE. Regulation of renal transport processes and hemodynamics by macrophages and lymphocytes. Am J Physiol 1990;258(4 Pt 2):F761–7.
[58] Sharma S, Kulkarni SK, Chopra K. Curcumin, the active principle of turmeric (Curcuma longa), ameliorates diabetic nephropathy in rats. Clin Exp Pharmacol Physiol 2006;33(10):940–5.
[59] Li Q, Verma IM. NF-kappaB regulation in the immune system. Nat Rev Immunol 2002;2(10):725–34.
[60] Karin M, Greten FR. NF-kappaB: linking inflammation and immunity to cancer development and progression. Nat Rev Immunol 2005;5(10):749–59.
[61] Ahn KS, Sethi G, Krishnan K, Aggarwal BB. Gamma-tocotrienol inhibits nuclear factor-kappaB signaling pathway through inhibition of receptor-interacting protein and TAK1 leading to suppression of antiapoptotic gene products and potentiation of apoptosis. J Biol Chem 2007;282(1):809–20.
[62] Allen DA, Harwood SM, Varagunam M, Raftery MJ, Yaqoob MM. High glucose-induced oxidative stress causes apoptosis in proximal tubular epithelial cells and is mediated by multiple caspases. Faseb J 2003;17(3):908–10.
[63] Osakada F, Hashino A, Kume T, Katsuki H, Kaneko S, Akaike A. Alpha-tocotrienol provides the most potent neuroprotection among vitamin E analogs on cultured striatal neurons. Neuropharmacology 2004;47(6):904–15.
[64] Mazlan M, Sue Mian T, Mat Top G, Zurinah Wan Ngah W. Comparative effects of alpha-tocopherol and gamma-tocotrienol against hydrogen peroxide induced apoptosis on primary-cultured astrocytes. J Neurol Sci 2006;243(1–2):5–12.

CHAPTER

15

Polyphenols, Oxidative Stress, and Vascular Damage in Diabetes

Raffaele Marfella, Nunzia D'Onofrio†, Ivana Sirangelo†, Maria Rosaria Rizzo*, Maria Carmela Capoluongo*, Luigi Servillo†, Giuseppe Paolisso*, Maria Luisa Balestrieri†*

*Department of Geriatrics and Metabolic Diseases, Naples, Italy, †Department of Biochemistry, Biophysics and General Pathology, Second University of Naples, Naples, Italy

List of Abbreviations

ADP Adenosine diphosphate
AGE Advanced glycation end products
BH4 Tetrahydrobiopterin
CVD Cardiovascular disease
eNOS Endothelial nitrogen monoxide synthase
EPCs Endothelial progenitor cells
ER Endoplasmic reticulum
GFAT Glutamine: fructose-6-phosphate amidotransferase
G-CSF Granulocyte colony-stimulating factor
GM-CSF Granulocyte macrophage colony-stimulating factor
GTPCH Guanosine 5'-triphosphate cyclohydrolase I
ICAM-1 Intercellular adhesion molecule-1
IL-6 Interleukin-6
iNOS Inducible nitric oxide synthase
MCP-1 Monocyte chemoattractant protein -1
MMP-2 Matrix mettalloproteinase-2
MnSOD Manganese superoxide dismutase
NADPH Nicotinamide adenine dinucleotide phosphate
NF-κB Nuclear factor kappa-light-chain-enhancer of activated B cells
NO Nitric oxide
NOS Nitrogen monoxide synthase
PAD Peripheral artery disease
PAF Platelet-activating factor
PAI Plasminogen activator inhibitor
PARP Poly (ADP ribose) polymerase
PBMC Peripheral blood mononuclear cells
p38MAPK p38 mitogen-activated protein kinase
PGI2 Prostaglandin I2
PI3K Phospoinositide3-kinase
PKC Protein kinase C
RNS Reactive nitrogen species
ROS Reactive oxygen species
SERCA2a Sarcoplasmic reticulum Ca(2+)-ATPase 2a
SIRT1 Silent information regulator 1
SOD Superoxide dismutase
SDF-1 Stromal cell-derived factor-1
TCA Tricarboxylic acid cycle
TGF-1 Transforming growth factor, beta 1
TNF α Tumor necrosis factor α
t-PA Tissue plasminogen activator
UCP-1 Uncoupling protein 1
UPS Ubiquitin proteasome system
VCAM-1 Vascular cell adhesion molecule-1
VEGF Vascular endothelial growth factor
vWF von Willebrand factor

INTRODUCTION

Oxidative stress plays a pivotal role in the pathogenesis of many diseases, including inflammatory, chronic, and progressive diseases. An excess of reactive oxygen species (ROS) and reactive nitrogen species (RNS) is a key mediator of cellular damage. ROS include free radicals such as superoxide ($O{\cdot}_2^-$), hydroxyl ($OH{\cdot}$), peroxyl ($RO_2{\cdot}$), hydroperoxyl ($HRO_2{\cdot}^-$), as well as non-radical species such as hydrogen peroxide (H_2O_2) and hypochlorous acid (HOCl) that can damage cellular components, such as lipids, proteins or DNA [1]. A correct balance between oxidants and antioxidants is necessary for the maintenance of biological functions. In fact, many proteins are sensitive to even mild changes in this balance. Major alterations of this equilibrium can lead to cell dysfunction, apoptosis, and necrosis. Pro-oxidant action may damage the cell by altering several components, such as membrane phospholipids, nucleic acids (causing mutations), and proteins (resulting in the loss of their function) [1].

Diabetes: Oxidative Stress and Dietary Antioxidants.
http://dx.doi.org/10.1016/B978-0-12-405885-9.00015-2

Diabetes mellitus is one of the diseases in which oxidative stress develops [2]. Both forms of diabetes mellitus, type 1 and type 2, are characterized by hyperglycemia, a relative or absolute lack of insulin action, and by pathway-selective insulin resistance. Evidence suggests that hyperglycemia plays a pivotal role on oxidative stress production in diabetic subjects [1]. Diabetes-related hyperglycemia exerts its harmful action through five mechanisms [3], all triggered by a single event, i.e., the increase in mitochondrial production of ROS. The five mechanisms are: increase of sugar flux through the polyol pathway; intracellular production of advanced glycation end products (AGE) and expression of receptors for AGE; increase in hexosamine pathway flux; increase of protein kinase C activation; and mitochondrial superoxide production [4].

Increase of sugar flux through polyol pathway. Aldose reductase is a key player in the polyol pathway. This is an antioxidant enzyme that reduces toxic aldehydes to alcohols in cells and is also responsible for the reduction of glucose to sorbitol, which is successively oxidized to fructose. This process determines the consumption of NADPH, an important cofactor essential for the regeneration of critical intracellular antioxidants. Therefore, since hyperglycemia causes the consumption of NADPH, it also causes an increase in oxidative stress [5].

Intracellular production of AGE and increased expression of AGE receptor. Another cause of oxidative stress is an increase in AGE, produced as a result of glycation through a non-enzymatic reaction due to the increased concentration of glucose in the blood [6]. Three mechanisms account for cellular dysfunctions: the first is protein modification and consequent loss of function, specifically for proteins involved in the regulation of gene transcription [7]. The second mechanism is the extracellular diffusion of AGE [8] and their interaction with extracellular matrix components, such as integrins. The third mechanism involves the interaction of AGE with plasma proteins, receptors of other cells, such as macrophages, vascular endothelial cells, and vascular smooth muscle cells. In addition to directly affecting protein structure and function, AGE also exert cellular effects mediated by AGE receptors. Indeed, glycation may be responsible for an increase in oxidative stress and inflammation through the formation of ROS and the activation of NF-κB, leading to pathological changes in gene expression.

Increase of hexosamine pathway flux. Hyperglycemia leads to an increase in the synthesis of diacylglycerol, which activates the protein kinase C (PKC) isoforms α, β, and δ [9]. The increased PKC activity causes a reduction in nitric oxide (NO) production [10] and inhibition of the expression of endothelial nitric oxide synthase (eNOS) [11]. Furthermore, PKC has been also implicated in the overexpression of the plasminogen activator inhibitor (PAI) [12,13], and in the activation of NF-κB in cultured endothelial cells and vascular smooth muscle cells [14].

Increase of protein kinase C activation. Hyperglycemia and insulin resistance cause an increase of fatty acid oxidation and fructose 6-phophate flux through the hexosamine pathway [15]. Actually, fructose-6-phosphate is deflected from glycolysis to provide support to the rate limiting glutamine-fructose-6-phosphate amidotransferase enzyme (GFAT), which converts fructose 6-phosphate into glucosamine 6-phosphate, which is subsequently converted into UDP-N-acetylglucosamine. Hyperglycemia causes a four-fold increase in O-linked N-acetylglucosamine transfer to proteins with inhibition of eNOS activity, reduction of SERCA2a (sarcoplasmic reticulum $Ca^{(2+)}$ATPase2) mRNA, reduction of protein expression, and decreased SERCA2a promoter activity.

Mitochondrial superoxide production. All the mechanisms described above derive from a single process; superoxide overproduction by the mitochondrial electron transport chain [16]. Superoxide is produced during hyperglycemia due to impairment of mitochondrial electron transport system and by other processes, such as redox changes and uncoupling of eNOS. However, the overexpression of manganese superoxide dismutase (SOD) and UCP-1 prevents the inhibition of eNOS. Furthermore, the increased expression of oxidative phosphorylation genes and electron transport system complex II genes seem to be associated with a more rapid evolution of diabetic nephropathy and then of diabetic complications [17].

OXIDATIVE STRESS, NITRIC OXIDE, AND ENDOTHELIAL DYSFUNCTION

Repeated exposure to hyperglycemia leads to endothelial dysfunction that may become irreversible over time [18]. It has been demonstrated that hyperglycemic spikes induce endothelial dysfunction in both diabetic and normal subjects [19]. The high-glucose-induced 'oxidative stress' and 'endoplasmic reticulum (ER) stress' of the endothelium may play major roles in the initiation and progression of cardiovascular clinical manifestations in diabetes [20]. Moreover, oxidative stress and ER stress appear in connection with the complications of diabetes [19]. Endothelial cells are responsible for the maintenance of blood fluidity and restoration of vessel wall integrity to avoid bleeding. In addition, they maintain the balance between vasoconstriction and vasodilatation by releasing a variety of contracting and relaxing substances, such as prostacyclin and NO, in response to neurohumoral mediators and mechanical forces. Endothelial dysfunction is a systemic pathological condition in which there is an imbalance between the production of vasoconstrictive and vasodilatator substances [20].

Various studies have been performed both in animal models and human to assess endothelial function in diabetic subjects. These studies showed impaired endothelial vasodilation and endothelial dysfunction in diabetic patients, probably due to hyperglycemia-dependent oxidative stress [20]. Endothelial dysfunction is responsible for diabetic complications, both microvascular (retinopathy, nephropathy and neuropathy) and macrovascular (ischemic heart disease, peripheral vascular disease (PAD), and stroke). Different molecular entities have been linked to endothelial dysfunction related to hyperglycemia but the cellular mechanisms underlying these processes are not yet clear. In type 2 diabetes, the endothelial dysfunction seems to be triggered by three mechanisms: hyperlipidemia, early hyperinsulinemia, and hyperinsulinemia followed by pancreatic β-cell failure leading to hyperglycemia [21]. Hyperglycemia also increases the oxidation of glucose and the production of mitochondrial superoxide anions, which leads to DNA damage and activation of poly (ADP ribose) polymerase (PARP) [21]. Also the ADP ribosylation of glyceraldehyde phosphate dehydrogenase, which is induced by PARP, then diverts glucose from its glycolytic pathway toward alternative biochemical pathways leading to increases in polyols, hexosamine flux, AGE, and activation of classical isoforms of protein kinase C[21]. All these pathways seem to converge in the production of ROS. The excessive ROS production appears to affect the endothelium-dependent vasodilation by inhibiting the activity of eNOS and NO synthesis. Thus, the vascular complications of diabetes are the result of diabetes-related oxidative stress and the resulting endothelial dysfunction [21]. Diabetes also produces an increase in inflammatory activity, which leads to increased expression of monocyte chemoattractant protein-1 (MCP-1), vascular cell adhesion molecule-1 (VCAM-1), intercellular adhesion molecule-1 (ICAM-1), interleukin-6 (IL-6), and inducible nitric oxide synthase (iNOS), which are associated with increased cardiovascular risk [22]. Generation of NO is mediated by NADPH oxidase, which is activated by high glucose and acts as the primary source of ROS. This event promotes eNOS uncoupling and production of more H_2O_2 and superoxide. The excess ROS production also appears to reduce the bioavailability of NO, hence reducing endothelium-dependent vasodilatation [23] (Figure 15.1). The increase in ROS is accompanied by an increase in NO which reacts to form peroxynitrite ($ONOO^-$). Peroxynitrite oxidizes tetrahydrobiopterin (BH4), which stabilizes the dimeric forms of NOS. BH4 is an essential cofactor in the regulation of eNOS and iNOS levels in endothelial cells, playing an important role in the genesis of endothelial dysfunction, in which the endothelium loses its physiological ability to promote vasodilation, fibrinolysis and antiaggregation (Figure 15.1).

Insulin resistance, diabetes, and endothelial dysfunction share a common deregulation of ubiquitin proteasome system (UPS), the major pathway for non-lysosomal intracellular protein degradation in eucaryotic cells [24]. In this context, it has been demonstrated that

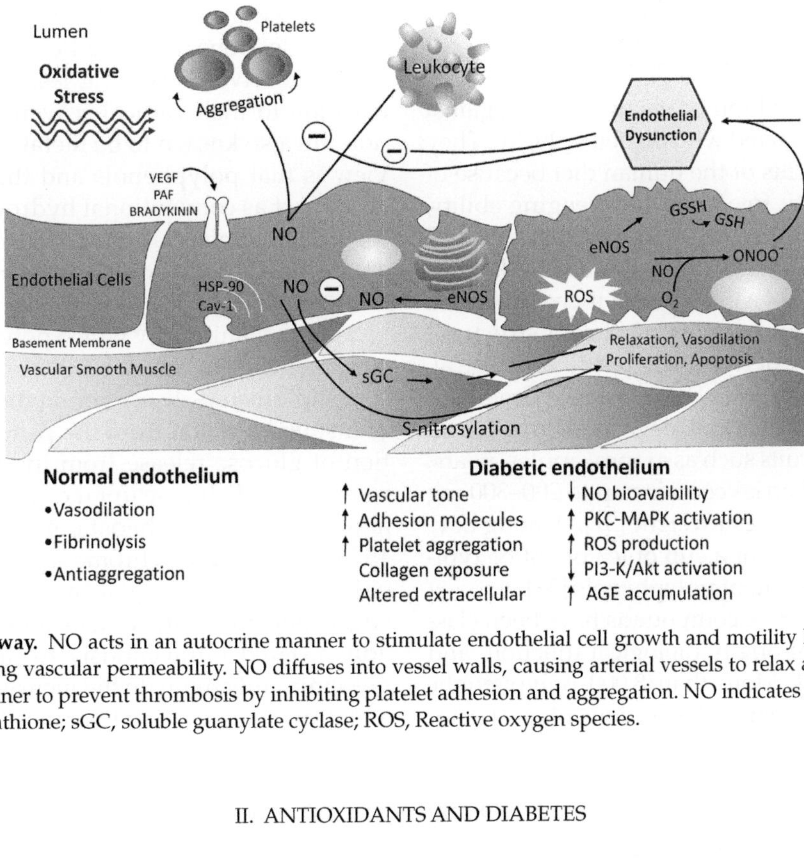

FIGURE 15.1 NO Pathway. NO acts in an autocrine manner to stimulate endothelial cell growth and motility leading to angiogenesis. NO also contributes to increasing vascular permeability. NO diffuses into vessel walls, causing arterial vessels to relax and increase blood flow. NO also acts in a paracrine manner to prevent thrombosis by inhibiting platelet adhesion and aggregation. NO indicates nitric oxide; eNOS, endothelial nitric oxide; GSH, Glutathione; sGC, soluble guanylate cyclase; ROS, Reactive oxygen species.

hyperglycemia reduces levels of BH4 via 26S proteasome-mediated degradation of guanosine 5'-triphosphate cyclohydrolase I (GTPCH), which is the rate limiting enzyme of BH4 synthesis [25]. Additionally, hyperglycemia significantly increases levels of superoxide anion and 3-nitrotyrosine-positive proteins [25]. Adenoviral overexpression of SOD was found to significantly attenuate hyperglycemia-induced 26S proteasome activation and GTPCH reduction [25]. BH4 deficiency in diabetes mellitus is due to a reduction in GTPCH, an enzyme critical to BH4 synthesis, via a process that is peroxynitrite mediated and proteasome dependent [26]. These studies uncover a possible novel mechanism underlying endothelial dysfunction in diabetic vascular diseases. On the other hand, hyperglycemic spikes may also cause endothelial dysfunction by reducing NO production through eNOS degradation. These effects of hyperglycemia may be mediated by oxidative stress, as both peroxynitrite and nitrotyrosine may induce eNOS degradation through UPS up-regulation [27]. Therefore, ubiquitin-proteasome pathways are the major proteolytic systems responsible for the regulated degradation of NOS isozymes [28], although their functional importance and potential implication for vascular physiology and pathophysiology need further study. However, the observation that eNOS is preferentially ubiquitinated suggests that the loss of endothelial function during hyperglycemia associated with impairment of eNOS activity could be due to a combination of excessive oxidative stress and UPS-dependent proteolysis.

POLYPHENOLS AND ANTIOXIDANT MECHANISMS IN DIABETES

Dietary polyphenols exhibit protective action against the oxidative stress associated with diabetes [29,30]. They are important components of the human diet because of their antioxidant activity, free radical scavenging ability, and capacity to ameliorate the oxidative stress-induced tissue damage associated with chronic disease [29,30]. The molecular structure of a polyphenol is characterized by the presence of a large number of phenol structural units, from which they derive their peculiar physical, chemical, and biological properties. Fruits, vegetables, cereals, legumes, chocolate, and beverages are rich in polyphenols. Indeed, fruits such as grapes, apples, pears, cherries, and different berries contains up to 200–300 mg polyphenols per 100 g of fresh weight [31]. Among beverages, a glass of red wine or a cup of tea or coffee typically contains about 100 mg of polyphenols [31].

These naturally occurring compounds have been classified by their source of origin, biological function, and chemical structure [31]. More than 8,000 polyphenolic compounds have been identified in various plant species (Table 15.1, Figure 15.2). The structural diversity of polyphenols extends from simple one-phenol hydroxybenzoic and hydroxycinnamic acids to large polymeric macromolecules like proanthocyanidins and ellagitannins. The flavonoids, including structural classes such as flavonols, are themselves distributed among several classes, i.e., flavones, flavanols, flavanones, anthocyanidins, and isoflavones (Table 15.1, Figure 15.2). The main classes of polyphenols include phenolic acids, flavonoids, stilbenes, and lignans. The two main types of polyphenols are flavonoids and phenolic acids. They are mostly derivatives, and/or isomers of flavones, isoflavones, flavonols, catechins, and phenolic acids. Quercetin is a common flavonol found in onions, tea, and apples; catechin is a flavanol found in tea and several fruits; hesperetin is a flavanone present in citrus fruits; cyanidinis is an anthocyanin giving its color to many red fruits (blackcurrant, raspberry, strawberry, etc.); daidzein is the main isoflavone in soybeans; proanthocyanidins are common in many fruits, such as apples, grapes, or cocoa. Caffeic acid is one of the most common phenolic acids present in many fruits and vegetables, most often esterified with quinic acid as in chlorogenic acid, which is the major phenolic compound in coffee. Another common phenolic acid is ferulic acid, which is present in cereals and is esterified to hemicelluloses in the cell wall.

Polyphenols neutralize free radicals by donating an electron or hydrogen atom; they suppress the generation of free radicals, thus reducing the rate of oxidation by inhibiting the formation of free radicals by deactivating their active species and precursors. They act as direct radical scavengers of lipid peroxidation chain reactions because they are chain breakers, which donate electrons to free radicals thus neutralizing them and themselves becoming less reactive radicals [1]. In addition to their radical scavenging activity, polyphenols are also known to be metal chelators. An emerging view is that polyphenols and their *in vivo* metabolites do not act as conventional hydrogen or electron-donating antioxidants, but may exert modulatory actions in cells by acting on protein kinase and lipid kinase signaling pathways [1].

The mechanisms by which polyphenols influence glucose metabolism are: inhibition of carbohydrate digestion and glucose absorption in the intestine, stimulation of insulin secretion from the pancreatic β cells, modulation of glucose release from liver, activation of insulin receptors and glucose uptake in insulin-sensitive tissues, and modulation of hepatic glucose output [1] (Figure 15.3). The acute or chronic administration of polyphenols may influence glycemia as shown by evidence suggesting that caffeic acid and isoferulic acid, when administered intravenously to rats, reduce the fasting glycemia and attenuate the increase of plasma glucose in an intravenous glucose tolerance test [1].

TABLE 15.1 Sources of Main Dietary Polyphenols

Polyphenols		Source
ANTHOCYANINS		
Chemical structure		
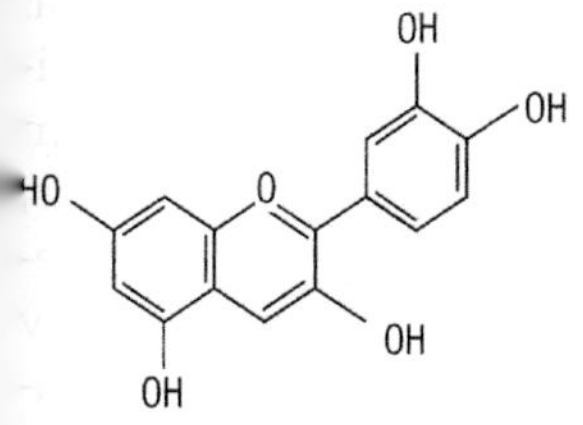 *Cyanidin*	Malvidin 3-glucoside	Red wine
	Cyanidine 3-glucoside	Orange juice
	Malvidin 3-glucoside	Red grape juice
	Cyanidine 3-glucoside	Red fruit extract
FLAVANONES		
Chemical structure		
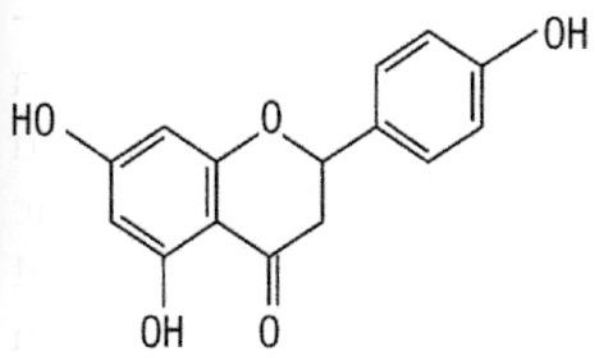 *Naringenin*	Hesperidin	Orange juice
	Hesperidin	Orange juice
	Hesperidin	Pure compound
	Naringenin	Grapefruit juice
	Naringenin	Pure compound
	Naringenin	Orange juice
FLAVONOLS		
Chemical structure		
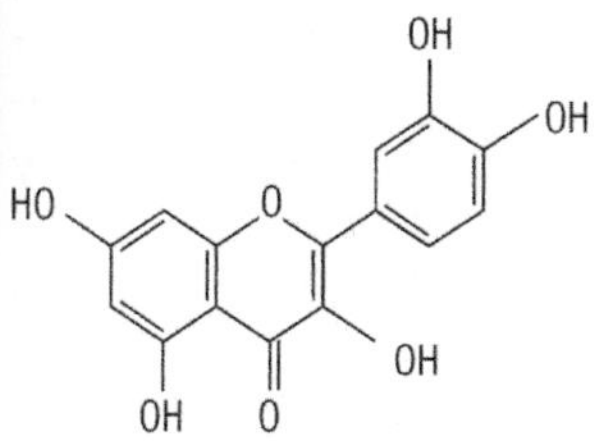 *Quercetin*	Daidzein	Soy milk
	Genistein	Soy milk
	Glycitein	Soy milk
	Daidzein	Soy nuts
	Genistein	Soy nuts
	Glycitein	Pure compound
	Daidzein	Soy extract
	Genistein	Soy extract
	Daidzein	Pure compound
	Genistein	Pure compound
HYDROXYBENZOIC ACIDS		
Chemical structure		
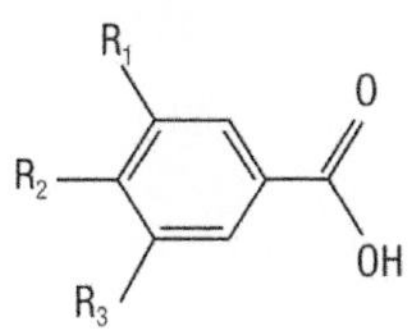 $R_1=R_2=R_3=OH$: Gallic acid; $R_1=R_2=OH$, $R_3=OH$: Protocatechuic acid	Gallic acid	Red wine
	Gallic acid	Assam black tea
	Gallic acid	Pure compound

(Continued)

TABLE 15.1 Sources of Main Dietary Polyphenols — cont'd

Polyphenols		Source
HYDROXYCINNAMIC ACIDS		
Chemical structure		
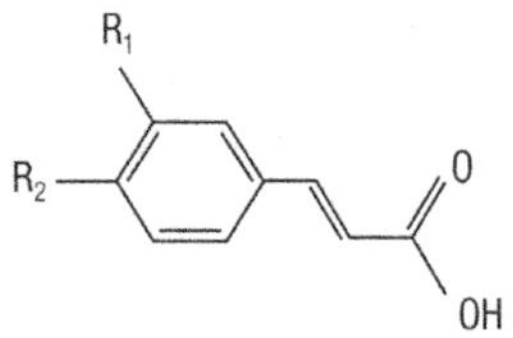	Caffeic acid	Red wine
	Caffeic acid	Red wine
	Chlorogenic acid	Caffee
	Hydrocinnamic acids	Apple cider
R_1=OH: Coumaric acid R_1=R_2=OH: Caffeic acid		
FLAVANOLS		
Chemical structure		
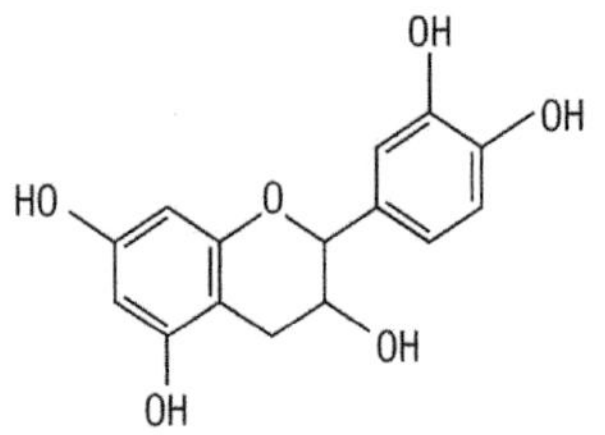	Catechin	Pure compound
	Catechin	Red wine
	Epicatechin	Chocolate
	Epigallocatechin gallate	Green tea infusion
	Epigallocatechin gallate	Pure compound
Catechins	Epigallocatechin gallate	Green tea extract
	Catechins	Black tea
	Procyanidin B1	Grapeseed extract

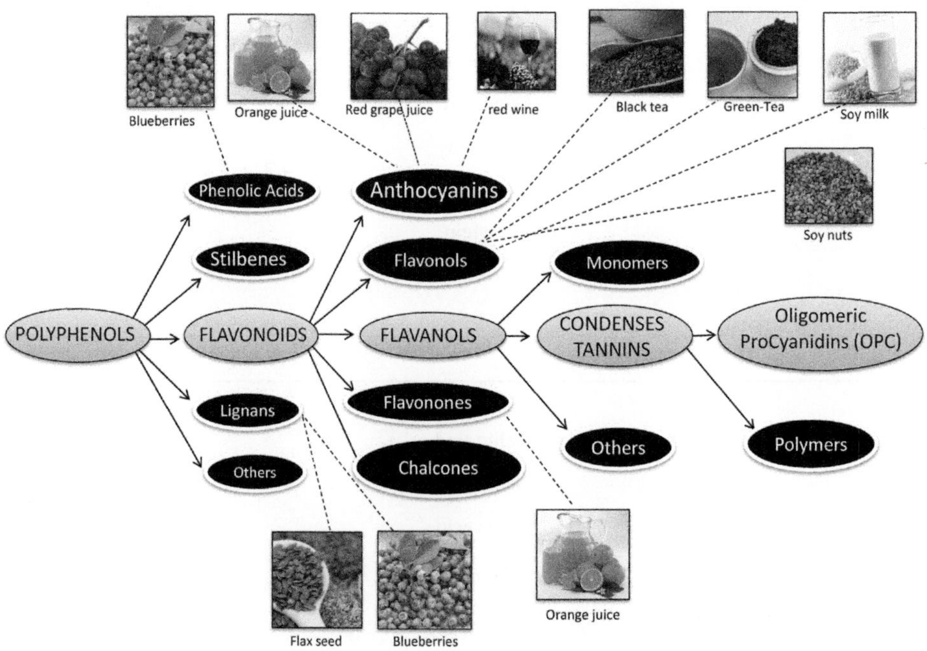

FIGURE 15.2 **Classification of polyphenols and main food sources.**

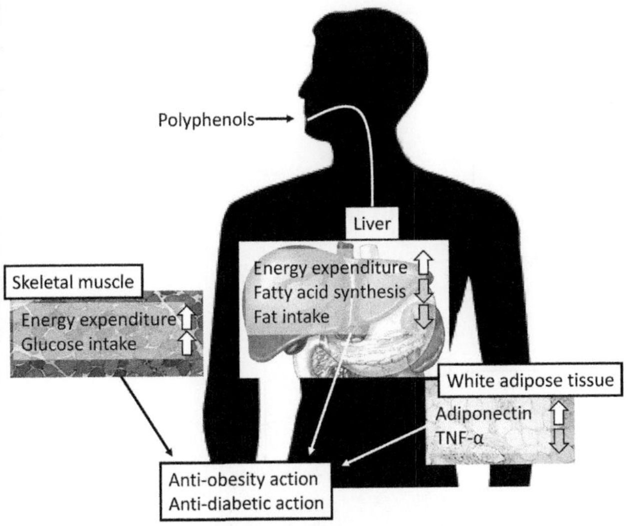

FIGURE 15.3 Sites of action of dietary polyphenols. Polyphenols act on the intestine by inhibition of digestion and absorption; protect β cells from glucotoxicity; act by suppression of glucose release from liver storage and by improvement of glucose uptake in peripheral tissues.

A consistent number of *in vitro*, animal, and epidemiological studies have described the effect of polyphenol consumption on glucose metabolism [29–35]. However, sometimes the studies showed conflicting results [29,34]. Cocoa proanthocyanidins and naringin prevented the increase of blood glucose in genetically diabetic obese mice, with no effects on body weight or total food consumption [34]. In streptozocin-induced diabetic rats, procyanidins and tea polyphenols showed an antihyperglycemic effect [34,36]. On the other hand, grape seed extract supplementation showed limited protective effect in the liver tissue of streptozocin-induced diabetic rats by affecting NO levels [37]. Naringenin, but not the glycoside naringin, inhibited glucose uptake in the intestine *in vitro* and also showed an antihyperglycemic action *in vivo* [34]. Intervention studies that have examined the effect of polyphenol-rich foods on postprandial blood glucose levels in volunteers showed a reduction in apparent glycemic index for red wine, sugar cane extract, coffee, berries and apple juice [30]. In another other study, procyanidin-rich chocolate prevented the unfavorable glucose response induced by the control polyphenol-free chocolate in a crossover study in volunteers [38]. A pilot study on the additive effects of berberine combined with a conventional oral regimen for patients with suboptimal glycemic control showed a positive effect on glycemic and lipid parameters [39]. Moreover, a significant reduction of glycosylated hemoglobin, basal insulin, homeostatic model assessment of insulin resistance, total and low-density lipoprotein cholesterol, and triglycerides was observed [39].

Epidemiological studies have pointed out that moderate wine consumption (one glass a day) is associated with decreased incidence of CVD, hypertension, and diabetes [40]. The health benefits have been ascribed to an increase in antioxidant capacity, changes in lipid profiles, and anti-inflammatory effects. However, to date it is still unclear whether the possible beneficial health effects of alcoholic beverages are due to the polyphenol content or to ethanol [40].

Several polyphenolic compounds contained in red wine are responsible for eNOS activation, trans-resveratrol having a greater effect and cinnamic and hydroxycinnamic acids, cyanidin, and some phenolic acids having smaller effects [33]. In smooth muscle cells, the mechanisms of the polyphenol effects involve redox-insensitive mechanisms and inhibition of the p38 mitogen-activated protein kinase (p38 MAPK) by a redox-sensitive pathway [33]. Several studies have reported the hypoglycemic effect of resveratrol [33]. However, the opposite effect has also been observed [41]. The mechanism of this effect is still unclear, although processes such as its binding effect on sulfonylurea receptors and its ability to block the pancreatic adenosine triphosphate-sensitive K^+ channels in β cell and voltage-gated K^+ channels have been reported [42]. It has also been reported that resveratrol strongly activates the silent information regulator 1 (SIRT1), known to mediate many of the effects of calorie restriction on metabolic pathways of organisms, and to modulate downstream pathways of energy restriction that produce beneficial effect on glucose homeostasis and insulin sensitivity [43].

Dietary polyphenols act by increasing the production of NO, endothelium-derived hyperpolarizing factor and prostacycline, and by inhibiting the synthesis of vasoconstrictor endothelin-1 in endothelial cells [33]. In particular, the activation of eNOS is due to two mechanisms; increased Ca^{2+} intracellular concentration and phosphorylation of eNOS by the PI3-kinase/Akt pathway (Figure 15.4). The beneficial effects of polyphenols may be attributed to their ability to scavenge free radicals, increase the production of NO, endothelium-derived hyperpolarizing factor and prostacycline, and to inhibit the synthesis of vasoconstrictor endothelin-1. Moreover, dietary polyphenols induce antioxidant enzymes such as glutathione peroxidase, catalase, and superoxide dismutase that decompose hydroperoxides, hydrogen peroxide, and superoxide anions, respectively (Figure 15.4).

POLYPHENOLS AND VASCULAR REGENERATION IN DIABETES

Diabetes mellitus is characterized by a three-to-four fold increase in cardiovascular risk [44]. The development of vascular complications in patients with diabetes is related to endothelial dysfunction and the diminished ability to form collateral vessels in response to ischemia

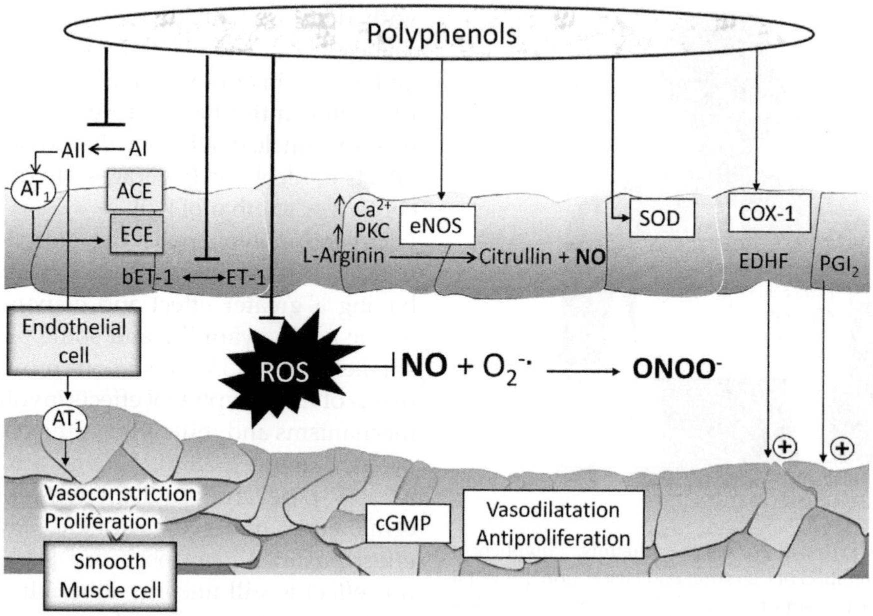

FIGURE 15.4 Antioxidant action of polyphenols. Plant polyphenols induce nitric oxide (NO)-mediated endothelium-dependent relaxations in isolated arteries. NO is synthesized by eNOS from L-arginine in the presence of the cofactor tetrahydrobiopterin. The activation of endothelial NO synthase (eNOS) is due to two mechanisms: 1) an increase in Ca^{2+} intracellular concentration; 2) a phosphorylation of eNOS by the PI3-kinase/Akt pathway. NO increases intracellular cGMP concentrations and, in turn, induces a relaxation of vascular smooth muscle cells. NO not only leads to vasodilation but also prevents leukocyte adhesion and migration, smooth muscle cell proliferation, and platelet adhesion and aggregation. Polyphenols may activate endothelium-derived hyperpolarizing factor (EDHF), increase endothelial prostacyclin release, or inhibit the synthesis of endothelin-1 (ET). Moreover, polyphenols may inhibit angiotensin-converting enzyme (ACE). AII indicates angiotensin II; AI, angiotensin I; PKC, protein kinase C; SOD, superoxide dismutase; ROS, reactive oxygen species; PGI_2, prostacyclin; ACE, angiotensin-converting enzyme; ECE, endothelin-converting enzyme; AT_1, angiotensin receptor; ET-1, endothelin 1; bET-1, big endothelin 1; cGMP, cyclic guanosine monophosphate.

in the heart and peripheral tissues [44]. Vasculopathies associated with diabetes involve increased blood vessel formation and accelerated atherosclerosis leading to coronary artery disease, PAD, and cerebrovascular disease. The severity of macrovascular complications in diabetes is due to profound impaired collateralization of vascular ischemic beds [44].

Neovascularization in adults is not solely the result of the proliferation of local endothelial cells (angiogenesis), but it also involves endothelial progenitor cells (EPCs), a subset of bone marrow-derived peripheral blood mononuclear cells capable of differentiating into mature endothelial cells and homing to sites of vascular damage [44]. In response to cytokine stimulation, these cells are mobilized from the bone marrow, act as 'repair' cells, and contribute to the maintenance of vascular integrity. Once in the bloodstream, EPCs home specifically to sites of vascular damage to repair the disrupted endothelium and to provide pro-angiogenic stimuli in an attempt to restore blood flow and counter any shortage in oxygen and nutrients (Figure 15.5).

EPCs identified as cells expressing CD34, CD133 and VEGFR-2 (KDR) are defined as 'early' EPCs. Cells that have lost CD133 and begun to express endothelial lineage cell markers, including von Willebrand factor (vWF), and eNOS are identified as 'late' EPCs. These two phenotypes display different proliferation potentials. The early EPCs have low proliferative capacity and express CD14 and CD45 antigens, whereas late EPCs show high proliferative capacity and seem to stem from $CD14^-/CD45^-$ subpopulation. However, contradictory findings have been reported concerning the real nature of EPCs and their contribution to the neovascularization of ischemic tissues and re-endothelization of injured vessels. Early EPCs phenotypically resembling monocytes have been found to strongly augment angiogenesis in a paracrine fashion. On the other hand, late EPCs, but not early EPCs, form tubules independently and incorporate into developing vascular networks *in vitro*. The homing of EPCs to the site of vascular damage is mediated by several factors, namley stromal cell-derived factor-1 (SDF-1), granulocyte colony-stimulating factor (G-CSF), granulocyte macrophage colony-stimulating factor (GM-CSF), and other cytokines and hormones. Once in the damaged area, EPCs form a patch, mediated by cell-cell interaction with mature EPCs and transforming growth factor-β1, which proceeds to vascular repair. The hypoxia of an ischemic area induces endothelial cells to produce SDF-1 and VEGF. These two signaling proteins bind on EPCs their respective receptors, i.e., C-X-C

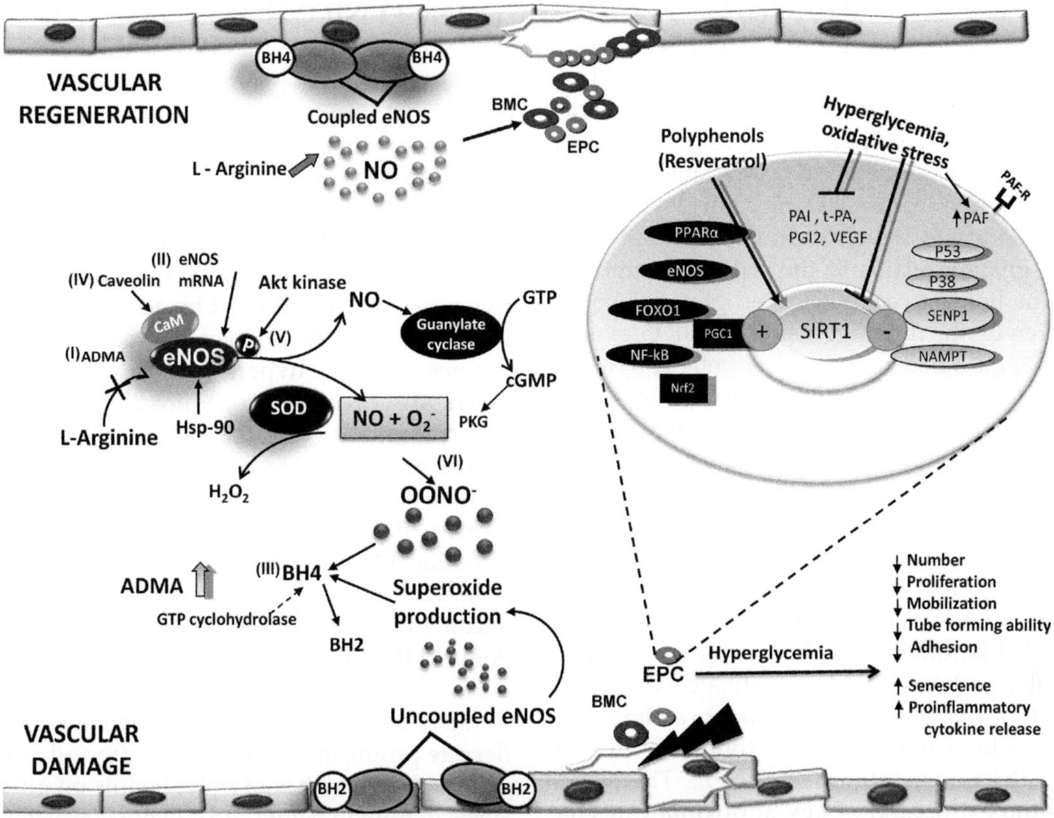

FIGURE 15.5 **Polyphenols in vascular repair.** In vascular disease states such as diabetes, superoxide production by oxidases is markedly increased. Several mechanisms can account for endothelial dysfunction and vascular damage, including: (I) decreased substrate availability; (II) changes in eNOS mRNA or protein levels; (III) decreased cofactor availability; (IV) improper subcellular localization; (V) abnormal phosphorylation; (VI) scavenging of NO by superoxide (O_2^-) to form peroxynitrite anion ($ONOO^-$). Peroxynitrite and other reactive oxygen species oxidize BH4, via the BH3 radical to BH2 and biopterin, which reduces the bioavailability of BH4 and promotes eNOS uncoupling. This form of eNOS no longer produces NO, but instead generates superoxide. In EPC, hyperglycemia down-regulates SIRT1 protein, thereby, affecting EPC survival through the acetylation/deacetylation status of a wide range of protein targets (SENP1, p53, NAMPT and RelA/p65, and PARP-1). SIRT1 down-regulation is responsible for high p53 acetylation and Jun NH2-terminal kinase (JNK) activation. Hyperglycemia and oxidative stress also determine an increased biosynthesis of PAF and expression of its receptor (PAF-R). Polyphenols, such as resveratrol, attenuate oxidative stress-mediated modification of SIRT1 either by increasing the activity of SIRT1 and reducing the ROS levels. ADMA, dimethylarginine; BH4, tetrahydrobiopterin; SOD, superoxide dismutase; PKG, protein kinase G; eNOS, endothelial nitric oxide synthase; TM, trombomodulin; VCAM-1, vascular cell adhesion molecule; BMC, bone marrow cell; EPC, endothelial progenitor cell; SIRT1, Silent information regulator 1; t-PA, Tissue plasminogen activator; VEGF, Vascular endothelial growth factor; PI3K, Phosphatidylinositol 3-kinases; PGI2, Prostaglandin I2; PGC-1α, Peroxisome proliferator-activated receptor-gamma coactivator-1α; PAI-1,Plasminogen activator inhibitor-1; PAF-R, Platelet-Activating Factor receptor; PAF, Platelet-Activating Factor; NAMPT, Nicotinamide phosphoribosyltransferase; NF-κB, Nuclear factor-κB.

chemokine receptor-4 (CXCR-4) and VEGF-Receptor-2, thus recruiting EPCs to the ischemic area.

The loss of EPC functionality in diabetes mellitus compromises the ability to counteract the damage caused by hyperglycemia [44] (Figure 15.5). Moreover, there is a negative correlation between the severity of vascular disease and the number of circulating EPCs (e.g., CD34+KDR+) in diabetic patients [45]. The reduction of EPC number in diabetes is thought to explain, at least in part, the high associated CVD risk, as these patients are less able to repair any endothelial injury. Moreover, the reduction in EPCs may also intervene as a pathogenic factor in microangiopathy, as clinically significant correlations have been found in the setting of retinopathy, nephropathy, and wound healing [45]. In addition, EPCs are not only reduced in number in the bloodstream of diabetic patients, but they also show functional defects, such as impaired adhesion, proliferation, and tubulogenesis [45] due to an enhanced senescence and reduced tube-forming ability of early and late EPCs via NO-related mechanisms [46] (Figure 15.5). Another cause of the development of vascular disease in diabetes can be ascribed to the impaired secretion from late EPCs of vasoactive substances such as NO, plasminogen activator inhibitor-1 (PAI-1), tissue plasminogen activator (t-PA), prostaglandin I2 (PGI2), and vascular endothelial growth factor (VEGF) [47]. It is also likely that the increased production of AGE impairs EPC functional properties through the inhibition of the PI3K/Akt/eNOS pathway [48,49]. Early outgrown EPCs, which release Platelet-Activating Factor (1-O-alkyl-2-acetyl-sn-glycero-3-phosphocholine, PAF), upon stimulation with TNF-α or high glucose concentration, respond to PAF signaling via a transient increase of cytoplasmic Ca^{2+} concentration, since they express PAF-receptor (PAF-R) [50]. Downregulation of EPC levels during short-term exposure to high glucose relates to the reduced activity of SIRT1 [51]. The link between SIRT1 and glucose homeostasis is proven by the downregulation of SIRT1 expression in peripheral blood mononuclear cells (PBMC) of subjects with pre-diabetes compared to subjects with normal glucose regulation [52] and in subjects with type 2 diabetes [53]. Notably, the down-regulation of SIRT1 in the early EPCs of type 2 diabetic patients occurs in a more marked fashion in those with poor glycemic control than in those with good glycemic control. There is also a relationship between SIRT1 down-regulation and a marked up-regulation of PAF-receptor protein expression [53].

Resveratrol, like other polyphenols, activates similar intracellular pathways to those activated by caloric restriction [54]. It activates SIRT1, leading to an improvement in mitochondrial function, followed by the activation of the transcription factor Nrf2. This factor coordinates the expression of key antioxidant mechanisms by binding to the antioxidant response elements [54] (Figure 15.5). Resveratrol treatment significantly reduces the blood glucose level in streptozocin-treated type 1 diabetic animals through insulin-dependent and insulin-independent pathways [54].

Improvement in endothelial function has been observed following cacao, red wine, and green tea consumption and this seems to be due to their polyphenol content [55]. In endothelial cells, red wine polyphenols activate NO production via redox-sensitive activation of the PI3-kinase/Akt pathway which in turn causes phosphorylation of eNOS [33] (Figure 15.5). Resveratrol determines an increase of estrogen receptor-caveolin-1-Src interaction in lipid rafts/caveolae at concentrations compatible with oral consumption, leading to NO production through a G-protein-coupled mechanism [56]. Moreover, the polyphenols of red wine prevented the reduction of human EPC number during *in vitro* treatment with TNF-α or high glucose concentrations, through an enhancement of NO levels, inhibition of p38 phosphorylation, and up-regulation of SIRT1 expression levels [57] (Figure 15.5). Finally, red wine ingestion enhanced blood flow recovery and new vessel formation in response to tissue ischemia in type 1 and type 2 diabetic mice. Intake of red wine up-regulated eNOS activity in ischemic tissues, promoted EPC mobilization, and improved c-kit positive bone marrow cell functions in streptozocin-induced diabetic mice [58].

CONCLUSIONS AND THE ROAD AHEAD

Oxidative stress plays a key role in the genesis of the damage induced by diabetes, which in turn increases the risk of cardiovascular diseases. Drugs and natural antioxidant compounds, such as polyphenols, aimed at reducing oxidative stress, may reduce cardiovascular risk factors and cardiovascular mortality. According to the current evidence, however, a reduction of the oxidative stress can be obtained by acting on the mechanisms involved in the initiation of its production, i.e., by reducing post-prandial hyperglycemia.

The discovery of progenitor cell reduction in diabetes represents a challenge for devising cell-based therapeutic strategies, which show promising results for both coronary and peripheral vascular disease, even if several aspects of EPC biology in diabetes still deserve special attention. Of these, monocyte plasticity and its disturbed polarization, which is thought to account for unbalanced EPCs, still need to be extensively investigated. Some of the EPC dysfunction found in diabetes mellitus is reversible following drug therapy and can be ameliorated with polyphenol supplementation. However, despite promising data from *in vitro* and animal studies, results on the effects of polyphenols on glucose homeostasis in human beings are still not consistent. Moreover, although epidemiological studies tend to support the protective effect of polyphenol-rich foods and beverages against development of type II diabetes, the effect on the risk of developing diabetes is not certain at the moment. Most likely, the action of polyphenols in reducing diabetes risk proceeds by multiple mechanisms; they include modification of post-prandial glycemic responses by inhibiting digestion or glucose transport, improving fasting blood glucose levels, enhanced insulin secretion, and improved insulin sensitivity. In order to clarify the health effects of polyphenols in glucose homeostasis and in vascular complications of diabetes, future clinical trials consistent in design and outcome measurements to help reproducibility are needed. Molecular pathways involved in glucose homeostasis that may translate into long-term health benefits, and which are not observed in short-term studies, will also be a future challenge in this field.

SUMMARY POINTS

- Hyperglycemia-induced oxidative stress plays a major role in the initiation and progression of diabetes.
- Repeated exposure to hyperglycemia leads to endothelial dysfunction.
- Hyperglycemia is associated with impaired EPC number and functional capacity.

- Reduced EPC levels during hyperglycemia relate to a reduced SIRT1 activity.
- Dietary polyphenols exhibit protection against the oxidative stress associated with diabetes.
- Dietary polyphenols modulate the generation of NO from vascular endothelium.
- Polyphenols have beneficial effects on endothelial function and EPC functional activities.

References

[1] Johansen JS, Harris AK, Rychly DJ, Ergul A. Oxidative stress and the use of antioxidants in diabetes: linking basic science to clinical practice. Cardiovasc Diabetol 2005;4:5.

[2] Norhammar A, Tenerz A, Nilsson G, Hamsten A, Efendíc S, Ryden L, et al. Glucose metabolism in patients with acute myocardial infarction and no previous diagnosis of diabetes mellitus: a prospective study. Lancet 2002;359:2140–4.

[3] Brownlee M. The pathobiology of diabetic complications: a unifying mechanism. Diabetes 2005;54:1615–25.

[4] Kaiser N, Sasson S, Feener EP, Boukobza-Vardi N, Higashi S, Moller DE, et al. Differential regulation of glucose transport and transporters by glucose in vascular endothelial and smooth muscle cells. Diabetes 1993;42:80–9.

[5] Lee AY, Chung SS. Contributions of polyol pathway to oxidative stress in diabetic cataract. FASEB J 1999;13:23–30.

[6] Wautier JL, Schmidt AM. Protein glycation: a firm link to endothelial cell dysfunction. Circ Res 2004;95:233–8.

[7] Giardino I, Edelstein D, Brownlee M. Non-enzymatic glycosylation *in vitro* and in bovine endothelial cells alters basic fibroblast growth factor activity: a model for intracellular glycosylation in diabetes. J Clin Invest 1994;94:110–7.

[8] McLellan AC, Thornalley PJ, Benn J, Sonksen PH. Glyoxalase system in clinical diabetes mellitus and correlation with diabetic complications. Clin Sci 1994;87:21–9.

[9] Goldin A, Beckman JA, Schmidt AM, Creager MA. Advanced glycation end products: sparking the development of diabetic vascular injury. Circulation 2006;114:597–605.

[10] Ganz MB, Seftel A. Glucose-induced changes in protein kinase C and nitric oxide are prevented by vitamin E. Am J Physiol Endocrinol Metab 2000;278:E146–52.

[11] Kuboki K, Jiang ZY, Takahara N, Ha SW, Igarashi M, Yamauchi T, et al. Regulation of endothelial constitutive nitric oxide synthase gene expression in endothelial cells and *in vivo*: a specific vascular action of insulin. Circulation 2000;101:676–81.

[12] Craven PA, Studer RK, Felder J, Phillips S, De Rubertis FR. Nitric oxide inhibition of transforming growth factor-beta and collagen synthesis in mesangial cells. Diabetes 1997;46:671–81.

[13] Feener EP, Xia P, Inoguchi T, Shiba T, Kunisaki M, King GL. Role of protein kinase C in glucose- and angiotensin II-induced plasminogen activator inhibitor expression. Contrib Nephrol 1996;118:180–7.

[14] Yerneni KK, Bai W, Khan BV, Medford RM, Natarajan R. Hyperglycemia induced activation of nuclear transcription factor kappaB in vascular smooth muscle cells. Diabetes 1999;48:855–64.

[15] Sayeski PP, Kudlow JE. Glucose metabolism to glucosamine is necessary for glucose stimulation of transforming growth factor-alpha gene transcription. J Biol Chem 1996;271:15237–43.

[16] Nishikawa T, Edelstein D, Du XL, Yamagishi S, Matsumura T, Kaneda Y, et al. Normalizing mitochondrial superoxide production blocks three pathways of hyperglycaemic damage. Nature 2000;404:787–90.

[17] Huang C, Kim Y, Caramori ML, Moore JH, Rich SS, Mychaleckyj JC, et al. Diabetic nephropathy is associated with gene expression levels of oxidative phosphorylation and related pathways. Diabetes 2006;55:1826–31.

[18] Del Prato S. Loss of early insulin secretion leads to post-prandial hyperglycemia. Diabetologia 2003;46:M2–8.

[19] Giugliano D, Marfella R, Coppola L, Verrazzo G, Acampora R, Giunta R, et al. Vascular effects of acute hyperglycemia in humans are reversed by L-arginine: evidence for reduced availability of nitric oxide during hyperglycemia. Circulation 1997;95:1783–90.

[20] Basha B, Samuel SM, Triggler CR, Ding H. Endothelial dysfunction in diabetes mellitus: possible involvement of endoplasmic reticulum stress? Exp Diabetes Res 2012; volume 2012, article ID 481840, 14 pages (1–14).

[21] Fowler MJ. Microvascular and macrovascular complications of diabetes. Clinical Diabetes 2008;26:77–82.

[22] Bakker W, Eringa EC, Sipkema P, Van Hinsbergh VWM. Endothelial dysfunction and diabetes: roles of hyperglycemia, impaired insulin signaling and obesity. Cell Tissue Res 2009;335:165–89.

[23] Inoguchi T, Li P, Umeda F, Yu HY, Kakimoto M, Imamura M, et al. High glucose level and free fatty acid stimulate reactive oxygen species production through protein kinase C-dependent activation of NAD(P)H oxidase in cultured vascular cells. Diabetes 2000;49:1939–45.

[24] Marfella R, D'Amico M, Di Filippo C, Siniscalchi M, Sasso FC, Ferraraccio F, et al. The possible role of the ubiquitin proteasome system in the development of atherosclerosis in diabetes. Cardiovasc Diabetol 2007;6:35.

[25] Xu J, Wu Y, Song P, Zhang M, Wang S, Zou MH. Proteasome dependent degradation of guanosine 5'-triphosphate cyclohydrolase I causes tetrahydrobiopterin deficiency in diabetes mellitus. Circulation 2007;116:944–53.

[26] Wei Q, Xia Y. Proteasome inhibition down-regulates endothelial nitric oxide synthase phosphorylation and function. J Biol Chem 2006;281:21652–9.

[27] Kone BC, Kuncewicz T, Zhang W, Yu ZY. Protein interactions with nitric oxide synthases: controlling the right time, the right place, and the right amount of nitric oxide. Am J Physiol Renal Physiol 2003;285:F178–90.

[28] Stangl V, Lorenz M, Meiners S, Ludwig A, Bartsch C, Moobed M. Long-term up-regulation of eNOS and improvement of endothelial function by inhibition of the ubiquitin-proteasome pathway. FASEB 2004;18:272–9.

[29] de Bock M, Derraik JG, Cutfield WS. Polyphenols and glucose homeostasis in humans. J Acad Nutr Diet 2012;112:808–15.

[30] Hanhineva K, Törrönen R, Bondia-Pons I, Pekkinen J, Kolehmainen M, Mykkänen H, et al. Impact of dietary polyphenols on carbohydrate metabolism. Int J Mol Sci 2010;11:1365–402.

[31] Scalbert A, Johnson IT, Saltmarsh M. Polyphenols: antioxidants and beyond. Am J Clin Nutr 2005;81:215S–7S.

[32] Bhatt JK, Thomas S, Nanjan MJ. Resveratrol supplementation improves glycemic control in type 2 diabetes mellitus. Nutr Res 2012;32:537–41.

[33] Ignarro LJ, Balestrieri ML, Napoli C. Nutrition, physical activity, and cardiovascular disease: an update. Cardiovasc Res 2007;73:326–40.

[34] Williamson G. Possible effects of dietary polyphenols on sugar absorption and digestion. Mol Nutr Food Res 2012;57:48–57.

[35] Pérez-Torres I, Ruiz-Ramírez A, Baños G, El-Hafidi M. Hibiscus Sabdariffa Linnaeus (Malvaceae), curcumin and resveratrol as alternative medicinal agents against metabolic syndrome. Cardiovasc Hematol Agents Med Chem 2012; 2012 Jun 20 [Epub ahead of print].

[36] Gao R, Wang Y, Wu Z, Ming J, Zhao G. Interaction of barley β-glucan and tea polyphenols on glucose metabolism in streptozotocin-induced diabetic rats. J Food Sci 2012;77:H128–34.

[37] Belviranli M, Gökbel H, Okudan N, Büyükbaş S. Oxidative stress and antioxidant status in diabetic rat liver: Effect of plant polyphenols. Arch Physiol Biochem 2012;118:237–43.

[38] Almoosawi S, Tsang C, Ostertag LM, Fyfe L, Al-Dujaili EA. Differential effect of polyphenol-rich dark chocolate on biomarkers of glucose metabolism and cardiovascular risk factors in healthy, overweight and obese subjects: a randomized clinical trial. Food Funct 2012;43:1035–43.

[39] Di Pierro F, Villanova N, Agostini F, Marzocchi R, Soverini V, Marchesini, et al. Pilot study on the additive effects of berberine and oral type 2 diabetes agents for patients with suboptimal glycemic control. Diabetes Metab Syndr Obes 2012;5:213–7.

[40] Arranz S, Chiva-Blanch G, Valderas-Martínez P, Medina-Remón A, Lamuela-Raventós RM, Estruch R. Wine, beer, alcohol and polyphenols on cardiovascular disease and cancer. Nutrients 2012;4:59–81.

[41] Ates O, Cayli SR, Yucel N, Altinoz E, Kocak A, Durak MA, et al. Central nervous system protection by resveratrol in streptozocin-induced diabetic rats. J Clin Neurosci 2007;14:256–60.

[42] Chen WP, Chi TC, Chuang LM, Su MJ. Resveratrol enhances insulin secretion by blocking KATP and KV channels of beta cells. Eur J Pharmacol 2007;568:269–77.

[43] Sharma S, Misra CS, Arumugam S, Roy S, Shah V, Davis JA, et al. Antidiabetic activity of resveratrol, a known SIRT1 activator in a genetic model for type 2 diabetes. Phytother Res 2011;25:67–73.

[44] Fadini GP, Agostini C, Avogaro A. Endothelial progenitor cells and vascular biology in diabetes mellitus: current knowledge and future perspectives. Curr Diabetes Rev 2005;1:41–58.

[45] Fadini GP, Avogaro A. It is all in the blood: the multifaceted contribution of circulating progenitor cells in diabetic complications. Exp Diabetes Res 2012; 2012:742976. Exp Diabetes Res.volume 2012 article ID 742976, 8 pages (1–8).

[46] Chen YH, Lin SJ, Lin FY, Wu TC, Tsao CR, Huang PH, et al. High glucose impairs early and late endothelial progenitor cells by modifying nitric oxide-related but not oxidative stress-mediated mechanisms. Diabetes 2007;56:1559–68.

[47] Zhan J, Zhang X, Li H, Cui X, Guan X, Tang K, et al. Hyperglycemia exerts deleterious effects on late endothelial progenitor cell secretion actions. Diab Vasc Dis Res 2012;10(1):49–56.

[48] Li H, Zhang X, Guan X, Cui X, Wang Y, Chu H, et al. Advanced glycation end products impair the migration, adhesion and secretion potentials of late endothelial progenitor cells. Cardiovasc Diabetol 2012;11:46.

[49] Chen J, Song M, Yu S, Gao P, Yu Y, Wang H, et al. Advanced glycation end products alter functions and promote apoptosis in endothelial progenitor cells through receptor for advanced glycation endproducts mediate overpression of cell oxidant stress. Mol Cell Biochem 2010;335:137–46.

[50] Balestrieri ML, Giovane A, Milone L, Servillo L. Endothelial progenitor cells express PAF receptor and respond to PAF via Ca(2+)-dependent signaling. Biochim Biophys Acta 2010;1801:1123–32.

[51] Balestrieri ML, Rienzo M, Felice F, Rossiello R, Grimaldi V, Milone L, et al. High glucose down-regulates endothelial progenitor cell number via SIRT1. Biochim Biophys Acta 2008;1784:936–45.

[52] de Kreutzenberg SV, Ceolotto G, Papparella I, Bortoluzzi A, Semplicini A, Dalla Man C, et al. Downregulation of the longevity-associated protein sirtuin 1 in insulin resistance and metabolic syndrome: potential biochemical mechanisms. Diabetes 2010;59:1006–15.

[53] Balestrieri ML, Servillo L, Esposito A, D'Onofrio N, Giovane A, Casale R, et al. Poor glycaemic control in type 2 diabetes patients reduces endothelial progenitor cell number by influencing SIRT1 signaling via platelet-activating factor receptor activation. Diabetologia 56:162–172.

[54] Turan B, Tuncay E, Vassort G. Resveratrol and diabetic cardiac function: focus on recent *in vitro* and *in vivo* studies. J Bioenerg Biomembr 2012;44:281–96; 2012.

[55] Landberg R, Naidoo N, van Dam RM. Diet and endothelial function: from individual components to dietary patterns. Curr Opin Lipidol 2012;23:147–55.

[56] Klinge CM, Wickramasinghe NS, Ivanova MM, Dougherty SM. Resveratrol stimulates nitric oxide production by increasing estrogen receptor alpha-Src-caveolin-1 interaction and phosphorylation in human umbilical vein endothelial cells. FASEB J 2008;22:2185–97.

[57] Balestrieri ML, Schiano C, Felice F, Casamassimi A, Balestrieri A, Milone L, et al. Effect of low doses of red wine and pure resveratrol on circulating endothelial progenitor cells. J Biochem 2008;143:179–86.

[58] Huang PH, Tsai HY, Wang CH, Chen YH, Chen JS, Lin FY, et al. Moderate intake of red wine improves ischemia-induced neovascularization in diabetic mice–roles of endothelial progenitor cells and nitric oxide. Atherosclerosis 2010;212:426–35.

CHAPTER

16

Vitamin E and Vascular Protection in Diabetes

Hagit Goldenstein, John Ward, Andrew P. Levy

The Ruth and Bruce Rappaport Faculty of Medicine, Technion-Israel Institute of Technology, Haifa, Israel

List of Abbreviations

DM Diabetes mellitus
CVD Cardiovascular disease
Hb Hemoglobin
Hp Haptoglobin
ROS Reactive oxygen species
LDL Low-density lipoprotein
HDL High-density lipoprotein
ApoA Apolipoprotein A
ApoE Apolipoprotein E
SOD Superoxide dismutase
H_2O_2 Hydrogen peroxide
LCAT Lecithin-cholesterol acetyl transferase
RCT Reverse cholesterol transport
LPL Lipoprotein lipase
PLTP Phospholipid transfer protein
DHR Dihydrorhodamine
MLD Minimum luminal diameter
HOPE Heart Outcomes Prevention Evaluation
EDC Epidemiology of Diabetes Complications
ICARE Israel Cardiovascular Atherosclerosis Risk and Vitamin E
CACTI Coronary Artery Calcification Type I
WAVE Women's Angiographic Vitamin and Estrogen

INTRODUCTION

Diabetes mellitus (DM) is a chronic progressive disease and a leading cause of cardiovascular (CV) complications, such as heart failure, stroke and atherosclerosis. In diabetes, decreased glucose metabolism results in glucose remaining in the plasma for longer. Hyperglycemia can cause endothelial dysfunction, leading to impairment of blood vessel wall integrity, hemolysis, and hemoglobin (Hb) leak into the plasma. Moreover, the circulating glucose glycates cell membranes and plasma proteins such as Hb. This non-enzymatic glycosylation of Hb allows it to mediate overproduction of reactive oxygen species (ROS) [1]. Newly formed radicals also react with plasma components, enhancing the oxidation of proteins and lipids, such as LDL. Oxidized LDL can penetrate the endothelial wall and accumulate in intimal macrophages, leading to the formation of foam cells, which comprise the core of atherosclerotic plaques. Oxidized LDL also triggers an inflammatory response that damages the blood vessel wall, and thereby accelerates the propagation of vascular disease [2].

HAPTOGLOBIN

Under normal conditions, Hb remains within red blood cells. Additionally, antioxidants in the red blood cells, such as catalase and superoxide dismutase (SOD), decrease the levels of hydrogen peroxide (H_2O_2) and superoxide anions ($O_2\cdot^-$), respectively. Thus, Hb is prevented from acting as an oxidizing reagent. However, during hemolysis, Hb is released from red blood cells and the protective effect of catalase and SOD is unavailable. In the plasma there are several components that act as antioxidants. Haptoglobin (Hp) is one of them and its specialty is to protect against the oxidative cascade associated with free Hb.

HAPTOGLOBIN GENE AND PROTEIN STRUCTURE

In humans, the Hp gene is located on chromosome 16q22 and has two major functional classes of alleles, known as 1 and 2. Allele 1 is alike in humans and animals. However, allele 2 was formed during evolution by unequal crossing-over between two Hp 1 alleles and is unique to humans (see Figure 16.1) [3].

The Hp protein is composed of α and β subunits, which are linked to each other by disulfide bonds. The β subunit is the same in both Hp 1 and Hp 2, but the α

Diabetes: Oxidative Stress and Dietary Antioxidants.
http://dx.doi.org/10.1016/B978-0-12-405885-9.00016-4

subunit is different due to duplication. Since the duplication site is located on the chain in the multidimerization domain, the polymeric structure of the proteins differ between Hp types. The α_1 subunit in Hp 1 has only one sulfhydryl group available for multidimerization, while the α_2 subunit in Hp 2 has two sulfhydryl groups. In humans, there are three different Hp genotypes and thus three different polymeric structures. The homozygous 1–1 genotype forms dimers with only one disulfide bond between two Hp 1 monomers. The homozygous 2–2 genotype forms cyclic polymers with several disulfide bonds between variable numbers of Hp 2 monomers. The heterozygous 2–1 genotype forms linear polymers with variable numbers of Hp 2 monomers in the middle and Hp 1 monomers at either end of the chain (see Figure 16.2A). Each Hp phenotype has a unique electrophoretic pattern

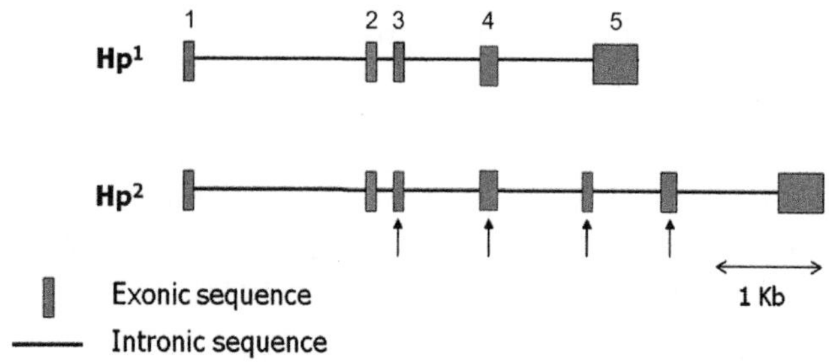

FIGURE 16.1 **The structure of haptoglobin (Hp) 1 and Hp 2 genes.** Hp 2 gene was formed by duplication of exons 3 and 4 of Hp 1 gene [10]. *Figure reproduced from Goldenstein et al. Haptoglobin genotype and its role in determining heme-iron mediated vascular disease published 2012 in Pharmacological Research 66(1): 1–6.*

that can be identified by using Hb starch gel (or polyacrylamide gel). The dimers of Hp 1–1 show one rapidly migrating band, while the bigger polymeric cyclic proteins of Hp 2–2 show a series of slower migrating bands. The linear polymeric proteins of Hp 2–1 show a pattern of intermediate-sized bands (see Figure 16.2B) [4].

GEOGRAPHICAL DISTRIBUTION

In most Western populations, the most common phenotype of Hp is Hp 2–1 (48%). The prevalence of Hp 2–2 is 36%, while that of Hp 1–1 is only 16%. This distribution differs in some geographical regions, such as Southeast Asia, where 90% of the population are Hp 2–2 [4].

HP ANTIOXIDANT FUNCTION

Hp/Hb Complex Formation and Binding to CD163

Each Hp monomer binds an Hb α-β dimer through a powerful noncovalent interaction with $K_d = 1x10^{-15}$. This interaction is irreversible, and allows a unique epitope on the Hp/Hb complex to be recognized by CD163, a scavenger receptor on macrophages and circulating monocytes. Within the macrophage, the heme is degraded by the heme oxygenase system. This clearance mechanism is especially important after hemolysis, when there is a need to clear the plasma of free Hb [3].

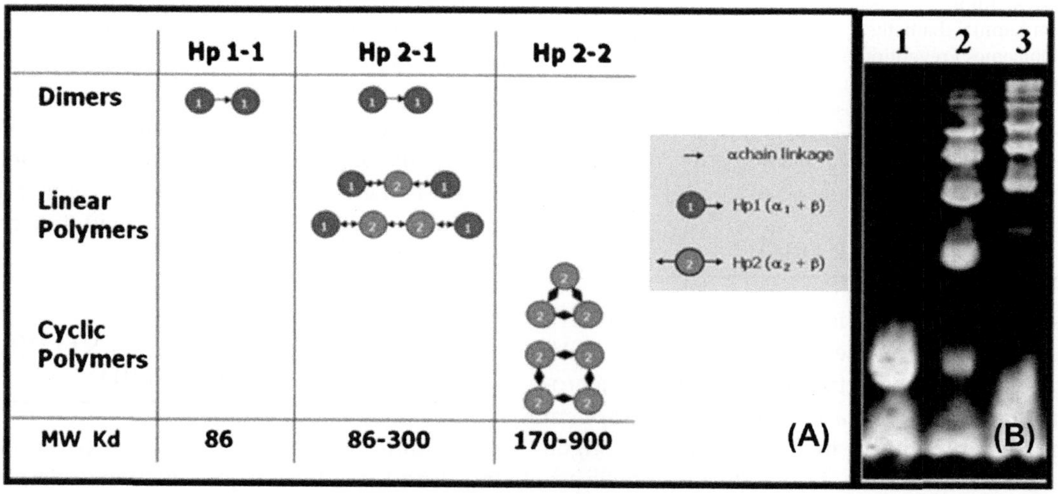

FIGURE 16.2 **Polymer structure of haptoglobin (Hp) in individuals with the different Hp genotypes.** (A) Disulfide bonds between the α chains form the subunits of the polymers. Individuals with Hp 1–1 phenotype form dimers only. Hp 2–1 individuals form linear polymers and Hp 2–2 individuals form cyclic polymers. (B) Hp typing from serum with excess amount of hemoglobin (Hb) by electrophoresis. Each Hp type has a unique banding pattern. The single band at the bottom of the gel is free Hb. Lane 1 contains Hp 1–1 dimers which run as a single band. Lane 2 contains Hp 2–1 linear polymers, which have different sizes and therefore run as a series of bands in the upper part of the gel, with a single band of Hp 1–1 dimers in the bottom of the gel. Lane 3 contains Hp 2–2 polymers, which form cyclic polymers of different sizes, running as a series of bands near the top of the gel [3]. *Figure adapted from Levy et al. Haptoglobin: basic and clinical aspects published 2010 in Antioxidants and Redox Signaling 12(2):293–304.*

However, in diabetes there is a reduction in the number of circulating monocytes that express CD163, and of macrophages expressing CD163 in atherosclerotic plaques. This reduction was especially prominent in Hp 2–2 diabetic individuals, who showed a greater reduction of macrophages expressing CD163 in atherosclerotic plaques than Hp 1–1 diabetic individuals. Moreover, a larger amount of plasma-soluble CD163 was found in Hp 2–2 diabetic individuals when compared to Hp 1–1 diabetic individuals [5].

As an indication of the clearance rate of Hp/Hb complexes from the plasma, ^{125}I labeled Hp/Hb complexes were injected into transgenic mice intravenously, and the loss of radioactivity in the blood was measured over time. In the absence of diabetes, it was found that the half-life of Hp2–2/Hb complexes was 2.5-fold greater than Hp1–1/Hb complexes (50 minutes versus 20 minutes, respectively). In the presence of diabetes, the half-life of Hp 2–2/Hb complexes was five-fold greater than Hp 1–1/Hb complexes (100 minutes versus 20 minutes, respectively [6]). In summary, the ability of Hp 2–2 diabetic individuals to clear the Hp/Hb complexes from the circulation is markedly inferior to that of Hp 1–1 diabetic individuals, resulting in increased opportunities for Hb to participate in oxidative reactions.

Another consequence of impaired clearance of Hp 2–2/Hb complexes in diabetic individuals is increased iron deposition in the kidneys and atherosclerotic plaques. The amount of iron in tissues can be qualified using a Perl stain. It was found that Hp 2–2 diabetic mice had higher levels of iron in their proximal tubules than Hp 1–1 diabetic mice. In Hp 2–2 diabetic mice bred on an apolipoprotein E (apoE) knockout background, a specific mouse model used to study atherosclerotic plaque development, higher levels of intraplaque iron were observed when compared to apoE knockout Hp 1–1 diabetic mice (see Figure 16.3) [7]. The same results were seen in diabetic patients with different Hp phenotypes [8].

Oxidation Reaction Catalyzed by Heme Iron

As mentioned above, free Hb can mediate the formation of ROS. The iron within the heme pocket can undergo oxidation by several oxidizing agents, such as H_2O_2. This pseudoperoxidase activity of Hb can yield ferrylhemoglobin (Fe^{4+}), a molecule with a high redox potential, which can react with another molecule of hydrogen peroxide to yield ferric Hb (Fe^{3+}) and a superoxide anion [9]. Another highly reactive radical that can be formed during the reaction of ferrous Hb (Fe^{2+}) with hydrogen peroxide is the hydroxyl radical. In this reaction, ferric Hb (Fe^{3+}) is also formed, which now can react with another molecule of hydrogen peroxide, as described previously [10]. Moreover, ferric Hb, also known as methemoglobin, can spontaneously release the heme moiety into the circulation. Heme, a hydrophobic molecule, immediately enters diverse lipophilic environments such as cell membranes or LDL. In these new lipid environments, Hb can react with adjacent lipid peroxides or mediate any of the reactions described above, and thereby amplify the production of free radicals, which can then oxidize lipids and proteins [11].

DIFFERENT HP TYPES DIFFER IN THEIR ABILITY TO INHIBIT HB REDOX ACTIVITIES

The binding of Hp to Hb stabilizes the heme moiety within the heme pocket and prevents it from mediating formation of radicals. However, several studies have shown that Hp 2–2 is inferior to Hp 1–1 in neutralizing the redox activity of heme iron. For example, in a study

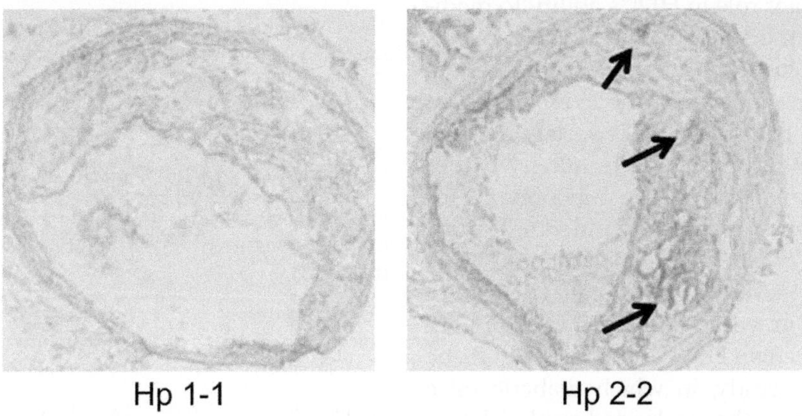

FIGURE 16.3 **Atherosclerotic plaques show higher levels of intraplaque iron in haptoglobin (Hp) 2–2 mice.** Hp 1–1 and Hp 2–2 diabetic mice bred on an apolipoprotein E (apoE) knockout background were studied for atherosclerotic plaque development. Aortic sections were isolated from the mice and stained for iron. The arrows point to deposits of iron in the plaque of Hp 2–2 ApoE mice [7]. *Figure reproduced from Levy et al. Haptoglobin genotype is a determinant of iron, lipid peroxidation, and macrophage accumulation in the atherosclerotic plaque published 2007 in Arteriosclerosis, Thrombosis and Vascular Biology 27(1):134–40.*

that investigated the ability of Hp types to prevent heme transfer from methemoglobin to LDL, it was shown that Hp 2–2 is less efficient than Hp 1–1 in preventing this transfer [12]. In another study, the redox activity of plasma iron was measured using an *in vitro* kinetic fluorometric assay with dihydrorhodamine (DHR) in the presence of an iron chelator. A marked increase in the amount of redox-reactive iron present was observed with Hp 2–2/Hb complexes as compared with Hp 1–1/Hb complexes, which was enhanced when using *in vitro* glycated Hb [1].

In a separate study, human macrophage cells (THP-1) were exposed to Hp/Hb complexes in the presence or absence of hyperglycemic medium. Using a substrate named 2,7-dichlorofluorescein, which fluoresces when oxidized, the amount of oxidation was measured by flow cytometry. Additionally, the effect of desferroxamine, a high affinity iron chelator, was tested. It was found that under hyperglycemic conditions, a greater amount of fluorescence was seen in cells that were exposed to Hp 2–2/Hb complexes compared to Hp 1–1/Hb complexes. Since the oxidation was inhibited by desferroxamine, the conclusion from this study was that in a hyperglycemic environment, the iron within the heme pocket has higher redox activity than in normal conditions. These results were repeated *in vivo* in another experiment on transgenic mice, which showed an increase in redox active iron in Hp 2–2 diabetic mice compared with Hp 1–1 diabetic mice [1].

HP AND HIGH-DENSITY LIPOPROTEIN (HDL)

Hp binds to apolipoprotein A (apoA), the main lipoprotein of HDL, at a site located near the binding site of lecithin-cholesterol acetyl transferase (LCAT). LCAT is an enzyme with a major role in HDL's ability to mediate reverse cholesterol transport (RCT). LCAT converts cholesterol on HDL to cholesterol ester, which is subsequently scavenged by receptor B1 in the liver. However, since the binding sites of Hp and LCAT overlap, binding of Hp displaces LCAT. In order to determine whether this displacement interfered with the functionality of LCAT, HDL from diabetic patients was added to human macrophages cultured *in vitro* with labeled cholesterol. It was found that the amount of tritiated cholesterol released into the medium was lower with HDL from Hp 2–2 diabetic individuals than HDL from Hp 1–1 diabetic individuals. In another study, in which diabetic mice were injected with macrophages loaded with labeled cholesterol, the amount of labeled cholesterol ester in the plasma, feces, and liver was significantly higher in Hp 1–1 diabetic mice than Hp 2–2 diabetic mice. These findings demonstrate that the RCT function of HDL is impaired in Hp 2–2 diabetic individuals [13].

Another explanation for the decrease in RCT in Hp 2–2 individuals might be the increased oxidation of lipids associated with HDL, which might interfere with antioxidant enzymes of HDL such as paraoxonase and glutathione peroxidase [14].

In conclusion, all of the studies mentioned above provide valid proof of the importance of oxidative stress in diabetes, and the role of Hp in preventing it. In order to investigate the relationship between Hp genotypes and cardiovascular complications, samples were collected from the Strong Heart Study [15]. About 400 people participated in this study, half of whom were diabetic. Their Hp phenotypes were determined and the prevalence of cardiovascular disease (CVD) was assessed. The results concluded that the Hp 2–2 phenotype is associated with a three-to-five-fold increased risk of developing cardiovascular complications. The Hp 1–1 phenotype has the least risk of cardiovascular complications and the Hp 2–1 phenotype had intermediate risk. In the following years, several clinical studies in the diabetic population were established to further investigate these findings (see Table 16.1). Those studies proved that the Hp genotype is a genetic marker for predicting the risk of developing cardiovascular complications in diabetic people.

TABLE 16.1 Clinical Studies Showing Increased Risk of Vascular Complications in Hp 2–2 Diabetic Individuals [10]

Research Study Name	Increased Risk in Hp 2–2 Genotype	Ref
Strong Heart Study	Three-to-five-fold increased incidence of cardiovascular disease (CVD)	[15]
Munich Stent Study	Increase in the incidence of major adverse cardiac events (MACE) in the one year period following percutaneous transluminal coronary angioplasty	[16]
The Rambam Myocardial Infarction Outcomes in Diabetes Study	Eightfold increased incidence of death and heart failure in the 30 day period after myocardial infarction	[17]
Israel Cardiovascular Vitamin E study (ICARE)	Two-to-three-fold increased risk of MACE	[18]
Epidemiology of Diabetes Complications Study (EDC)	Twofold increased risk of CVD in type 1 diabetic individuals	[19]
Coronary Artery Calcification Type I (CACTI) Study	Increased risk of development of coronary artery calcification in type 1 diabetic individuals	[20]
Epidemiology of Diabetes Complications Study (EDC)	Twofold increased risk for estimated glomerular filtration rate decline and end stage renal disease	[21]

Table reproduced from Goldenstein et al. Haptoglobin genotype and its role in determining heme-iron mediated vascular disease published 2012 in Pharmacological Research 66(1): 1–6.

Due to the increased incidence of CVD in Hp 2–2 diabetic individuals and the oxidative stress mechanism involved, which cannot be prevented by Hp 2–2, it was postulated that supplementation with antioxidants, specifically in this subgroup of patients, might help. Several epidemiological studies were designed to study this theory, and in the next part of the chapter, the therapeutic role of vitamin E in the prevention of cardiovascular complications in Hp 2–2 diabetic patients will be discussed.

VITAMIN E

Vitamin E is a lipophilic molecule with many biological functions, but it is best known as an antioxidant. In the body, vitamin E can be found in the plasma in the lipid phase compartment, like lipoproteins, or within the cellular compartment, such as the cell membrane, the Golgi, and the lysosome where it is most abundant [22].

Vitamin E can be consumed in the diet by eating foods such as milk, eggs, and green vegetables. In the circulation, vitamin E is transferred to lipoproteins and cells by phospholipid transfer protein (PLTP) and lipoprotein lipase (LPL) [23]. In a lipophilic environment, vitamin E can act as an antioxidant due to its ability to scavenge lipid radicals, such as lipid peroxyl radical. This interaction terminates the oxidative lipid chain reaction, but turns vitamin E into a radical. Thus, in the circulation, there are other soluble antioxidants that can recycle vitamin E back to its non-oxidized form [24].

Although vitamin E can be consumed in a regular diet, therapeutic doses of vitamin E (400 mg/day) were prescribed routinely by cardiologists as a preventive treatment for CVD for the entire population, due to its role as an antioxidant. However, in the past two decades, several epidemiological studies [25–27] concluded that supplementation of vitamin E did not have a beneficial effect on cardiovascular complications, and also increased the risk of CVD and even mortality [28]. Thus, vitamin E treatment has been stopped. However, another group of epidemiological studies were recently established to investigate the association between vitamin E and Hp polymorphism in the diabetic population. Those studies demonstrated that in contrast to previous studies on the entire population, vitamin E has a beneficial effect on the specific subgroup of diabetic individuals who carry the Hp 2–2 genotype. Those studies will be discussed below.

EPIDEMIOLOGICAL STUDIES OF VITAMIN E SUPPLEMENTATION FOR HP 2–2 DIABETIC INDIVIDUALS

The first study to investigate this theory was the Heart Outcomes Prevention Evaluation (HOPE) study, published in 2000 [29]. In this study, about 10,000 diabetic individuals with diagnosed CVD and another risk factor were randomized to receive vitamin E (400 IU/day) or placebo, and were followed for 4.5 years. The statistically significant results showed a 50% decrease in the occurrence of myocardial infarctions and cardiovascular death in Hp 2–2 diabetic individuals who received vitamin E treatment. The same results were shown by Milman and colleagues in 2008, in the prospective placebo controlled double blinded clinical trial, known as the Israel Cardiovascular Atherosclerosis Risk and Vitamin E (ICARE) study [18]. Hp 2–2 diabetic individuals who received vitamin E had a 50% reduction in the risk of developing cardiovascular disease compared to the placebo group (see Figure 16.4). In another study involving Hp 2–2 diabetic patients, it was found that statin therapy is less effective than a dual therapy of statins and vitamin E in decreasing the risk of developing cardiovascular complications [30]. As mentioned before, HDL dysfunction is a common complication in diabetic individuals, and is increased in Hp 2–2 diabetic individuals. Asleh and colleagues formed a trial to investigate whether vitamin E supplementation can restore HDL-mediated cholesterol efflux to normal levels, as seen in Hp 1–1 diabetic individuals [6]. In this study, serum samples were collected from participants at the beginning of the experiment as a baseline, and again after the completion of either treatment (vitamin E) or placebo. Another serum sample was collected two months after cessation of vitamin E supplementation. The serum was added to human macrophage cells (THP-1) that were loaded with labeled cholesterol, and the ability of HDL to promote cholesterol efflux from the cells was measured. The results were as expected, showing vitamin E improved the RCT

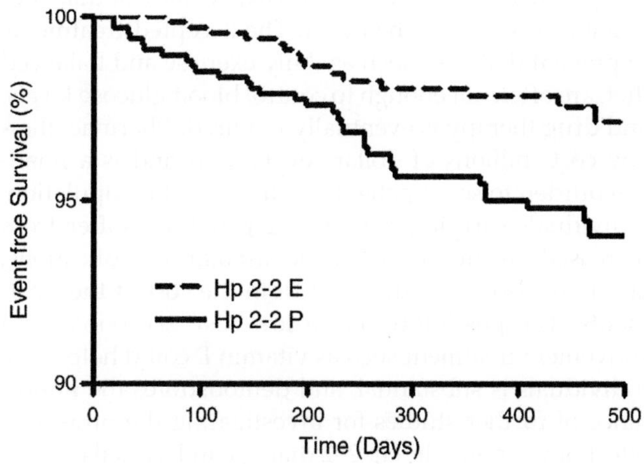

FIGURE 16.4 **Kaplan-Meier plot of the effect of vitamin E on the survival of haptoglobin (Hp) 2–2 diabetic patients who suffered from cardiovascular disease.** In Hp 2–2 individuals who were randomized to vitamin E treatment (E) compared with those randomized to placebo (P), there was a significant decrease in cardiovascular events such as cardiovascular death, myocardial infarction or stroke (p=0.01 by log rank) [3]. *Figure adapted from Levy et al. Haptoglobin: basic and clinical aspects published 2010 in Antioxidants and Redox Signaling 12(2):293–304.*

function of HDL in Hp 2–2 diabetic individuals. Moreover, the protective effect of vitamin E on HDL function stopped after the cessation of treatment. Another study, performed with similar methodology, showed nearly the same results but with one unexpected finding: not only did vitamin E supplementation not improve HDL function in Hp 2–1 diabetic individuals, it made HDL function worse [31]. This finding may explain why vitamin E treatment should be given to Hp 2–2 diabetic individuals only.

However, the Women's Angiographic Vitamin and Estrogen (WAVE) trial showed different results. In this study, diabetic postmenopausal women carrying the Hp 1–1 genotype, with one or more coronary vessel stenosis at 15–75% occlusion, showed greater improvement in the minimum luminal diameter (MLD) after receiving vitamin E or vitamin C than Hp 2–2 individuals with the same characteristics [32]. Another study, which investigated HDL function in diabetic individuals who received both vitamin E and vitamin C, showed the opposing effects these vitamins have on HDL function. *In vitro* studies of these vitamins showed that vitamin C caused an increase in oxidative stress in the presence of glycated Hb/Hp 2–2 complexes while vitamin E blocked the oxidative stress (see Figure 16.5). Moreover, in Hp 2–2 diabetic mice, vitamin E improved HDL function, but vitamin C did not. Thus it is suggested that co-administration of vitamin C and vitamin E in Hp 2–2 diabetic individuals might cause vitamin C to interfere with the protective effect of vitamin E [33].

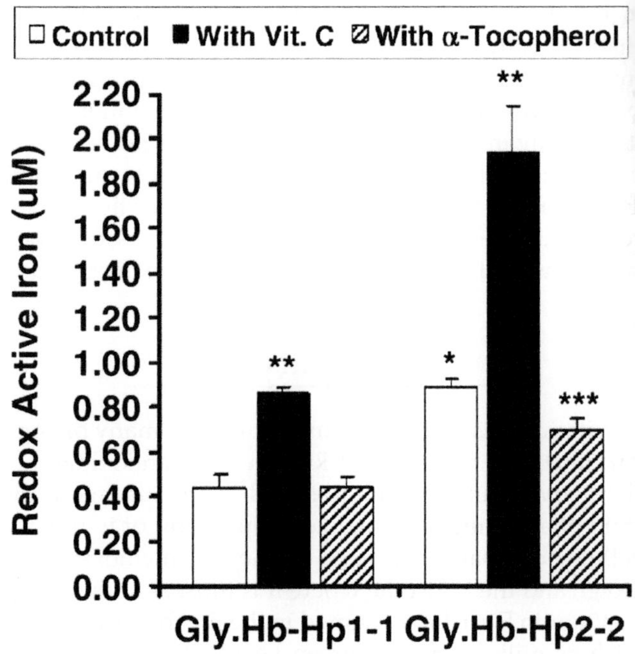

FIGURE 16.5 **Vitamin C and vitamin E differ in their effect on the reactivity of heme iron.** In glycated hemoglobin-haptoglobin 2–2 (Gly.Hb-Hp2–2) complexes versus glycated hemoglobin-haptoglobin 1–1 (Gly.Hb-Hp1–1) complexes, there was a significant increase (*) in redox active iron. Vitamin C resulted in a significant increase (**) of the reactivity of heme iron. Vitamin E resulted in a significant decrease (***) of the reactivity of heme iron associated with Hp 2–2 [33]. Data are presented as mean±SEM. *Figure adapted from Asleh and Levy Divergent effects of α-tocopherol and vitamin C on the generation of dysfunctional HDL associated with diabetes and the Hp 2–2 genotype published 2010 in Antioxidants and Redox Signaling 12(2):209–217.*

IN CONCLUSION

Cardiovascular complications are the leading cause of death in diabetic patients. Despite the intensive care this population receives, the life expectancy of diabetics remains lower than the norm. The accepted treatments to prevent diabetes, such as daily exercise and balanced diet, are often not enough to control blood glucose levels, and drug therapy is eventually required. Pharmacotherapy costs billions of dollars every year and is a financial burden to some patients. In the diabetic population, individuals carrying the Hp 2–2 genotype suffer from increased incidence of cardiovascular complications, and may also suffer the most from the cost of the treatments. The possibility that a low-cost, accessible, and convenient treatment such as vitamin E could help these individuals is substantial, and demonstrates the importance of further studies for investigating the protective effect of vitamin E in Hp 2–2 diabetic individuals.

SUMMARY POINTS

- In diabetes there is an increased risk of developing cardiovascular complications such as atherosclerosis, myocardial infarction, and stroke.
- In diabetes, there is an increased rate of oxidative stress mediated by the iron within the heme pocket of hemoglobin.
- Haptoglobin (Hp) is a plasma protein that binds hemoglobin and prevents it from mediating free radical formation.
- Haptoglobin phenotypes differ in their antioxidant abilities.
- Diabetic individuals carrying the haptoglobin 2–2 phenotype suffer from increased risk of oxidative stress, HDL dysfunction, and iron accumulation in atherosclerotic plaques.
- Due to the increased levels of oxidative stress, Hp 2–2 diabetic individuals suffer from a higher incidence of cardiovascular complications as compared to diabetic individuals with different Hp phenotypes.
- Supplementation of vitamin E, an antioxidant, improved HDL function and decreased cardiovascular complication occurrence in Hp 2–2 diabetic individuals in several epidemiological studies.
- Further investigation is needed to understand the mechanism by which vitamin E protects Hp 2–2 diabetic individuals against increased oxidative stress.

Acknowledgments and Disclosure

This work was supported by grants from the NIH (RO1DK085226) and the Israeli Science Foundation. Professor Levy's institution owns a patent which claims that the Hp genotype can predict the risk of diabetic vascular complications.

References

[1] Asleh R, Guetta J, Kalet-Litman S, Miller-Lotan R, Levy AP. Haptoglobin genotype and diabetes dependent differences in iron mediated oxidative stress *in vitro* and *in vivo*. Circ Res 2005 Mar 4;96(4):435–41. Epub 2005 Jan 20.

[2] Kita T, Kume N, Minami M, Hayashida K, Murayama T, Sano H, et al. Role of oxidized LDL in atherosclerosis. Ann N Y Acad Sci 2001 Dec;947:199–205; discussion 205–206.

[3] Levy AP, Asleh R, Blum S, Levy NS, Miller-Lotan R, Kalet-Litman S, et al. Haptoglobin: basic and clinical aspects. Antioxid Redox Signal 2010 Feb;12(2):293–304.

[4] Langlois MR, Delanghe JR. Biological and clinical significance of haptoglobin polymorphism in humans. Clin Chem 1996 Oct;42(10):1589–600.

[5] Levy AP, Purushothaman KR, Levy NS, Purushothaman M, Strauss M, Asleh R, et al. Downregulation of the hemoglobin scavenger receptor in individuals with diabetes and the hp 2–2 genotype: implications for the response to intraplaque hemorrhage and plaque vulnerability. Circ Res 2007 Jul 6;101(1):106–10.

[6] Asleh R, Blum S, Kalet-Litman S, Alshiek J, Miller-Lotan R, Asaf R, et al. Correction of HDL dysfunction in individuals with diabetes and the haptoglobin 2–2 genotype. Diabetes 2008 Oct;57(10):2794–800.

[7] Levy AP, Levy JE, Kalet-Litman S, Miller-Lotan R, Levy NS, Asaf R, et al. Haptoglobin genotype is a determinant of iron, lipid peroxidation, and macrophage accumulation in the atherosclerotic plaque. Arterioscler Thromb Vasc Biol 2007 Jan;27(1):134–40.

[8] Moreno PR, Purushothaman KR, Purushothaman M, Muntner P, Levy NS, Fuster V, et al. Haptoglobin genotype is a major determinant of the amount of iron in the human atherosclerotic plaque. J Am Coll Cardiol 2008 Sep 23;52(13):1049–51.

[9] Rifkind JM, Ramasamy S, Manoharan PT, Nagababu E, Mohanty JG. Redox reactions of hemoglobin. Antioxid Redox Signal 2004 June;6(3):657–66.

[10] Goldenstein H, Levy NS, Levy AP. Haptoglobin genotype and its role in determining heme-iron mediated vascular disease. Pharmacol Res 2012 Jul;66(1):1–6.

[11] Belcher JD, Beckman JD, Balla G, Balla J, Vercellotti G. Heme degradation and vascular injury. Antioxid Redox Signal 2010 Feb;12(2):233–48.

[12] Bamm VV, Tsemakhovich VA, Shaklai M, Shaklai N. Haptoglobin phenotypes differ in their ability to inhibit heme transfer from hemoglobin to LDL. Biochemistry 2004 Apr 6;43(13):3899–906.

[13] Asleh R, Miller-Lotan R, Aviram M, Hayek T, Yulish M, Levy JE, et al. Haptoglobin genotype is a regulator of reverse cholesterol transport in diabetes *in vitro* and *in vivo*. Circ Res 2006 Dec 8;99(12): 1419–25.

[14] Navab M, Anantharamaiah GM, Reddy ST, Van Lenten BJ, Ansell BJ, Fogelman AM. Mechanisms of disease: Proatherogenic HDL – an evolving field. Nat Clin Pract Endocrinol Metab 2006 Sep;2(9):504–11.

[15] Levy AP, Hochberg I, Jablonski K, Resnick HE, Lee ET, Best L, et al. Strong Heart Study. Haptoglobin phenotype is an independent risk factor for cardiovascular disease in individuals with diabetes: the strong heart study. J Am Coll Cardiol 2002 Dec 4;40(11):1984–90.

[16] Roguin A, Koch W, Kastrati A, Aronson D, Schomig A, Levy AP. Haptoglobin genotype is predictive of major adverse cardiac events in the 1-year period after percutaneous transluminal coronary angioplasty in individuals with diabetes. Diabetes Care 2003 Sep;26(9):2628–31.

[17] Suleiman M, Aronson D, Asleh R, Kapeliovich MR, Roguin A, Meisel SR, et al. Haptoglobin polymorphism predicts 30-day mortality and heart failure in patients with diabetes and acute myocardial infarction. Diabetes 2005 Sep;54(9):2802–6.

[18] Milman U, Blum S, Shapira C, Aronson D, Miller-Lotan R, Anbinder Y, et al. Vitamin E supplementation reduces cardiovascular events in a subgroup of middle-aged individuals with both type 2 diabetes mellitus and the haptoglobin 2–2 genotype: a prospective double-blinded clinical trial. Arterioscler Thromb Vasc Biol 2008 Feb;28(2):341–7.

[19] Costacou T, Ferrell RE, Orchard TJ. Haptoglobin genotype: a determinant of cardiovascular complication risk in type 1 diabetes. Diabetes 2008 Jun;57(6):1702–6.

[20] Simpson M, Snell-Bergeon JK, Kinney GL, Lache O, Miller-Lotan R, Anbinder Y, et al. Haptoglobin genotype predicts development of coronary artery calcification in a prospective cohort of patients with type 1 diabetes. Cardiovasc Diabetol 2011 Nov 20;10:99.

[21] Costacou T, Ferrell RE, Ellis D, Orchard TJ. Haptoglobin genotype and renal function decline in type 1 diabetes. Diabetes 2009 Dec;58(12):2904–9.

[22] Farbstein D, Kozak-Blickstein A, Levy AP. Antioxidant vitamins and their use in preventing cardiovascular disease. Molecules 2010 Nov 9;15(11):8098–110.

[23] Kostner GM, Oettl K, Jauhiainen M, Ehnholm C, Esterbauer H, Dieplinger H. Human plasma phospholipid transfer protein accelerates exchange/transfer of alpha-tocopherol between lipoproteins and cells. Biochem J 1995 Jan 15;305(2):659–67.

[24] Brigelius-Flohé R. Vitamin E: the shrew waiting to be tamed. Free Radic Biol Med 2009 Mar 1;46(5):534–54.

[25] Sesso HD, Buring JE, Christen WG, Kurth T, Belanger C, MacFadyen J, et al. Vitamins E and C in the prevention of cardiovascular disease in men: the Physicians' Health Study II randomized controlled trial. JAMA 2008 Nov 12;300(18):2123–33.

[26] Lee IM, Cook NR, Gaziano JM, Gordon D, Ridker PM, Manson JE, et al. Vitamin E in the primary prevention of cardiovascular disease and cancer: the Women's Health Study: a randomized controlled trial. JAMA 2005 Jul 6;294(1):56–65.

[27] Stephens NG, Parsons A, Schofield PM, Kelly F, Cheeseman K, Mitchinson MJ. Randomised controlled trial of vitamin E in patients with coronary disease: Cambridge Heart Antioxidant Study (CHAOS). JAMA 1996 Mar 23;347(9004):781–6.

[28] Boaz M, Smetana S, Weinstein T, Matas Z, Gafter U, Iaina A, et al. Secondary prevention with antioxidants of cardiovascular disease in endstage renal disease (SPACE): randomised placebo-controlled trial. Lancet 2000 Oct 7;356(9237):1213–8.

[29] Yusuf S, Dagenais G, Pogue J, Bosch J, Sleight P. Vitamin E supplementation and cardiovascular events in high-risk patients the heart outcomes prevention evaluation study investigators. N Engl J Med 2000 Jan 20;342(3):154–60.

[30] Blum S, Milman U, Shapira C, Miller-Lotan R, Bennett L, Kostenko M, et al. Dual therapy with statins and antioxidants is superior to statins alone in decreasing the risk of cardiovascular disease in a subgroup of middle-aged individuals with both diabetes mellitus and the haptoglobin 2–2 genotype. Arterioscler Thromb Vasc Biol 2008 Mar;28(3):e18–20.

[31] Farbstein D, Blum S, Pollak M, Asaf R, Viener HL, Lache O, et al. Vitamin E therapy results in a reduction in HDL function in individuals with diabetes and the haptoglobin 2–1 genotype. Atherosclerosis 2011 Nov;219(1):240–4.

[32] Levy AP, Friedenberg P, Lotan R, Ouyang P, Tripputi M, Higginson L, et al. The effect of vitamin therapy on the progression of coronary artery atherosclerosis varies by haptoglobin type in postmenopausal women. Diabetes Care 2004 Apr;27(4):925–30.

[33] Asleh R, Levy AP. Divergent effects of alpha-tocopherol and vitamin C on the generation of dysfunctional HDL associated with diabetes and the Hp 2–2 genotype. Antioxid Redox Signal 2010 Feb;12(2):209–17.

CHAPTER

17

The Use of *Ginkgo biloba* Extract in Cardiovascular Protection in Patients with Diabetes

Soo Lim[*,†], *Kyong Soo Park*[*]

*Department of Internal Medicine, Seoul National University College of Medicine, Seoul, South Korea, †Seoul National University Bundang Hospital, Seoul, Republic of Korea

List of Abbreviations

T2D Type 2 diabetes
DSHEA Dietary Supplement Health and Education Act
SOD Superoxide dismutase
ROS Reactive oxygen species
MMP-9 Matrix metalloproteinase-9
BAEC Bovine aortic endothelial cell
LDL Low density lipoprotein
oxLDL Oxidized low density lipoprotein
TUNEL Terminal deoxynucleotidyl transferase-mediated dUTP nick and labeling
H_2O_2 Hydrogen peroxide
PAD Peripheral arterial disease
PDX-1 Pancreatic and duodenal homeobox-1
VSMC Vascular smooth muscle cell
CVD Cardiovascular disease

INTRODUCTION

In 2010, the world prevalence of diabetes among adults (aged 20–79 years) was 6.4%, affecting 285 million people, and these figures will increase to 7.7% and 439 million people by 2030 [1]. This increase in diabetes has associated socio-economic problems as well as individual health disorders, because of the various complications of diabetes: as an example, diabetic retinopathy is the number one cause of blindness in people of working age. In addition, diabetic nephropathy has become the number one cause of renal replacement therapy. Most of all, cardiovascular complications are directly associated with morbidity and mortality in patients with diabetes.

Thus, the primary prevention of vascular complications in people with diabetes is now an important public health priority worldwide [2]. Nearly 80% of patients with type 2 diabetes (T2D) die from cardiovascular diseases (CVD), such as myocardial infarction or stroke. Primary coronary intervention with stent implantation is now widely performed in patients with symptomatic coronary artery disease. Although the development of drug-eluting stents has reduced the incidence of restenosis after coronary intervention, restenosis of the intervened vessel is still a critical issue [3]. The risk of restenosis is particularly high in patients with diabetes mellitus and might be partly associated with metabolic derangements that cause endothelial dysfunction [4].

Although glucose control is fundamental in preventing and reducing the complications of diabetes, recent clinical trials have indicated that intensive blood glucose control might not be sufficient to reduce macrovascular complications [5,6]. Lipid-lowering agents and aspirin have been widely used to prevent or delay vascular complications in subjects with diabetes, but residual risk remains. Therefore, new pharmacotherapeutic agents other than those that directly affect glucose levels are required to prevent or delay the macrovascular complications of diabetes. Several agents that are involved in inflammatory processes or anti-oxidative pathways have been used in clinical trials for this purpose [7,8].

Ginkgo biloba L. (Ginkgoaceae), known as the 'Maidenhair Tree', is a best-selling source of herbal remedies in the USA and Europe [9]. Traditionally, the fruits and seeds of Ginkgo have been used in Oriental medicine to improve chronic cough or enuresis [10]. In 1994, the USA Dietary Supplement Health and Education Act (DSHEA) classified Ginkgo as a dietary supplement. Since then,

Diabetes: Oxidative Stress and Dietary Antioxidants.
http://dx.doi.org/10.1016/B978-0-12-405885-9.00017-6

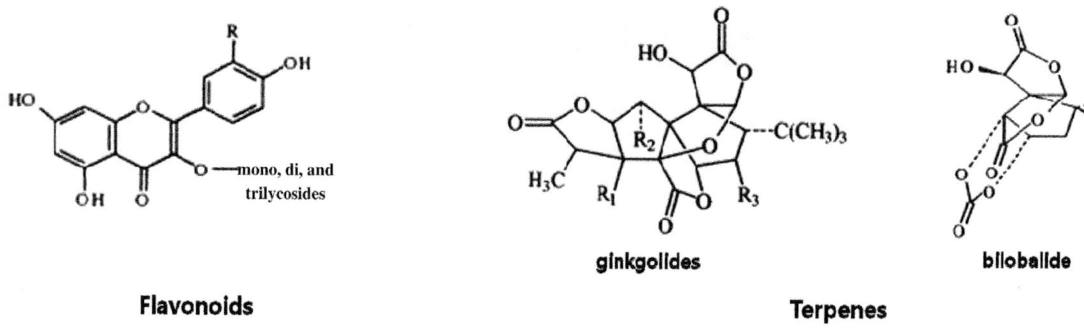

FIGURE 17.1 **The major compounds in *Ginkgo biloba* leaves.** Flavonoids (derivatives of quercetin, kaempferol and isorhamnetin) and terpenes (bilobalide and ginkgolides) are the major chemicals extracted.

various forms of Ginkgo have been introduced into the market after their pharmacological quality has been enhanced [11]. *Ginkgo biloba* extracts have been found to have a broad spectrum of pharmacological activities, which allows them to be used in numerous potential therapeutic applications, including conditions associated with cognitive impairment, depression, liver and kidney injury, cerebrovascular insufficiency, myocardial ischemia, and peripheral arterial occlusive disease.

CHARACTERISTICS OF *GINKGO BILOBA* EXTRACT

Ginkgo leaves were used to treat skin infections in traditional Chinese medicine [12]. During recent decades, several different *Ginkgo* extracts have been introduced to the market. However, in the early 1990s, EGb761, a standardized extract of Ginkgo leaves, became the most popularly used dietary supplement for treating vascular circulation problems and improving memory. There are two major fractions in *Ginkgo biloba* leaves (Figure 17.1); flavonoids and terpenes, each with distinct pharmaceutical properties. The flavonoid fraction has an antioxidant effect by reducing reactive oxygen species (ROS), promoting the expression of antioxidant proteins and increasing the levels of antioxidant metabolites such as glutathione [13–15]. Flavonoids react preferentially with hydroxyl radicals because of their aromatic ring and double bond [16]. The terpene lactones include bilobalide and ginkgolides A, B, C, J and M [17]. Sub-compounds of EGb761 are described in Table 17.1. This composition is responsible for giving EGb761 its exceptionally diverse pharmacological activities.

TABLE 17.1 Components of EGb761, a Standardized Extract of *Gingko* Leaves

Component		Content (%)
Flavonoids	Quercetin	11.71
	Kaempferol	10.70
	Isorhamnetin	2.20
	Total	24.61
Terpenes	Bilobalide	2.65
	Ginkgolide A	1.11
	Ginkgolide B	0.78
	Ginkgolide C	0.88
	Total	5.42
Proanthocyanidins		7.0
Carboxylic acid		13.0
Catechins		2.0
Non-flavone glycosides		20.0
Others (high molecules, inorganic, water, etc.)		28.0

EFFECTS OF *GINKGO BILOBA* EXTRACT ON GLUCOSE METABOLISM

Chronic hyperglycemia and hyperlipidemia cause pancreatic β-cell apoptosis and dysfunction, thereby contributing to the pathogenesis of T2D. There have been reports showing that Ginkgo extract improves glucose homeostasis [18,19]. A recent study proved that treatment with EGb761 induced insulin secretion mediated by increased intracellular calcium transients in a rat β-cell line [20]. Another group reported that EGb761 ingestion increased plasma insulin levels in response to oral glucose loading in patients with T2D [21]. Our group also found that EGb761 treatment reduced glucose excursions after glucose loading significantly in an animal model of T2D [22]. These data thus suggest that EGb761 has the potential to enhance pancreatic β-cell function.

Among the various compounds in *Ginkgo biloba* extract, kaempferol has been found to play a role in pancreatic β-cell protection [23]. Kaempferol treatment promoted β-cell viability, inhibited β-cell apoptosis and reduced caspase-3 activity in hyperglycemic conditions. Kaempferol also prevented the lipotoxicity-induced down-regulation of the anti-apoptotic proteins Akt and Bcl-2. In another study, the β-cell protective effects of kaempferol were associated with increased pancreatic and duodenal homeobox-1 (PDX-1) expression [24].

Oxidative stress is one of the main factors contributing to the development of diabetes [25]. The flavonoid fraction in *Ginkgo biloba* extract has antioxidant potential, resulting in increases in the expression levels of antioxidant proteins such as superoxide dismutase (SOD) and the attenuation of ROS production [26,27]. Taken together, these findings suggest that kaempferol has protective properties for pancreatic β-cells in conditions with high risks associated with T2D.

PROTECTIVE EFFECTS OF GINKGO BILOBA EXTRACTS ON CARDIOVASCULAR HEALTH

Heart and Coronary Artery Diseases

Ginkgo biloba extracts have several major biochemical/pharmacological effects on cardiovascular health, including free radical scavenger activity, provision of mitochondrial protection, anti-platelet activity, anti-inflammatory effects, and anti-apoptotic properties [28–32].

Oxidative stress induced by mitochondrial damage is involved in the development of atherosclerosis [33]. In fact, ROS have been shown to mediate vascular smooth muscle cell (VSMC) proliferation and increase the proliferative response to platelet-derived growth factor (PDGF) and thrombin [34,35]. A study involving treatment with *Ginkgo biloba* extract for two months showed a direct antiatherosclerotic effect among cardiovascular high-risk patients by up-regulating the free radical scavenging enzymes and attenuating the risk factors, such as oxidized LDL and lipoprotein small (a) [36]. In another study, EGb761 was able to protect mitochondria from ROS-induced damage [37] and to reduce ROS levels and ROS-induced apoptosis in experimental animals [38].

Pietri and colleagues showed that treatment of patients with Ginkgo leaf extract before cardiac surgery helped in reducing reperfusion-induced lipid peroxidation and prevented tissue necrosis and cardiac dysfunction. Moreover, they also showed that ginkgolide B reduced the post-ischemic production of ROS by 60% [39]. The same group also showed that reperfused hearts treated with terpene constituents recovered their function [40]. These data suggest that among the many constituents of Ginkgo, terpenoid compounds help to protect against the myocardial damage associated with ischemic reperfusion.

Ginkgolide B, another compound in *Ginkgo biloba* extract, is known to improve coronary blood flow through anti-platelet activity and improvements in vascular contractility, which occur in response to the increased release of catecholamines from endogenous tissue reserves caused by flavonoids (quercetin, kaempferol and isorhamnetin) [41,42].

Recently, more direct evidence supporting the anti-atherosclerotic effects of *Ginkgo biloba* has emerged. Treatment with a *Ginkgo biloba* extract decreased the homocysteine-induced intimal thickening resulting from balloon injury in the abdominal aorta of rabbits [43]. This antiatherosclerotic effect was possibly associated with the suppression of matrix metalloproteinase-9 (MMP-9) expression and the promotion of endogenous p21 expression by *Ginkgo biloba* extract. We also found that treatment with EGb761 reduced restenosis in obese rats with T2D after balloon injury to the carotid artery (Figure 17.3) [22]. EGb761 significantly suppressed the proliferation and migration of VSMCs, promoted apoptosis and reduced inflammatory processes [22].

Several studies have proved the vasodilatory effect of *Ginkgo biloba* extract. A study with bovine aortic endothelial cells (BAECs) showed a protective effect of EGb761 against the cell damage induced by hydrogen peroxide (H_2O_2) [44]. Pretreatment of BAECs with EGb761 (from 10 mg/l to 100 mg/l) for 10 min decreased intracellular free calcium ion concentrations by up to 20.6%. Pretreatment of BAECs with EGb761 (100 mg/l) also reduced the rate of apoptosis, decreased the percentage of terminal deoxynucleotidyl transferase-mediated dUTP nick end labeling (TUNEL)-positive cells and inhibited the caspase-3 activity induced by oxidative stress.

Most recently, in hamsters fed a high cholesterol diet, EGb761 was seen to improve endothelial function, as deduced from lowered total plasma cholesterol levels and atherosclerotic plaque formation in the thoracic aorta [45]. However, there has been no human study on this issue, so whether *Ginkgo biloba* extracts can induce a further stabilization of plaque formation among individuals who are already on statin treatment remains to be revealed.

Cerebrovascular Diseases

One of the most well-recognized standardized extracts of *Ginkgo biloba* leaves, EGb761, has been shown to have neuroprotective and antioxidant properties [46] that can act against various cerebrovascular and neurological disorders such as ischemia, Alzheimer's disease and depression [47,48]. Its actions are thought to be mediated mainly via phenolic and terpenoid compounds. EGb761 has been shown to reduce the neuronal death induced by brain ischemia [49,50]. It has also been shown to be effective in reducing the cognitive dysfunctions associated with aging or dementia [51]. Thus, the beneficial effects of *Ginkgo biloba* extract have been revealed mostly in situations of ischemic brain damage or cognitive dysfunction, whereas direct evidence of its

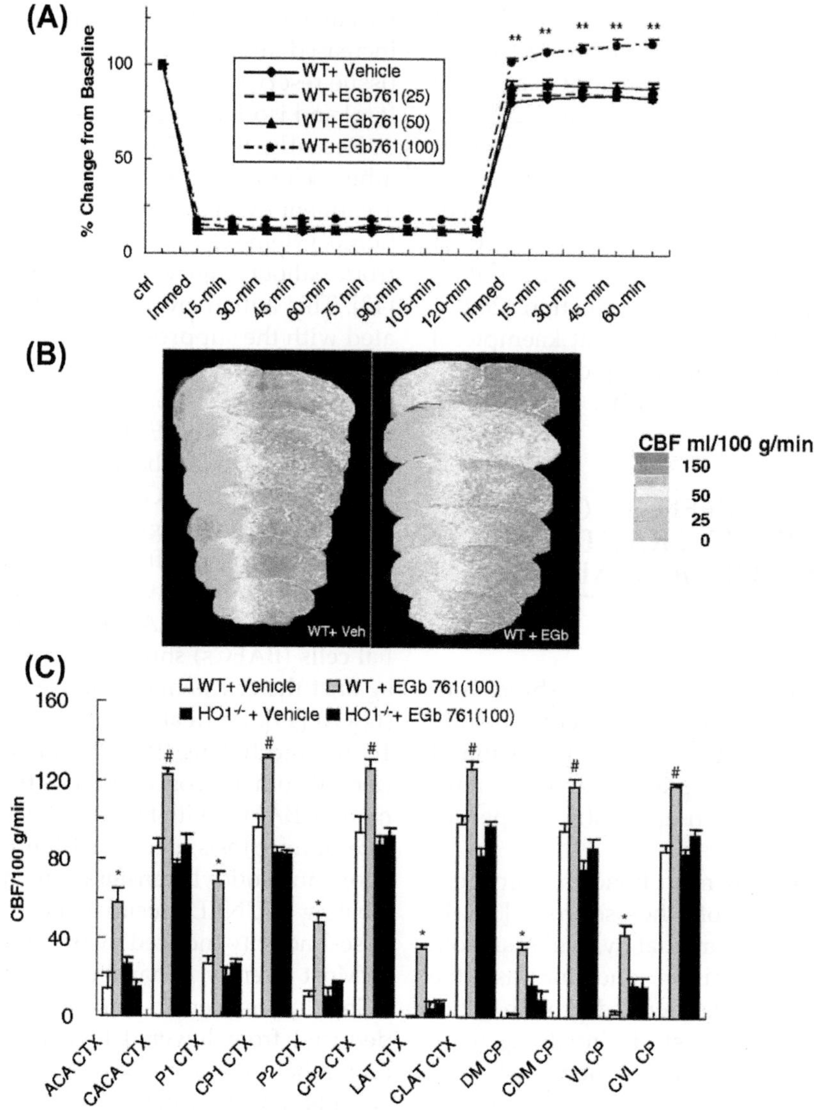

FIGURE 17.2 Effects of EGb761 on cerebral blood flow. (A) Relative cerebral blood flow (CBF) was recorded at baseline, at the induction of ischemia and at 15-min intervals during ischemia and 1 h of reperfusion. $^{**}p<0.01$. (B) ^{14}C-IAP autoradiographic images of a wild-type (WT) mouse and an EGb761-treated mouse. Red represents areas of higher blood flow whereas blue represents areas of lower blood flow. (C) Mean CBF of each mouse group; $^{*}p<0.05$; $\#p<0.01$. Key: ACA CTX, anterior cerebral artery cortex; CACA, contralateral anterior cerebral artery; P1, parietal 1; CP1&2, contralateral parietal 1&2; LAT CTX, lateral cortex; CLAT CTX, contralateral lateral cortex; DM, dorsomedial; CDM, contralateral dorsomedial; VL, ventrolateral; CVL, contralateral ventrolateral; CP, caudate putamen. *Reproduced with permission from Saleem et al. [69].* This figure is reproduced in color in the color section.

anti-atherosclerotic properties in the cerebrovascular system is limited.

The mechanism of action of EGb761 in protecting against ischemia-induced brain injury is not clearly known, but it has been postulated that the heme oxygenase pathway is involved. It has been demonstrated that EGb761 induces heme oxygenase-1 expression in a time- and dose-dependent manner [52]. In another study, pretreatment with EGb761 for one week protected against ischemia/reperfusion-induced brain injury in an animal model in a dose-dependent manner [53].

Acute ischemic stroke is associated with oxidative stress and inflammatory responses [54]. EGb761, with its free radical scavenging activity, has been shown to reduce the size of cerebral infarctions in animal models [55]. In another animal model, mice pretreated with EGb761 showed less neurological dysfunction and smaller infarct volumes than vehicle-treated mice. These data demonstrate the neuroprotective effect of EGb761 against free radical damage and excitotoxicity (Figure 17.2) [56].

A recent study of patients with ischemic stroke showed that therapy with a *Ginkgo biloba* extract (1500 mg/day) reduced oxidative stress and inflammatory responses, supporting a potential role for *Ginkgo* in humans [57]. Besides a direct scavenging effect on ROS, *Ginkgo biloba*

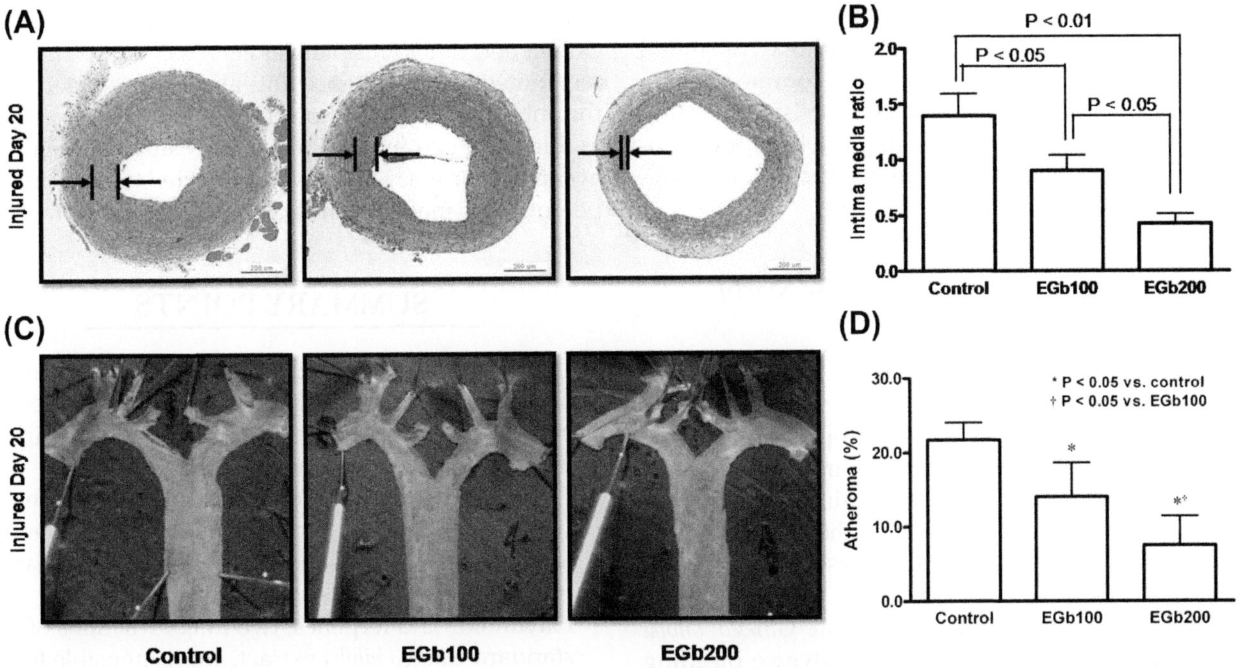

FIGURE 17.3 ***In vivo* inhibition of neointimal formation after 6 weeks of treatment with EGb761 (EGb100 group, 100mg/kg; EGb200 group, 200mg/kg).** (A) Haematoxylin and eosin-stained sections. (B) Intima-to-media ratios (IMRs; n=10 in each group) are shown. Treatment with EGb761 produced a lower IMR than in controls in a dose-dependent manner (the higher the dose of EGb761, the lower the IMR; $p<0.05$). (C) Representative examples of aortas from ApoE$^{-/-}$gene knock-out mice stained *en-face* with Oil Red O. Red staining indicates the aortic arch where plaque accumulation is the highest. (D) Quantification of aortic arch plaque in the three groups, expressed as the mean ± SEM (percentage). A dose-dependently decreased plaque volume was found in the EGb761 treatment groups. *Reproduced with permission from Lim et al. [22].* This figure is reproduced in color in the color section.

extract exerts an anti-inflammatory effect on inflammatory cells by suppressing the production of ROS and radical nitrogen species [58].

Peripheral Vascular Diseases

Ginkgo biloba extracts have been reported to have beneficial effects on the peripheral vascular system. A meta-analysis of the efficacy of *Ginkgo biloba* extract for the treatment of intermittent claudication showed a significant difference in the increase in pain-free walking distance after treatment with *Ginkgo biloba* extracts (EGb761 and others) compared with controls (weighted mean difference 34 m; 95% confidence interval [CI] 26–43 m) [59]. These results suggest that *Ginkgo biloba* extracts are superior to placebos in the symptomatic treatment of intermittent claudication. However, the treatment effect is modest, and its clinical relevance is questionable.

In another study, a *Ginkgo biloba* extract and cilostazol were evaluated alone or in combination for anti-platelet activity using *in vitro* and *in vivo* models [60]. The combination of a *Ginkgo biloba* extract with cilostazol showed better inhibition of both the shear- and collagen-induced platelet aggregation than did either treatment alone. In accordance with these enhanced *in vitro* anti-platelet activities, the combined treatment provided enhanced anti-thrombotic effects in *in vivo* models of pulmonary embolism and arterial thrombosis [61]. Another study using co-treatment with a *Ginkgo biloba* extract and cilostazol demonstrated a more potent anti-atherosclerotic effect than treatment with cilostazol alone in hyperlipidemic apolipoprotein E (ApoE)-null mice, suggesting a potential therapeutic strategy for the treatment of atherosclerosis [62].

In conclusion, *Ginkgo biloba* extracts might be a good therapeutic option for treating patients with peripheral vascular diseases, because no optimal treatment for intermittent claudication has been identified yet.

Data Showing No Protective Role of *Ginkgo biloba* Extract in Cardio- or Cerebrovascular Diseases

There are studies demonstrating no protective role of *Ginkgo biloba* extract in cardiovascular disease. One study using animal models of stroke did not prove any beneficial effect of EGb761 in reducing brain infarct size [63]. In a double-blind trial with 3,069 randomly assigned participants over 75 years of age and with a 6.1-year follow-up, there were no differences in the incidences of myocardial infarction, angina pectoris or stroke between groups treated with *Ginkgo biloba* extract and placebo [64]. However, there were fewer peripheral vascular disease events in the group treated with *Ginkgo biloba* extract. From this study, the authors concluded that *Ginkgo biloba* extract could not be recommended for preventing CVD. Thus, controversy persists regarding the role of *Ginkgo biloba* in mediating cerebro- or cardiovascular incidents, although there have been some positive data.

Bleeding Issues in *Ginkgo biloba* Use With/Without Aspirin

Thrombosis and thromboembolic occlusions of blood vessels are major complications in various peripheral vascular diseases. Therefore, anti-platelet agents – key tools in the treatment of atherothrombosis – have become essential medications for treating a broad spectrum of vascular diseases. However, there are concerns about uncontrolled bleeding with the use of anti-platelet agents.

Several reports have suggested that *Ginkgo biloba* extracts may play a role in clinically adverse bleeding disorders. In elderly participants with peripheral arterial disease or risk factors for CVD, EGb761 (300 mg/day) was compared with a placebo for its effects on measures of platelet aggregation among adults taking aspirin (325 mg/day) in a randomized, double-blind, placebo-controlled, parallel design trial lasting four weeks [65]. There were no clinically or statistically significant differences in either platelet function or platelet aggregation between treatment groups. *Ginkgo biloba* extract combined with 325 mg/day of aspirin did not have a clinically or statistically detectable impact on the indices of coagulation, compared with the effect of aspirin alone.

In another study, a *Ginkgo biloba* extract or cilostazol were evaluated alone or in combination for their anti-platelet activity and bleeding risk using *in vitro* and *in vivo* models [66]. Notably, the combination of cilostazol and a *Ginkgo biloba* extract did not have a significant effect on the bleeding time or prothrombin time, and did not increase the activated partial thromboplastin time. This result and other study findings suggest that *Ginkgo biloba* extracts might potentiate the anti-platelet effect of cilostazol without the prolongation of bleeding time or coagulation time [67,68].

CONCLUSIONS

Ginkgo biloba has a broad spectrum of pharmacological activities that could be useful for cardiovascular protection as well as ameliorating cognitive impairment, depression and liver and kidney injury. The cardioprotective effects of *Ginkgo biloba* act via antioxidant and anti-platelet activities and increased blood flow through the release of nitric oxide and prostaglandins. Therefore, combination therapy using a *Ginkgo biloba* extract and other anti-platelet agents or statins might be recommended to enhance anti-atherosclerotic and anti-thrombotic efficacy without increasing side effects such as bleeding tendency. Prospective studies with CVD events as a primary objective are needed to confirm these potentially beneficial effects of *Ginkgo biloba* extracts.

SUMMARY POINTS

- *Ginkgo biloba* has a broad spectrum of pharmacological activities that could be useful for cardiovascular protection as well as combating cognitive impairment, depression and liver and kidney injury.
- *Ginkgo biloba* extracts show cardioprotective effects via their antioxidant and anti-platelet actions, and lead to increases in blood flow through the release of nitric oxide and prostaglandins.
- Flavonoids and terpenes, two major fractions of the standard *Ginkgo biloba* extract, are responsible for its exceptionally diverse pharmacological activities.
- Although there is no direct evidence that *Ginkgo biloba* extracts can reduce cardiovascular morbidity and mortality, they might be considered as an adjuvant to aspirin or statin because of their anti-atherosclerotic properties.
- To confirm the cardioprotective effects of *Ginkgo biloba* extracts against CVD, prospective studies with a cardiovascular endpoint as a primary objective are warranted.

References

[1] Shaw JE, Sicree RA, Zimmet PZ. Global estimates of the prevalence of diabetes for 2010 and 2030. Diabetes Res Clin Pract 2010 January;87(1):4–14.

[2] Zhang P, Zhang X, Brown J, Vistisen D, Sicree R, Shaw J, et al. Global healthcare expenditure on diabetes for 2010 and 2030. Diabetes Res Clin Pract 2010 March;87(3):293–301.

[3] Rodriguez AE, Maree AO, Mieres J, Berrocal D, Grinfeld L, Fernandez-Pereira C, et al. Late loss of early benefit from drug-eluting stents when compared with bare-metal stents and coronary artery bypass surgery: three year follow-up of the ERACI III registry. Eur Heart J 2007 September;28(17):2118–25.

[4] Aronson D, Bloomgarden Z, Rayfield EJ. Potential mechanisms promoting restenosis in diabetic patients. J Am Coll Cardiol 1996 March 1;27(3):528–35.

[5] Patel A, MacMahon S, Chalmers J, Neal B, Billot L, Woodward M, et al. Intensive blood glucose control and vascular outcomes in patients with type 2 diabetes. N Engl J Med 2008 June 12;358(24):2560–72.

[6] Gerstein HC, Miller ME, Byington RP, Goff Jr DC, Bigger JT, Buse JB, et al. Effects of intensive glucose lowering in type 2 diabetes. N Engl J Med 2008 June 12;358(24):2545–59.

[7] Gennaro G, Menard C, Michaud SE, Deblois D, Rivard A. Inhibition of vascular smooth muscle cell proliferation and neointimal formation in injured arteries by a novel, oral mitogen-activated protein kinase/extracellular signal-regulated kinase inhibitor. Circulation 2004 November 23;110(21):3367–71.

[8] Ashley EA, Ferrara R, King JY, Vailaya A, Kuchinsky A, He X, et al. Network analysis of human in-stent restenosis. Circulation 2006 December 12;114(24):2644–54.
[9] Valli G, Giardina EG. Benefits, adverse effects and drug interactions of herbal therapies with cardiovascular effects. J Am Coll Cardiol 2002 April 3;39(7):1083–95.
[10] Zimmermann M, Colciaghi F, Cattabeni F, Di LM. *Ginkgo biloba* extract: from molecular mechanisms to the treatment of Alzheimer's disease. Cell Mol Biol 2002 September;48(6):613–23.
[11] Kressmann S, Muller WE, Blume HH. Pharmaceutical quality of different *Ginkgo biloba* brands. J Pharm Pharmacol 2002 May;54(5):661–9.
[12] DeFeudis FV, Drieu K. *Ginkgo biloba* extract (EGb 761) and CNS functions: basic studies and clinical applications. Curr Drug Targets 2000 July;1(1):25–58.
[13] Smith JV, Luo Y. Elevation of oxidative free radicals in Alzheimer's disease models can be attenuated by *Ginkgo biloba* extract EGb 761. J Alzheimers Dis 2003 August;5(4):287–300.
[14] Gohil K, Packer L. Global gene expression analysis identifies cell and tissue specific actions of *Ginkgo biloba* extract, EGb 761. Cell Mol Biol 2002 September;48(6):625–31.
[15] Oken BS, Storzbach DM, Kaye JA. The efficacy of *Ginkgo biloba* on cognitive function in Alzheimer disease. Arch Neurol 1998 November;55(11):1409–15.
[16] Zimmermann M, Colciaghi F, Cattabeni F, Di LM. *Ginkgo biloba* extract: from molecular mechanisms to the treatment of Alzheimer's disease. Cell Mol Biol 2002 September;48(6):613–23.
[17] Smith JV, Luo Y. Studies on molecular mechanisms of *Ginkgo biloba* extract. Appl Microbiol Biotechnol 2004 May;64(4):465–72.
[18] Choi SE, Shin HC, Kim HE, Lee SJ, Jang HJ, Lee KW, et al. Involvement of Ca^{2+}, CaMK II and PKA in EGb 761-induced insulin secretion in INS-1 cells. J Ethnopharmacol 2007 March 1;110(1):49–55.
[19] Kudolo GB. The effect of three-month ingestion of *Ginkgo biloba* extract (EGb 761) on pancreatic beta-cell function in response to glucose loading in individuals with non-insulin-dependent diabetes mellitus. J Clin Pharmacol 2001 June;41(6):600–11.
[20] Choi SE, Shin HC, Kim HE, Lee SJ, Jang HJ, Lee KW, et al. Involvement of Ca^{2+}, CaMK II and PKA in EGb 761-induced insulin secretion in INS-1 cells. J Ethnopharmacol 2007 March 1;110(1):49–55.
[21] Kudolo GB. The effect of 3-month ingestion of *Ginkgo biloba* extract (EGb 761) on pancreatic beta-cell function in response to glucose loading in individuals with non-insulin-dependent diabetes mellitus. J Clin Pharmacol 2001 June;41(6):600–11.
[22] Lim S, Yoon JW, Kang SM, Choi SH, Cho BJ, Kim M, et al. EGb761, a *Ginkgo biloba* extract, is effective against atherosclerosis *in vitro*, and in a rat model of type 2 diabetes. PLoS One 2011;6(6):e20301.
[23] Zhang Y, Liu D. Flavonol kaempferol improves chronic hyperglycemia-impaired pancreatic beta-cell viability and insulin secretory function. Eur J Pharmacol 2011 November 16;670(1): 325–32.
[24] Zhang Y, Zhen W, Maechler P, Liu D. Small molecule kaempferol modulates PDX-1 protein expression and subsequently promotes pancreatic beta-cell survival and function via CREB. J Nutr Biochem 2012 July 20.
[25] Tiedge M, Lortz S, Drinkgern J, Lenzen S. Relation between antioxidant enzyme gene expression and antioxidative defense status of insulin-producing cells. Diabetes 1997 November;46(11): 1733–42.
[26] Smith JV, Luo Y. Elevation of oxidative free radicals in Alzheimer's disease models can be attenuated by *Ginkgo biloba* extract EGb 761. J Alzheimers Dis 2003 August;5(4):287–300.
[27] Gohil K, Packer L. Global gene expression analysis identifies cell and tissue specific actions of *Ginkgo biloba* extract, EGb 761. Cell Mol Biol (Noisy -le-grand) 2002 September;48(6):625–31.
[28] DeFeudis FV, Drieu K. *Ginkgo biloba* extract (EGb 761) and CNS functions: basic studies and clinical applications. Curr Drug Targets 2000 July;1(1):25–58.
[29] Smith PF, Maclennan K, Darlington CL. The neuroprotective properties of the *Ginkgo biloba* leaf: a review of the possible relationship to platelet-activating factor (PAF). J Ethnopharmacol 1996 March;50(3):131–9.
[30] Haines DD, Varga B, Bak I, Juhasz B, Mahmoud FF, Kalantari H, et al. Summative interaction between astaxanthin, *Ginkgo biloba* extract (EGb761) and vitamin C in suppression of respiratory inflammation: a comparison with ibuprofen. Phytother Res 2011;25(1):128–36.
[31] Smith JV, Burdick AJ, Golik P, Khan I, Wallace D, Luo Y. Anti-apoptotic properties of *Ginkgo biloba* extract EGb 761 in differentiated PC12 cells. Cell Mol Biol (Noisy -le-grand) 2002 September;48(6):699–707.
[32] Eckert A, Keil U, Kressmann S, Schindowski K, Leutner S, Leutz S, et al. Effects of EGb 761 *Ginkgo biloba* extract on mitochondrial function and oxidative stress. Pharmacopsychiatry 2003 June;36(Suppl. 1):S15–23.
[33] Libby P, Theroux P. Pathophysiology of coronary artery disease. Circulation 2005 June 28;111(25):3481–8.
[34] Patterson C, Ruef J, Madamanchi NR, Barry-Lane P, Hu Z, Horaist C, et al. Stimulation of a vascular smooth muscle cell NAD(P)H oxidase by thrombin. Evidence that p47(phox) may participate in forming this oxidase *in vitro* and *in vivo*. J Biol Chem 1999 July 9;274(28):19814–22.
[35] Madamanchi NR, Moon SK, Hakim ZS, Clark S, Mehrizi A, Patterson C, et al. Differential activation of mitogenic signaling pathways in aortic smooth muscle cells deficient in superoxide dismutase isoforms. Arterioscler Thromb Vasc Biol 2005 May;25(5):950–6.
[36] Rodriguez M, Ringstad L, Schafer P, Just S, Hofer HW, Malmsten M, et al. Reduction of atherosclerotic nanoplaque formation and size by *Ginkgo biloba* (EGb 761) in cardiovascular high-risk patients. Atherosclerosis 2007 June;192(2):438–44.
[37] Sastre J, Millan A, Garcia de la AJ, Pla R, Juan G, Pallardo, et al. A *Ginkgo biloba* extract (EGb 761) prevents mitochondrial aging by protecting against oxidative stress. Free Radic Biol Med 1998 January 15;24(2):298–304.
[38] Eckert A, Keil U, Kressmann S, Schindowski K, Leutner S, Leutz S, et al. Effects of EGb 761 *Ginkgo biloba* extract on mitochondrial function and oxidative stress. Pharmacopsychiatry 2003 June;36(Suppl. 1):S15–23.
[39] Pietri S, Seguin JR, d'Arbigny P, Drieu K, Culcasi M. *Ginkgo biloba* extract (EGb 761) pretreatment limits free radical-induced oxidative stress in patients undergoing coronary bypass surgery. Cardiovasc Drugs Ther 1997 April;11(2):121–31.
[40] Pietri S, Maurelli E, Drieu K, Culcasi M. Cardioprotective and antioxidant effects of the terpenoid constituents of *Ginkgo biloba* extract (EGb 761). J Mol Cell Cardiol 1997 February;29(2): 733–42.
[41] Auguet M, DeFeudis FV, Clostre F. Effects of *Ginkgo biloba* on arterial smooth muscle responses to vasoactive stimuli. Gen Pharmacol 1982;13(2):169–71.
[42] Mahady GB. *Ginkgo biloba* for the prevention and treatment of cardiovascular disease: a review of the literature. J Cardiovasc Nurs 2002 July;16(4):21–32.
[43] Liu F, Zhang J, Yu S, Wang R, Wang B, Lai L, et al. Inhibitory effect of *Ginkgo biloba* extract on hyperhomocysteinemia-induced intimal thickening in rabbit abdominal aorta after balloon injury. Phytother Res 2008 April;22(4):506–10.
[44] Ren DC, Du GH, Zhang JT. Protective effect of *Ginkgo biloba* extract on endothelial cell against damage induced by oxidative stress. J Cardiovasc Pharmacol 2002 December;40(6): 809–14.

[45] Gautam J, Kushwaha P, Swarnkar G, Khedgikar V, Nagar GK, Singh D, et al. EGb 761 promotes osteoblastogenesis, lowers bone marrow adipogenesis and atherosclerotic plaque formation. Phytomedicine 2012 September 15;19(12):1134–42.
[46] Clark WM, Rinker LG, Lessov NS, Lowery SL, Cipolla MJ. Efficacy of antioxidant therapies in transient focal ischemia in mice. Stroke 2001 April;32(4):1000–4.
[47] Ahlemeyer B, Krieglstein J. Neuroprotective effects of *Ginkgo biloba* extract. Cell Mol Life Sci 2003 September;60(9):1779–92.
[48] Chandrasekaran K, Mehrabian Z, Spinnewyn B, Chinopoulos C, Drieu K, Fiskum G. Neuroprotective effects of bilobalide, a component of *Ginkgo biloba* extract (EGb 761) in global brain ischemia and in excitotoxicity-induced neuronal death. Pharmacopsychiatry 2003 June;36(Suppl. 1):S89–94.
[49] Clark WM, Rinker LG, Lessov NS, Lowery SL, Cipolla MJ. Efficacy of antioxidant therapies in transient focal ischemia in mice. Stroke 2001 April;32(4):1000–4.
[50] Chandrasekaran K, Mehrabian Z, Spinnewyn B, Chinopoulos C, Drieu K, Fiskum G. Neuroprotective effects of bilobalide, a component of *Ginkgo biloba* extract (EGb 761) in global brain ischemia and in excitotoxicity-induced neuronal death. Pharmacopsychiatry 2003 June;36(Suppl. 1):S89–94.
[51] van DM, van RE, Kessels A, Sielhorst H, Knipschild P. Ginkgo for elderly people with dementia and age-associated memory impairment: a randomized clinical trial. J Clin Epidemiol 2003 April;56(4):367–76.
[52] Zhuang H, Pin S, Christen Y, Dore S. Induction of heme oxygenase 1 by *Ginkgo biloba* in neuronal cultures and potential implications in ischemia. Cell Mol Biol (Noisy -le-grand) 2002 September;48(6):647–53.
[53] Erbil G, Ozbal S, Sonmez U, Pekcetin C, Tugyan K, Bagriyanik A, et al. Neuroprotective effects of selenium and *Ginkgo biloba* extract (EGb761) against ischemia and reperfusion injury in rat brain. Neurosciences (Riyadh) 2008 July;13(3):233–8.
[54] Lo EH, Dalkara T, Moskowitz MA. Mechanisms, challenges and opportunities in stroke. Nat Rev Neurosci 2003 May;4(5):399–415.
[55] Zhang Z, Peng D, Zhu H, Wang X. Experimental evidence of *Ginkgo biloba* extract EGB as a neuroprotective agent in ischemia stroke rats. Brain Res Bull 2012 February 10;87(2–3):193–8.
[56] Saleem S, Zhuang H, Biswal S, Christen Y, Dore S. *Ginkgo biloba* extract neuroprotective action is dependent on heme oxygenase 1 in ischemic reperfusion brain injury. Stroke 2008 December;39(12):3389–96.
[57] Thanoon IA, bdul-Jabbar HA. Taha DA. Oxidative stress and c-reactive protein in patients with cerebrovascular accident (ischaemic stroke): The role of *Ginkgo biloba* extract. Sultan Qaboos Univ Med J 2012 May;12(2):197–205.
[58] Chen C, Wei T, Gao Z, Zhao B, Hou J, Xu H, et al. Different effect of the constituents of EGb761 on apoptosis in rat cerebellar granule cells induced by hydroxyl radicals. Biochem Mol Biol Int 1999 March;47(3):397–405.
[59] Pittler MH, Ernst E. *Ginkgo biloba* extract for the treatment of intermittent claudication: a meta-analysis of randomized trials. Am J Med 2000 March;108(4):276–81.
[60] Ryu KH, Han HY, Lee SY, Jeon SD, Im GJ, Lee BY, et al. *Ginkgo biloba* extract enhances anti-platelet and antithrombotic effects of cilostazol without prolongation of bleeding time. Thromb Res 2009 July;124(3):328–34.
[61] Ryu KH, Han HY, Lee SY, Jeon SD, Im GJ, Lee BY, et al. *Ginkgo biloba* extract enhances antiplatelet and antithrombotic effects of cilostazol without prolongation of bleeding time. Thromb Res 2009 July;124(3):328–34.
[62] Jung IH, Lee YH, Yoo JY, Jeong SJ, Sonn SK, Park JG, et al. *Ginkgo biloba* extract (GbE) enhances the anti-atherogenic effect of cilostazol by inhibiting ROS generation. Exp Mol Med 2012 May 31;44(5):311–8.
[63] de Lima KC, Schilichting CL, Junior LA, da Silva FM, Benetoli A, Milani H. The *Ginkgo biloba* extract, EGb 761, fails to reduce brain infarct size in rats after transient, middle cerebral artery occlusion in conditions of unprevented, ischemia-induced fever. Phytother Res 2006 June;20(6):438–43.
[64] Kuller LH, Ives DG, Fitzpatrick AL, Carlson MC, Mercado C, Lopez OL, et al. Does *Ginkgo biloba* reduce the risk of cardiovascular events? Circ Cardiovasc Qual Outcomes 2010 January;3(1):41–7.
[65] Gardner CD, Zehnder JL, Rigby AJ, Nicholus JR, Farquhar JW. Effect of *Ginkgo biloba* (EGb 761) and aspirin on platelet aggregation and platelet function analysis among older adults at risk of cardiovascular disease: a randomized clinical trial. Blood Coagul Fibrinolysis 2007 December;18(8):787–93.
[66] Ryu KH, Han HY, Lee SY, Jeon SD, Im GJ, Lee BY, et al. *Ginkgo biloba* extract enhances antiplatelet and antithrombotic effects of cilostazol without prolongation of bleeding time. Thromb Res 2009 July;124(3):328–34.
[67] Le Bars PL, Katz MM, Berman N, Itil TM, Freedman AM, Schatzberg AF. A placebo-controlled, double-blind, randomized trial of an extract of *Ginkgo biloba* for dementia. North American EGb Study Group. JAMA 1997 October 22;278(16):1327–32.
[68] Pittler MH, Ernst E. *Ginkgo biloba* extract for the treatment of intermittent claudication: a meta-analysis of randomized trials. Am J Med 2000 March;108(4):276–81.
[69] Saleem S, Zhuang H, Biswal S, Christen Y, Dore S. *Ginkgo biloba* extract neuroprotective action is dependent on heme oxygenase 1 in ischemic reperfusion brain injury. Stroke 2008 December;39(12):3389–96.

CHAPTER

18

The Protective Role of Taurine in Cardiac Oxidative Stress under Diabetic Conditions

Joydeep Das, Parames C. Sil

Division of Molecular Medicine, Bose Institute, Kolkata, India

List of Abbreviations

AGE Advanced glycation endproducts
AT-II Angiotensin type 2
CaMKII Ca^{2+}/calmodulin-dependent protein kinases II
CAT Catalase
DAG Diacylglycerol
DM Diabetes mellitus
ETC Electron transport chain
FFA Free fatty acid
GAPDH Glyceraldehyde-3-phosphate dehydrogenase
Glut-2 Glucose transporter type 2
GSH Reduced glutathione
GR Glutathione reductase
GPx Glutathione peroxidase
HOCl Hypochlorous acid
IR Insulin receptor
IRS Insulin receptor substrate
MAPKs Mitogen activated protein kinases
MCP-1 Monocyte chemotactic protein-1
$NADP^+$ Nicotinamide adenine dinucleotide phosphate
NADH/NAD^+ Nicotinamide adenine dinucleotide (reduced)/Nicotinamide adenine dinucleotide (oxidized)
NADPH Nicotinamide adenine dinucleotide phosphate-oxidase
NAD^+ Nicotinamide adenine dinucleotide
NF-κB Nuclear factor κB
NOX2 Nicotinamide adenine dinucleotide phosphate-oxidase 2
Pdx1 Pancreatic and duodenal homeobox 1
PKC Protein kinase c
RAS Renin-angiotensin system
ROS Reactive oxygen species
SOD Superoxide dismutase
TNF-α Tumor necrosis factor-alpha

INTRODUCTION

The World Health Organization has declared diabetes mellitus (DM) to be a global endemic associated with an increasing occurrence of coronary artery disease, heart failure, and cardiovascular mortality [1–3]. The relationship between diabetes and cardiac disease has been the subject of intensive investigation over the last few decades, although it is still far from being fully elucidated.

Among several presumed mechanisms responsible for the effects of DM on myocardial dysfunction, the role of the reactive oxygen (ROS) and reactive nitrogen species (RNS) has been well established [4]. It has been reported that hyperglycemia-induced oxidative stress plays a critical role in the development of pathogenesis in the diabetic myocardium, including cardiomyocyte death, hypertrophy, fibrosis, abnormalities of calcium homeostasis, endothelial dysfunction and subsequent diabetic cardiomyopathy and heart failure [5–8]. ROS (such as superoxide radical, hydroxyl radical and hydrogen peroxide) act as intracellular signaling molecules at moderate levels. They are generated by oxygen metabolism under physiological conditions and their levels are regulated by a number of antioxidant enzymes as well as non-enzymatic antioxidants [9]. On the other hand, elevated level of ROS induces oxidative stress, which imposes harmful effects on the functional integrity of biological tissues, including cardiomyocytes, leading to cell death [10].

Antioxidant treatment has raised the possibility of new therapeutic tools for diabetic cardiovascular complications. Taurine (Figure 18.1) could be considered as a potent therapeutic candidate in this regard due to its anti-hyperglycemic and potent antioxidant properties [11–15]. Besides, taurine also displays osmoregulatory, membrane stabilizing, and cytoprotective effects, and it can also control blood pressure and intracellular Ca^{2+} concentration, and modulate the movement of ions and neurotransmitters [16–18]. This chapter discusses emerging evidence regarding oxidative stress and signaling mechanisms in the pathogenesis of the cardiovascular complications under diabetic conditions. In addition, we also highlight the anti-hyperglycemic and antioxidant mechanisms of taurine in combating oxidative stress-induced myocardial dysfunctions in diabetes.

Diabetes: Oxidative Stress and Dietary Antioxidants.
http://dx.doi.org/10.1016/B978-0-12-405885-9.00018-8

DIABETES-INDUCED OXIDATIVE STRESS

Under diabetic conditions, oxidative stress occurs via multiple mechanisms, such as disruption of the electron transport chain in the mitochondria [19], increased activity of the polyol/sorbitol pathway [20], auto-oxidation of glucose [21], and non-enzymatic glycation of proteins [22]. However, the possible mechanisms of ROS production in the diabetic heart are: mitochondrial dysfunction due to mitochondrial fragmentation [23], disruption of the electron transport chain [24], impaired insulin signaling [25], glycated protein-induced activation of Nicotinamide adenine dinucleotide phosphate-oxidase (NADPH) oxidase [26], increased PKC isoform expression, increased pathways of polyol and hexosamine flux [27], and enhanced xanthine oxidase activity [11,28] (Figure 18.2).

THE ROLE OF MITOCHONDRIA IN ROS PRODUCTION

In cardiomyocytes, mitochondria are the key source of ROS production. These are mainly superoxides, which then generate peroxynitrite which causes damage to mitochondria [24,29,30]. Ye et al. [24] showed that overproduction of mitochondrial ROS in OVE26 diabetic mouse cardiomyocytes can be eliminated by treatment with mitochondrial electron transport chain inhibitors, rotenone and thenoyltrifluoroacetone. Yu et al. [23] showed that mitochondrial fission mediated by DLP1 (dynamin-like protein) is necessary for mitochondrial fragmentation leading to the increase in ROS levels and cardiomyocyte death under hyperglycemic conditions. Boudina et al. [25] also reported that genetic deletion of insulin receptors in mouse cardiomyocytes promotes oxidative stress in mitochondria which might directly cause mitochondrial dysfunction in obesity and diabetes mellitus.

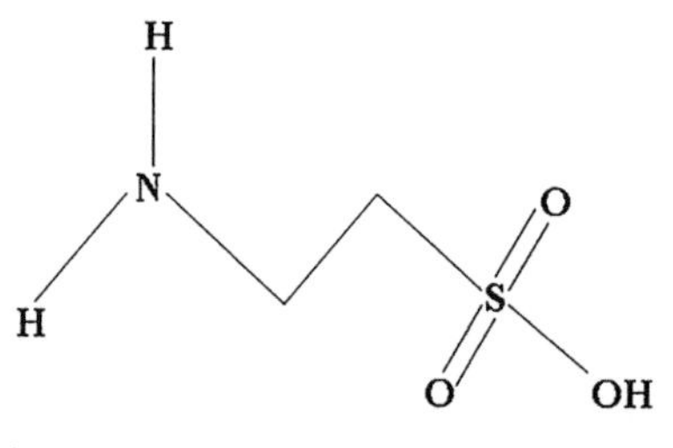

FIGURE 18.1 **Structure of taurine.** 2-amino ethane sulphonic acid.

ADVANCED GLYCATION END PRODUCTS (AGE) MEDIATED ROS PRODUCTION

Under hyperglycemic conditions, AGEs are produced when reducing sugars react non-enzymatically with the amino groups of proteins and other macromolecules, forming irreversible Schiff bases and more stable Amadori products. This leads to the formation of AGEs via auto-oxidation of the Amadori products. The AGEs thus formed bind with their receptors (RAGE) and lead to ROS production. Besides, glycation can also inactivate antioxidant enzymes and impair antioxidant defense. It has also been reported that glycated proteins stimulate ROS production in neonatal rat cardiomyocytes, largely by means of PKC-mediated activation of a Nicotinamide adenine dinucleotide phosphate-oxidase 2 (NOX 2)-containing NADPH oxidase [26].

THE ROLE OF NADPH OXIDASE IN ROS PRODUCTION

NADPH oxidase, a multi-subunit complex, contains a membrane-bound cytochrome b558 which is made up of the subunits p22*phox* and one of several NOX isoforms. Of the five NOX isoforms, the major ones expressed in cardiomyocytes are NOX 2 and NOX 4 [31]. NOX 2 is regulated by four cytosolic subunits (p40*phox*, p47*phox*, p67*phox* and Rac1 or Rac2) and translocates to the membrane upon enzyme activation. Nishio et al. [32] showed that in streptozotocin-induced diabetic rat hearts, ROS

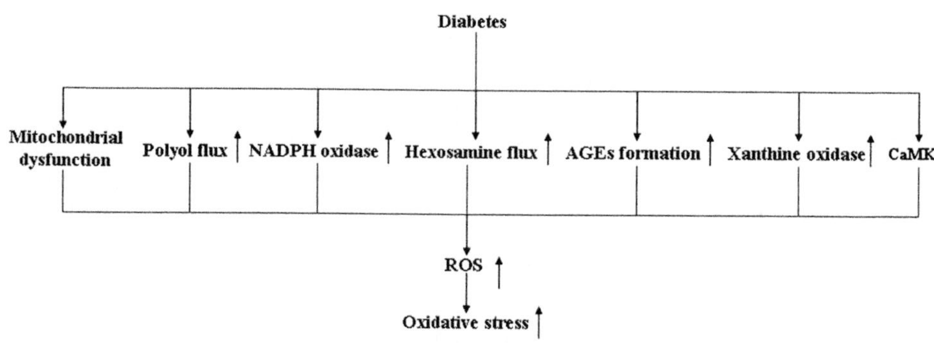

FIGURE 18.2 **Schematic diagram of the possible sources of ROS leading to cardiac oxidative stress under diabetic conditions.** The possible sources of ROS in the diabetic heart are: mitochondrial dysfunction, advanced glycation endproducts (AGEs) formation, activation of NADPH oxidase and CaMKII (Ca^{2+}/calmodulin-dependent protein kinases II) increased pathways of polyol and hexosamine flux, as well as enhanced xanthine oxidase activity.

and p47phox as well as p67phox protein expressions were increased, thereby suggesting the contribution of NADPH oxidase to ROS formation.

THE ROLE OF CAMKII IN ROS PRODUCTION

CaMKII, Ca^{2+}/calmodulin-dependent protein kinase, a multifunctional serine/threonine protein kinase, is activated on Ca^{2+}-calmodulin complex formation and is known to increase ROS production in streptozotocin-induced diabetic rat hearts [32]. Nishio et al. [32] also showed that in cardiomyocytes exposed to high glucose, phosphorylation of CaMKII was increased because of increased intracellular Ca^{2+}, at least in part by activation of Na^+–Ca^{2+} exchangers (NCX) and Na^+–H^+ exchangers (NHE), respectively [32]. Upon activation, CaMKII further activates NADPH oxidases and increases ROS production. Moreover, a number of recent studies have demonstrated that CaMKII can be activated in a Ca^{2+}-independent and ROS-dependent fashion [33]. The activation of CaMKII also enhances the activity of NHE [34], which further increase ROS.

THE ROLE OF FATTY ACIDS IN ROS PRODUCTION

Studies using several human and animal diabetic models have demonstrated that increased fatty acid (FA) uptake in cardiomyocytes enhances mitochondrial and cytosolic ROS generation [35]. Elevation of circulating and tissue FAs is caused by both adipose tissue lipolysis and hydrolysis of augmented myocardial triglyceride stores. After entering into the mitochondria, the FA is oxidized and forms ROS. Besides a large quantity of mitochondrial ROS formation, FA also generates ROS in the cytosol via activation of NADPH oxidase [35].

THE ROLE OF THE POLYOL PATHWAY IN ROS PRODUCTION

Under hyperglycemic conditions, excess glucose enters into the polyol pathway and induces ROS production. Ramasamy et al. [36] showed that sorbitol and fructose levels as well as the Nicotinamide adenine dinucleotide (reduced)/Nicotinamide adenine dinucleotide (oxidized) ($NADH/NAD^+$) ratio and AR (aldose reductase) activity were increased in diabetic rat hearts. In the diabetic state, due to increased activation of polyol pathway, the availability of NADPH (cofactor of GSH) is decreased and this depletes GSH. It has also been reported that NADH produced in this pathway translocates into the mitochondria and is oxidized by the respiratory chain, thus generating superoxide radicals [37].

THE ROLE OF NRF2 IN ROS PRODUCTION

The nuclear factor (erythroid-derived 2)-related factor 2 (Nrf2) related antioxidant response signaling pathway is known to be the primary cellular defense mechanism against oxidative stress. Tan et al. [38] reported that cardiac Nrf2 expression was down-regulated in both diabetic animals and in patients. They demonstrated that in the early stage of diabetes, Nrf2 is adaptively trying to remain functional to overcome oxidative damage. On the other hand, the decrease in cardiac Nrf2 expression in the late stages of diabetes confirms the further impairment of cardiac antioxidant function.

THE ROLE OF XANTHINE OXIDASE IN ROS PRODUCTION

Xanthine oxidase is responsible for the production of ROS under diabetic conditions. It catalyzes the production of uric acid via the oxidation of hypoxanthine and xanthine, and produces H_2O_2 and superoxide under some circumstances. Increased xanthine oxidase activity could initiate the ROS mediated damage in the cardiac tissues of alloxan-induced diabetic rats [11,28].

THE ROLE OF INCREASED HEXOSAMINE FLUX IN ROS PRODUCTION

Increased hexosamine pathway flux is an important non-mitochondrial source of ROS in the diabetic heart [27]. Hyperglycemia increases the hexosamine pathway flux and provides more fructose-6-phosphate for glutamine to produce glucosamine-6 phosphate. Fructose-6-phosphate amidotransferase (GFAT) is the rate limiting enzyme in this pathway. Glucosamine-6-phosphate inhibits the activity of glucose-6-phosphate dehydrogenase (G6PD), the rate limiting enzyme in the pentose phosphate pathway which maintains the level of NADPH. Under hyperglycemic conditions, increased mitochondrial ROS (superoxide) causes inhibition of GAPDH (glyceraldehyde-3-phosphate dehydrogenase) leading to the accumulation of glycolytic intermediates upstream of GAPDH [39]. As a result, flux along the hexosamine pathway is increased due to increased fructose-6-phosphate levels (Figure 18.3). Inhibition of G6PD or activation of NADPH oxidase decreases $NADPH/NADP^+$ ratios and induces oxidative stress by two mechanisms; first by decreasing the rejuvenation of GSH from oxidized glutathione GSSG, and second by decreasing the activity of catalase due to decreased availability of NADPH.

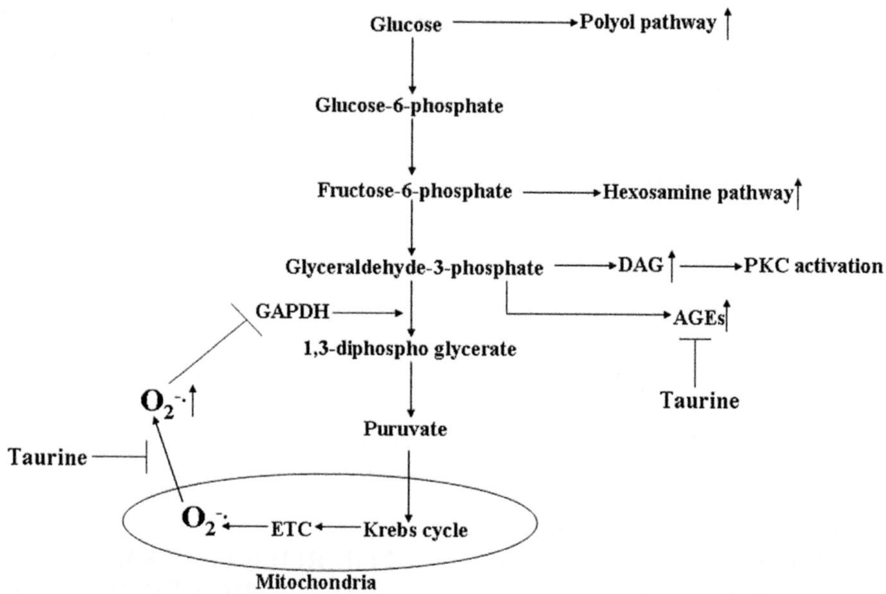

FIGURE 18.3 **Schematic diagram of the pathway that contributes to oxidative stress in response to increased glucose flux, and the anti-oxidant role of taurine.** The metabolism of glucose by mitochondria produces superoxides via disruption of the electron transport chain and inhibition of GAPDH (glyceraldehyde-3-phosphate dehydrogenase), resulting in the accumulation of glycolytic intermediates upstream of GAPDH. Accumulation of these intermediates stimulates pathological pathways, such as the hexosamine, polyol and AGE (advanced glycation endproducts) biosynthetic pathways. In addition, substrate-directed activity of the *de novo* DAG (diacylglycerol) synthetic pathway is increased which is the activator of protein kinase C. Taurine improves mitochondrial function and minimizes glucose-mediated oxidant formation by the mitochondria, as well as diminishing AGE formation.

THE ROLE OF PKC ACTIVATION IN ROS PRODUCTION

Under hyperglycemic conditions, excess glucose activates protein PKC directly by several mechanisms, e.g., through *de novo* synthesis of diacylglycerol (DAG) as indicated in Figure 18.3, by inhibition of DAG kinase and by activation of phospholipase C [40,41]. It can also be activated indirectly via increased activity of the polyol pathway and ligation of AGE receptors [19]. PKC activates NADPH oxidase and induces oxidative stress, thereby provoking diabetic cardiomyopathy [19,27].

THE ROLE OF ANGIOTENSIN II ACTIVATION IN ROS PRODUCTION

Of the several sources of ROS in hyperglycemia, angiotensin II (AT-II) is known to play a major role in the diabetic heart [42]. Hyperglycemia up-regulates the local rennin-angiotensin system (RAS), and that leads to the formation of AT-II. It has been demonstrated experimentally and clinically that AT-II induces oxidative damage through the NADPH oxidase system [42–44]. However, the AT-1 receptor is responsible for such effects in the heart [42].

ENDOGENOUS ANTIOXIDANT MECHANISMS

Under diabetic conditions, a number of protective enzymatic as well as non-enzymatic antioxidants constitute an antioxidant reserve that counteracts the damaging effects of ROS. The action of some important antioxidant enzymes (SOD, CAT, GR and GPx) are summarized in Figure 18.4.

THE BENEFICIAL ROLE OF TAURINE

Taurine, the most abundant free amino acid in the human body (0.1% of total body weight) is neither metabolized nor incorporated into cellular proteins in mammals, and modulates a variety of physiological functions. Moreover, it is found in moderately high concentrations in the heart compared to other organs, at approximately 50% in rodents and 25% in humans. The requirement for taurine in mammals is fulfilled via endogenous syntheses from methionine and cysteine, as well as dietary intake, especially from meats and sea food. Rodents have a high biosynthetic capacity for taurine, but the biosynthetic capacity in humans is very low. It is highly abundant in human breast milk and plays an important role in infant brain and retinal development.

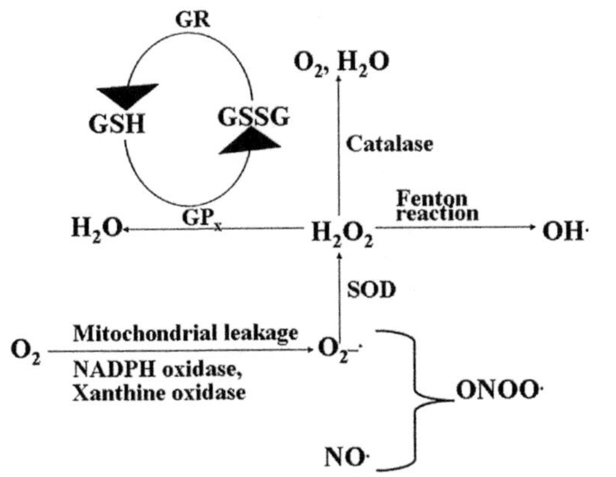

FIGURE 18.4 Endogenous stimuli leading to ROS generation in the diabetic heart, and the function of the endogenous antioxidant enzymes in maintaining the redox equilibrium. Superoxide (O_2–) is formed due to mitochondrial leakage and enhanced activities of NADPH oxidase and xanthine oxidase. SOD catalyzes the dismutation of superoxide to hydrogen peroxide (H_2O_2). This H_2O_2 is then converted to water via the action of both catalase and glutathione peroxidase (GPx), thereby preventing the formation of highly reactive OH·. Glutathione reductase (GR) reduces oxidized glutathione (GSSG) to GSH. GSH, the major endogenous antioxidant in the cells, functions as a direct scavenger of free radicals and as a co-substrate for GPx.

Taurine is found to be beneficial against diabetes, its associated complications, and other pathophysiological situations [11,12,45,46]. Taurine levels in plasma and tissue are known to decrease in both diabetic patients and animals as well as in other pathophysiological situations. Since taurine deficiency is associated with various organ dysfunctions, this decrease in taurine level in diabetic subjects might cause diabetic complications.

MECHANISMS OF THE ANTI-HYPERGLYCEMIC ACTION OF TAURINE

The main mechanisms that account for the anti-diabetic role of taurine have been summarized as follows:

1) Taurine confers protection to the pancreatic β-cells (Figure 18.5) [11,15], and modulates insulin sensitivity [11,47] and insulin secretion [48]. It does this by modulating the phosphorylation states of IRS-1/2 and Akt in peripheral tissues, and by interacting with IRs directly [11,47]. Taurine also affects the secretion of insulin elevating the expression levels of genes that stimulate this process (e.g., Glut-2, glucokinase, sulfonylurea receptor-1 and Pdx-1) and by inhibiting ATP-sensitive K^+ channels [48,49].
2) Taurine exerts antioxidant properties by reducing excessive superoxide production by the mitochondria by conjugating with the key uridine moiety of mitochondrial tRNA [50]. The detailed antioxidant mechanistic pathway will be discussed later.
3) Taurine exhibits anti-inflammatory activities by repressing the secretion of diabetes-related cytokines (TNF-α and MCP-1) [51].

THE ANTIOXIDANT MECHANISM OF TAURINE AGAINST CARDIAC OXIDATIVE STRESS UNDER DIABETIC CONDITIONS

The main mechanisms that account for the antioxidant role of taurine have been summarized as follows:

1) As an anti-hyperglycemic agent, taurine can reduce blood glucose levels (as discussed above) and thereby block the subsequent ROS formation induced by high glucose.
2) Taurine is unable to scavenge classical ROS such as superoxide radical, hydroxyl radical and hydrogen peroxide, but it inhibits excess ROS production by restoring the levels of endogenous antioxidants such as GSH (Table 18.1) and antioxidant enzymes (Table 18.2). It has been reported that taurine treatment of diabetic rats significantly increased the activities of SOD, CAT, GST, GR as well as GPx (Table 18.2) and reduced the intracellular ROS level (Table 18.1) in cardiac tissue [11]. However, the GSH level in cardiac tissue did not change significantly, because even though more GSH was biosynthesized, it was distributed to several tissues, including the heart, in diabetic conditions [11]. So, as GSH became depleted, more GSH was supplied to the heart, and consequently GSSG levels increased significantly due to its oxidation via reactive free radicals. In the hearts of diabetic rats, taurine increased the GSH/GSSG ratio by normalizing the GSSG content (Table 18.1), which resulted from the elevated GR activity [11]. On the other hand, taurine can only directly detoxify HOCl as an antioxidant.
3) Taurine is present at high concentrations within the mitochondria, and its depletion causes mitochondrial ROS formation. Mitochondrial DNA encodes the electron transport chain proteins. Suzuki et al. [50] showed the occurrence of two modified uridines in mitochondrial tRNAs for leucine and lysine. These two modified uridines have a sulfonic acid group contributed by taurine, and they play a vital role in the translation of the electron transport proteins, suggesting that diminished taurine levels might lead to defective tRNAs, and this impairs electron transport capacity. This in turn leads to a drop in the transport of electrons through the electron transport chain, and a diversion of these electrons from the respiratory chain to forming superoxide

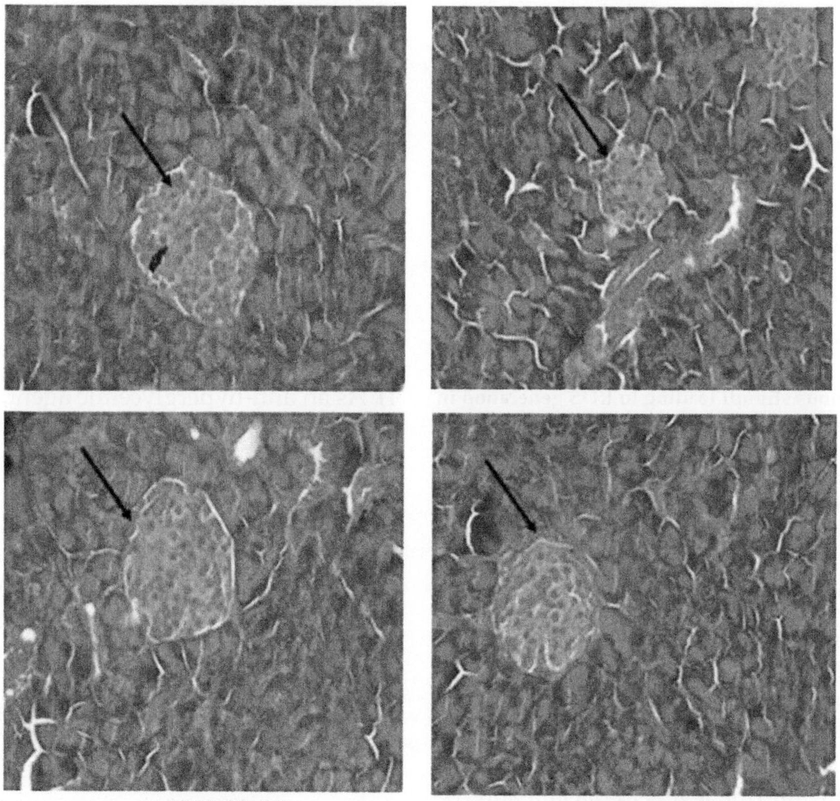

FIGURE 18.5 **Effect of taurine on diabetic pancreatic tissue (stained with hematoxylin and eosin dye).** Normal: pancreatic section of normal rat pancreas; ALX: pancreatic section from the diabetic group (single i.p. dose of alloxan at 120 mg/kg body weight); ALX&TAU: pancreatic tissue section from the taurine simultaneous (1% w/v taurine in water, orally for 21 days, 1 hr before alloxan injection); and ALX+TAU: taurine post treated rats (1% w/v taurine in water, orally for 21 days, after diabetic onset) respectively (x 200). Arrows indicate islets of Langerhans. The pancreatic islets of Langerhans were smaller with decreased number of β-cells in the ALX-induced diabetic rats than the normal group. However, treatment with taurine prevented the development of ALX-induced changes. *(Reprinted from Toxicol Appl Pharmacol, 258 (2012) 296–308 with the permission from Elsevier.)*

anions [52]. Since mitochondria are the major source of glucose-mediated oxidative stress, it would be expected that increased taurine levels would improve mitochondrial function, minimize glucose-mediated oxidant formation by the mitochondria, and diminish the PKC inactivation pathway and AGE formation due to inactivation of GAPDH via mitochondria derived superoxides (Figure 18.3).

4) NADPH oxidase is activated via several pathways, such as PKC, CaMKII, fatty acids and AT-II, and is an important source of ROS in diabetic heart (Figure 18.6). Taurine has been shown to inhibit NADPH oxidase in cardiomyocytes [53], and hence it can be considered as a potential cardiovascular therapeutic. Besides, taurine also down-regulates AT-II in the diabetic rat heart [54], hence it might block AT-II-induced NADPH oxidase activation (Figure 18.7).

5) Intracellular Ca^{2+} concentrations have been shown to be increased in diabetic rat hearts [32]. This impaired calcium metabolism activates CaMKII and produces ROS in cardiomyocytes [32]. However, taurine has been shown to prevent this intracellular calcium overload and to maintain calcium homeostasis [55], suggesting that taurine treatment might inhibit ROS formation via maintenance of calcium homeostasis (Figure 18.7).

6) Taurine can form an amide bond with the carbonyl group of reducing sugars via its amino group. However, in the absence of taurine, these carbonyls accumulate in the diabetic heart and form extensively cross-linked glycation end products (AGEs). These AGEs can further activate RAGE receptors and stimulate the formation of ROS. Therefore, it has been suggested that taurine may alter the effect of glucose-mediated oxidative stress via conjugation reactions with carbonyls [56].

7) Another important source of ROS in the diabetic heart is xanthine oxidase, which produces H_2O_2 and superoxide. Taurine can effectively reduce xanthine

TABLE 18.1 Effect of Alloxan and Taurine on the Status of the Thiol Based Antioxidants and Intracellular ROS (Reactive Oxygen Species) in Cardiac Tissue of Rats

Parameters	Normal Control	Taurine Treated	Alloxan Treated	Alloxan & Taurine	Alloxan + Taurine
GSH (nmol/mg protein)	18.68± 0.734	18.44± 0.722	16.80 ± 0.640	17.92± 0.796	17.98± 0.799
GSSG (nmol/mg protein)	0.64± 0.022	0.62± 0.021	0.99± 0.039 ^{a*,b*}	0.65± 0.022 ^{c*}	0.67± 0.024 ^{c*}
Redox ratio (GSH/GSSG)	29.19± 1.359	29.74± 1.387	16.92± 0.746^{a***,b***}	27. 56± 1.278^{c***}	26.84± 1.242^{c***}
Intracellular ROS (% over control)	100± 4	67± 2.35	210± 9.5 ^{a***,b***}	102± 4.1 ^{b**,c***}	107± 4.35 ^{b**,c***}

In the heart of diabetic rats the intracellular ROS level ($p < 0.001$) was increased compared to normal rats. On the other hand, the GSH:GSSG ratio ($p < 0.001$) was decreased in the cardiac tissue of the diabetic rats compared to normal rats. The decrease of intracellular GSH content in diabetic rat heart was not significant, whereas diabetes increased GSSG ($p < 0.05$) content in diabetic rats compared to normal. However, treatment with taurine significantly increased the GSH:GSSG ratio ($p < 0.001$) and decreasd the ROS level ($p < 0.001$) compared to a alloxan-exposed group. Values are expressed as mean ± SD, for 6 animals in each group. "a" indicates differs significantly from normal; "b" indicates differs significantly from taurine; "c" indicates differs significantly from alloxan. ($p^* < 0.05$), ($p^{**} < 0.01$), ($p^{***} < 0.001$).
(Reprinted from Toxicol Appl Pharmacol, 258 (2012) 296–308 with the permission from Elsevier.)

oxidase activity (Table 18.2) and thereby inhibit ROS production (Figure 18.7) [11].

8) Enhanced FFAs cause both mitochondrial and cytoplasmic ROS level. Due to the unique lipid lowering effect of taurine, it can reduce the triglyceride level [11]. Therefore, taurine treatment might also reduce FFAs and the subsequent ROS formation (Figure 18.7).
9) Taurine may indirectly affect lipid peroxidation by limiting their availability, and it could interact with cell membranes, possibly by electrostatic interaction between its sulphonic acid and amino groups and the phosphate and amino or ammonium groups of membrane phospholipids [57]. Taurine also inhibits the enzyme phospholipids N-methyltransferase which catalyzes the conversion of phosphatidylethanolamine (PE) to phosphatidylcholine (PC) [58]. As a result, taurine elevates the PE/PC ratio, alters the cellular membrane fluidity and thereby might enhance its ability to resist toxic insults. Taurine has been shown to reduce lipid peroxidation in diabetic rat hearts [11].

TABLE 18.2 Effect of Alloxan and Taurine on the Activities of Antioxidant Enzymes and Xanthine Oxidase in Cardiac Tissue of Rats

Name of the Parameters	Normal Control	Taurine Treated	Alloxan Treated	Alloxan & Taurine	Alloxan + Taurine
SOD (Unit/mg protein)	16.8± 0.74	17.4± 0.67	5.2± 0.16 ^{a***,b***}	14.8± 0.64 ^{b*,c***}	15.2± 0.66 ^{c***}
CAT (μmol/min/mg protein)	136.85± 5.842	140.25± 6.998	83.85± 3.193 ^{a***,b***}	134.63± 5.732 ^{b*,c***}	125.97± 5.298 ^{a*,b*,c***}
GST (μmol/min/mg protein)	3.66± 0.173	3.41± 0.169	1.91± 0.085 ^{a**,b**}	3.74± 0.176 ^{c**}	3.69± 0.174 ^{c**}
GR (nmol/min/mg protein)	6.014± 0.299	6.635± 0.232	1.792± 0.079 ^{a***,b***}	7.835± 0.292 ^{a**,b*,c***}	7.659± 0.283 ^{a*,b*,c***}
GPx (nmol/min/mg protein)	119.94± 4.79	122.14± 4.99	78.41± 2.92 ^{a***,b***}	112.43± 4.64 ^{c***}	109.20± 4.29 ^{b*,c***}
Xanthine oxidase activity (mU/mg protein)	0. 48± 0.032	0.47± 0.02650.	0.80± 0.055 ^{a**,b**}	0.53± 0.0445 ^{c**}	0.55± 0.045 ^{c**}

In the diabetic rats the cardiac anti-oxidant enzymes activities, e.g., SOD ($p < 0.001$), CAT ($p < 0.001$), GST ($p < 0.01$), GR ($p < 0.001$) and GPx ($p < 0.001$) were decreased, and xanthine oxidase activity was increased ($p < 0.01$) compared to normal rats. However, treatment with taurine significantly decreased the xanthine oxidase activity ($p < 0.01$) and increased the anti-oxidant enzymes activities; SOD ($p < 0.001$), CAT ($p < 0.001$), GST ($p < 0.01$), GR ($p < 0.001$) and GPx ($p < 0.001$) compared to the alloxan-exposed group. Values are expressed as mean ± SD, for 6 animals in each group. "a" indicates differs significantly from normal; "b" indicates differs significantly from taurine; "c" indicates differs significantly from alloxan. ($p^* < 0.05$), ($p^{**} < 0.01$), ($p^{***} < 0.001$).
(Reprinted from Toxicol Appl Pharmacol, 258 (2012) 296–308 with the permission from Elsevier).

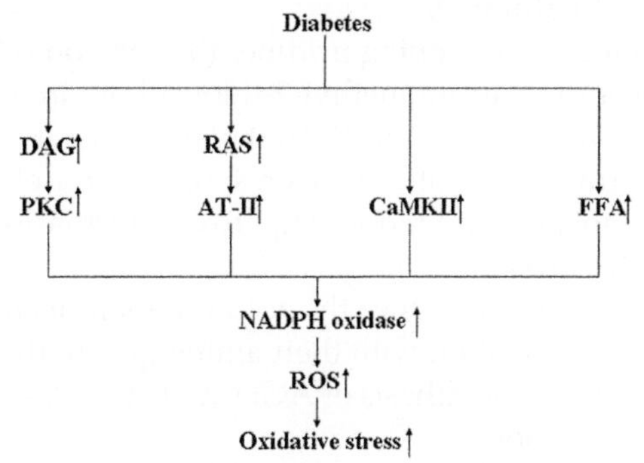

FIGURE 18.6 Schematic diagram of the possible route of activation of NADPH oxidase in cardiac tissue under diabetic conditions. In diabetic heart, NADPH oxidase is activated via several mechanistic pathways, such as DAG (diacylglycerol) induced protein kinase C activation, CaMKII (Ca^{2+}/calmodulin-dependent protein kinases II) activation, increased level of (FFA) free fatty acids and RAS (rennin-angiotensin system) induced formation of AT-II (angiotensin II) leading to ROS formation.

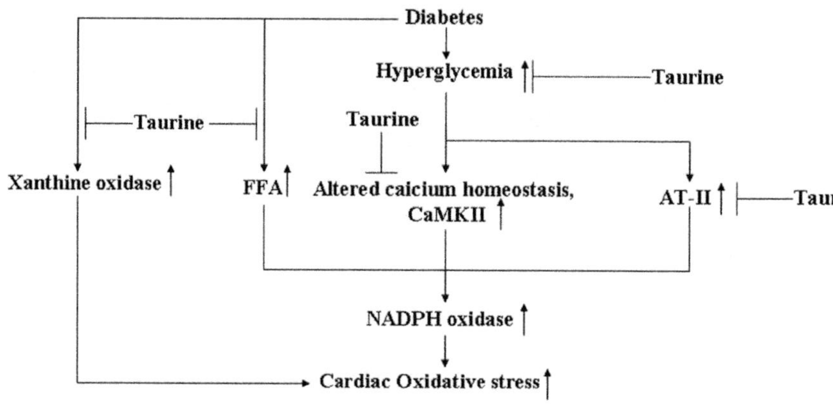

FIGURE 18.7 Schematic diagram of the possible route of inactivation of NADPH oxidase via taurine in cardiac tissue under diabetic conditions. Taurine confers protection against diabetic cardiac oxidative stress via down-regulating AT-II (angiotensin II), reducing xanthine oxidase activity and FFA (free fatty acids) levels. The anti-hyperglycemic effect of taurine also prevents intracellular calcium overload and maintains calcium homeostasis, thereby inactivating CaMKII (Ca^{2+}/calmodulin-dependent protein kinases II) and subsequent ROS formation.

SUMMARY POINTS

- Hyperglycemia-induced oxidative stress is a well-known risk factor for cardiovascular disease, cardiomyopathy and heart failure.
- The important sources of ROS (reactive oxygen species) in diabetic hearts are defective mitochondrial transport chain proteins, activation of NADPH oxidase and xanthine oxidase as well as accumulation of AGEs (advanced glycation end products).
- The other sources of cardiac oxidative stress under diabetic conditions are activation of the Ca^{+2}/CaMKII (Ca^{2+}/calmodulin-dependent protein kinases II) pathway, increased hexosamine and polyol pathway flux as well as increased levels of free fatty acids.
- Taurine, being a hypoglycemic agent, directly reduces blood glucose level and subsequent ROS formation.
- Taurine can reduce oxidative stress in the diabetic heart by restoring levels of antioxidant enzymes and GSH (glutathione).
- Two taurine-containing uridines (5-taurinomethyluridine and 5-taurinomethyl-2-thiouridine) in mitochondrial tRNAs (trans RNAs) play a crucial role in the translation of proteins responsible for electron transport and reduce superoxide formation in mitochondria.
- Taurine can also reduce the accumulation of carbonyls via conjugation with their amino group, thereby inhibiting the synthesis of AGEs and subsequent ROS formation.
- Taurine is capable of reducing ROS via maintaining the altered calcium homeostasis and inhibiting xanthine oxidase as well NADPH oxidase.
- Taurine is worthy of future research as a potential antioxidant, as it helps reduce the risk of cardiovascular complications in diabetic condition.

References

[1] Adeghate E. Molecular and cellular basis of the aetiology and management of diabetic cardiomyopathy:ashortreview. Mol Cell Biochem 2004;261:187–91.
[2] Le Winter MM. Diabetic cardiomyopathy: an overview. Coron Artery Dis 1996;7:95–8.
[3] Kannel WB, McGee DL. Diabetes and cardiovascular disease. The Framingham study. J Am Med Ass 1979;241:2035–8.
[4] Stevens MJ. Oxidative-nitrosative stress as a contributing factor to cardiovascular disease in subjects with diabetes. Curr Vasc Pharmacol 2005;3:253–66.
[5] Boudina S, Abel ED. Diabetic cardiomyopathy revisited. Circulation 2007;115:3213–23.
[6] Haidara MA, Yassin HZ, Rateb M, Ammar H, Zorkani MA. Role of oxidative stress in development of cardiovascular complications in diabetes mellitus. Curr Vasc Pharmacol 2006;4:215–27.
[7] Fang ZY, Prins JB, Marwick TH. Diabetic cardiomyopathy: evidence, mechanisms, and therapeutic implications. Endocr Rev 2004;25:543–67.
[8] Cai L, Kang YJ. Cell death and diabetic cardiomyopathy. Cardiovasc Toxicol 2003;3:219–28.
[9] Hool LC. Reactive oxygen species in cardiac signaling: frommitochondria to plasma membrane ion channels. Clin Exp Pharmacol Physiol 2006;33:146–51.
[10] Li C, Jackson RM. Reactive species mechanisms of cellular hypoxia-reoxygenation injury. Am J Physiol Cell Physiol 2002;282:C227–41.
[11] Das J, Vasan V, Sil PC. Taurine exerts hypoglycemic effect in alloxan-induced diabetic rats, improves insulin-mediated glucose transport signaling pathway in heart and ameliorates cardiac oxidative stress and apoptosis. Toxicol Appl Pharmacol 2012;258:296–308.
[12] Das J, Ghosh J, Manna P, Sil PC. Taurine suppresses doxorubicin-triggered oxidative stress and cardiac apoptosis in rat via up-regulation of PI3-K/Akt and inhibition of p53, p38-JNK. Biochem Pharmacol 2011;81:891–909.
[13] Roy A, Manna P, Sil PC. Prophylactic role of taurine on arsenic mediated oxidative renal dysfunction via MAPKs/ NF-κB and mitochondria dependent pathways. Free Radic Res 2009;43:995–1007.
[14] Winiarska K, Szymanski K, Gorniak P, Dudziak M, Bryla J. Hypoglycaemic, antioxidative and nephroprotective effects of taurine in alloxan diabetic rabbits. Biochimie 2009;91; 261e270.

[15] Gavrovskaya LK, Ryzhova OV, Safonova AF, Matveev AK, Sapronov NS. Protective effect of taurine on rats with experimental insulin-dependent diabetes mellitus. Bull Exp Biol Med 2008;146:226–8.
[16] Huxtable RJ. Physiological actions of taurine. Physiol Rev 1992;72:101–63.
[17] Satoh H. Cardiac actions of taurine as a modulator of the ion channels. Adv Exp Med Biol 1998;442:121–8.
[18] Schaffer S, Takahashi K, Azuma J. Role of osmoregulation in the actions of taurine. Amino Acids 2000;19:527–46.
[19] Nishikawa T, Edelstein D, Du XL, Yamagishi S, Matsumura T, Kaneda Y, et al. Normalizing mitochondrial superoxide production blocks three pathways of hyperglycemic damage. Nature 2000;404:787–90.
[20] Ciuchi E, Odetti P, Prando R. Relationship between glutathione and sorbitol concentrations in erythrocytes from diabetic patients. Metabolism 1996;45:611–3.
[21] Wolff SP, Dean RT. Glucose autoxidation and protein modification. The potential role of 'autoxidative glycosylation' in diabetes. Biochem J 1987;245:243–50.
[22] Mullarkey CJ, Edelstein D, Brownlee M. Free radical generation by early glycation products: a mechanism for accelerated atherogenesis in diabetes. Biochem Biophys Res Commun 1990;173:932–9.
[23] Yu T, Sheu SS, Robotham JL, Yoon Y. Mitochondrial fission mediates high glucose induced cell death through elevated production of reactive oxygen species. Cardiovasc Res 2008;79:341–51.
[24] Ye G, Metreveli NS, Donthi RV, Xia S, Xu M, Carlson EC, et al. Catalase protects cardiomyocyte function in models of type 1 and type 2 diabetes. Diabetes 2004;53:1336–43.
[25] Boudina S, Bugger H, Sena S, O'Neill BT, Zaha VG, Ilkun O, et al. Contribution of impaired myocardial insulin signaling to mitochondrial dysfunction and oxidative stress in the heart. Circulation 2009;119:1272–83.
[26] Zhang M, Kho AL, Anilkumar N, Chibber R, Pagano PJ, Shah AM, et al. Glycated proteins stimulate reactive oxygen species production in cardiacmyocytes: involvement of Nox2 (gp91phox)-containing NADPH oxidase. Circulation 2006;113:1235–43.
[27] Wold LE, Ceylan-Isik AF, Ren J. Oxidative stress and stress signaling: menace of diabetic cardiomyopathy. Acta Pharmacologica Sinica 2005;26:908–17.
[28] Akhileshwar V, Patel SP, Katyare SS. Diabetic cardiomyopathy and reactive oxygen species (ROS) related parameters in male and female rats: a comparative study. Ind J Clin Biochem 2007;22:84–90.
[29] Song Y, Du Y, Prabhu SD, Epstein PN. Diabetic cardiomyopathy in OVE26 mice shows mitochondrial ROS production and divergence between *in vivo* and *in vitro* contractility. Rev Diabet Stud 2007;4:159–68.
[30] Turko IV, Li L, Aulak KS, Stuehr DJ, Chang JY, Murad F. Protein tyrosine nitration in the mitochondria from diabetic mouse heart. Implications to dysfunctional mitochondria in diabetes. J Biol Chem 2003;278:33972–7.
[31] Griendling KK. Novel NAD(P)H oxidases in the cardiovascular system. Heart 2004;90:491–3.
[32] Nishio S, Teshima Y, Takahashi N, Thuc LC, Saito S, Fukui A, et al. Activation of CaMKII as a key regulator of reactive oxygen species production in diabetic rat heart. J Mol Cell Cardiol 2012;52:1103–11.
[33] Erickson JR, Joiner ML, Guan X, Kutschke W, Yang J, Oddis CV, et al. A dynamic pathway for calcium-independent activation of CaMKII by methionine oxidation. Cell 2008;133:462–74.
[34] Vila-Petroff M, Mundina-Weilenmann C, Lezcano N, Snabaitis AK, Huergo MA, Valverde CA, et al. Ca^{2+}/calmodulin-dependent protein kinase II contributes to intracellular pH recovery from acidosis via Na^{+}/H^{+} exchanger activation. J Mol Cell Cardiol 2010;49:106–12.
[35] Boudina S, Abel ED. Diabetic cardiomyopathy, causes and effects. Rev. Endocr. Metab. Disord 2010;11:31–9.
[36] Ramasamy R, Oates PJ, Schaefer S. Aldose reductase inhibition protects diabetic and nondiabetic rat hearts from ischemic injury. Diabetes 1997;46:292–300.
[37] Ceriello A, Russ P, Amstael P, Cerutt P. High glucose induces antioxidants enzymes in humans endothelial cells in culture: Evidence linking hyperglycemia and oxidative stress. Diabetes 1996;45:471–7.
[38] Tan Y, Ichikawa T, Li J, Si Q, Yang H, Chen X, et al. Diabetic Down-regulation of Nrf2 Activity via ERK contributes to oxidative stress–induced insulin resistance in cardiac cells *in vitro* and *in vivo*. Diabetes 2011;60:625–33.
[39] Du XL. Hyperglycemia-induced mitochondrial superoxide overproduction activates the hexosamine pathway and induces plasminogen activator inhibitor-1 expression by increasing Sp1 glycosylation. Proc Natl Acad Sci USA 2000;97:12222–6.
[40] Keogh RJ, Dunlop ME, Larkins RG. Effect of inhibition of aldose reductase on glucose flux, diacylglycerol formation, protein kinase C, and phospholipase A2 activation. Metabolism 1997;46:41–7.
[41] Xia P, Inoguchi T, Kern TS, Engerman RL, Oates PJ, King GL. Characterization of the mechanism for the chronic activation of diacylglycerol-protein kinase C pathway in diabetes and hypergalactosemia. Diabetes 1994;43:1122–9.
[42] Frustaci A, Kajstura J, Chimenti C, Jakoniuk I, Leri A, Maseri A, et al. Myocardial cell death in human diabetes. Circ Res 2000;87:1123–32.
[43] Fiordaliso F, Li B, Latini R, Sonnenblick EH, Anversa P, Leri A, et al. Myocyte death in streptozotocin-induced diabetes in rats in angiotensin II- dependent. Lab Invest 2000;80:513–27.
[44] Kajstura J, Fiordaliso F, Andreoli AM, Li B, Chimenti S, Medow MS, et al. IGF-1 overexpression inhibits the development of diabetic cardiomyopathy and angiotensin II-mediated oxidative stress. Diabetes 2001;50:1414–24.
[45] Das J, Ghosh J, Manna P, Sil PC. Taurine protects rat testes against doxorubicin-induced oxidative stress as well as p53, Fas and caspase 12-mediated apoptosis. Amino Acids 2012;42:1839–55.
[46] Das J, Ghosh J, Manna P, Sil PC. Acetaminophen induced acute liver failure via oxidative stress and JNK activation: Protective role of taurine by the suppression of cytochrome P450 2E1. Free Radic Res 2010;44:340–55.
[47] Wu N, Lu Y, He B, Zhang Y, Lin J, Zhao S, et al. Taurine prevents free fatty acid-induced hepatic insulin resistance in association with inhibiting JNK1 activation and improving insulin signaling *in vivo*. Diabetes Res Clin Pract 2010;90:288–96.
[48] Carneiro EM, Latorraca MQ, Araujo E, Beltra M, Oliveras MJ, Navarro M, et al. Taurine supplementation modulates glucose homeostasis and islet function. J Nutr Biochem 2009;20:503–11.
[49] Park EJ, Bae JH, Kim SY, Lim JG, Baek WK, Kwon TK, et al. Inhibition of ATP-sensitive K+ channels by taurine through a benzamido-binding site on sulfonylurea receptor 1. Biochem Pharmacol 2004;67:1089–96.
[50] Suzuki T, Suzuki T, Wada T, Saigo K, Watanabe K. Novel taurine- containing uridine derivatives and mitochondrial human diseases. Nucleic Acids Res Suppl 2001;1:257–8.
[51] Park E, Quinn MR, Wright CE, Schuller-Levis G. Taurine chloramine inhibits the synthesis of nitric oxide and the release of tumor necrosis factor in activated RAW 264.7 cells. J Leukoc Biol 1993;54:119–24.
[52] Franconi F, Di Leo MA, Bennardini F, Ghirlanda G. Is Taurine Beneficial in Reducing Risk Factors for Diabetes Mellitus? Neurochem Res 2004;29:143–50.
[53] Li Y, Arnold JMO, Pampillo M, Babwah AV, Peng T. Taurine prevents cardiomyocyte death by inhibiting NADPH oxidase-mediated calpain activation. Free Radic Biol Med 2009;46:51–61.

[54] Li C, Cao L, Zeng Q, Liu X, Zhang Y, Dai T, et al. Taurine May Prevent Diabetic Rats from Developing Cardiomyopathy also by Downregulating Angiotensin II Type2 Receptor Expression. Cardiovas. Drugs Ther 2005;18:105–12.

[55] Schaffer S, Takahashi K, Azuma J. Role of osmoregulation in the actions of taurine. Amino Acids 2000;19:527–46.

[56] Schaffer S, Jong CJ, Ramila KC, Ito T, Azuma J. In: El Idrissi A, L'Amoreaux W, editors. Physiological and therapeutic roles of taurine in the heart. Taurine in Health and Disease; 2012. p. 23–51: ISBN: 978–81–7895–520–9.

[57] Schaffer SW, Azuma J, Madura JD. Mechanisms underlying taurine-mediated alterations in membrane function. Amino Acid 1995;8:231–46.

[58] Hamaguchi T, Azuma J, Schaffer S. Interaction of taurine wit methionine: inhibition of myocardial phospholipid methyltransferase. J Cardiovasc Pharmacol 1991;18:224–30.

CHAPTER

19

Statins, Diabetic Oxidative Stress and Vascular Tissue

Jonathan R. Murrow

Georgia Regents University – University of Georgia Medical Partnership, Athens, GA, USA

List of Abbreviations

BH4 Tetrahydrobiopterin
eNOS Endothelial nitric oxide synthase
FMD Flow mediated dilation
GTPCH-I Guanosine triphosphate cyclohydrolase I
HMG CoA Hydroxymethyl-glutaryl CoA
hs-CRP High sensitivity C-reactive protein
LDL Low density lipoprotein
NADPH Nicotinamide adenine dinucleotide phosphate
NF-κB Nuclear factor κB
NO Nitric oxide
ROS Reactive oxygen species
VEGF Vascular endothelial growth factor

INTRODUCTION

Controversy surrounds the current understanding of diabetic vascular disease with regard to the role of glucose. While the hallmark abnormality of diabetes is hyperglycemia, vascular complications bear the greatest clinical impact [1]. The link between these two phenomena remains the subject of much research, with a central theme of oxidative stress uniting these two strands of knowledge. This chapter aims to summarize the evidence supporting the central role of oxidative stress pathways in linking hyperglycemia to vascular disorders in diabetes. Several sources of oxidative stress will be highlighted. In addition to exploring the etiology and consequences of oxidative stress in diabetes, this chapter will focus on an important class of therapeutics in mitigating the effects of oxidative stress in diabetes. Hydroxymethyl-glutaryl (HMG) coA reductase inihibitors (or 'statins') will be scrutinized for their impact on oxidative stress in diabetes – especially in their effects independent of lowering plasma lipids. The impact of statins on differing sources of oxidative stress will be explored. Finally, this chapter will summarize the key clinical trials of statins that have been shown to influence the development or progression of diabetic macrovascular and microvascular disease.

OXIDATIVE STRESS AND DIABETES

High plasma glucose relative to normal, homeostatic levels elicits a pathologic compensatory response. Several metabolic and signaling pathways are perturbed in the setting of hyperglycemia – including enhanced nuclear factor κB and enhanced advanced glycation end product production [2]. Importantly, one compensatory response is the increased production of reactive oxygen species (ROS), and therefore the increase in vascular oxidative stress. Vascular tissue contains several potential reservoirs for the generation of oxidative stress, the most important of which are endothelial cell cytosolic sources, endothelial mitochondria, and monocytes. Exposing cultured aortic endothelial cells to high concentrations of glucose will elicit production of reactive oxygen species [3]. In human aortic endothelial cells, Piga and coworkers demonstrated that short term high glucose exposure resulted in enhanced adhesion and migration molecule expression as well as pro-inflammatory NF-κB expression [4]. Importantly, intracellular ROS production as measured by fluorescence probes increased after exposure of aortic endothelial cells to high glucose solutions in what appeared to be an upstream event of NF-κB activation. Other experiments implicate mitochonidral oxidases in hyperglycemia-induced ROS generation. Blockade of the mitochondrial electron transport chain uncouples oxidative phosphorylation while attenuating glucose-induced production of ROS [3]. By a different mechanism, Venugopal and coworkers demonstrated that under hyperglycemic conditions, monocytes release superoxide via NADPH pathways [5] (Figure 19.1).

Diabetes: Oxidative Stress and Dietary Antioxidants.
http://dx.doi.org/10.1016/B978-0-12-405885-9.00019-X

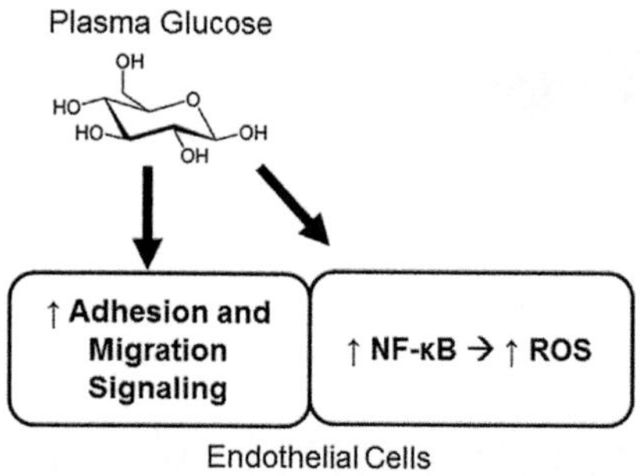

FIGURE 19.1 **Impact of hyperglycemia on oxidative stress.** High plasma glucose up-regulates adhesion and migration signaling molecules. In addition, pro-inflammatory NF-κB expression increases and results in increased release of reactive oxygen species (ROS).

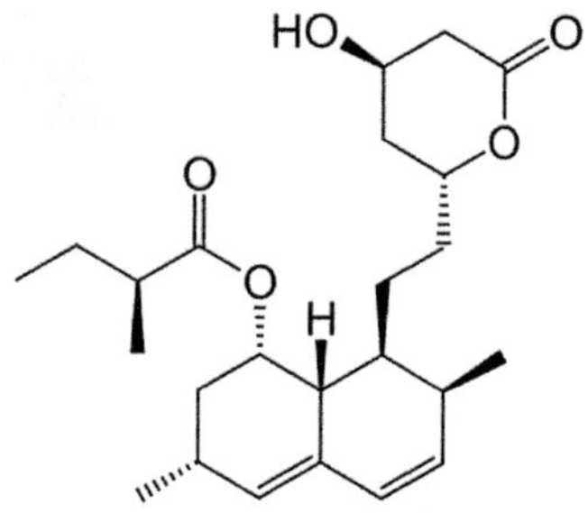

FIGURE 19.2 **Molecular structure of lovastatin.**

TABLE 19.1 Summary of Available Statin Agents and Doses

Compound	Dose
Lovastatin	20 mg, 40 mg
Pravastatin	10 mg, 20 mg, 40 mg, 80 mg
Simvastatin	5 mg, 10 mg, 20 mg, 40 mg
Atorvastatin	10 mg, 20 mg, 40 mg, 80 mg
Rosuvastatin	5 mg, 10 mg, 20 mg, 40 mg
Pitavastatin	1 mg, 2 mg, 4 mg

As stated, control of hyperglycemia alone in experimental models and in human subjects does not attenuate the development of diabetic vascular disease. Here an important intersection between hyperglycemia, oxidative stress and lipoprotein metabolism must be considered. Activation of hyperglycemic-dependent oxidative stress pathways certainly promotes atherogenesis; clinical macrovascular disease in diabetes does not arise completely independently of the dysregulation of lipoprotein metabolism. Renard and coworkers have demonstrated in a mouse model of type 1 diabetes that the acceleration of pathologic precursors to aggressive atherosclerosis lesions required concomitant dyslipoproteinemia [6]. Clinical trials of glucose-lowering therapies have failed to similarly reduce cardiovascular events. In the UKPDS trial, aggressive glycemic control with oral hypoglycemic agents failed to reduce the incidence of macrovascular complications relative to less aggressive glycemic control over a 10 year period [7]. Only after a prolonged followup period (averaging 17 years) was glycemic control with oral hypoglycemic agents associated with risk reduction for myocardial infarction (15% to 33%) [8]. By contrast, cholesterol-lowering therapy among diabetics with and without known vascular disease has demonstrated a 22% to 33% relative risk reduction in cardiovascular events over a five year treatment period [9]. Importantly, diabetic subjects with known dyslipidemia derive the greatest reduction in clinical events. Although in these trials a reduction in mean lipoprotein levels was achieved, the full benefit may be disproportional to the level of lipids achieved – suggesting a 'pleiotropic' benefit to statin therapy.

STATINS: DISCOVERY AND MECHANISMS

The synthesis of plasma cholesterol involves a series of enzymatic reactions that includes three serial condensations of acetyl-CoA subunits to form 3-hydroxy-3-methylglutaryl coenzyme A (HMG CoA) [10]. This compound is then reduced to mevalonate and undergoes several steps en route to the final product: cholesterol. Recognizing that high plasma cholesterol is a potent risk condition for the development of atherosclerosis, a key therapeutic target in cardiovascular risk reduction over the past several decades has been disruption of the cholesterol metabolic pathway. In 1976, Endo and coworkers reported the discovery of a compound capable of competitively inhibiting the reduction of HMG CoA (Figure 19.2). Subsequently, similar compounds were identified, the first of which to be used in human studies was lovastatin. Similar drugs in current use are synthetic derivatives with unique molecular properties (Table 19.1).

IMPACT OF STATINS ON OXIDATIVE STRESS

The clinical benefits of statins may in part be attributed to mechanisms independent of their cholesterol-lowering effects [11]. Importantly, statins impact vascular oxidative stress and endothelial dysfunction by a mechanism that is independent of cholesterol reduction [12]. Recent large clinical trials have highlighted the possible benefit of treating subjects with high dose statins even though they enjoy controlled lipid levels, regardless of age or the presence of stable or unstable coronary artery disease [13–16]. Several studies have shown a dose response effect in the influence of statin therapy on

TABLE 19.2 Sources of Oxidative Stress

Source	Abnormality in Type 2 Diabetes	Impact from Statin Therapy
NADPH oxidases	Increased expression	Decreased expression via Rac-1
Xanthine oxidases	Limited data in diabetes	Scavenge superoxide produced by xanthine oxidases
Mitochondrial oxidases	Limited data in diabetes	Impacts mitochondrial membrane enzymes
Cellular thiol redox circuits	Limited data in diabetes	Improves aminothiol levels
Uncoupled nitric oxide synthase	Increased superoxide production	Increased NOS cofactor production

measures of endothelial dysfunction. Ky and coworkers examined the effect of a panel of markers of oxidative stress in hypercholesterolemic subjects at 16 weeks followup, finding variable effects depending on statin and dose [17]. Singh and coworkers found that high dose atorvastatin (80 mg daily) versus low dose (10 mg daily) was associated with improvements in oxidized LDL, as well as inflammatory markers hs-CRP, matrix metalloproteinase-9 and NF-κB activity [18]. Improvements in FMD were observed in high dose (40mg/d) but not low dose (20mg/d) atorvastatin in hyperlipidemic subjects [19]. In subjects with stable coronary artery disease, high dose statin therapy was associated with improved endothelial function in explanted internal mammary arteries [20]. By contrast, Mulder and coworkers failed to find a benefit of high dose atorvastatin versus moderate dose simvastatin in improving oxidized LDL, CRP, or other inflammatory markers after 16 weeks of therapy [21].

Statins have been shown to be protective in subjects at high risk and appear to also reduce oxidative stress in experimental studies, possibly by reversing the inhibitory effect of oxidized LDL on endothelial nitric oxide synthase (eNOS). In addition, statins may exert direct antioxidant effects on LDL *in vitro* and *ex vivo* by inhibiting the production of an isoprenoid critical for NADPH oxidase-mediated vascular ROS [22]. Reactive oxygen species, the arbiters of tissue damage in oxidative stress, arise primarily from pertubations of NADPH oxidase; however, xanthine oxidase, mitochondrial oxidases, and uncoupled endothelial nitric oxide synthases have all been implicated as sources of oxidative stress in vascular tissue [23] (Table 19.2).

NADPH Oxidases

Several lines of evidence in animal and human vascular models support the notion that NADPH oxidases are a key source of oxidative stress in atherosclerosis-risk conditions such as diabetes [24]. Inducing diabetes in streptozotocin-treated rats results in activation of NADPH oxidases and increased expression of mRNA precursors [25]. In the explanted saphenous veins of patients with coronary artery disease, Guzik and coworkers demonstrated that vascular superoxide primarily arose from NADPH-dependent oxidases that had a negative effect on NO-dependent vasodilation [26]. Diabetes among these subjects was strongly associated with increased NADH-dependent superoxide production.

Atorvastatin reduced the expression of NADPH oxidase subunits and subsequent superoxide production in diabetic rodents, improving endothelial vasomotor function [27,28]. These effects are mediated by suppression of Rac-1 signaling, and are thought to rely on direct effects from hydroxymethyl-CoA inhibition [29]. In human subjects treated with atorvastatin versus controls, the NADPH oxidase subunit $gp91^{phox}$ levels were significantly reduced over a 30 day period in a mechanism mediated by adiponectin [30]. Other studies have confirmed a reduction in plasma $gp91^{phox}$ in hypercholesterolemic subjects treated with statin therapy [31]. Subjects undergoing coronary bypass grafting treated with atorvastatin exhibited a reduction in NADPH-stimulated superoxide production in explanted saphenous vein segments independent of LDL-lowering effects [32].

In addition to effects on large vessels, basic work suggests an attenuation of deleterious NADPH oxidase-mediated oxidative stress in the microvasculature. Qian and coworkers demonstrated that statin therapy attenuated oxidant-induced damage in cultured human retinal cells by blocking the activation of NADPH oxidases [33]. Others have demonstrated that statins attenuate the blood-retinal barrier breakdown that contributes to diabetic retinopathy via similar mechanisms [34,35]. As for the renal microcirculation, in diabetic dyslipidemic mice, statin therapy is associated with reduced expression of NADPH oxidases, with reduction of oxidative stress-induced filtration barrier injury, and albuminuria [36–39].

Xanthine Oxidases

Xanthine oxidases are a source of ROS in vascular tissue [23]. *In vitro* assays of oxidative DNA damage have demonstrated that statins scavenge superoxide anions in the hypoxanthine-xanthine oxidase system [40]. In a heart failure cohort, inhibition of the xanthine oxidase system with allopurinol resulted in no additional reduction of oxidative stress markers, endothelial function, and functional capacity when compared to atorvastatin therapy alone [41]. Though the body of evidence is limited, these findings suggest that statins likely impact the oxidative stress mediated by xanthine oxidases.

Mitochondrial Oxidases

Basic work suggests that statins influence mitochondrial function in myocytes. Studies suggest that mitochondrial oxidases contribute to the development of oxidative stress that is harmful to vascular function [42,43]. Jones and coworkers found that simvastatin attenuated rat mitochondrial membrane depolarization – thus improving myocyte survival – in the setting of oxidant stress [44]. Other work has shown an increase in mitochonidral oxidative capacity – reflecting increased mitochondrial biogenesis – in the atrial tissue of human subjects treated with statins [45]. By contrast, in skeletal myocytes there may be a reduction of respiratory chain enzyme activities with statin treatment [45,46]. This pathway has been implicated in statin-inducted myopathy [47].

Non-ROS Oxidative Stress

One pathway of oxidative stress in vascular tissue operates independent of the generation of ROS. Disruption of cellular thiol redox circuits results in cellular injury independent of free radical production [48]. Higher levels of oxidized aminothiol metabolites are associated with worse endothelial dysfunction [49]. Other studies, however, have not demonstrated a clear link to elevated oxidized aminothiol metabolites in diabetes [50]. In subjects with metabolic syndrome or diabetes, the impact of lipophilic atorvastatin versus hydrophilic pravastatin on oxidative stress was compared [51]. On the whole, statin therapy improved aminothiol oxidative stress only in those with increased oxidative stress and reduced endothelial function (measured by flow mediated dilation or FMD) at baseline. These findings suggest that the mechanism of benefit of statins may well involve attenuating this non-free radical component of oxidative stress.

NOS Uncoupling

One important source of vascular oxidative stress in diabetes is the generation of ROS from vascular nitric oxide synthases [52]. In response to the presence of peroxynitrite, these enzymes can become 'uncoupled' from their beneficial production of nitric oxide and begin generating superoxide. Basic work has shown an important impact of statins on this pathway (independent of cholesterol lowering) by increasing the expression and activity of endothelial nitric oxide synthase (eNOS) as well as by enhancing levels of the eNOS cofactor tetrahydrobiopterin (BH4) [53]. Laufs and coworkers demonstrated an increase in eNOS expression via Rho geranylgeranylation in endothelial cells treated with a statin [54]. NO-inhibiting caveolin-1 expression is attenuated by atorvastatin in endothelial cells [55]. Moreover, statins promote NO-enhancing Akt signaling in endothelial cells in response to vascular endothelial growth factor (VEGF) and shear stress [56]. Cofactor BH4 levels are enhanced in endothelial cells exposed to statins via increased expression of GTP cyclohydrolase I (GTPCH-I) – a promoter of eNOS cofactor BH4 [57]. In diabetic rats treatment with atorvastatin has been shown to increase the expression of GTPCH-I, with the downstream effect of improved endothelial function due to decreased vascular superoxide and attenuated eNOS uncoupling [58]. In renal vascular beds of mice with experimental diabetes, pitavastatin likewise decreased nitrotyrosine levels – a marker of NO mediated oxidative stress – and improved proteinuria [59]. Further evidence that statins favorably impact eNOS uncoupling arises from endothelial cell studies in which NO levels improve relative to peroxynitrite after atorvastatin or simvastatin exposure [60].

In human subjects with diabetes, statin therapy reduces plasma nitrotyrosine and other myeloperoxidase-derived and nitric oxide-derived markers, suggesting a mechanism of impact involving this pathway [61]. Moreover, diabetic subjects treated with atorvastatin demonstrate improvement in flow-mediated dilation, as well as decreases in vasoconstrictor endothelin-1 expression, plasminogen activator inhibitor-1, and tissue plasminogen activator [62]. Other studies demonstrate a decrease in the inflammatory markers interleukin-6, and C-reactive protein among diabetic subjects treated with statins [63]. In other measures of diabetic endothelial dysfunction, atorvastatin therapy was associated with attenuating the impairment of high glucose on endothelial-dependent vasodilation in diabetic subjects [64]. This work in total supports the notion that statins imbue a benefit to favorable nitric oxide signaling in vascular tissue, independent of impacting cholesterol levels.

DIABETIC MACROVASCULAR DISEASE: CLINICAL EVIDENCE

Large clinical trials have been conducted to evaluate the clinical impact of statin therapy on patients with known cardiovascular disease, as well in those at increased risk of developing atherosclerosis. None have specifically enrolled subjects with type 2 diabetes alone, although in three major trials large groups of diabetics were randomized to statin versus placebo treatment arms (Table 19.3). From post-hoc analyses of these subjects, insights into the impact of statin therapy on cardiovascular risk reduction can be derived. Given the nature of these studies, however, limited direct conclusions can be drawn about the mechanism of benefit – including the impact on oxidative stress.

TABLE 19.3 Summary of Clinical Trials of Statins in Diabetes

Clinical Trial Name	Study Population	Intervention	Outcome
Heart Protection Study (HPS) [9]	20536 subjects with cardiovascular risk factors, including 5963 diabetics	Simvastatin 40 mg daily versus placebo	22% relative risk reduction in simvastatin-treated diabetics versus placebo
Scandinavian Simvastatin Survival Trial (4S) [65]	4444 subjects with coronary heart disease, including 458 with metabolic syndrome	Simvastatin 40 mg daily versus placebo	48% relative risk reduction versus placebo for metabolic syndrome subjects
Cholesterol and Recurrent Events (CARE) [66]	4159 subjects with coronary heart disease, including 586 diabetics	Pravastatin 40 mg daily versus placebo	25% relative risk reduction versus placebo for diabetics subjects

The Heart Protection Study provided insight into the clinical impact of statin on diabetic vascular disease [9]. Among the 20,536 subjects enrolled in HPS, 5,963 were diabetic. The reduction in the first coronary event, stroke, or revascularization was similar in diabetics allocated to simvastatin therapy in comparison to non-diabetics in the statin arm. Even in the absence of previously diagnosed obstructive atherosclerosis or hypercholesterolemia, diabetics subjects allocated to the simvastatin arm demonstrated a 22% reduction in events versus placebo allocated groups ($p<0.0001$). Simvastatin reduced the incidence of major coronary events by 27% ($p<0.001$), a 25% reduction in strokes, and a 24% reduction in the incidence of revascularization when compared to placebo therapy. Considered differently, simvastatin therapy prevented one major first vascular event for every 20 subjects treated over five years. Notably, statin therapy prevented one recurrent vascular event for every 11 subjects treated over five years. In addition, statin therapy among diabetics was associated with a reduced rate of increase in serum creatinine over the study followup period.

A subgroup analysis of the Scandinavian Simvastatin Survival Study examined the impact of statins in 458 subjects with metabolic syndrome (the hallmark of which is insulin resistance and a predisposition to type 2 diabetes mellitus) [65]. Subjects treated with simvastatin 40 mg daily versus placebo were followed for a mean of 4.9 years for cardiovascular outcomes. The baseline risk of events in this subgroup was higher than that of the study population as a whole, but the benefit of risk reduction was more pronounced (52% versus 14%, $p=0.03$). In the Cholesterol and Recurrent Events study, 40 mg pravastatin daily was associated with a 25% relative reduction in recurrent coronary events over five years in a subgroup of 586 diabetic subjects relative to the larger cohort (which experienced a relative risk reduction of 23%) [66].

DIABETIC MICROVASCULAR DISEASE: CLINICAL EVIDENCE

Diabetic Retinopathy

Building on basic idea that statins attenuate pathologic neovascularization in animal models of diabetic retinopathy, clinical trials have examined the impact of statins on the ophthalmologic complications of diabetes [67]. The Fenofibrate Intervention and Event Lowering in Diabetes study failed to demonstrate a significant reduction in diabetic retinopathy among subjects taking simvastatin alone, although in combination with fenofibrate statin therapy may impact disease progression [68].

Diabetic Nephropathy

Rosuvastatin therapy has been associated with a reduction in albuminuria and oxidative stress as measured by malondialdehyde-modified LDL [69]. Other studies show mixed results with regard to reduction in albuminuria progression [70]. Little efficacy has been shown for statin therapy in reducing progression of diabetic nephropathy in randomized clinical trials of human subjects [71].

Diabetic Neuropathy

Basic work in animal models suggests that statin therapy can attenuate the effects of oxidative stress in diabetic neuropathy and improve NO signaling [72,73]. Observational studies report that statin use is associated with less incident neuropathy in diabetes [74]. A short term improvement in motor conduction velocity has been observed in a small trial of atorvastatin versus placebo among diabetic patients with neuropathy [75]. Other small studies show a benefit for statin therapy versus placebo in subjects with diabetic foot ulcers [76].

SUMMARY AND FUTURE DIRECTIONS

Research from the past several decades has revealed that vascular complications of type 2 diabetes are in large part mediated by oxidative stress. These findings help to account for why therapies that reduce oxidative stress reduce adverse cardiovascular events more than therapeutic strategies of glycemic control alone.

Among these therapies, a central role is presently held by statins. Through direct lowering of plasma cholesterol, statins appear to reduce the burden of oxidative stress exerted by hyperlipidemia. In addition, current work has illustrated mechanisms by which statins influence oxidative stress pathways independently to cholesterol lowering. This includes influencing NADPH oxidases, xanthine oxidases, mitochondrial oxidases, aminothiol metabolism, as well as the important phenomenon of NO uncoupling. Clinical trials of statins have demonstrated the impact of these agents in reducing macrovascular events such as myocardial infarction or stroke. Meanwhile, attenuation of microvascular complications by statins has been modest. Remaining questions include accounting for the lack of robust benefit in retinal, renal, and neurologic microvascular beds. In addition, current work suggests that although statins exhibit a potent class effect in plasma cholesterol reduction, there may be important differences between different statins with regard to their non-cholesterol lowering or 'pleiotropic' effects [77]. Determining the magnitude of these differences and distinguishing whether some statins are uniquely capable of influencing deleterious oxidative stress may yield the next important benefit to patients at risk for diabetic vascular disease.

SUMMARY POINTS

- The pathobiology of vascular disease in type 2 diabetes is likely mediated in part by oxidative stress.
- Sources of oxidative stress are varied and all may not contribute equally to the pathophysiology of diabetic vascular disease.
- Statin drugs exert direct and indirect oxidant effects, independently of their lipid lowering action.
- Subgroups of diabetics in large clinical trials of lipid lowering therapy benefit from statins.
- Evidence is modest supporting an influence of statin therapy on diabetic microvascular disease.

References

[1] Reusch JE, Wang CC. Cardiovascular disease in diabetes: where does glucose fit in? J Clin Endocrinol Metab 2011;96(8):2367–76.

[2] Orasanu G, Plutzky J. The pathologic continuum of diabetic vascular disease. J Am Coll Cardiol 2009;53(5 Suppl.):S35–42.

[3] Nishikawa T, Edelstein D, Du XL, Yamagishi S, Matsumura T, Kaneda Y, et al. Normalizing mitochondrial superoxide production blocks three pathways of hyperglycaemic damage. Nature 2000;404(6779):787–90.

[4] Piga R, Naito Y, Kokura S, Handa O, Yoshikawa T. Short-term high glucose exposure induces monocyte-endothelial cells adhesion and transmigration by increasing VCAM-1 and MCP-1 expression in human aortic endothelial cells. Atherosclerosis 2007;193(2):328–34.

[5] Venugopal SK, Devaraj S, Yang T, Jialal I. Alpha-tocopherol decreases superoxide anion release in human monocytes under hyperglycemic conditions via inhibition of protein kinase C-alpha. Diabetes 2002;51(10):3049–54.

[6] Renard CB, Kramer F, Johansson F, Lamharzi N, Tannock LR, von Herrath MG, et al. Diabetes and diabetes-associated lipid abnormalities have distinct effects on initiation and progression of atherosclerotic lesions. J Clin Invest 2004;114(5):659–68.

[7] Intensive blood-glucose control with sulphonylureas or insulin compared with conventional treatment and risk of complications in patients with type 2 diabetes (UKPDS 33). UK Prospective Diabetes Study (UKPDS) Group. Lancet 1998;352(9131):837–53.

[8] Holman RR, Paul SK, Bethel MA, Matthews DR, Neil HA. 10-year follow-up of intensive glucose control in type 2 diabetes. N Engl J Med 2008;359(15):1577–89.

[9] Collins R, Armitage J, Parish S, Sleigh P, Peto RCINLA. Pmid. MRC/BHF Heart Protection Study of cholesterol-lowering with simvastatin in 5,963 people with diabetes: a randomised placebo-controlled trial. Lancet 2003;361(9374):2005–16.

[10] Alberts AW. Discovery, biochemistry and biology of lovastatin. Am J Cardiol 1988;62(15):10J–5J.

[11] Davignon J. Beneficial cardiovascular pleiotropic effects of statins. Circulation 2004(23 Suppl. 1):III39–43.

[12] Yasunari K, Maeda K, Minami M, Yoshikawa J. HMG-CoA reductase inhibitors prevent migration of human coronary smooth muscle cells through suppression of increase in oxidative stress. Arterioscler Thromb Vasc Biol 2001;21(6):937–42.

[13] LaRosa JC, Grundy SM, Waters DD, Shear C, Barter P, Fruchart JC, et al. Intensive lipid lowering with atorvastatin in patients with stable coronary disease. N Engl J Med 2005;352(14):1425–35.

[14] Wenger NK, Lewis SJ, Herrington DM, Bittner V, Welty FK. Outcomes of using high- or low-dose atorvastatin in patients 65 years of age or older with stable coronary heart disease. Ann Intern Med 2007;147(1):1–9.

[15] Cannon CP, Braunwald E, McCabe CH, Rader DJ, Rouleau JL, Belder R, et al. Intensive versus moderate lipid lowering with statins after acute coronary syndromes. N Engl J Med 2004;350(15):1495–504.

[16] Murphy SA, Cannon CP, Wiviott SD, de Lemos JA, Blazing MA, McCabe CH, et al. Effect of intensive lipid-lowering therapy on mortality after acute coronary syndrome (a patient-level analysis of the Aggrastat to Zocor and Pravastatin or Atorvastatin Evaluation and Infection Therapy-Thrombolysis in Myocardial Infarction 22 trials). Am J Cardiol 2007;100(7):1047–51.

[17] Ky B, Burke A, Tsimikas S, Wolfe ML, Tadesse MG, Szapary PO, et al. The influence of pravastatin and atorvastatin on markers of oxidative stress in hypercholesterolemic humans. J Am Coll Cardiol 2008;51(17):1653–62.

[18] Singh U, Devaraj S, Jialal I, Siegel D. Comparison effect of atorvastatin (10 versus 80 mg) on biomarkers of inflammation and oxidative stress in subjects with metabolic syndrome. Am J Cardiol 2008;102(3):321–5.

[19] Taneva E, Borucki K, Wiens L, Makarova R, Schmidt-Lucke C, Luley C, et al. Early effects on endothelial function of atorvastatin 40 mg twice daily and its withdrawal. Am J Cardiol 2006;97(7):1002–6.

[20] van der Harst P, Wagenaar LJ, Buikema H, Voors AA, Plokker HW, Morshuis WJ, et al. Effect of intensive versus moderate lipid lowering on endothelial function and vascular responsiveness to angiotensin II in stable coronary artery disease. Am J Cardiol 2005;96(10):1361–4.

[21] Mulder DJ, van Haelst PL, Wobbes MH, Gans RO, Zijlstra F, May JF, et al. The effect of aggressive versus conventional lipid-lowering therapy on markers of inflammatory and oxidative stress. Cardiovasc Drugs Ther 2007;21(2):91–7.

[22] Martinez-Gonzalez J, Badimon L. Influence of statin use on endothelial function: from bench to clinics. Curr Pharm Des 2007;13(17):1771–86.
[23] Munzel T, Gori T, Bruno RM, Taddei S. Is oxidative stress a therapeutic target in cardiovascular disease? Eur Heart J 2010;31(22):2741–8.
[24] Antonopoulos AS, Margaritis M, Shirodaria C, Antoniades C. Translating the effects of statins: From redox regulation to suppression of vascular wall inflammation. Thromb Haemost 2012;108(5):840–8.
[25] Hink U, Li H, Mollnau H, Oelze M, Matheis E, Hartmann M, et al. Mechanisms underlying endothelial dysfunction in diabetes mellitus. Circ Res 2001;88(2):E14–22.
[26] Guzik TJ, West NE, Black E, McDonald D, Ratnatunga C, Pillai R, et al. Vascular superoxide production by NAD(P)H oxidase: association with endothelial dysfunction and clinical risk factors. Circ Res 2000;86(9):E85–90.
[27] Tian XY, Wong WT, Xu A, Chen ZY, Lu Y, Liu LM, et al. Rosuvastatin improves endothelial function in db/db mice: role of angiotensin II type 1 receptors and oxidative stress. Br J Pharmacol 2011;164(2b):598–606.
[28] Riad A, Du J, Stiehl S, Westermann D, Mohr Z, Sobirey M, et al. Low-dose treatment with atorvastatin leads to anti-oxidative and anti-inflammatory effects in diabetes mellitus. Eur J Pharmacol 2007;569(3):204–11.
[29] Vecchione C, Gentile MT, Aretini A, Marino G, Poulet R, Maffei A, et al. A novel mechanism of action for statins against diabetes-induced oxidative stress. Diabetologia 2007;50(4):874–80.
[30] Carnevale R, Pignatelli P, Di Santo S, Bartimoccia S, Sanguigni V, Napoleone L, et al. Atorvastatin inhibits oxidative stress via adiponectin-mediated NADPH oxidase down-regulation in hypercholesterolemic patients. Atherosclerosis 2010;213(1):225–34.
[31] Pignatelli P, Carnevale R, Cangemi R, Loffredo L, Sanguigni V, Stefanutti C, et al. Atorvastatin inhibits gp91phox circulating levels in patients with hypercholesterolemia. Arterioscler Thromb Vasc Biol 2010;30(2):360–7.
[32] Antoniades C, Bakogiannis C, Tousoulis D, Reilly S, Zhang MH, Paschalis A, et al. Preoperative atorvastatin treatment in CABG patients rapidly improves vein graft redox state by inhibition of Rac1 and NADPH-oxidase activity. Circulation 2010;122(11 Suppl.):S66–73.
[33] Qian J, Keyes KT, Long B, Chen G, Ye Y. Impact of HMG-CoA reductase inhibition on oxidant-induced injury in human retinal pigment epithelium cells. J Cell Biochem 2011;112(9):2480–9.
[34] Li J, Wang JJ, Yu Q, Chen K, Mahadev K, Zhang SX. Inhibition of reactive oxygen species by Lovastatin downregulates vascular endothelial growth factor expression and ameliorates blood-retinal barrier breakdown in db/db mice: role of NADPH oxidase 4. Diabetes 2010;59(6):1528–38.
[35] Al-Shabrawey M, Bartoli M, El-Remessy AB, Ma G, Matragoon S, Lemtalsi T, et al. Role of NADPH oxidase and Stat3 in statin-mediated protection against diabetic retinopathy. Invest Ophthalmol Vis Sci 2008;49(7):3231–8.
[36] Giunti S, Calkin AC, Forbes JM, Allen TJ, Thomas MC, Cooper ME, et al. The pleiotropic actions of rosuvastatin confer renal benefits in the diabetic Apo-E knockout mouse. Am J Physiol Renal Physiol 2010;299(3):F528–35.
[37] Whaley-Connell A, Habibi J, Nistala R, Cooper SA, Karuparthi PR, Hayden MR, et al. Attenuation of NADPH oxidase activation and glomerular filtration barrier remodeling with statin treatment. Hypertension 2008;51(2):474–80.
[38] Whaley-Connell A, DeMarco VG, Lastra G, Manrique C, Nistala R, Cooper SA, et al. Insulin resistance, oxidative stress, and podocyte injury: role of rosuvastatin modulation of filtration barrier injury. Am J Nephrol 2008;28(1):67–75.
[39] Fujii M, Inoguchi T, Maeda Y, Sasaki S, Sawada F, Saito R, et al. Pitavastatin ameliorates albuminuria and renal mesangial expansion by downregulating NOX4 in db/db mice. Kidney Int 2007;72(4):473–80.
[40] Imaeda A, Tanigawa T, Aoki T, Kondo Y, Nakamura N, Yoshikawa T. Antioxidative effects of fluvastatin and its metabolites against oxidative DNA damage in mammalian cultured cells. Free Radic Res 2001;35(6):789–801.
[41] Greig D, Alcaino H, Castro PF, Garcia L, Verdejo HE, Navarro M, et al. Xanthine-oxidase inhibitors and statins in chronic heart failure: effects on vascular and functional parameters. J Heart Lung Transplant 2011;30(4):408–13.
[42] Rojas A, Figueroa H, Morales MA, Re L. Facing up the ROS labyrinth – Where to go? Curr vasc pharmacol 2006;4(3):277–89.
[43] Ramachandran A, Levonen AL, Brookes PS, Ceaser E, Shiva S, Barone MC, et al. Mitochondria, nitric oxide, and cardiovascular dysfunction. Free radic biol med 2002;33(11):1465–74.
[44] Jones SP, Teshima Y, Akao M, Marban E. Simvastatin attenuates oxidant-induced mitochondrial dysfunction in cardiac myocytes. Circ Res 2003;93(8):697–9.
[45] Bouitbir J, Charles AL, Echaniz-Laguna A, Kindo M, Daussin F, Auwerx J, et al. Opposite effects of statins on mitochondria of cardiac and skeletal muscles: a 'mitohormesis' mechanism involving reactive oxygen species and PGC-1. Eur Heart J 2012;33(11):1397–407.
[46] Paiva H, Thelen KM, Van Coster R, Smet J, De Paepe B, Mattila KM, et al. High-dose statins and skeletal muscle metabolism in humans: a randomized, controlled trial. Clin Pharmacol Ther 2005;78(1):60–8.
[47] Duncan AJ, Hargreaves IP, Damian MS, Land JM, Heales SJ. Decreased ubiquinone availability and impaired mitochondrial cytochrome oxidase activity associated with statin treatment. Toxicol mech methods 2009;19(1):44–50.
[48] Jones DP. Radical-free biology of oxidative stress. Am J Physiol Cell Physiol 2008;295(4):C849–68.
[49] Ashfaq S, Abramson JL, Jones DP, Rhodes SD, Weintraub WS, Hooper WC, et al. Endothelial function and aminothiol biomarkers of oxidative stress in healthy adults. Hypertension 2008;52(1):80–5.
[50] Houze P, Gamra S, Madelaine I, Bousquet B, Gourmel B. Simultaneous determination of total plasma glutathione, homocysteine, cysteinylglycine, and methionine by high-performance liquid chromatography with electrochemical detection. J clin lab anal 2001;15(3):144–53.
[51] Murrow JR, Sher S, Ali S, Uphoff I, Patel R, Porkert M, et al. The differential effect of statins on oxidative stress and endothelial function: atorvastatin versus pravastatin. J clin lipidol 2012;6(1):42–9.
[52] Forstermann U. Nitric oxide and oxidative stress in vascular disease. Pflugers Arch 2010;459(6):923–39.
[53] Forstermann U, Sessa WC. Nitric oxide synthases: regulation and function. Eur Heart J 2012;33(7):829–37; 37a-37d.
[54] Laufs U, Liao JK. Post-transcriptional regulation of endothelial nitric oxide synthase mRNA stability by Rho GTPase. J biol chem 1998;273(37):24266–71.
[55] Feron O, Dessy C, Desager JP, Balligand JLCINCJ. Pmid. Hydroxy-methylglutaryl-coenzyme A reductase inhibition promotes endothelial nitric oxide synthase activation through a decrease in caveolin abundance. Circulation 2001;103(1):113–8.
[56] Kureishi Y, Luo Z, Shiojima I, Bialik A, Fulton D, Lefer DJ, et al. The HMG-CoA reductase inhibitor simvastatin activates the protein kinase Akt and promotes angiogenesis in normocholesterolemic animals. Nat Med 2000;6(9):1004–10.
[57] Hattori Y, Nakanishi N, Akimoto K, Yoshida M, Kasai K. HMG-CoA reductase inhibitor increases GTP cyclohydrolase I mRNA and tetrahydrobiopterin in vascular endothelial cells. Arterioscler Thromb Vasc Biol 2003;23(2):176–82.

[58] Wenzel P, Daiber A, Oelze M, Brandt M, Closs E, Xu J, et al. Mechanisms underlying recoupling of eNOS by HMG-CoA reductase inhibition in a rat model of streptozotocin-induced diabetes mellitus. Atherosclerosis 2008;198(1):65–76.
[59] Matsumoto M, Tanimoto M, Gohda T, Aoki T, Murakoshi M, Yamada K, et al. Effect of pitavastatin on type 2 diabetes mellitus nephropathy in KK-Ay/Ta mice. Metabolism 2008;57(5):691–7.
[60] Heeba G, Hassan MK, Khalifa M, Malinski T. Adverse balance of nitric oxide/peroxynitrite in the dysfunctional endothelium can be reversed by statins. J Cardiovasc Pharmacol 2007;50(4):391–8.
[61] Shishehbor MH, Brennan ML, Aviles RJ, Fu X, Penn MS, Sprecher DL, et al. Statins promote potent systemic antioxidant effects through specific inflammatory pathways. Circulation 2003;108(4):426–31.
[62] Economides PA, Caselli A, Tiani E, Khaodhiar L, Horton ES, Veves A. The effects of atorvastatin on endothelial function in diabetic patients and subjects at risk for type 2 diabetes. J Clin Endocrinol Metab 2004;89(2):740–7.
[63] Tousoulis D, Antoniades C, Vasiliadou C, Kourtellaris P, Koniari K, Marinou K, et al. Effects of atorvastatin and vitamin C on forearm hyperaemic blood flow, asymmentrical dimethylarginine levels and the inflammatory process in patients with type 2 diabetes mellitus. Heart (British Cardiac Society) 2007;93(2):244–6.
[64] Tousoulis D, Koniari K, Antoniades C, Miliou A, Noutsou M, Nikolopoulou A, et al. Impact of 6 weeks of treatment with low-dose metformin and atorvastatin on glucose-induced changes of endothelial function in adults with newly diagnosed type 2 diabetes mellitus: A single-blind study. Clin Ther 2010;32(10):1720–8.
[65] Ballantyne CM, Olsson AG, Cook TJ, Mercuri MF, Pedersen TR, Kjekshus JCINCJ, et al. Influence of low high-density lipoprotein cholesterol and elevated triglyceride on coronary heart disease events and response to simvastatin therapy in 4S. Circulation 2001;104(25):3046–51.
[66] Goldberg RB, Mellies MJ, Sacks FM, Moye LA, Howard BV, Howard WJ, et al. Cardiovascular events and their reduction with pravastatin in diabetic and glucose-intolerant myocardial infarction survivors with average cholesterol levels: subgroup analyses in the cholesterol and recurrent events (CARE) trial. The Care Investigators. Circulation 1998;98(23):2513–9.
[67] Medina RJ, O'Neill CL, Devine AB, Gardiner TA, Stitt AW. The pleiotropic effects of simvastatin on retinal microvascular endothelium has important implications for ischaemic retinopathies. PloS one 2008;3(7):e2584.
[68] Klein BECONNEJMJ. Pmid. Reduction in risk of progression c diabetic retinopathy. N Engl J Med 2010;363(3):287–8.
[69] Abe M, Maruyama N, Okada K, Matsumoto S, Matsumoto K Soma M. Effects of lipid-lowering therapy with rosuvastatin on kidney function and oxidative stress in patients with diabetic nephropathy. J Atheroscler Thromb 2011;18(11):1018–28.
[70] Tonolo G, Ciccarese M, Brizzi P, Puddu L, Secchi G, Calvia P, et al Reduction of albumin excretion rate in normotensive microalbuminuric type 2 diabetic patients during long-term simvastatin treatment. Diabetes Care 1997;20(12):1891–5.
[71] Rutter MK, Prais HR, Charlton-Menys V, Gittins M, Roberts C Davies RR, et al. Protection Against Nephropathy in Diabetes with Atorvastatin (PANDA): a randomized double-blind placebo-controlled trial of high- vs. low-dose atorvastatin(1). Diabet Med 2011;28(1):100–8.
[72] Gurpinar T, Ekerbicer N, Harzadin NU, Barut T, Tarakci F, Tuglu MI. Statin treatment reduces oxidative stress-associated apoptosis of sciatic nerve in diabetes mellitus. Biotech Histochem 2011;86(6):373–8.
[73] Ii M, Nishimura H, Kusano KF, Qin G, Yoon YS, Wecker A, et al. Neuronal nitric oxide synthase mediates statin-induced restoration of vasa nervorum and reversal of diabetic neuropathy. Circulation 2005;112(1):93–102.
[74] Davis TM, Yeap BB, Davis WA, Bruce DG. Lipid-lowering therapy and peripheral sensory neuropathy in type 2 diabetes: the Fremantle Diabetes Study. Diabetologia 2008;51(4):562–6.
[75] Zangiabadi N, Shafiee K, Alavi KH, Assadi AR, Damavandi M. Atorvastatin treatment improves diabetic polyneuropathy electrophysiological changes in non-insulin dependent diabetic patients: a double blind, randomized clinical trial. Minerva endocrinologica 2012;37(2):195–200.
[76] Johansen OE, Birkeland KI, Jorgensen AP, Orvik E, Sorgard B, Torjussen BR, et al. Diabetic foot ulcer burden may be modified by high-dose atorvastatin: A 6-month randomized controlled pilot trial. J diabetes 2009;1(3):182–7.
[77] Mason RP, Walter MF, Day CA, Jacob RF. Intermolecular differences of 3-hydroxy-3-methylglutaryl coenzyme a reductase inhibitors contribute to distinct pharmacologic and pleiotropic actions. Am J Cardiol 2005;96(5A):11F–23F.

CHAPTER

20

Resveratrol and Cerebral Arterioles during Type 1 Diabetes

William G. Mayhan, Denise M. Arrick

Department of Cellular Biology and Anatomy, and Center of Excellence in Cardiovascular Diseases and Sciences, Louisiana State University Health Sciences Center-Shreveport, Shreveport, LA, USA

List of Abbreviations

ADP Adenosine 5′-diphosphate
BH_4 Tetrahydrobiopterin
eNOS Endothelial nitric oxide synthase
GADPH glyceraldehyde 3-phosphate dehydrogenase
NADPH nicotinamide adenine dinucleotide phosphate
NMDA N-methyl-D-aspartic acid
nNOS Neuronal nitric oxide synthase
NOS nitric oxide synthase
Nrf2 NFE2-related factor 2
PARP Poly(ADP-ribose) polymerase
SIRT1 Silent information regulator 2/Sirtuin-1
SOD-1 Superoxide dismutase 1
Copper/zinc superoxide dismutase
SOD-2 Superoxide dismutase 2
Manganese superoxide dismutase
T1D Type 1 diabetes
T2D Type 2 diabetes

INTRODUCTION

Based upon statistics released in the 2011 National Diabetes Fact Sheet, diabetes (type 1 and type 2) affects nearly 26 million children and adults in the United States [1]. In addition, close to 80 million people exhibit signs of pre-diabetes. Diabetes is listed as the seventh leading cause of death, with over 71,000 death certificates listing diabetes as the underlying cause of death and another 160,000 death certificates listing diabetes as a contributing factor in premature death. Predictions suggest that 300 million people will be diagnosed with diabetes by the year 2025, making diabetes a major pandemic worldwide. The estimated cost of diabetes in the United States is $174 billion per year, with $116 billion per year for direct medical costs and $58 billion per year for disability, work loss and premature mortality related to diabete [1,2]. Although the incidence of type 1 diabetes (T1D) is less than type 2 diabetes (T2D), estimates suggest that over 3 million people in the United States have T1D, with an additional 30,000 individuals per year being diagnosed with it [2]. While the number of individuals with T1D is less than that for T2D, the economic burden per case of diabetes is greater for T1D than for T2D. Although T1D accounts for less than 6% of diagnosed cases, it accounts for about 9% of excess medical costs associated with diagnosed diabetes and about 8% of excess loss of productivity costs [2]. In addition, the average total cost per case for T2D per year is relatively constant (in a range of $9,200 to $9,700). However, this average total cost per case for T1D per year increases dramatically with age (from about $4,000 in young individuals to well over $35,000 for individuals 65 and older) [2]. Thus, the average economic burden per person with diabetes appears to be much greater for T1D than for T2D.

Hyperglycemia associated with T1D produces long-term damage to many organ systems including the heart, kidneys, brain, eyes and nerves, and is a major cause of morbidity and mortality in children and adults. The damaging effects of T1D appear to be related to the formation of reactive oxygen species, i.e., an increase in oxidative stress. Many studies have shown that T1D affects endothelial cell function in peripheral blood vessels by influencing the generation of nitric oxide via nitric oxide synthase (NOS), and/or via the formation of reactive oxygen species to inactivate nitric oxide [3,4]. In addition to peripheral organ systems and peripheral blood vessels, the brain and blood vessels within the

Diabetes: Oxidative Stress and Dietary Antioxidants.
http://dx.doi.org/10.1016/B978-0-12-405885-9.00020-6

brain are very susceptible to the damaging effects of hyperglycemia-induced increases in oxidative stress in T1D [5]. Further, the risk of stroke is significantly higher in diabetics than in non-diabetics and the mortality following a stroke is significantly higher in diabetics compared to non-diabetics [6]. We suggest that alterations in reactivity of cerebral resistance blood vessels may have important implications for the pathogenesis of cognitive decline and/or stroke during a variety of disease states, including T1D.

Many naturally occurring compounds are capable of ameliorating oxidative stress in blood vessels to produce an increase in overall vascular health during a variety of disease states, including T1D. One such compound is resveratrol. Resveratrol (3,4′,5-trihydroxystilbene) is found in many dietary plants, and it is a phytoalexin present in grapes and red wines. It has been reported to have a variety of pharmacological effects, including anti-inflammatory, anticarcinogenic, and antioxidant properties, and inhibition of platelet aggregation/adherence [7–10]. Several investigators have shown that resveratrol has both acute and chronic influences on organ systems [11,12] and the endothelial function of large peripheral blood vessels during T1D [13,14]. The mechanisms that account for the effects of resveratrol on vascular function are varied, but appear to involve an increase in the expression of eNOS, an increase in the expression of antioxidant pathways and pathways that might regulate antioxidant responses in cells (including silent information regulator 2/sirtuin-1 [SIRT1] and NFE2-related factor 2 [Nrf2]), and/or a decrease in the expression of endothelin (ET-1) [8,14–17]. Thus, resveratrol can limit oxidative stress and restore nitric oxide bioavailability, to preserve NOS-dependent reactivity of large peripheral blood vessels.

This review will focus on the influence of T1D on the eNOS- and nNOS-dependent responses of cerebral arterioles, the role of oxidative stress in impairing the function of cerebral arterioles, and the influence of resveratrol on cerebral arterioles in T1D. We suggest that the findings presented in this review may indicate an important therapeutic potential for resveratrol in treating T1D-induced cerebrovascular dysfunction, including vascular cognitive impairment and/or stroke.

OXIDATIVE STRESS AND IMPAIRED CEREBROVASCULAR FUNCTION IN T1D

While it is well beyond the scope of this review to discuss all of the cellular pathways/networks that could potentially contribute to cerebrovascular dysfunction in T1D, it is important to comment on a few of them, since resveratrol may directly or indirectly influence the formation of oxidants via their action. Numerous studies have reported that T1D induces oxidative stress in a variety of tissues, including the brain. In addition, impaired NOS-dependent dilation of peripheral blood vessels [3] and cerebral blood vessels [18] in T1D can be alleviated, and in some cases restored, by treatment with agents that scavenge oxygen radicals, in particular superoxide anions. However, the void in our knowledge centers upon an understanding of the potential cellular pathways/networks that may be responsible for the formation of superoxide anions during T1D and the potential influence of resveratrol on these oxidant-producing pathways/networks.

There are several cellular pathways/networks that produce superoxide and/or are activated by superoxide, and thus could potentially contribute to vascular dysfunction during T1D; including mitochondrial respiration, the arachidonic acid cascade (lipoxygenase and cyclooxygenase pathways), poly(ADP-ribose) polymerase (PARP), protein kinase C, eNOS, and nicotinamide adenine dinucleotide phosphate (NADPH) oxidase. Although the precise role of each of these pathways/networks has not been extensively examined for cerebral resistance blood vessels during T1D, several lines of evidence, from our laboratory and others, have suggested that many of them may play a critical role in cerebrovascular dysfunction in T1D. In early studies, we [19] found that inhibition of the cyclooxygenase pathway with indomethacin and inhibition of the thromboxane A_2-prostaglandin H_2 receptor with SQ 29548 could restore impaired eNOS-dependent responses of cerebral arterioles observed in diabetic rats towards that observed in non-diabetic rats. These findings suggested a role for the activation of the cyclooxygenase pathway, via the formation of oxidative stress and/or the production of a constrictor substance, in impaired cerebrovascular function during T1D.

Other studies, by Pelligrino et al. [20], report that impaired eNOS-dependent reactivity of pial arterioles in diabetic rats could be alleviated by acute treatment with staurosporine, suggesting a potential role for the activation of protein kinase C and/or the production of superoxide anion via activation of protein kinase C. Under certain conditions eNOS can become uncoupled, leading to the production of superoxide anion and peroxynitrite [21,22]. Once formed, peroxynitrite can oxidize tetrahydrobiopterin (BH_4) to produce dihydrobiopterin. Under conditions of BH_4 deficiency eNOS is in an uncoupled state and electrons flowing from the eNOS reductase domain to the oxygenase domain are diverted to molecular oxygen rather than to L-arginine [21], resulting in the production of superoxide rather than nitric oxide. Treatment of diabetic rats and type II diabetic humans with BH_4 improves impaired NOS-dependent dilation of peripheral blood vessels [23], but no studies that we are aware of have examined the benefits of BH_4 supplementation on reactivity of cerebral blood vessels in T1D. Thus, while an uncoupling of eNOS may be a viable source of superoxide, there is a lack of information regarding whether such an uncoupling is relevant to impaired NOS-dependent reactivity of cerebral vessels in T1D.

Poly(ADP-ribose) polymerase (PARP) is a nuclear enzyme that participates in DNA repair [24]. An increase in oxidant production, as seen in T1D, can induce cell injury and lead to the activation of PARP [25], thereby resulting in a cascade of events leading to cellular dysfunction [24,25]. Investigators [26] have reported an increase in the activation of PARP in hearts of diabetic rats and mice. This increased activity was associated with cardiac dysfunction and a decrease in NOS-dependent reactivity of the thoracic aorta. Others [25,27] also report that T1D-induced endothelial dysfunction of the thoracic aorta could be prevented by treatment with an inhibitor of PARP (PJ-34). We also found that inhibition of PARP with PJ-34 could restore impaired NOS-dependent reactivity of cerebral arterioles in T1D [28]. Thus, it appears that activation of PARP via an increase in oxidative stress may be a viable mechanism by which T1D impairs the NOS-dependent reactivity of cerebral arterioles.

NADPH oxidase is a multi-component enzyme complex that includes membrane- and cytosolic-associated subunits, and activation of NADPH oxidase contributes to the production of reactive oxygen species. Activation of NADPH has been implicated in a variety of disease states, including T1D and T2D. In a previous study [29] we found that inhibition of NADPH oxidase with apocynin alleviated impaired eNOS-dependent reactivity of cerebral arterioles in T1D, and inhibited superoxide formation in parietal cortex tissue obtained from diabetic rats. Thus, NADPH oxidase may be a viable source of superoxide formation in cerebral arterioles during T1D. However, the precise cellular pathway underlying increased NADPH oxidase subunit expression in T1D remains uncertain. One possibility is that angiotensin II plays a critical role. Stimulation of vascular smooth muscle cells with angiotensin II, thrombin, lipopolysaccharide and cytokines increases the activity of NADPH oxidase and the production of oxygen radicals [30–32]. Tissue and plasma levels of angiotensin converting enzyme, and thus angiotensin II, are elevated in diabetics [33,34], and since angiotensin II has been shown to activate NADPH oxidase [35], it seems reasonable that the formation of superoxide in T1D may be related to angiotensin II-induced stimulation of NADPH oxidase. In support of this concept, studies have shown that treatment of diabetic subjects with angiotensin-converting enzyme inhibitors improve impaired NOS-dependent responses of large peripheral blood vessels [36]. In addition, we have shown that treatment of diabetic rats with enalapril and losartan can alleviate impaired NOS-dependent responses of cerebral arterioles [37,38].

In summary, there are numerous cellular pathways/networks that can be activated by T1D to produce an increase in oxidative stress. Further, increases in oxidative stress can, in turn, activate or inactivate other cellular pathways/networks that could contribute to dysfunction of cerebral arterioles during T1D. We suggest that a dysfunction in dilator and constrictor properties of cerebral arterioles, vessels that directly regulate blood flow to various regions of the brain, via an increase in oxidative stress may be a contributing factor in the pathogenesis of T1D-induced complications of the brain, including vascular cognitive impairment and/or stroke. We speculate that resveratrol may exert an influence on one or more of these cellular pathways/networks (as outlined below) to protect a number of organ systems, including the brain, from the damaging effects of T1D.

INFLUENCE OF RESVERATROL ON VASCULAR FUNCTION

Many studies have reported that resveratrol can provide protection for the heart [17], kidney [39], and may inhibit carcinogenesis [40]. Others also have reported that resveratrol may alleviate or restore impaired vascular function of large peripheral blood vessels during type 1 [13,14] and type 2 [41] diabetes. Silan [13] reported that treatment of diabetic rats with resveratrol prevented impaired relaxation of the aorta to acetylcholine, presumably via an influence of resveratrol on oxidative stress.

In order to examine whether the protective effects of resveratrol extended to resistance arterioles in the brain, we examined the responses of cerebral (pial) arterioles *in vivo* to an NOS-dependent agonists (adenosine 5′-diphosphate [ADP] and N-methyl-D-aspartic acid [NMDA]) in non-diabetic and diabetic rats [42]. ADP appears to dilate cerebral arterioles via activation of eNOS [43]. However, others have suggested that relaxation of the rat middle cerebral artery to purines is related, in part, to nitric oxide and to the synthesis/release of an endothelium derived hyperpolarizing factor (EDHF) [44]. We found that dilation of cerebral arterioles in response to ADP (Figure 20.1) was less in diabetic rats than in non-diabetic rats [42]. In addition, although treatment with resveratrol (10 mg/kg/day for 4–6 weeks) did not influence the reactivity of cerebral arterioles to ADP in non-diabetic rats, resveratrol restored the impaired responses of cerebral arterioles observed in diabetic rats to ADP.

Our findings with ADP may have important clinical significance. Platelets contain large amounts of ADP, serotonin and thromboxane. When a thrombus forms in the lumen of a cerebral blood vessel and platelets aggregate on the thrombus, the release of ADP would normally produce vasodilation, so that cerebral blood

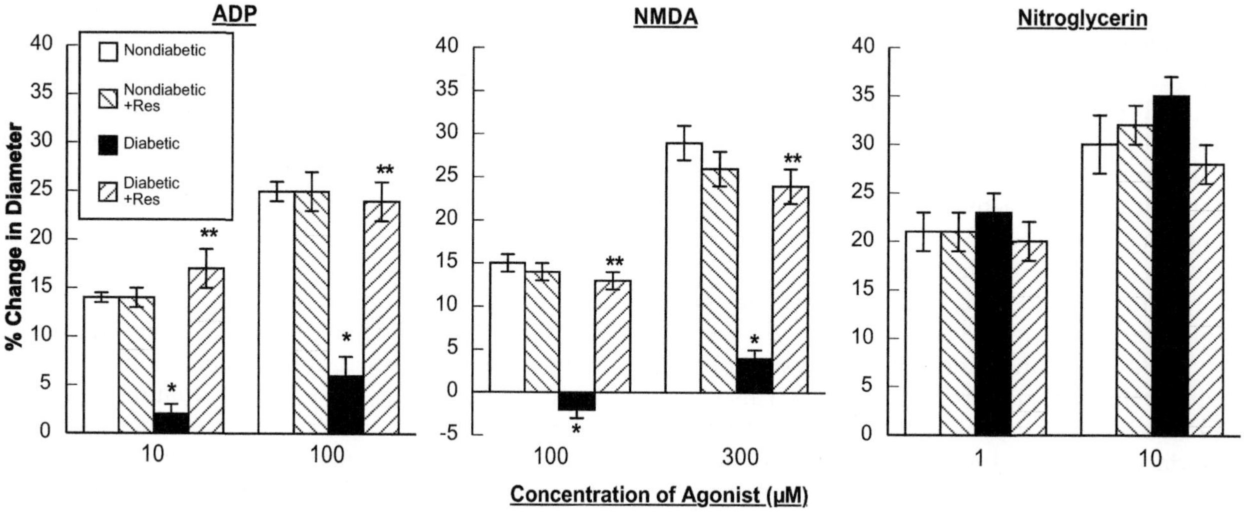

FIGURE 20.1 **Reactivity of cerebral arterioles.** Responses of cerebral (pial) arterioles to ADP, NMDA and nitroglycerin in non-diabetic, resveratrol-treated non-diabetic, diabetic and resveratrol-treated diabetic rats. Values are means ± SE. * $p<0.05$ versus response in control non-diabetic rats. ** $p<0.05$ versus response in control diabetic rats. *With permission from [42].*

flow could increase or at least be maintained in spite of the thrombus. However, in the case of T1D, when endothelial function is impaired, the release of ADP by aggregating platelets would not produce vasodilation, and cerebral blood flow would not be maintained and/or increased during potential changes in metabolic demand. This concept is supported by findings from a previous study showing that platelets from diabetic subjects have an impaired ability to produce relaxation of the carotid artery in rabbits [45]. Further, since vasoconstriction in response to serotonin and thromboxane would presumably be maintained, or more likely increased, cerebral blood flow would suffer. This scenario would lead to cerebral ischemic injury and perhaps stroke.

Next, we examined responses to NMDA. We and others have shown that NMDA dilates cerebral arterioles via the activation of nNOS and the subsequent release of nitric oxide [46,47]. We found that NMDA produced dilation of cerebral arterioles in non-diabetic and diabetic rats (Figure 20.1). However, the magnitude of vasodilation was less in diabetic than in non-diabetic rats. In addition, while resveratrol did not influence reactivity of cerebral arterioles to NMDA in non-diabetic rats, it restored impaired responses in diabetic rats to that observed in non-diabetic rats. In contrast to findings with ADP and NMDA, responses of cerebral arterioles to nitroglycerin were not different between the various groups of rats, and were not influenced by treatment with resveratrol (Figure 20.1). Since NMDA activates glutamate receptor subtypes to produce dilation of cerebral arteries and arterioles to increase cerebral blood flow, our finding that T1D impairs responses to NMDA may have important clinical significance. Diabetes leads to cognitive impairment [48]. Although the mechanisms by which this occurs are not clear, it is possible that altered vascular function may be a key predictor in its development. An understanding of the coupling between cerebral blood vessels, cerebral blood flow, neurons and astrocytes, i.e., neurovascular coupling, appears to be a critical step in the treatment of altered brain function during disease states, including diabetes. Thus, our studies depicting impaired eNOS- and nNOS-dependent vascular function in T1D may have important translational significance to mechanisms responsible for cerebral functional impairment in patients with T1D.

Studies have been conducted to examine the metabolic/cellular/molecular mechanisms by which resveratrol may play a protective role in blood vessels and organ systems. Roghani and Baluchnejadmojarad [14] found that chronic resveratrol treatment prevented T1D-induced impairment in relaxation of the thoracic aorta in rats via its metabolic (hypoglycemic and/or hypolipidemic) and/or antioxidant properties. In addition, others have reported that resveratrol decreases blood glucose concentration and oxidant status in diabetic rats [49]. In our study, we [42] found a small but significant decrease in blood glucose concentration in diabetic rats treated with resveratrol (Figure 20.2). However, we did not find an influence of resveratrol on blood glucose concentration in non-diabetic rats. In addition, treatment with resveratrol did not influence baseline diameter of pial arterioles in or between non-diabetic and diabetic rats. We also examined superoxide levels in brain tissue obtained from rats treated with resveratrol [42]. We found that basal superoxide levels were higher in brain tissue obtained from diabetic compared to non-diabetic rats (Figure 20.3). In addition, in non-diabetic rats we found that basal levels of superoxide in cortex

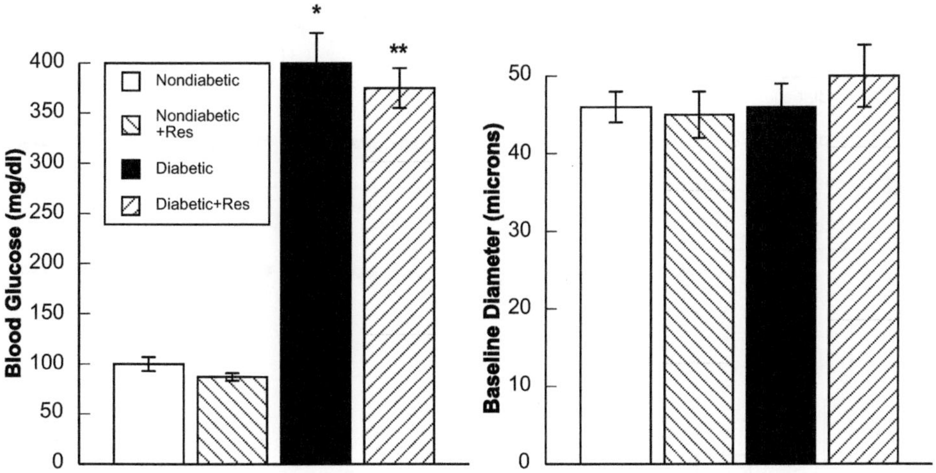

FIGURE 20.2 **Blood glucose and vascular diameter.** Blood glucose concentration and baseline diameter of cerebral (pial) arterioles in non-diabetic, resveratrol-treated non-diabetic, diabetic and resveratrol-treated diabetic rats. Values are means ± SE. * $p<0.05$ versus non-diabetic rats. ** $p<0.05$ versus diabetic rats. *With permission from [42].*

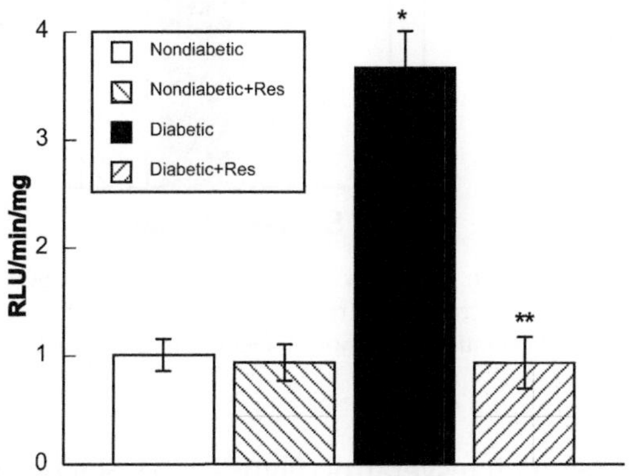

FIGURE 20.3 **Oxidative stress status.** Superoxide production by brain cortex tissue in non-diabetic, resveratrol-treated non-diabetic, diabetic and resveratrol-treated diabetic rats under basal conditions. Values are means ± SE. * $p<0.05$ versus control non-diabetic rats. ** $p<0.05$ versus diabetic rats. *With permission from [42].*

tissue were not influenced by treatment with resveratrol. In contrast, treatment with resveratrol restored basal levels of superoxide in diabetic rats to that observed in non-diabetic rats. Thus, superoxide levels are elevated by T1D and resveratrol is able to inhibit this increase in superoxide.

We suggest that, although it is conceivable that the small change in blood glucose concentration produced by resveratrol in diabetic rats could contribute to the improvement in eNOS- and nNOS-dependent responses of cerebral arterioles, it is more likely that the beneficial influence of resveratrol may be related to its ability to limit oxidative stress. This would restore nitric oxide bioavailability and preserve NOS-dependent reactivity of cerebral arterioles. However, what remains to be determined is the precise mechanism by which resveratrol may limit oxidative damage to cerebral arterioles and which cellular pathway(s)/network(s) in the neurovascular unit are influenced by resveratrol.

Others are beginning to examine the influence of resveratrol on various cellular pathways/networks and transcription factors that may regulate oxidant/antioxidant pathways/networks and/or nitric oxide bioavailability in peripheral organ systems. Some workers [50] have shown that resveratrol has significant anti-inflammatory properties. Since diabetes may increase pro-inflammatory agents, such as TNF-α, it is possible that it may decrease the activity of pro-inflammatory pathways to influence vascular function. Support for this concept can be found in a recent study [41] which reported that resveratrol inhibited TNF-α-induced activation of NADPH oxidase and improved endothelial function in the aorta of T2D mice.

Since an increase in oxidative stress via activation of several cellular pathways may be critical for vascular dysfunction in T1D, investigators have examined the influence of resveratrol on pathways that lead to an increase in oxidative stress. Studies have shown that resveratrol can reduce the activation of PARP, thereby decrease oxidative stress and cellular DNA damage [51]. In addition, resveratrol has been shown to reduce protein kinase C activity [52]. Thus, if T1D stimulates the production of superoxide via the activation of PARP and/or protein kinase C, it may act by inhibiting the hyperglycemia-induced activation of these key pathways/networks. Some studies have suggested that T1D (i.e., hyperglycemia) may increase the formation of reactive oxygen species via an effect on mitochondria and the electron transport chain [53,54]. Resveratrol has been shown to inhibit complex III of the electron transport chain [8], reduce mitochondrial production of reactive oxygen species [55] and improve MnSOD (SOD 2) function in T2D [56]. Thus, since the damaging influence of

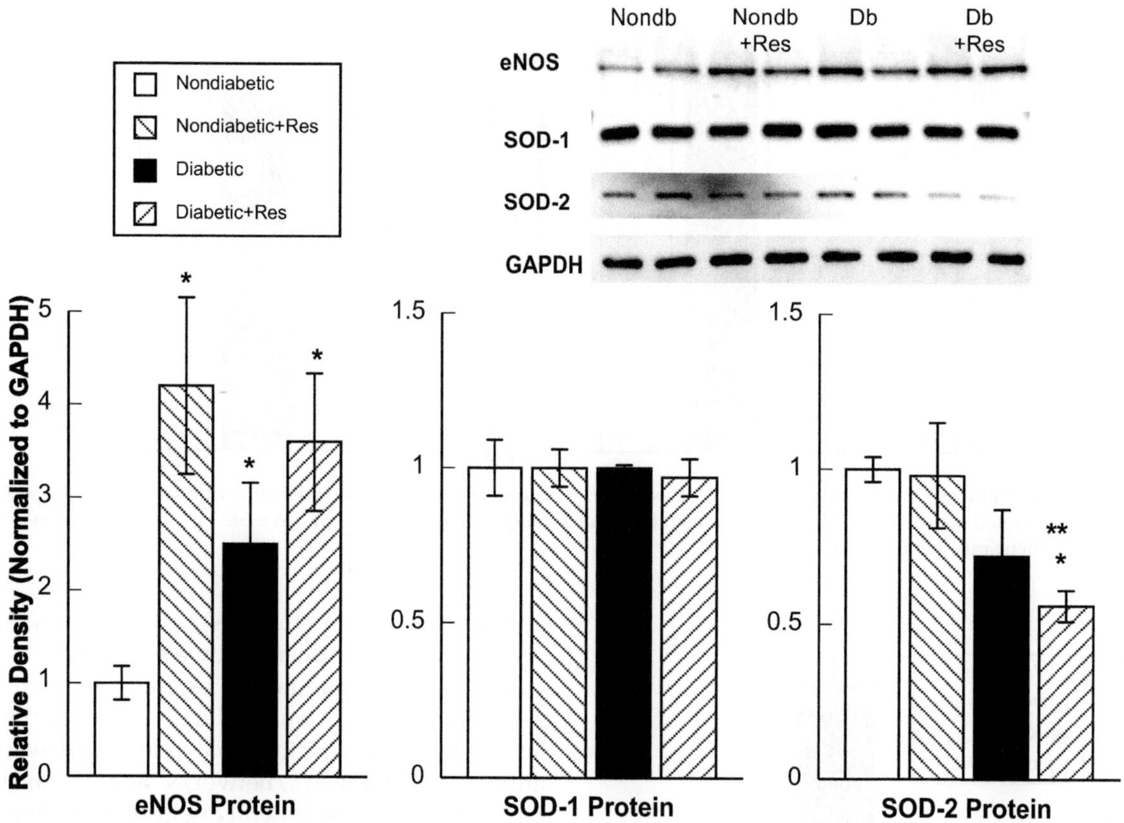

FIGURE 20.4 **Protein levels of eNOS and antioxidants in cerebral microvessels.** Western blot analysis of eNOS, SOD-1 and SOD-2 proteins (normalized to glyceraldehyde 3-phosphate dehydrogenase GAPDH) from cerebral microvessels from non-diabetic, resveratrol-treated non-diabetic, diabetic and resveratrol-treated diabetic rats. Values are means ± SE. * $p < 0.05$ versus control non-diabetic rats and ** $p < 0.05$ versus resveratrol-treated non-diabetic rats. *With permission from [42].*

oxidative stress during T1D may be the result of superoxide produced via the mitochondrial electron transport chain, it is conceivable that resveratrol may be beneficial by inhibiting superoxide generation via this pathway.

Finally, resveratrol may play a beneficial role during T1D by influencing a transcription factor that could alter the expression of eNOS and pathways that might regulate antioxidant responses in cells (including SIRT1 and Nrf2) [15,57]. This concept is supported by studies that have shown that T1D leads to a decrease in Nrf2, which would promote a decrease in nitric oxide production via eNOS and a decrease in the expression of several antioxidant enzymes including superoxide dismutase, catalase, heme oxygenase-1 and NADPH quinone oxireductase [58,59].

In our studies [42], we have begun to examine the role of various enzyme systems in impaired cerebrovascular function in T1D and the influence of resveratrol on these enzyme systems. We examined eNOS, nNOS, SOD-1 and SOD-2 protein levels in cerebral arterioles and brain tissue in non-diabetic and diabetic rats treated with resveratrol. Regarding cerebral arterioles, we found that eNOS protein was elevated by resveratrol in non-diabetic rats, elevated in diabetic rats, and elevated in diabetic rats treated with resveratrol (Figure 20.4). SOD-1 protein was not altered by T1D or treatment with resveratrol. SOD-2 protein expression was similar in non-diabetic rats, regardless of treatment with resveratrol. However, SOD-2 protein expression was significantly decreased in diabetic rats treated with resveratrol when compared to non-diabetic rats and non-diabetic rats treated with resveratrol, but not to diabetic rats. Thus, T1D and treatment of non-diabetic rats with resveratrol produce an increase in eNOS protein expression, there is no change in SOD-1 protein expression by resveratrol or T1D, and resveratrol treatment decreases SOD-2 protein expression in diabetic rats when compared to non-diabetic rats and non-diabetic rats treated with resveratrol.

Finally, we [42] examined nNOS, SOD-1 and SOD-2 protein levels in parietal cortex tissue in the four groups of rats (Figure 20.5). We found that nNOS protein was increased by resveratrol treatment in non-diabetic rats, was increased in control diabetic rats, and was increased in diabetic rats treated with resveratrol when compared to control non-diabetic rats. However, the increase in nNOS protein in diabetic rats treated with resveratrol was not significantly different to that observed in diabetic rats. Similar to our findings using cerebral

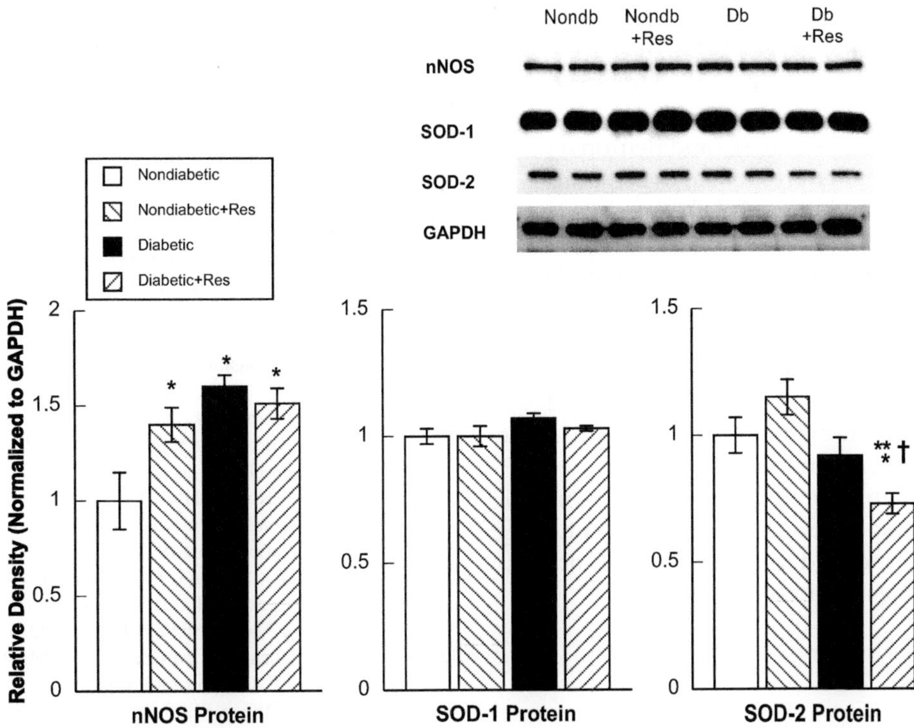

FIGURE 20.5 **Protein levels of nNOS and antioxidants in brain tissue.** Western blot analysis of nNOS, SOD-1 and SOD-2 proteins (normalized to GAPDH) from brain tissue from non-diabetic, resveratrol-treated non-diabetic, diabetic and resveratrol-treated diabetic rats. Values are means ± SE. * $p<0.05$ versus control non-diabetic rats, ** $p<0.05$ versus resveratrol-treated non-diabetic rats and † $p<0.05$ versus diabetic rats. *With permission from [42].*

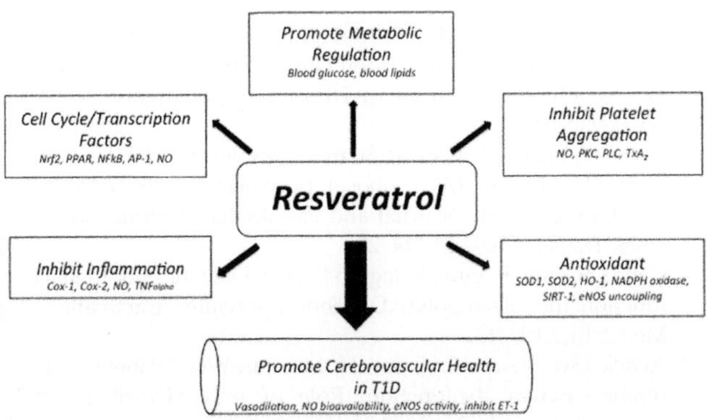

FIGURE 20.6 **Influence of resveratrol on oxidant/antioxidant pathways.** Schematic representing the potential influences of resveratrol on various cellular pathways/networks. Resveratrol may promote cerebrovascular health in T1D by influencing metabolic regulation, influencing cellular pathways that regulate platelet function, regulating the formation of oxidants via up-regulation of antioxidant pathways/networks, by influence cellular transcription factors and/or by inhibition of vascular inflammation.

arterioles, we did not find a difference in SOD-1 protein expression between the various groups of rats. We found that SOD-2 protein expression was similar in non-diabetic rats, non-diabetic rats treated with resveratrol and diabetic rats. However, SOD-2 protein expression was significantly decreased in diabetic rats treated with resveratrol when compared to the other groups of rats. Thus, T1D and treatment of non-diabetic rats with resveratrol produce an increase in nNOS protein expression, there is no change in SOD-1 protein expression by resveratrol treatment or T1D, and resveratrol treatment decreases SOD-2 protein expression in parietal cortex tissue in diabetic rats when compared to non-diabetic rats.

Thus, it appears that resveratrol may have multiple and overlapping influences on a number of key cellular pathways/networks to influence oxidant status and nitric oxide bioavailability that could account for its protective influence during T1D (Figure 20.6). Although, it was beyond the scope of our study to examine all such possibilities, we have provided some key data with regards to the influence of resveratrol on impaired vascular function of cerebral arterioles in T1D, and its potential influence on oxidative stress.

SUMMARY POINTS

- Type 1 diabetes is a major cause of morbidity and mortality, and a major economic burden throughout the world.
- The damaging effects of type 1 diabetes appear to be related to an influence of hyperglycemia on various cellular pathways/networks that influence the formation of reactive oxygen species.

- Alteration in vascular function of large cerebral arteries and small cerebral arterioles may contribute to the progression of vascular cognitive impairment and/or stroke.
- Endothelial nitric oxide synthase- and neuronal nitric oxide synthase-dependent responses of cerebral arterioles are impaired in type 1 diabetes.
- Impaired cerebrovascular function in type 1 diabetes is associated with an increase in oxidative stress, presumably an increase in superoxide anion.
- Resveratrol prevented an increase in superoxide anion in brain tissue and prevented impaired endothelial nitric oxide synthase- and neuronal nitric oxide synthase-dependent vascular function.
- Resveratrol, through its antioxidant influence, may be a potential therapeutic agent for the prevention of type 1 diabetes-induced cerebrovascular function, including cognitive impairment and stroke.

References

[1] Association AD. Diabetes statistics. Available at http:www.diabetes.org/diabetes-basics/diabetes-statistics; 2011.

[2] Dall TM, Mann SE, Zhang Y, et al. Distinguishing the economic costs associated with type 1 and type 2 diabetes. Popul Health Manag 2009;12:103–10.

[3] Ohishi K, Carmines PK. Superoxide dismutase restores the influence of nitric oxide on renal arterioles in diabetes mellitus. J Am Soc Nephrol 1995;5:1559–66.

[4] Coppey LJ, Gellett JS, Davidson EP, Yorek MA. Preventing superoxide formation in epineurial arterioles of the sciatic nerve from diabetic rats restores endothelium-dependent vasodilation. Free Radic Res 2003;37:33–40.

[5] Sun H, Molacek E, Zheng H, Fang Q, Patel KP, Mayhan WG. Alcohol-induced impairment of neuronal nitric oxide synthase (nNOS)-dependent dilation of cerebral arterioles: role of NAD(P)H oxidase. J Mol Cell Cardiol 2006;40:321–8.

[6] Baird TA, Parsons MW, Barber PA, et al. The influence of diabetes mellitus and hyperglycaemia on stroke incidence and outcome. J Clin Neurosci 2002;9:618–26.

[7] Vilar S, Quezada E, Santana L, et al. Design, synthesis, and vasorelaxant and platelet antiaggregatory activities of coumarin-resveratrol hybrids. Bioorg Med Chem Lett 2006;16:257–61.

[8] Zini R, Morin C, Bertelli A, Bertelli AA, Tillement JP. Effects of resveratrol on the rat brain respiratory chain. Drugs Exp Clin Res 1999;25:87–97.

[9] Bertelli AA, Giovannini L, Bernini W, et al. Antiplatelet activity of cis-resveratrol. Drugs Exp Clin Res 1996;22:61–3.

[10] Fulgenzi A, Bertelli AA, Magni E, Ferrero E, Ferrero ME. *In vivo* inhibition of TNF-α-induced vascular permeability by resveratrol. Transplant Proc 2001;33:2341–3.

[11] Bertelli AA, Migliori M, Panichi V, et al. Resveratrol, a component of wine and grapes, in the prevention of kidney disease. Ann N Y Acad Sci 2002;957:230–8.

[12] Bradamante S, Barenghi L, Piccinini F, et al. Resveratrol provides late-phase cardioprotection by means of a nitric oxide- and adenosine-mediated mechanism. Eur J Pharmacol 2003;465:115–23.

[13] Silan C. The effects of chronic resveratrol treatment on vascular responsiveness of streptozotocin-induced diabetic rats. Biol Pharm Bull 2008;31:897–902.

[14] Roghani M, Baluchnejadmojarad T. Mechanisms underlyin vascular effects of chronic resveratrol in streptozotocin-diabeti rats. Phytother Res 2009;10:1–7.

[15] Hasko G, Pacher P. Endothelial Nrf2 activation: a new target fc resveratrol? Am J Physiol Heart Circ Physiol 2010;299:H10–2.

[16] Csiszar A, Labinskyy N, Pinto JT, et al. Resveratrol induce mitochondrial biogenesis in endothelial cells. Am J Physiol Hear Circ Physiol 2009;297:H13–20.

[17] Thirunavukkarasu M, Penumathsa SV, Koneru S, et al. Resveratrol alleviates cardiac dysfunction in streptozotocin-induced diabetes: Role of nitric oxide, thioredoxin, and heme oxygenase. Fre Radic Biol Med 2007;43:720–9.

[18] Mayhan WG. Superoxide dismutase partially restores impaired dilatation of the basilar artery during diabetes mellitus. Brain Res 1997;760:204–9.

[19] Mayhan WG, Simmons LK, Sharpe GM. Mechanism of impaired responses of cerebral arterioles during diabetes mellitus. Am J Physiol 1991;260:H319–26.

[20] Pelligrino DA, Koenig HM, Wang Q, Albrecht RF. Protein kinase C suppresses receptor-mediated pial arteriolar relaxation in the diabetic rat. Neuroreport 1994;5:417–20.

[21] Vasquez-Vivar J, Kalyanaraman B, Martasek P, et al. Superoxide generation by endothelial nitric oxide synthase: the influence of cofactors. Proc Natl Acad Sci 1998;95:9220–5.

[22] Stroes E, Hijmering M, van Zandvoort M, Wever R, Rabelink TJ, van Faassen EE. Origin of superoxide production by endothelial nitric oxide synthase. FEBS Letters 1998;438:161–4.

[23] Heitzer T, Krohn K, Albers S, Meinertz T. Tetrahydrobiopterin improves endothelium-dependent vasodilation by increasing nitric oxide activity in patients with Type II diabetes mellitus. Diabetologia 2000;43:143–8.

[24] Pieper AA, Verma A, Zhang J, Snyder SH. Poly (ADP-ribose) polymerase, nitric oxide and cell death. Trends Pharmacol Sci 1999;20:171–81.

[25] Garcia Soriano F, Pacher P, Mabley J, Liaudet L, Szabo C. Rapid reversal of the diabetic endothelial dysfunction by pharmacological inhibition of poly (ADP-ribose) polymerase. Circ Res 2001;89:684–91.

[26] Pacher P, Liaudet L, Garcia Soriano F, Mabley JG, Szabo E, Szabo C. The role of poly (ADP-ribose) polymerase activation in the development of myocardial and endothelial dysfunction in diabetes. Diabetes 2002;51:514–21.

[27] Garcia Soriano F, Virag L, Jagtap P, et al. Diabetic endothelial dysfunction: the role of poly(ADP-ribose) polymerase activation. Nat Med 2001;7:108–13.

[28] Arrick DM, Sharpe GM, Sun H, Mayhan WG. Diabetes-induced cerebrovascular dysfunction: Role of poly(ADP-ribose) polymerase. Microvasc Res 2007;73:1–6.

[29] Mayhan WG, Arrick DM, Sharpe GM, Patel KP, Sun H. Inhibition of NAD(P)H oxidase alleviates impaired NOS-dependent responses of pial arterioles in Type 1 diabetes mellitus. Microcirculation 2006;13:567–75.

[30] Alexander JS, Elrod JW. Extracellular matrix, junctional integrity and matrix metalloproteinase interactions in endothelial permeability regulation. J Anat 2002;200:561–74.

[31] Burkey JL, Campanale KM, O'Bannon DD, Cramer JW, Farid NA. Disposition of LY333531, a selective protein kinase C beta inhibitor, in the Fischer 344 rat and beagle dog. Xenobiotica 2002;32:1045–52.

[32] Landmesser U, Cai H, Dikalov S, et al. Role of p47(phox) in vascular oxidative stress and hypertension caused by angiotensin II. Hypertension 2002;40:511–5.

[33] Duntas L, Keck FS, Haug C, et al. Serum angiotensin-converting enzyme activity and active renin plasma concentrations in insulin-dependentdiabetesmellitus. DiabetesResClinPract1992;16:203–8.

[34] Schernthaner G, Schwarzer C, Kuzmits R, Muller MM, Klemen U, Freyler H. Increased angiotensin-converting enzyme activities in diabetes mellitus: analysis of diabetes type, state of metabolic control and occurrence of diabetes vascular disease. J Clin Pathol 1984;37:307–12.
[35] Griendling KK, Minieri CA, Ollerenshaw JD, Alexander RW. Angiotensin II stimulates NADH and NADPH oxidase activity in cultured vascular smooth muscle cells. Circ Res 1994;74:1141–8.
[36] Cheetham C, Collis J, O'Driscoll G, Stanton K, Taylor R, Green D. Losartan, an angiotensin type 1 receptor antagonist, improves endothelial function in non-insulin-dependent diabetes. J Am Coll Cardiol 2000;36:1461–6.
[37] Trauernicht AK, Sun H, Patel KP, Mayhan WG. Enalapril prevents impaired nitric oxide synthase-dependent dilatation of cerebral arterioles in diabetic rats. Stroke 2003;34:2698–703.
[38] Arrick DM, Sharpe GM, Sun H, Mayhan WG. Losartan improves impaired nitric oxide synthase-dependent dilatation of cerebral arterioles in type 1 diabetic rats. Brain Res 2008;1209:128–35.
[39] Sharma S, Anjaneyulu M, Kulkarni SK, Chopra K. Resveratrol, a polyphenolic phytoalexin, attenuates diabetic nephropathy in rats. Pharmacology 2006;76:69–75.
[40] Ho SM. Estrogens and anti-estrogens: key mediators of prostate carcinogenesis and new therapeutic candidates. J Cell Biochem 2004;91:491–503.
[41] Zhang H, Zhang J, Ungvari Z, Zhang C. Resveratrol improves endothelial function: role of TNF-α and vascular oxidative stress. Arterioscler Thromb Vasc Biol 2009;29:1164–71.
[42] Arrick DM, Sun H, Patel KP, Mayhan WG. Chronic Resveratrol Treatment Restores Vascular Responsiveness of Cerebral Arterioles in Type 1 Diabetic Rats. Am J Physiol Heart Circ Physiol 2011;301:H696–703.
[43] Mayhan WG. Endothelium-dependent responses of cerebral arterioles to adenosine 5′-diphosphate. J Vasc Res 1992;29:353–8.
[44] Marrelli SP, Khorovets A, Johnson TD, Childres WF, Bryan Jr RM. P2 purinoceptor-mediated dilations in the rat middle cerebral artery after ischemia-reperfusion. Am J Physiol 1999;276: H33–41.
[45] Oskarsson HJ, Hofmeyer TG. Platelets from patients with diabetes mellitus have impaired ability to mediate vasodilation. J Am Coll Cardiol 1996;27:464–70.
[46] Faraci FM, Breese KR. Nitric oxide mediates vasodilatation in response to activation of N-methyl-D-aspartate receptors in brain. Circ Res 1993;72:476–80.
[47] Sun H, Patel KP, Mayhan WG. Impairment of neuronal nitric oxide synthase-dependent dilatation of cerebral arterioles during chronic alcohol consumption. Alcoholism 2002;26:663–70.
[48] Mogi M, Horiuchi M. Neurovascular coupling in cognitive impairment associated with diabetes mellitus. Circ J 2011;75: 1042–1048.
[49] Su HC, Hung LM, Chen JK. Resveratrol, a red wine antioxidant, possesses an insulin-like effect in streptozotocin-induced diabetic rats. Am J Physiol Endocrinol Metab 2006;290:E1339–46.
[50] Das S, Das DK. Anti-inflammatory responses of resveratrol. Inflamm Allergy Drug Targets 2007;6:168–73.
[51] Ku CR, Lee HJ, Kim SK, Lee EY, Lee MK, Lee EJ. Resveratrol prevents streptozotocin-induced diabetes by inhibiting the apoptosis of pancreatic beta-cell and the cleavage of poly (ADP-ribose) polymerase. Endocr J 2012;59:103–9.
[52] Yang YM, Wang XX, Chen JZ, Wang SJ, Hu H, Wang HQ. Resveratrol attenuates adenosine diphosphate-induced platelet activation by reducing protein kinase C activity. Am J Chin Med 2008;36:603–13.
[53] Nishikawa T, Edelstein D, Du XL, et al. Normalizing mitochondrial superoxide production blocks three pathways of hyperglycaemic damage. Nature 2000;404:787–90.
[54] Dong L, Xie MJ, Zhang P, et al. Rotenone partially reverses decreased BK Ca currents in cerebral artery smooth muscle cells from streptozotocin-induced diabetic mice. Clin Exp Pharmacol Physiol 2009;36:e57–64.
[55] Morin C, Zini R, Albengres E, Bertelli AA, Bertelli A, Tillement JP. Evidence for resveratrol-induced preservation of brain mitochondria functions after hypoxia-reoxygenation. Drugs Exp Clin Res 2003;29:227–33.
[56] Kitada M, Kume S, Imaizumi N, Koya D. Resveratrol improves oxidative stress and protects against diabetic nephropathy through normalization of Mn-SOD dysfunction in AMPK/SIRT1-independent pathway. Diabetes 2011;60:634–43.
[57] Ungvari Z, Bagi Z, Feher A, et al. Resveratrol confers endothelial protection via activation of the antioxidant transcription factor Nrf2. Am J Physiol Heart Circ Physiol 2010;299:H18–24.
[58] Li B, Liu S, Miao L, Cai L. Prevention of diabetic complications by activation of Nrf2: diabetic cardiomyopathy and nephropathy. Exp Diabetes Res 2012;2012:216512.
[59] Cui W, Bai Y, Miao X, et al. Prevention of diabetic nephropathy by sulforaphane: possible role of nrf2 upregulation and activation. Oxid Med Cell Longev 2012;2012:821936.

CHAPTER

21

Herbal Chrysanthemi Flos, Oxidative Damage and Protection against Diabetic Complications

Sung-Jin Kim

Department of Pharmacology and Toxicology, School of Dentistry, Kyung Hee University, Seoul, Republic of Korea

List of Abbreviations

1,3-DPG 1,3-diphosphoglycerate
$^1O_2$ Singlet oxygen
AGEs Advanced glycation end products
ALP Alkaline phosphatase
ALT Alanine transaminase
AR Aldose reductase
AST Aspartate transaminase
ATP Adenosine triphosphate
CAT Catalase
CF Chrysanthemi Flos
DM Diabetes mellitus
DPPH 2,2-Diphenyl-1-picrylhydrazyl
eNOS Endothelial nitric oxide synthase
FFA Free fatty acids
GAPDH Glyceraldehyde 3-phosphate dehydrogenase
GFPT Glucosamine:fructose acetyl transferase
GPx Glutathione peroxidase
GR Glutathione reductase
GSH Glutathione, reduced
GSSG Glutathione, oxidized
H_2O Water
H_2O_2 Hydrogen peroxide
HK Hexokinase
HNO_2 Nitrous acid
HOCl Hypochlorous acid
LDL Low density lipoprotein
LPO Lipid peroxidation
MAPKs Mitogen-activated protein kinase
MDA Malondialdehyde
N_2O_3 Dinitrogen trioxide
NAD^+ Nicotinamide adenine dinucleotide
NADH Nicotinamide adenine dinucleotide, reduced
$NADP^+$ Nicotinamide adenine dinucleotide phosphate
NADPH Nicotinamide adenine dinucleotide phosphate, reduced
NBT Nitroblue tetrazolium
NF-κB Nuclear factor-κB
NO Nitric oxide
NO· Nitric oxide radical
NO_2 Nitric dioxide
NOS Nitric oxide synthase
O_2 Oxygen
$O_2\cdot^-$ Superoxide anion radical
OCl^- Hypochlorite
OH· Hydroxyl radical
ONOO· Peroxynitrite radical
PARP Poly(ADP-ribose) polymerase
PKC Protein kinase C
RAGEs Receptors of AGEs
RNS Reactive nitrogen species
ROS Reactive oxygen species
SD Sprague Dawley
SDH Sorbitol dehydrogenase
SOD Superoxide dismutase
STZ Streptozotocin
TBARS Thiobarbituric acid reactive substances
TBE Tris-Borate-EDTA.

DIABETES

Diabetes mellitus (DM) is one of the most significant lifelong metabolic disorders in the world [1,2]. In the Asia-Pacific region there are already over 30 million people with diabetes, and it is estimated that this number will double by 2025 [3]. DM is characterized by hyperglycemia and insufficient secretion or action of endogenous insulin, and it is associated with macro- and microvascular complications [1]. Biochemical alterations in glucose and lipid metabolism result in high levels of free radicals, either reactive oxygen species (ROS) or reactive nitrogen species (RNS), which cause damage to cellular proteins, membrane lipids and nucelic acids, and eventually cell death [4] (Figure 21.1). When glucose is high, disturbances in various metabolic pathways such as the polyol pathway, glycolytic pathway, hexosamine pathway, protein kinase C (PKC) pathway, and the methylglyoxal and advanced glycation end products (AGEs) pathways have been suggested to contribute to the

Diabetes: Oxidative Stress and Dietary Antioxidants.
http://dx.doi.org/10.1016/B978-0-12-405885-9.00021-8

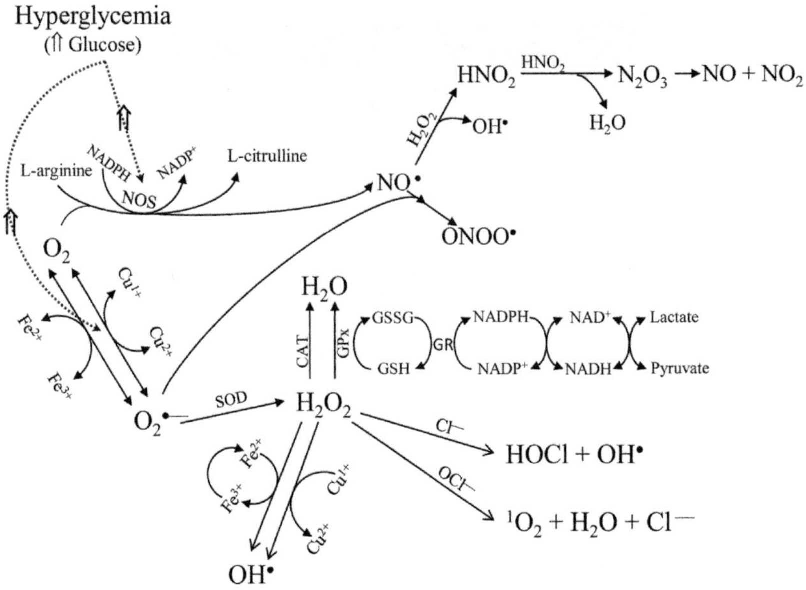

FIGURE 21.1 **Formation of reactive oxygen and nitrogen species (ROS/RNS) induced by hyperglycemia in diabetes mellitus (DM).**

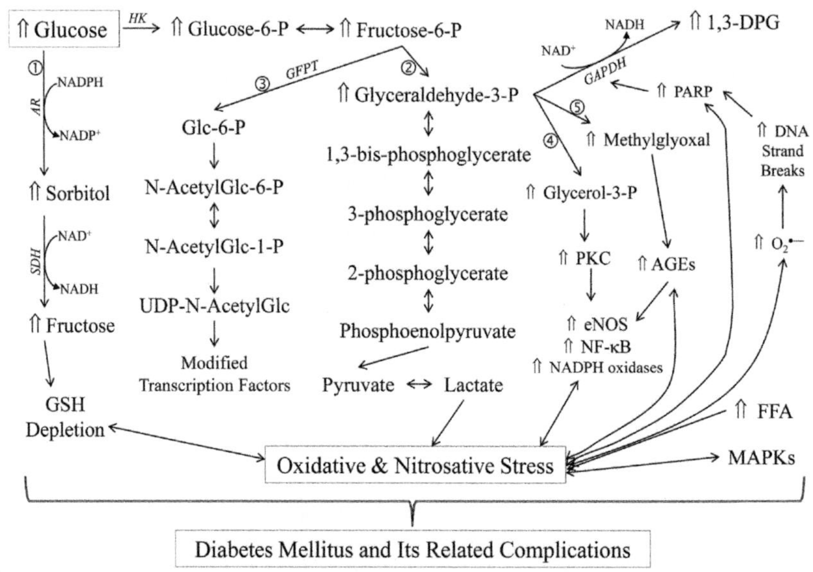

FIGURE 21.2 **Hyperglycemia induced metabolic pathways involved in diabetes mellitus (DM).** 1 Polyol pathway; 2 Glycolysis; 3 Hexosamine pathway; 4 Protein kinase C (PKC) pathway; 5 Advanced glycation end-product pathway.

development of diabetic complications (Figure 21.2). In contrast, healthy dietary habits are effective in managing DM, insulin resistance, and in the prevention and management of hyperglycemia.

CHRYSANTHEMI FLOS

Chrysanthemi Flos (CF) is the flower of *Chrysanthemum indicum Linne* or *Chrysanthemum morifolium Ramatuelle* [2]. It is a member of the genus *Chrysanthemum*, which consists of about 30 species and belongs to the family Asteraceae (Compositae). These species were previously classified under the genus name *Dendranthema. Chrysanthemum* are herbaceous perennial plants, of which *C. indicum*, is one of the most widespread species ranging from the north of Russia to the southeastern part of Asia, Korea, China and Europe [5]. It is a cross-pollination species, which can reproduce both sexually by out-crossed seeds and asexually through rhizomes [6].

The CF harvest starts in early November, when the petals are flat and stamens are 60–70% spread [7]. This flower has been widely used as a health food for thousands of years, and also in traditional medicine in Korea and Southeast Asia for the treatment of a wide spectrum of ailments requiring analgesic, antipyretic, anti-inflammatory, antihypertensive action, and also for neurasthenic head-ache and eye diseases [8]. CF is also very common in traditional Chinese medicine, in which it is used as a heat clearing and detoxification herb.

EFFECTS OF CF ON DIABETES AND ITS COMPLICATIONS

Effect of CF on Body Weight Changes

The body weight was significantly reduced in STZ-induced diabetic mice [2]. Studies have indicated that, in diabetes, loss of body weight may be related to significant levels of chronic hyperglycemia and loss or degradation of structural proteins [2]. Diabetic patients also demonstrate weight loss alongside increased water/food consumption [9]. The average body weight of the normal rats increased significantly more than that of the diabetic rats, which increased only slightly over eight weeks [10]. On the other hand, CF treatment showed a tendency to delay body weight loss. Exogenous administration of CF extract to diabetic mice showed a gradual but significant increase in body weight during the 30 days of the experiment, compared with untreated diabetic mice (Table 21.1) [2]. Similarly, the body weights of CF treated rats were significantly higher than that of the diabetic group in the fifth week after STZ induction [9]. The capability of CF to protect the body weight loss seems to be related to its ability to reduce oxidative damage and may be due to the retained levels of glucose and insulin levels in CF treated animals.

Effect of CF on Serum Marker Enzymes

Measurements of the activities of serum aspartate transaminase (AST), alanine transaminase (ALT) and alkaline phosphatase (ALP) is the most sensitive test employed in the diagnosis of organ damage. AST, ALT, and ALP activities were significantly elevated in STZ-induced diabetic mice compared with controls [2]. An increase in serum AST, ALT, or ALP activity is an indicator of liver and kidney destruction, probably due to lipid peroxidation subsequent to free radical production. Administration of CF to diabetic mice showed decreased levels of serum AST, ALT, and ALP. This proves that CF treatment can preserve the structural integrity of the liver and kidney from the adverse effects of diabetes mellitus (Figure 21.3) [2].

TABLE 21.1 Effect of CF on Body Weight

	Control	Diabetic	Diabetic + CF
Initial Bodyweight (g)	23.08 ± 1.91	24.03 ± 1.55^{NS}	24.02 ± 1.60^{NS}
Final Bodyweight (g)	28.38 ± 3.39	24.92 ± 1.66*	27.95 ± 2.19*

Values are expressed as mean ± SD (n=6). Diabetic mice were compared with control group. CF treated mice were compared with diabetic group. $^{*}p<0.05$ and ^{NS} – Non-significant.
Source: Kim et al., 2012; 6(4): 622–630 [2].

Effect of CF on Lipid Peroxidation

Increased oxidative stress is a widely accepted factor in the development and progression of diabetes and its complications [1]. Diabetes is usually accompanied by increased production of free radicals or impaired antioxidant defenses [1]. Lipid peroxidation (LPO) is a marker of cellular damage initiated by reactive oxygen species. Hyperglycemia can induce oxidative stress through AGE formation and increased flux along the polyol and hexosamine pathways. AGEs produce ROS and superoxide and the subsequent increase in oxidative stress may lead to endothelial dysfunction and ultimately cardiovascular disease through several different mechanisms. The increased levels of lipid peroxidation induce oxidative damage by increasing the levels of peroxy and hydroxyl radicals. Hydroxyl radicals may react with transition metals like iron or copper to form stable aldehydes such as malondialdehyde, which will damage cell membranes [1]. Peroxy radicals can remove hydrogen from lipids, producing hydroperoxides that further propagate the free radical pathway. The mechanisms by which increased oxidative stress is involved in the diabetic complications are partly understood, and include the activation of transcription factors, AGEs, and protein kinase C [1].

LPO is one of the cellular features of chronic diabetes. Increased LPO impairs membrane function by decreasing membrane fluidity and changing the activity of membrane-bound enzymes and receptors. LPO end products are commonly detected by the measurement of thiobarbituric acid reactive substances (TBARS) [4]. The use of TBARS as an index of lipid peroxidation has been increased in DM [11]. TBARS are produced during lipoperoxidation oxidative stress induced damage of lipids,

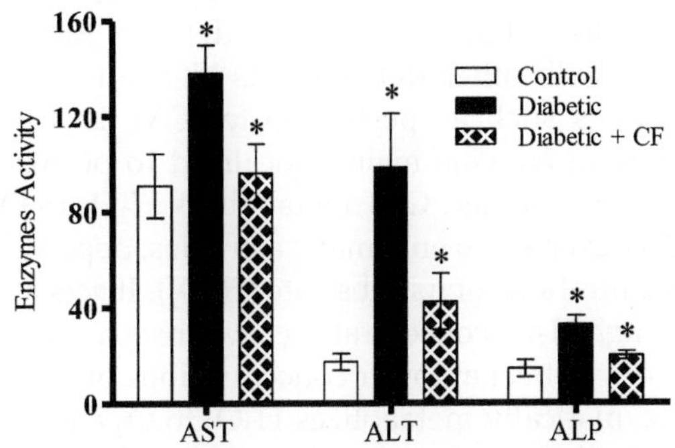

FIGURE 21.3 **Effect of CF on serum marker enzymes.** AST and ALT – IU/L; ALP – KA units. Values are expressed as mean ± SD (n=6). Diabetic mice were compared with control group. CF treated mice were compared with diabetic group. $*p<0.05$. *Source: Kim et al., 2012; 6(4): 622–630 [2].*

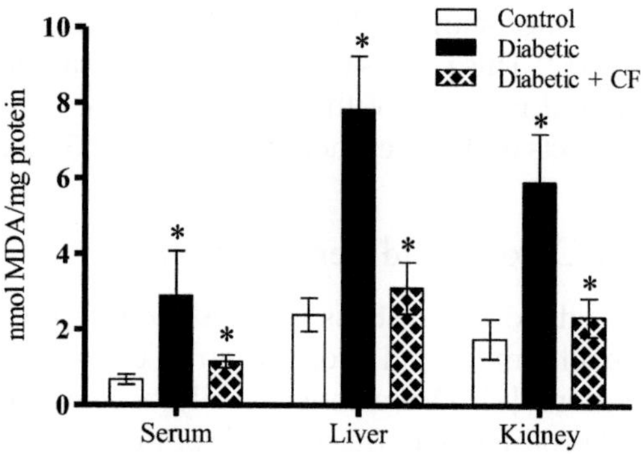

FIGURE 21.4 **Effect of CF on MDA levels.** Values are expressed as mean ± SD (n=6). Diabetic mice were compared with control group. CF treated mice were compared with diabetic group. *$p<0.05$. *Source: Kim et al., 2012; 6(4): 622–630 [2].*

TABLE 21.2 Effect of CF on Enzymatic Antioxidants

	Control	Diabetic	Diabetic + CF
LIVER			
SOD	3.94 ± 0.37	2.05 ± 0.48*	3.06 ± 0.36*
CAT	7.59 ± 0.77	4.47 ± 0.52*	6.49 ± 0.59*
GPx	5.72 ± 0.38	3.31 ± 0.37*	4.77 ± 0.46*
KIDNEY			
SOD	3.75 ± 0.55	2.08 ± 0.40*	3.08 ± 0.27*
CAT	3.90 ± 0.47	2.63 ± 0.42*	3.26 ± 0.45*
GPx	3.08 ± 0.40	1.34 ± 0.30*	2.24 ± 0.51*

Values are expressed as mean ± SD (n=6). Diabetic mice were compared with control group. CF treated mice were compared with diabetic group. *$p<0.05$. SOD – 50% inhibition of nitroblue tetrazolium (NBT) reduction/min/mg protein; CAT – μM of H_2O_2 consumed/min/mg protein; GPx – μM of GSH consumed/min/mg protein. *Source: Kim et al., 2012; 6(4): 622–630 [2].*

and are thus a widely used marker of oxidative stress [4,11]. However, they represent a heterogenous group of compounds of which the best known is malondialdehyde (MDA). In diabetics induced by streptozotocin (STZ) there was a significant elevation in serum, liver and kidney MDA levels. Administration of CF extract significantly decreased these levels in diabetic mice as compared to untreated diabetic mice (Figure 21.4) [2].

Effect of CF on Enzymic Antioxidants

Antioxidant enzymes scavenge or eliminate a variety of free radicals, including those generated during biological processes. The main antioxidant enzymes are superoxide dismutase (SOD), catalase (CAT) and glutathione peroxidase (GPx). SOD exists in three different isoforms; Cu,Zn-SOD is mostly found in the cytosol, extracellular SOD is found in the plasma and extracellular space, and Mn-SOD is located in the mitochondria. SOD maintains cellular levels of superoxide anions within physiological concentrations by converting it to hydrogen peroxide (H_2O_2). H_2O_2 can cross cell membranes and may oxidize a number of compounds, giving rise to hydroxyl radicals within the cell. Thus the removal of H_2O_2 is very important for cellular antioxidant defense. Superoxide may react with other ROS such as NO to form highly toxic species such as peroxynitrite. CAT is an H_2O_2-decomposing enzyme mainly localized to peroxicomes or microperoxicomes. CAT metabolizes H_2O_2 to O_2 and H_2O. CAT exerts two enzymatic activities, depending on the concentrations of its substrate (H_2O_2). It acts as a catalyst at high H_2O_2 concentrations, whereas it produces a peroxidative effect at lower concentrations of H_2O_2 [12]. GPx enzymatically metabolizes H_2O_2 to O_2 and H_2O by using a hydrogen donor, reduced glutathione (GSH), which is oxidized to glutathione disulfide (GSSG) [12].

Reports regarding the activities of antioxidant enzymes in diabetes are very contradictory, with increases, decreases or no change of antioxidant activity being observed [13]. In our study, there was a significant reduction in the activities of SOD, CAT and GPx in the liver and kidney of diabetic mice compared with the controls [2]. The decreased efficiency of antioxidant defenses seems to correlate with the severity of pathological tissue changes during diabetes. The major reason for the decrease of enzymatic antioxidant activities may be increased glycation and inactivation of these enzymes and/or deleterious effects of increased oxygen radicals by glycated proteins in diabetic hyperglycemia [11,13]. The decreased activities of SOD, CAT and GPx in the diabetic mice were significantly restored by CF treatment as compared with untreated diabetic mice (Table 21.2) [2].

Effect of CF on Non-Enzymic Antioxidants

GSH is a ubiquitous tripeptide that functions as a direct free radical scavenger, as a co-substrate for GPx activity, and as a co-factor for many enzymes, and it acts as a conjugate in endo- and xenobiotic reactions. GSH is essential in maintaining the structural and functional integrity of erythrocytes. When H_2O_2 and lipid peroxides are detoxified by GPx, the GSH is simultaneously converted to its oxidized form (GSSG) [4,13]. Glutathione reductase (GR) catalyzes the NAD(P)H-dependent reduction of oxidized glutathione, serving to maintain intercellular glutathione stores and a favorable redox status.

During hyperglycemia, ROS bind to receptors that promote oxidative stress and generate intracellular oxidants. Aldose reductase (AR) is reported to metabolize GSH-lipid derived aldehyde adducts, which results in a decrease in GSH and a subsequent increase in oxidative stress. An increased polyol pathway flux during hyperglycemia is due to increase in AR activity in tissues which reduces glucose to sorbitol by consuming NADPH. In DM, altered activities of AR [1] and reduced

TABLE 21.3 Effect of CF on Non-Enzymatic Antioxidants

	Control	Diabetic	Diabetic + CF
SERUM			
GSH (mg/dL)	30.75 ± 3.46	18.70 ± 1.49*	27.01 ± 3.56*
Vitamin C (mg/dL)	0.97 ± 0.22	0.31 ± 0.09*	0.76 ± 0.12*
Vitamin E (mg/dL)	4.68 ± 1.19	13.10 ± 1.84*	6.49 ± 1.22*
LIVER			
GSH (nmol/mg protein)	3.99 ± 1.93	1.17 ± 0.44*	3.09 ± 0.34*
Vitamin C (mg/100g tissue)	0.67 ± 0.07	0.38 ± 0.07*	0.60 ± 0.09*
Vitamin E (mg/100g tissue)	0.72 ± 0.16	1.26 ± 0.31*	0.99 ± 0.14*
KIDNEY			
GSH (nmol/mg protein)	1.65 ± 0.41	0.74 ± 0.13*	1.25 ± 0.15*
Vitamin C (mg/100g tissue)	0.49 ± 0.08	0.27 ± 0.06*	0.42 ± 0.08*
Vitamin E (mg/100g tissue)	0.20 ± 0.09	0.80 ± 0.15*	0.30 ± 0.09*

Values are expressed as mean μ SD (n=6). Diabetic mice were compared with control group. CF treated mice were compared with diabetic group. $^{*}p < 0.05$.
Source: Kim et al., 2012; 6(4): 622–630 [2].

levels of GSH [2] are thought to occur because oxidative stress consumes some naturally occurring local antioxidants such as GSH, and this reflects the overwhelming adaptive response to the challenge of oxidative stress in the diabetic state, with or without complications [11]. CF treatment showed a significant elevation in GSH levels in CF-treated diabetic mice (Table 21.3) [2].

Vitamin C and E are diet-derived [1] and probably have an important role in reducing the oxidative damage caused by nitric oxide and other free radicals [11]. Estimation of vitamin levels could provide insight into how well the body is coping with oxidative stress [11]. They also interact with recycling processes to generate reduced forms of the vitamins. Vitamin E, a component of the total peroxyl radical-trapping antioxidant system, reacts directly with peroxyl and superoxide radicals and singlet oxygen and protects the membranes from lipid peroxidation [1]. α-Tocoperol is reconstituted when ascorbic acid recycles the tocopherol radical. The dihydroascorbic acid thus generated is recycled by glutathione [1]. Plasma vitamin C levels increase the insulin action mainly due to reduction of oxidative stress with an improvement in nonoxidative glucose metabolism [14]. The vitamin E level was significantly elevated, and the vitamin C level markedly reduced in diabetic mice as compared with those of the controls. Elevated vitamin E levels in diabetics protects against increased peroxidation. The ability of vitamin C to preserve the levels of other antioxidants also regenerates vitamin E from its oxidized form [15]. The decreased vitamin C might be because it is being utilized to regenerate vitamin E. CF treatment showed significant amelioration in ascorbic acid and GSH concentrations, and caused a significant reduction in vitamin E in diabetic mice as compared with untreated diabetic mice (Table 21.3) [2].

Effect of CF on DNA Fragmentation

Hyperglycemia generates increased ROS levels by reducing equivalents formed from mitochondrial ETC and results in cellular dysfunction and mutations in mitochondrial DNA [12]. It is probable that the cytotoxic effects are also dependent upon DNA alkylation by site-specific reaction with DNA bases, and by free radical generation [16]. DNA damage induces the activation of poly ADP-ribosylation, which leads to a depletion in cellular NAD^+ and adenosine triphosphate (ATP) [17]. Enhanced ATP dephosphorylation supplies a substrate for xanthine oxidase, resulting in the formation of superoxide radicals [17]. Furthermore, hydrogen peroxide, hydroxyl radicals and nitric oxide also participate in DNA damage. A DNA fragmentation pattern examined in liver and kidney of STZ-induced diabetic mice showed defective DNA subunits in both organs [2]. Diabetic mice treated with CF showed a significant decrease in DNA fragmentation compared with untreated diabetic mice and controls. These observations suggest that CF treatment appears to significantly suppress the progression of apoptosis in the liver and kidney of diabetic mice (Figure 21.5) [2].

Effect of CF on Retina

Functional changes in the retina were examined via electroretinogram (ERG). A-wave amplitudes were reduced in diabetic and in CF-treated diabetic animals eight weeks after the induction of diabetes. These results suggest that CF treatment does not prevent a decrease in a-wave amplitude after diabetes induction. Treatment with a mixture of Lycium and CF showed a significant protective effect. and prevented the a-wave amplitude loss caused by diabetes to a similar extent to that achieved by insulin treatment. The results indicate that a mixture of extracts of Lycium and CF have protective effects which are similar to insulin treatment in preventing retinal function loss in diabetic rats [9].

Effect of CF on Glucosidase Inhibition

α-glucosidase inhibitor has been recognized as a therapeutic approach to the modulation of postprandial hyperglycemia [18]. Consumption of high-carbohydrate diets causes elevated postprandial hyperglycemia that can progress to full symptomatic

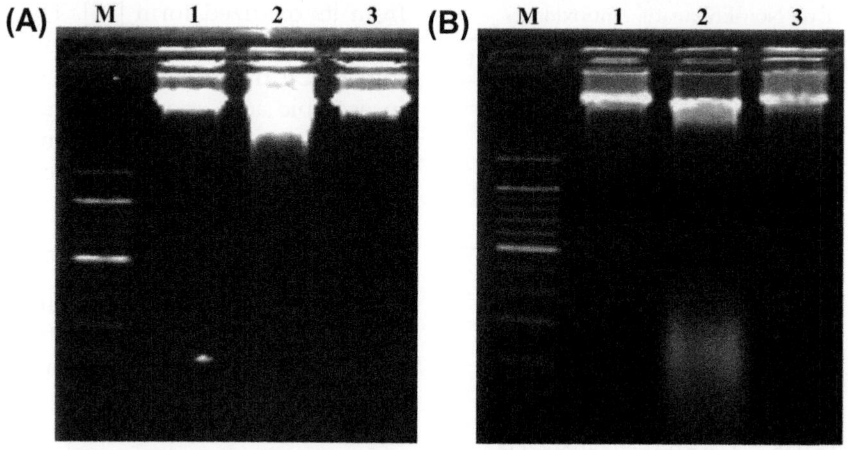

FIGURE 21.5 **Effect of CF on DNA fragmentation in diabetic liver (A) and kidney (B).** DNA samples were electrophoresed on 1.5% agarose in tris-borate-EDTA (TBE) buffer, ethidium bromide stained gel represent as lane M is a DNA size marker, lane 1 showing intact DNA (Control group), lane 2 showing fragmented DNA (diabetic group) and lane 3 showing fragmentation reverted to similar control (CF treated diabetic group). *Source: Kim et al., 2012; 6(4): 622–630 [2].*

type 2 diabetes [19]. The current therapeutic strategy for controlling postprandial hyperglycemia is the inhibition of α-glucosidase and α-amylase, resulting in aggressive delay of carbohydrate digestion to absorbable monosaccharide [20] as well as micro- and macrovascular complications including diabetic retinopathy, nephropathy, and neuropathy [21].

IC50 values for CF inhibition of intestinal maltase, intestinal sucrase and pancreatic α-amylase have been reported [18]. The percentage of intestinal maltase inhibition by CF was increased upon addition of mulberry extract. The inhibition activity of CF on pancreatic α-amylase was increased when roselle extract was added, indicating that CF and roselle synergistically inhibit pancreatic α-amylase. These additive and synergistic effects may have health implications for increasing the inhibition of intestinal maltase and pancreatic α-amylase activities [18]. The long-term inhibitory action of α-glucosidase inhibitors contributes to decreasing the level of HbA1c in diabetic patients, resulting in a significant reduction in the incidence of chronic vascular complications such as macro- and micro-vascular disease [22].

Effect of CF on Aldose Reductase Inhibition

Efforts to understand cataract formation have produced various hypotheses [1]. The polyol pathway consists of two enzymes [11]. The first of these, aldose reductase (AR), reduces glucose to sorbitol along with its co-factor NADPH, and the second, sorbitol dehydrogenase (SDH), with its co-factor NAD^+, converts sorbitol to fructose [11]. Increased non-enzymatic glycation and AGEs are also postulated to contribute to cataract formation [1]. Increased utilization of NADPH caused by enhanced activity of AR reduces intracellular concentration of GSH [12]. Reduced levels of GSH will impair the activity of GPx and GR activities. This impairs the antioxidant defense network and increases cellular susceptibility to oxidative stress [4].

Normally, AR has low affinity for glucose, so that the conversion of glucose to sorbitol only proceeds to a small extent [23]. However, in diabetes mellitus, the increased availability of glucose in insulin-insensitive tissues such as the lens, nerves, and retina leads to the increased formation of sorbitol through the polyol pathway. The resultant increase in water influx leads to the generation of osmotic stress, and hence to cataract formation [23,24]. Sorbitol does not readily diffuse across cell membranes [23]. Inefficient metabolism [24] and the intracellular accumulation of sorbitol has been implicated in the chronic complications of diabetes such as cataract, neuropathy, retinopathy [23], nephropathy and Alzheimer's disease [24].

The inhibitory activity of methanolic extracts of *C. indicum* and *C. morifolium* and isolated compounds from *C. indicum* such as apigenin-7-*O*-β-D-glucopyranoside, acacetin-7-*O*-(6′-α-L-rhamnopyranosyl)-β-D-glucopyranoside, luteolin, luteolin 7-*O*-β-D-glucopyranoside, luteolin 7-*O*-β-D-glucopyranosiduronic acid, diosmetin 7-*O*-β-D-glucopyranoside, quercetin 3,7-di-*O*-β-D-glucopyranoside, (2S)- and (2R)-eriodictyol 7-*O*-β-D-glucopyranosiduronic acids [23], (2*S*,3*S*)-1-phenyl-2,3-butanediol 3-*O*-β-D-glucopyranoside and eriodictyol, were reported on rat lens aldose reductase [10]. Treatment with AR inhibitors prevents the conversion of glucose to sorbitol, and this has been shown to be effective in preventing the development of various diabetic complications, including cataract, neuropathy, and nephropathy.

Effect of CF on Vasorelaxation

The endothelium plays an important role in maintaining normal vascular tone and blood fluidity, and the function of this layer is altered in certain cardiovascular diseases including diabetes [25]. Intracellular oxidative stress is mainly caused by an imbalance between the activity of endogenous pro-oxidants and antioxidants, and this disturbs vascular cell functions and alters the release of vasodilator substances. Factors that can modify ROS release have the potential to protect against endothelial dysfunction [26]. CF attenuates the decrease in contractile function and coronary flow caused by ischemia-reperfusion injury in the isolated rat heart [27], and causes vasodialatation in rat thoracic aortae [28].

EFFECT OF CF ON OTHER BIOLOGICAL ACTIVITIES

Free Radical Scavenging Activity

The antioxidant effect of *C. indicum* and *C. morifolium* on 2,2-diphenyl-1-picrylhydrazyl (DPPH) radical scavenging and ascorbic acid equivalent antioxidant capacity have been reported [29]. The DPPH radical scavenging activity, SOD activity, ABTS radical scavenging activity and total phenolic contents were reported for CF extracts prepared by hot-air drying at different temperatures, and by far-infrared drying methods [30]. CF possesses hydroxyl radical scavenging properties [31]. The DPPH free radical scavenging capacities of n-BuOH, petroleum ether and water extracts of CF were reported [7].

Antibacterial and Antimutagenic Activities

Chitosan was reported for its antibacterial activity by 99.9% of the bacterial reduction rate tested for *Staphylococcus aureus* and *Klebsiella pneumoniae* [32]. The antimutagenic activity of CF was also reported [33].

Osteoporosis and Inflammatory Bone Diseases

CF extract significantly increased the growth of MC3T3-E1 cells and caused a significant elevation of ALP activity, and the deposition of collagen and calcium in the cells suggesting that CF might be partly involved in estrogen-related activities [34].

Anti-Inflammatory Activity

CF inhibits nitric oxide (NO) production in lipopolysaccharide-activated macro-phages [28,35,36]. CF extract inhibits inflammatory responses by suppressing NF-κB-IκBα phosphorylation and the MAPK dependent pathway in lipopolysaccharide-induced RAW 264.7 macrophages [37]. CF strongly inhibited NO, PGE_2, TNF-α, and IL-1β production, and also significantly inhibited mRNA and the expression of iNOS and COX-2 in a dose-dependent manner [37]. An ethanol extract of CF inhibited topical edema in the mouse ear leading to substantial reductions in skin thickness and tissue weight, inflammatory cytokine production, neutrophil-mediated myeloperoxidase activity, and various histopathological indicators in a murine model of phorbol ester-induced dermatitis [38].

Hepatoprotective Activity

The antioxidant activity of EtOAc, n-hexane, n-BuOH, water and chloroform extracts of CF decreased in the order given [36]. In rats, the body weight increase ratio and feed efficiency ratio were decreased by ethanol treatment, but were gradually restored to levels similar to those of the normal group by administering CF EtOAc fraction. The whole blood concentrations of total cholesterol and LDL-cholesterol, and the activities of ALT and AST were elevated by ethanol, but were significantly decreased in the CF treated groups [36]. It was also observed that the activities of SOD, CAT, XO and GPx elevated by ethanol in rat livers were markedly decreased in the CF-treated group compared to the control group. These results suggest that CF has a possible protective effect against ethanol-induced hepatotoxicity in the rat liver. CF can effectively prevent hyperlipidemia [36].

Cardioprotective Activity

CF has a beneficial effect on coronary heart disease [27]. It reduces the agglutination of blood platelets and enhances myocardial blood circulation and white cell phagocytosis, which has been used to cure diseases, such as furuncle and skin nodules [39]. CF also possesses blood pressure reducing effects, and regulates blood lipid levels [40]. The total flavonoids in CF have been studied for their vasodilatory effect, and they were seen to protect EDHF-mediated vasorelaxation to acetylcholine in the mesenteric artery of rats [41].

Effect on Urinary Infection

CF is also used for the treatment of prostatitis and chronic pelvic inflammation [42].

Neuroprotective Activity

CF possesses potent neuroprotective abilities against 1-methyl-4-phenylpridinium ions (MPP+), a Parkinsonian toxin, in human SH-SY5Y neuroblastoma cells. It effectively inhibited cytotoxicity, improved cell viability, attenuated ROS level elevation, and increased Bax/Bcl-2 ratio, caspase-3 cleavage, and PARP proteolysis [43].

CHEMICAL CONSTITUENTS OF CF AND THEIR ACTIVITIES

Modern pharmacological research has demonstrated that extracts containing flavonoids, terpenoids, phenolic compounds and several other chemical constituents of CF posses certain biological properties. Due to their different habitats and varieties, CF plants have a range of characteristic chemical compositions [44]. A genetic diversity evaluation found that CF from different origins had significant differences in bioactive content, indicating that environmental and genetic factors may play an essential role in determining the bioactive value of CF [45]. *Chrysanthemum* contains a variety of flavonoids, essential oils, phenolics, lactones, and sesquiterpenes [46,47]. Phenolic compounds are known to act as antioxidants, not only because they are able to donate hydrogen or electrons, but also because they form stable radical intermediates, which prevent the oxidation of various food ingredients, particularly fatty acids and oils [48]. The total phenoic and flavonoid content of a water extract of CF has been reported [18].

The DPPH radical scavenging ability and ascorbic acid equivalent antioxidant capacity volatile compounds in *C. indicum* and *C. morifolium* have been reported [29]. The DPPH radical scavenging ability, SOD activity, ABTS radical scavenging and total phenolic contents were reported for CF extracts prepared by hot-air drying at different temperatures and by far-infrared drying [30]. The active components in the ethyl-acetate soluble portion of CF have been investigated for their ability to inhibit NO production in LPS-activated macrophages [35]. The flavonoids such as acacetin, apigenin, luteolin and quercetin were reported as potent bio-antimutagens by inhibition of chemical mutagen and ultraviolet (UV) irradiation-induced Son of Sevenless (SOS) genes response to DNA damage [33]. Rutin, quercetin-3-glucoside, myricetin, quercitrin, and luteolin [8] extracted from CF showed pancreatic α-amylase inhibition and slightly inhibited intestinal maltase and sucrase activities [18]. One new disesquiterpenoid and two new sesquiterpenoids were also recently isolated from the dry flos of *C. indicum* [5]. Thirteen volatile compounds known to have antimicrobial and anti-cancer activities were isolated from CF [30].

Acacetin (5,7-dihydroxy-4′-methoxyflavone) is an *O*-methylated flavone reported to have neuroprotective effects in Parkinson's disease (PD) models [49]. It has long been considered to have anti-cancer and anti-inflammatory activities [49]. Luteolin (3′,4′,5,7-tetrahydroxyflavone) and apigenin (4′,5,7-trihydroxyflavone) are two common flavones and bioactive components in CF [50]. Superoxide anion-induced impairmen[t] of vasodialation is greatly improved by oral admin[istration] of luteolin and apigenin [51]. Total flavo[noids] and main component of the flavonoids from CF including luteolin-7-*O*-β-D-glucoside, apigenin-7-*O*-β-D-glucoside and acacetin-7-*O*-β-D-glucoside have a hypotensive effect on rat under normal condition [52].

Apigenin, a cell-permeable flavone [53] found in CF, evoked vasorelaxation in endothelium-intact aortic rings in a concentration dependent manner, and protected against relaxation dysfunction caused by superoxide anion radicals. It is suggested that apigenin causes endothelium-independent vasorelaxation by inhibiting both L-and T-type voltage-gated Ca^{2+} currents in the rat thoracic aorta [54]. The vascular protective effect of apigenin may be mediated by its antioxidative ability and attenuation of NO reduction [26].

Camphor and borneol, the main active components constituted in the essential oil of Flos Chrysanthemi [55], have been reported to have shown significant antimicrobial activity [56]. Essential oils from CF containing 1,8-cineole, camphor, borneol and bornyl acetate as their major constituents showed significant antimicrobial effects. However, some difference in antimicrobial activity between oils was found, and was attributed to variations in levels of these components. Camphor exhibited greater bacteriostatic activity [56].

Caffeoylquinic acids (CQAs) are also regarded as major constituents of CF. Their antioxidant mechanism involves hydroxyl groups combining with oxygen-centered free radicals, which form semiquinoid free radicals and terminate chain reactions. The activities of the caffeoylquinic acids differ because of the different numbers and positions of the hydroxyl groups [57]. This was corroborated by the detection of standards using off-line DPPH assay [7]. CQAs, especially 5-CQA, possessed stronger hydroxyl radical scavenging activities than the flavonoids apigenin and luteolin and their glucosides, which were isolated from CF [7,44].

The inhibitory activity against rat lens aldose reductase of three eudesmane-type sesquiterpenes, called kikkanol A, B, and C, along with luteolin, acacetin and their flavone glycosides, and chlorogenic acid were reported [46]. Studies showed that an extract of CF showed antibacterial and dephlogisticate activity, and three active phenolic compounds; chlorogenic acid, linarin, and luteolin, were identified in this extract [2].

Chlorogenic acid, a functional ingredient found in CF, has reported to prevent high glucose-induced cytotoxicity in human lens epithelial cells, and also to inhibit xylose-induced lens opacity and cytotoxicity in HLE-B3 cells under cultured diabetic conditions. These results suggest the usefulness of chlorogenic acid, particularly in the treatment of diabetic cataracts [58].

TOXIC EFFECTS OF CF

CF extract is very safe and there are few side effects. It has been reported that oral administration (10–20 g/kg/day) of an ethanolic extract of the root of CF for three days did not show any toxicity in mice [59]. Oral administration (300 mg/kg/day) of an ethanolic extract of CF flowers to dogs for three weeks did not cause any significant toxic reactions and intraperitoneal administration of the ethanolic extract at up to 36 g per kg body weight did not change the echocardiography (ECG) and activities of the animal [59]. In subacute toxicological studies on rabbits it was found that oral administration of crude extract of CF (20 g/kg/day) for 14 days did not show any significant change in ECG [59]. More recently, it was reported that oral administration of etheric extract of CF (15 g/kg) to Sprague Dawley (SD) rats does not cause any mortality, or behavioral changes over two weeks for both male and female rats; in addition, the CF extract did not show any genotoxicity [60]. Taken together, CF extracts could be safely used by diabetic patients and healthy people as a healthy and functional food.

CONCLUSIONS

Diabetologists are seeking new and better therapeutic management of diabetes mellitus and its associated complications from alternative and/or complementary therapies. In the management of DM, the administration of antioxidants will help to scavenge free radicals and eliminate them from metabolic pathways. This will help to improve glycemic control by targeting both hyperglycemia and oxidative stress simultaneously. The identified activities of CF could offer a benefit in the treatment of diabetes mellitus and prevention of its complications (Figure 21.6). Thus, CF could be developed as a functional food for diabetic patients.

SUMMARY POINTS

- Diabetes mellitus (DM) is now one of the most significant lifelong metabolic disorders in the world and its occurrence in Asian countries is disproportionately high.
- Diabetologists are seeking new and better therapeutic management of DM and its associated complications from alternative and/or complementary therapies.
- In the management of DM, administration of antioxidants will help to scavenge free radicals and eliminate them from metabolic pathways. This is especially useful in targeting both hyperglycemia and oxidative stress simultaneously.
- Chrysanthemi Flos (CF) is the flower of *Chrysanthemum indicum Linne* or *C. morifolium Ramatuelle.*
- CF has been widely used thousands of years as a functional food or botanical with therapeutic properties for head-ache, eye diseases, heat clearing, detoxification and other ailments. It is reported to have wide ranging activities, including analgesic, antipyretic, anti-inflammatory, antihypertensive properties.
- Hyperglycemia can induce oxidative stress, and lipid peroxidation is a marker of cellular damage. CF administration significantly decreased lipid peroxidation and subsequently increased antioxidants levels.
- Hyperglycemia generates an increased production of reducing equivalents from mitochondrial respiration and results in cellular dysfunction and mutations in mitochondrial DNA. CF treatment appears to significantly suppress the progression of apoptosis.
- The detailed identification of the activities of CF offers a potential benefit in the treatment of DM and prevention of its complications.
- Thus, CF could be developed as a functional food for diabetic patients.

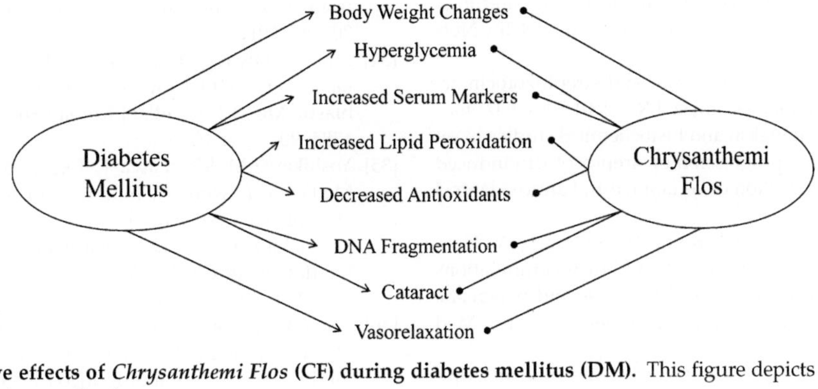

FIGURE 21.6 Protective effects of *Chrysanthemi Flos* (CF) during diabetes mellitus (DM). This figure depicts various useful effects of CF against diabetes and diabetic complications.

References

[1] Maritim AC, Sanders RA, Watkins 3rd JB. Diabetes, oxidative stress, and antioxidants: a review. J Biochem Mol Toxicol 2003;17(1):24–38.

[2] Kim J-J, Ramesh T, Kim S-J. Protective effects of Chrysanthemi Flos extract against streptozotocin-induced oxidative damage in diabetic mice. J Med Plants Res 2012;6(4):622–30.

[3] Cockram CS. Diabetes mellitus: perspective from the Asia-Pacific region. Diabetes Res Clin Pract 2000;50(Suppl. 2):S3–7.

[4] Ramalingam M, Kim S-J. Reactive oxygen/nitrogen species and their functional correlations in neurodegenerative diseases. J Neural Transm 2012;119(8):891–910.

[5] Zhou J, Wang JS, Zhang Y, Wang PR, Guo C, Kong LY. Disesquiterpenoid and sesquiterpenes from the flos of *Chrysanthemum indicum*. Chem Pharm Bull (Tokyo) 2012;60(8):1067–71.

[6] Fang H-l, Guo Q-s, Shen H-j, Shao Q-s. Phylogeography of *Chrysanthemum indicum* L. (Compositae) in China based on trnL-F sequences. Biochem Syst Ecol 2010;38(6):1204–11.

[7] Cui G, Niu Y, Wang H, Dong J, Yuki H, Chen S. Rapid isolation and identification of active antioxidant ingredients from Gongju using HPLC-DAD-ESI-MS(n) and postcolumn derivatization. J Agric Food Chem 2012;60(21):5407–13.

[8] Wu L-Y, Gao H-Z, Wang X-L, Ye J-H, Lu J-L, Liang Y-R. Analysis of chemical composition of *Chrysanthemum indicum* flowers by GC/MS and HPLC. J Med Plants Res 2010;4(5):421–6.

[9] Hu CK, Lee YJ, Colitz CM, Chang CJ, Lin CT. The protective effects of *Lycium barbarum* and *Chrysanthemum morifolum* on diabetic retinopathies in rats. Vet Ophthalmol 2012;15(Suppl. 2):65–71.

[10] Matsuda H, Morikawa T, Toguchida I, Harima S, Yoshikawa M. Medicinal flowers. VI. Absolute stereostructures of two new flavanone glycosides and a phenylbutanoid glycoside from the flowers of *Chrysanthemum indicum* L.: their inhibitory activities for rat lens aldose reductase. Chem Pharm Bull (Tokyo) 2002;50(7):972–5.

[11] Al-Rawi NH. Diabetes, Oxidative Stress, Antioxidants and Saliva: A Review. In: Lushchak VI, Gospodaryov DV, editors. Oxidative Stress and Diseases: InTech; 2012. p. 303–10.

[12] Erejuwa OO. Oxidative Stress in Diabetes Mellitus: Is there a role for hypoglycemic drugs and/or antioxidants? In: Lushchak VI, Gospodaryoy DV, editors. Oxidative Stress and Diseases: InTech; 2012. p. 217–246.

[13] Kumawat M, Singh I, Singh N, Singh V, Kharb S. Lipid peroxidation and lipid profile in type II diabetes mellitus. WebmedCentral BIOCHEMISTRY 2012;3(3): WMC003147.

[14] Paolisso G, D'Amore A, Balbi V, Volpe C, Galzerano D, Giugliano D, et al. Plasma vitamin C affects glucose homeostasis in healthy subjects and in non-insulin-dependent diabetics. Am J Physiol 1994;266(2 Pt 1):E261–8.

[15] Frei B. Ascorbic acid protects lipids in human plasma and low-density lipoprotein against oxidative damage. Am J Clin Nutr 1991;54(6 Suppl.); 1113S-8S.

[16] Szkudelski T. The mechanism of alloxan and streptozotocin action in B cells of the rat pancreas. Physiol Res 2001;50(6):537–46.

[17] Waer HF, Helmy SA. Cytological and histochemical studies in rat liver and pancreas during progression of streptozotocin induced diabetes and possible protection of certain natural antioxidants. J Nutr Food Sci 2012;2:9.

[18] Adisakwattana S, Ruengsamran T, Kampa P, Sompong W. *In vitro* inhibitory effects of plant-based foods and their combinations on intestinal inverted question mark-glucosidase and pancreatic inverted question mark-amylase. BMC Complement Altern Med 2012;12(1):110.

[19] Gerrits PM, Tsalikian E. Diabetes and fructose metabolism. Am J Clin Nutr 1993;58(5 Suppl.):796S–9S.

[20] Raptis SA, Dimitriadis GD. Oral hypoglycemic agents: insulin secretagogues, alpha-glucosidase inhibitors and insulin sensitizers. Exp Clin Endocrinol Diabetes 2001;109(Suppl. 2):S265–87.

[21] Sudhir R, Mohan V. Postprandial hyperglycemia in patients with type 2 diabetes mellitus. Treat Endocrinol 2002;1(2): 105–16.

[22] Scorpiglione N, Belfiglio M, Carinci F, Cavaliere D, De Curtis A, Franciosi M, et al. The effectiveness, safety and epidemiology of the use of acarbose in the treatment of patients with type II diabetes mellitus. A model of medicine-based evidence. Eur J Clin Pharmacol 1999;55(4):239–49.

[23] Matsuda H, Morikawa T, Toguchida I, Yoshikawa M. Structural requirements of flavonoids and related compounds for aldose reductase inhibitory activity. Chem Pharm Bull (Tokyo) 2002;50(6):788–95.

[24] Patel DK, Kumar R, Sairam K, Hemalatha S. Pharmacologically tested aldose reductase inhibitors isolated from plant sources – A concise report. Chin J Nat Med 2012;10(5):388–400.

[25] Rodriguez-Manas L, Angulo J, Vallejo S, Peiro C, Sanchez-Ferrer A, Cercas E, et al. Early and intermediate Amadori glycosylation adducts, oxidative stress, and endothelial dysfunction in the streptozotocin-induced diabetic rats vasculature. Diabetologia 2003;46(4):556–66.

[26] Jin BH, Qian LB, Chen S, Li J, Wang HP, Bruce IC, et al. Apigenin protects endothelium-dependent relaxation of rat aorta against oxidative stress. Eur J Pharmacol 2009;616(1–3):200–5.

[27] Jiang H, Xia Q, Xu W, Zheng M. Chrysanthemum morifolium attenuated the reduction of contraction of isolated rat heart and cardiomyocytes induced by ischemia/reperfusion. Pharmazie 2004;59(7):565–7.

[28] Jiang HD, Cai J, Xu JH, Zhou XM, Xia Q. Endothelium-dependent and direct relaxation induced by ethyl acetate extract from Flos Chrysanthemi in rat thoracic aorta. J Ethnopharmacol 2005;101 (1–3):221–6.

[29] Woo KS, Yu JS, Hwang IG, Lee YR, Lee CH, Yoon H-S, et al. Antioxidative activity of volatile compounds in flower of *Chrysanthemum indicum, C. morifolium* and *C. zawadskii*. J Korean Soc Food Sci Nutr 2008;37(6):805–9.

[30] Bae S-M, Na A-S, Seo H-K, Lee S-C. Effects of drying conditions on the antioxidant activities and volatile compounds of *Chrysanthemi flos* flowers. J Food Sci Nutr 2009;14:329–34.

[31] Chen GP, Wang S. Scavenging action of Huangshan Gongju extracts to hydroxyl radicals. Chemical Industry Times 2005;19(5): 14–7.

[32] Hong B-S, Chu Y-J, Lee E-J. Natural dyeing absorption properties of Chitosan and nano silver composite non-woven fabrics – Focus on *Chrysanthemum indicum* Linn. J Korean Soc Cloth Text 2010;34(5):775–83.

[33] Miyazawa M, Hisama M. Antimutagenic activity of flavonoids from *Chrysanthemum morifolium*. Biosci Biotechnol Biochem 2003;67(10):2091–9.

[34] Yun J, Hwang E-S, Kim G-H. Effects of *Chrysanthemum indicum* L. extract on the growth and differentiation of osteoblastic MC3T3-E1 cells. J Korean Soc Food Sci Nutr 2011;40(10): 1384–90.

[35] Yoshikawa M, Morikawa T, Toguchida I, Harima S, Matsuda H. Medicinal flowers. II. Inhibitors of nitric oxide production and absolute stereostructures of five new germacrane-type sesquiterpenes, kikkanols D, D monoacetate, E, F, and F monoacetate from the flowers of *Chrysanthemum indicum* L. Chem Pharm Bull (Tokyo) 2000;48(5):651–6.

[36] Choo MH, Jeong Y, Lee MY. Effects of an ethylacetate fraction of Chrysanthemi Flos on the antioxidative system and lipid profile in rats with ethanol-induced liver damage. J Food Sci Nutr 2004;9(4):352–60.

[37] Cheon MS, Yoon T, Lee do Y, Choi G, Moon BC, Lee AY, et al. *Chrysanthemum indicum* Linne extract inhibits the inflammatory response by suppressing NF-kappaB and MAPKs activation in lipopolysaccharide-induced RAW 264.7 macrophages. J Ethnopharmacol 2009;122(3):473–7.
[38] Lee DY, Choi G, Yoon T, Cheon MS, Choo BK, Kim HK. Anti-inflammatory activity of *Chrysanthemum indicum* extract in acute and chronic cutaneous inflammation. J Ethnopharmacol 2009;123(1):149–54.
[39] Zhang FK. Measurement of chemical components in common Chinese herbs. Beijing, China: People Sanitary Press; 1997, 606–610.
[40] Pan Z-J, Wang X-F, Zhou X-R. Effects of HuangShan GongJu decoction on blood pressures and blood lipids of hypertensive mice. Lishizhen Medicine and Materia Medica Research 2008;19(3):669–70.
[41] He D, Ru X, Wen L, Wen Y, Jiang H, Bruce IC, et al. Total flavonoids of *Flos Chrysanthemi* protect arterial endothelial cells against oxidative stress. J Ethnopharmacol 2012;139(1):68–73.
[42] National Commission of Chinese Pharmacopeia. In: The Pharmacopoeia of the People's Republic of China. vol. 1. Beijing: Chemical Industry Press; 2005, p. 596.
[43] Kim IS, Koppula S, Park PJ, Kim EH, Kim CG, Choi WS, et al. Chrysanthemum morifolium Ramat (CM) extract protects human neuroblastoma SH-SY5Y cells against MPP+-induced cytotoxicity. J Ethnopharmacol 2009;126(3):447–54.
[44] Niu Y, Yin L, Luo S, Dong J, Wang H, Hashi Y, et al. Identification of the Anti-oxidants in *Flos Chrysanthemi* by HPLC–DAD–ESI/MSn and HPLC Coupled with a Post-column Derivatisation System. Phytochem Anal 2013;24(1):59–68.
[45] Fang H-l, Guo Q-s, Shen H-j, Li Y-c. Genetic diversity evaluation of *Chrysanthemum indicum* L. by medicinal compounds and molecular biology tools. Biochem Syst Ecol 2012;41(0):26–34.
[46] Yoshikawa M, Morikawa T, Murakami T, Toguchida I, Harima S, Matsuda H. Medicinal flowers. I. Aldose reductase inhibitors and three new eudesmane-type sesquiterpenes, kikkanols A, B, and C, from the flowers of *Chrysanthemum indicum* L. Chem Pharm Bull (Tokyo) 1999;47(3):340–5.
[47] Shin YJ, Jeon JR, Park GS. Physiocochemical properties of Gamgug (*Chrysanthemum indicum* L.). J Korean Soc Food Sci Nutr 2004;33(1):146–51.
[48] Cuvelier ME, Richard H, Berset C. Comparison of the antioxidant activity of some acid phenols: structure-activity relationship. Biosci Biotechnol Biochem 2002;56:324–5.
[49] Kim HG, Ju MS, Ha SK, Lee H, Kim SY, Oh MS. Acacetin protects dopaminergic cells against 1-methyl-4-phenyl-1,2,3,6-tetrahydropyridine-induced neuroinflammation *in vitro* and *in vivo*. Biol Pharm Bull 2012;35(8):1287–94.
[50] Chen Z, Kong S, Song F, Li L, Jiang H. Pharmacokinetic study of luteolin, apigenin, chrysoeriol and diosmetin after oral administration of *Flos Chrysanthemi* extract in rats. Fitoterapia 2012;83(8):1616–22.
[51] Ma X, Li YF, Gao Q, Ye ZG, Lu XJ, Wang HP, et al. Inhibition of superoxide anion-mediated impairment of endothelium by treatment with luteolin and apigenin in rat mesenteric artery. Life Sci 2008;83(3–4):110–7.
[52] Dai M, Liu Q, Li D, Liu L. Research of material bases on antifebrile and hypotensive effects of *Flos Chrysanthemi*. Zhong Yao Cai 2001;24(7):505–6.
[53] Choi JS, Choi YJ, Park SH, Kang JS, Kang YH. Flavones mitigate tumor necrosis factor-alpha-induced adhesion molecule upregulation in cultured human endothelial cells: role of nuclear factor-kappa B. J Nutr 2004;134(5):1013–9.
[54] Ko FN, Huang TF, Teng CM. Vasodilatory action mechanisms of apigenin isolated from *Apium graveolens* in rat thoracic aorta. Biochim Biophys Acta 1991;1115(1):69–74.
[55] Ye Q, Deng C. Determination of camphor and borneol in *Flos Chrysanthemi* Indici by UAE and GC-FID. J Chromatogr Sci 2009;47(4):287–90.
[56] Shunying Z, Yang Y, Huaidong Y, Yue Y, Guolin Z. Chemical composition and antimicrobial activity of the essential oils of *Chrysanthemum indicum*. J Ethnopharmacol 2005;96(1–2):151–8.
[57] Chen S. The antioxidant activity and structure activity relationship of flavonoids. Strait Pharm 1998;10(4):4–6.
[58] Kim YS, Kim NH, Lee YM, Kim JS. Preventive effect of chlorogenic acid on lens opacity and cytotoxicity in human lens epithelial cells. Biol Pharm Bull 2011;34(6):925–8.
[59] Wang YS. Pharmacology and applications of Chinese Materia Medica. Beijing: People's Health Publisher; 1983.
[60] Shen H-J, Guo Q-S, Fang H-L. Toxicological evaluation of carotenoid-type extracts from *Flos Chrysanthemi Indici*. J Med Plants Res 2011;5(23):5507–12.

CHAPTER

22

Antioxidant Supplements and Diabetic Retinopathy

Jose Javier Garcia-Medina, Monica del-Rio-Vellosillo†, Vicente Zanon-Moreno**, Manuel Garcia-Medina‡, Maria Dolores Pinazo-Duran§, Roberto Gallego-Pinazo****

*Department of Ophthalmology, University General Hospital Reina Sofía and Department of Ophthalmology and Optometry, School of Medicine, University of Murcia, Murcia, Spain, †Department of Anesthesiology, University Hospital La Arrixaca, El Palmar, Murcia, Spain, **Genetic and Molecular Epidemiology Unit, Department of Preventive Medicine and Public Health, School of Medicine, University of Valencia and CIBER Fisiopatología de la Obesidad y Nutrición, ISCIII, Valencia, Spain, ‡Department of Ophthalmology, Torrecardenas Hospital, Almeria, Spain, §Ophthalmology Research Unit 'Santiago Grisolia' and Department of Surgery, School of Medicine, University of Valencia, Valencia, Spain, ***Department of Ophthalmology, University and Polytechnic Hospital La Fe, Valencia, Spain

List of Abbreviations

ALA α-linolenic acid
AREDS Age-related eye disease study
BP Blood pressure
BRECs Bovine retinal microvascular endothelial cells
Ca Dob Calcium dobesilate
CBD Cannabidiol
CD Conjugated dienes
CSME Clinically significant macular edema
DHA Docosahexaenoic acid
DR Diabetic retinopathy
EPA Eicosapentaenoic acid
ERG Electroretinogram
GR Glutathione reductase
GSH Glutathione
GSH-px Glutathione peroxidase
iBRB Internal blood-retinal barrier
ICAM Intercellular cell adhesion molecule
LP Lipid hydroperoxides
MDA Malondialdehyde
MnSOD Mitochondrial-specific superoxide dismutase
mtDNA Mitochondrial DNA
NO Nitric oxide
NOS Nitric oxide synthase
PEDF Pigment-epithelium-derived factor
PMS Postmarketing surveillance
POAG Primary open-angle glaucoma
ROS Reactive oxygen species
RPE Retinal pigmented epithelial
SOD Superoxide dismutase
TAS Total antioxidant status
TBARS Thiobarbituric acid-reactive substances
VCAM 1 Vascular cell adhesion molecule
VEGF Vascular endothelial growth factor

INTRODUCTION

Diabetic retinopathy (DR) is one of the major causes of blindness in older (65 years of age and older) and working age adults (20–70 years of age). Several studies have shown the importance of glycemic control or blood pressure (BP) control in reducing the incidence and progression of DR [1a–c]. However, it is remarkable that some patients may still develop DR or its complications, even with tight glycemic and/or BP control, and that standard treatments for DR, which include laser photocoagulation, vitrectomy, intravitreal corticosteroids and intravitreal anti-vascular endothelial growth factor (VEGF) agents, have not proved capable of arresting progression in all cases.

This resistance to halting DR is commonly known as 'metabolic memory', and it has been related to oxidative stress [1d]. All these facts reveal the need to develop alternative treatment methods, possibly to be used in combination with standard therapies, and antioxidant

Diabetes: Oxidative Stress and Dietary Antioxidants.
http://dx.doi.org/10.1016/B978-0-12-405885-9.00022-X

TABLE 22.1 *In Vitro* Studies in Retinal cells Cultured Under Hyperglycemic Conditions

Authors	Publication Date	Sample Type	Antioxidant(s) Used	Results
Ansari et al. [2]	1998	Cultured rat retina	Trolox	Decrease of TBARS (marker of oxidative stress)
Kowluru et al. [3]	2002	Bovine perycites and endothelial cells	Different antioxidants	Inhibition of increase of caspase-3 (apoptosis enzyme)
Amano et al. [4]	2005	Bovine retinal isolated perycites	PEDF	Reduction of apoptosis of pericytes; increased glutathione peroxidase; prevention of activation of caspase-3
Madsen-Bouterse et al. [5]	2010	Endothelial cells isolated from bovine retina and cultured	MnTBAP	Prevention of mitochondrial DNA damage
Zeng et al. [6]	2010	Müller cells cultures	Taurine	Decrease of TBARS, ROS; increase of the catalase, SOD and GSH-px activities in a dose-dependent manner
Dutot et al. [8]	2011	Human RPE cells cultured	EPA and DHA	Decrease of ROS overproduction
Li et al. [7]	2011	Cultured human retinal endothelial cells	SS31	Decrease of ROS production; decrease of the expression of caspase-3
Shen et al. [9]	2012	Rhesus macaque choroids-retinal endothelial cells cultured	α-linolenic acid (ALA), linoleic acid and Zinc	Abrogation of excess proliferation of retinal vascular endothelial cells. ALA suppresses ROS generation and increases SOD activity. ALA suppresses VEGF secretion by cultured cells
Wu et al. [10]	2012	BRECs with insuline stimulation	Ascorbic acid, α-lipoic acid, and α-tocopherol	Decreased superoxide anion production

therapy is one of the proposed options. A series of studies has been conducted on retinal cells *'in vitro'* (under hyperglycemic conditions), diabetic animals and diabetic patients to evaluate the effects of antioxidant agents on the different structural and functional abnormalities found in DR (Tables 22.1, 22.2, and 22.3, respectively).

IN VITRO STUDIES

In vitro studies have been performed by subjecting different types of retinal tissues or cells to hyperglycemic conditions. Then antioxidants agents have been included in the medium and the effects have been measured.

A range of studies have demonstrated that hyperglycemic conditions in cultured retinal tissues or cells trigger oxidative stress, characterized by an increase in reactive oxygen species (ROS). ROS production depletes endogenous antioxidants, leading to ROS accumulation and causing cellular damage. Such ROS overproduction can be prevented by exogenous antioxidants. Otherwise a medium high in glucose decreases antioxidant enzyme activities compared with a normal glucose medium. In addition, the exogenous antioxidants included in hyperglycemic media are related to an increase in several kinds of endogenous antioxidant agents. Increased oxidative stress in diabetes has been implicated, among with other mechanisms, in damaging mitochondrial DNA (mtDNA), activation of retinal caspase-3, and apoptosis of retinal cells. Some antioxidants *in vitro* also diminish the overexpression of caspase-3 and cellular apoptosis, and prevent damage to mtDNA (Table 22.1).

Thiobarbituric acid-reactive substances (TBARS), formed as a byproduct of lipid peroxidation, undergo several-fold increases in rat retinas cultured in a hyperglycemic medium, which decreases significantly when Trolox, a water soluble analog of vitamin E, is included in the medium [2].

Caspase-3 (an apoptosis execution enzyme) activity is inhibited in isolated retinal capillary cells by different antioxidants, such as N-acetyl cysteine, lipoic acid, a-tocopherol acetate, Trolox, ascorbic acid or b-carotene [3].

The pigment-epithelium-derived factor (PEDF), a multifunctional protein with antioxidant properties, blocks high-glucose-induced intracellular ROS generation and activation of caspase-3 in pericytes. In addition, PEDF protects high glucose-induced pericyte apoptosis [4].

Mitochondrial dysfunction induced by high glucose levels in retinal cells is related to mtDNA damage. mtDNA damage induces increased ROS production within the mitochondria. This effect can be counterbalanced by mitochondrial superoxide dismutase (MnSOD). An MnSOD mimic, MnTBAP, prevents mtDNA damage [5].

Incubation of Müller cells in hyperglycemic medium with taurine, a non-essential amino acid with antioxidant properties, induces a significant decrease in TBARS nd increases antioxidant defenses, such as catalase, uperoxide dismutase (SOD) and glutation peroxidase GSH-px) activity, in a dose-dependent manner [6]. Furhermore, a mitochondria-targeted antioxidant peptide, alled SS31, diminishes ROS production and the expresion of caspase-3 in cultured human retinal endothelial ells [7].

Recently it has been shown that omega-3 fatty acids rom fish oil, docosahexaenoic acid (DHA), and eicosaentaenoic acid (EPA) decrease ROS overproduction in uman retinal pigmented epithelial (RPE) cells cultured at a high glucose concentration [8]. Other polyunsaturated fatty acids found mainly in vegetables, such as α-linolenic (ALA) acid and α-linoleic acid, can abrogate the excess proliferation of retinal vascular endothelial cells. ALA also induces the inhibition of ROS generation and enhances SOD activity [9]. Moreover, bovine retinal microvascular endothelial cells (BRECs) cultured in a hyperglycemic medium display reduced oxidative stress, measured as superoxide anion production, when exposed to antioxidant agents such as ascorbic acid, α-lipoic acid or α-tocopherol [10].

ANIMAL STUDIES

The use of antioxidants to inhibit the development of DR in animal models appears to be promising (Table 22.2).

Nicanartine, an antioxidant and lipid-lowering compound, inhibits pericyte loss in diabetic rats, but has no effect on the formation of acellular capillaries or microaneurysms [11]. Similarly, Trolox also helps partially restore diminished pericytes in retinal vessels in diabetic rodents [2].

Vitamins C (ascorbic acid) and E (α-tocopherol) can individually prevent abnormalities of ocular blood hemodynamics and leukostasis in diabetic rats [12–14].

Vitamin E + selenium and taurine reduce retinal conjugated dienes (CD) and lipid hydroperoxides (LP) [15]. The VEGF protein concentration is high in diabetic rats if compared with control rats. Taurine and α-lipoic acid attenuate VEGF levels in diabetic rats [16–17]. In addition, α-lipoic acid preserves the number of pericytes and prevents the formation of acellular capillaries [18–19]. This effects the α-lipoic acid, which might be related to the inhibition of lipid peroxidation, the normalization of nuclear transcriptional factor and the restoration of antioxidant defenses observed in the retinas of diabetic rats [18–20]. Moreover, lipoic acid restores the electroretinogram b-wave amplitude of diabetic animals to control values [20].

In other studies it was seen that supplementation by long-term administration of both vitamins C and E prevents the development of acellular capillaries and pericyte ghosts in diabetic rats [21–23]. In addition, when vitamins C and E are supplemented with other antioxidants (vitamin C, α-tocopherol, Trolox, *N*-acetyl cysteine, β-carotene and selenium), the benefits relating to the survival of retinal cells are more obvious, and not only diminish the activation of retinal protein kinase C and lipid peroxidation indicators, but prevent a decrease in SOD, glutathione reductase (GR) and catalase [21]. The nuclear transcriptional factor and the apoptosis execution enzyme, caspase-3, are also inhibited by this antioxidant mixture [3,3b]. Green tea, highly antioxidant and rich in polyphenols, induces reductions in acellular capillaries and pericyte ghosts [23].

Curcumin, a natural yellow pigment, decreases oxidative stress and seems to have an anti-inflammatory effect on DR [24]. Another antioxidant, Ca Dob, inhibits pericyte loss and acellular capillaries formation [25], and protects iBRB by restoring tight junction production [26]. Alternatively, age-related eye disease study (AREDS)-based micronutrients (ascorbic acid, vitamin E, β-carotene, zinc, and copper) prevent retinal acellular capillaries from increasing. Additionally, this multiantioxidant complex diminishes oxidative and nitrative damage to retinas in diabetic rodents [27].

Carotenoids, such as lutein or zeaxanthin, also seem to have preventive effects on DR in diabetic rats. Lutein normalizes markers of retinal oxidative stress, avoids ganglion cell loss and decreases apoptosis markers (caspase-3) [28–30]. Lutein also attenuates the loss of ganglion cells and prevents impairment in ERGs [29]. Zeaxanthin not only inhibits oxidative damage, but also performs anti-inflammatory action [31].

MnSOD mimetics, such as tempol, can counterbalance the overproduction of superoxide radicals in DR, thus protecting vascular cells. Tempol partially improves the retinal microvascular hemodynamics in DR [32]. Moreover, this compound prevents oxidative damage and the accumulation of glial fibrillary acidic protein and fibronectin, early molecular markers of DR in diabetic mice [33].

Other agents that may affect the redox balance or can protect diabetic rats from DR are fidarestat [34], ebselen [28], cannabidiol [35], topical nepafenac [36], DHA [29], PEDF [37], carnosine [38] and curmicum [39] (Table 22.2).

CLINICAL STUDIES

Animal studies have shown that antioxidants have beneficial effects on the development of retinopathy, but the results of clinical trials are somewhat variable (Table 22.3). Several types of interventions in diabetic patients using a range of antioxidants, either singly or in combination, have been carried out by the corresponding authors. Some of these studies are described below.

Pycnogenol®, a French maritime pine bark extract, is a unique blend of natural, powerful antioxidants.

TABLE 22.2 *In Vivo* Studies in Diabetic Laboratory Animals

Author	Date Published	Antioxidant(s) Used	Results
Hammes et al. [11]	1997	Nicanartine	Prevention of increase in endothelial cells and reduction in pericyte numbers. No effects on the formation of acellular capillaries or microaneurysms.
Kunisaki et al. [12]	1998	Vitamin E	Prevention of abnormalities of retinal blood hemodynamics.
Ansari et al. [2]	1998	Trolox	Partial conservation of pericytes.
Kowluru et al. [21]	2001	Vitamins C and E	Less acellular capillaries and pericyte ghosts in supplemented diabetic rats.
Kowluru et al. [21]	2001	Multi-antioxidant diet	Less cellular capillaries and pericyte ghosts in supplemented galactosemic and diabetic rats. Parameters of retinal oxidative stress normalized by multi-antioxidant diet.
Obrosova et al. [17]	2001	α-lipoic acid or taurine	VEGF level was attenuated by taurine and prevented by α-lipoic acid.
Kowluru et al. [3]	2002	Multi-antioxidant diet	Prevent increase of caspase-3 (apoptosis enzyme).
Di Leo et al. [15]	2003	Taurine and vitamin E + selenium	Reduction of retinal conjugated dienes and lipid hydroperoxides.
Obrosova et al. [34]	2003	fidarestat	Arrested diabetes-induced retinal lipid peroxidation indirectly through aldose reductase inhibition.
Abiko et al. [13]	2003	α-lipoic acid or D-α-tocopherol	D-α-tocopherol prevents the increases in leukostasis and decreases in retinal blood flow; α-lipoic acid only prevents the increases in leukostasis.
Kowluru et al. [3b]	2003	Multi-antioxidant diet	Prevention of increase of nuclear transcriptional factor (proinflammatory and apoptosis factor).
Miranda et al. [28]	2004	Ebselen or lutein	Normalization of markers of retinal oxidative stress.
Kowluru et al. [18]	2004	α-lipoic acid	Prevention of capillary cell apoptosis and formation of acellular capillaries. Inhibition of retinal lipid peroxidation.
Padilla et al. [25]	2005	Calcium dobesilate	Attenuation of vascular tortuosity, acellular capillaries, focal accumulations of capillaries and reduction of the number of pericytes.
Mustata et al. [23]	2005	Green tea or Vitamin C and E	Prevention of acellular capillaries, and pericyte ghost. Decrease of superoxide production.
El-Remessy et al. [35]	2006	Cannabidiol (CBD)	CBD treatment reduces oxidative stress; it also decreases the levels of tumor necrosis factor-α, vascular endothelial growth factor, and ICAM-1; and it prevents retinal cell death and vascular hyperpermeability in the diabetic retina.
Yatoh et al. [22]	2006	Vitamins C and E	Amelioration of the increase of apoptosis of pericytes and endothelial cells and also inhibit acellular capillaries.
Lin et al. [19]	2006	α-lipoic acid	Preservation of pericytes. Reduction of oxidative stress and VEGF. Normalization of nuclear transcriptional factor and angiopoietin-2.
Jariyapongskul et al. [14]	2007	Vitamin C	Increase of adherent leukocytes and reduction of iris blood flow.
Kerns et al. [36]	2007	Topical nepafenac	Decrease of retinal prostaglandin E(2), superoxide, cyclooxygenase-2, and leukostasis. Reduction of acellular capillaries, and pericyte ghosts. Inhibition of oscillatory potential latency. No effect in retinal ganglion cell survival.
Kowluru et al. [39]	2007	Curmicum	Decrease of oxidative stress and proinflammatory.
Kowuluru et al. [31]	2008	Zeaxanthin	Inhibition of oxidative damage and anti-inflammatory action.
Johnsen-Soriano et al. [20]	2008	α-lipoic acid	Prevention of the decreases of GSH content and GSH-px activity and normalized MDA concentration. Moreover, lipoic acid restores ERG b-wave amplitude of diabetic animals to control values.

'ABLE 22.2 *In Vivo* Studies in Diabetic Laboratory Animals — cont'd

uthor	Date Published	Antioxidant(s) Used	Results
owuluru et al. [27]	2008	AREDS-based micronutrients	Prevention of oxidative and nitrative stress. Prevention of formation of acellular capillaries.
rnal et al. [29]	2009	DHA or lutein	Avoidance of reduction in retinal thickness. Prevention of impairment of the electroretinogram. Inhibition of lipidic peroxidation and apoptosis markers (caspase-3).
'oshida et al. [37]	2009	PEDF	Restoration of the decrease in amplitudes of a- and b-wave of ERG; reduced retinal VEGF; inhibition of retinal vascular hyperpermeability; reduction of retinal 8-hydroxydeoxyguanosine, a marker of oxidative stress.
Leal et al. [26]	2010	Calcium dobesilate	Prevention of the iBRB breakdown by restoring tight junction protein. Decrease of leukocyte adhesion to retinal vessels.
Sasaki et al. [30]	2010	Lutein	Avoidance of ganglion cell loss and decrease of caspase-3.
Pfister et al. [38]	2011	Carnosine	Prevention of retinal vascular damage; reduction of photoreceptors.
Yadav et al. [32]	2011	Tempol	Increase of blood flow rates and red blood cell velocity (the antioxidant tempol provides partial improvements in retinal microvascular hemodynamics early).
Rosales et al. [33]	2011	Tempol	Prevention of oxidative damage, glial fibrillary acidic protein and fibronectin accumulation (early molecular markers of DR).

TABLE 22.3 Clinical Studies in Diabetic Patients

Author	Date	Sample Size and Duration of Supplementation	Antioxidant(s) Used	Results
Larsen et al. [52]	1977	18 (8 months)	Calcium Dobesilate	No effects on the capillary resistance in the course of diabetic retinopathy.
Stamper et al. [53]	1978	42 (6 months) 36 (1 year)	Calcium dobesilate	No clinical effect found in non-proliferative diabetic retinopathy.
Vojnikovic [54]	1984	50 (3 months)	Calcium dobesilate	Reduction in the capillary fragility, microvascular hyperpermeability, and blood viscosity in the course of diabetic retinopathy.
Benarroch et al. [56]	1985	37 (3 months)	Calcium dobesilate	Reduction in whole blood viscosity and capillary fragility.
Leydhecker et al. [40]	1986	32 (6 months)	Calcium dobesilate (Dexium®) or Pycnogenol®	Pycnogenol® improved exudates in both eyes of five patients, whereas this was the case in only one Dexium-treated patient. Both drugs showed good effect on automated visual field (particularly Pycnogenol®).
Vojnikovic [55]	1991	79 (6 months)	Calcium dobesilate	Reduced both the surface area of retinal hemorrhages and whole blood and plasma viscosity in non-insulin-dependent diabetics.
Kähler et al. [43]	1993	80 (3 months)	α-lipoic acid or Selenium or Vit. E	Diminished serum concentrations of TBARS and of urinary albumin excretion rates in all treated groups.
Faure et al. [44]	1995	18 (3 months)	Zinc	Decrease of TBARS in all patients. Increase of plamatic GSH-px activity in patients with retinopathy.

(Continued)

TABLE 22.3 Clinical Studies in Diabetic Patients — cont'd

Author	Date	Sample Size and Duration of Supplementation	Antioxidant(s) Used	Results
Bursell et al. [45]	1999	45 (8 moths:4 months of treatment or placebo + crossover + 4 months of treatment or placebo)	Vitamin E	Baseline retinal blood flow was decreased in diabetic patients. After treatment, diabetic patient retinal blood flow was comparable with that of nondiabetic subjects.
Spadea et al. [41]	2001	30 (2 months)	Pycnogenol®	In placebo group retinopathy progressively worsened and the visual acuity decreased; Pycnogenol-treated patients showed no deterioration of retinal function and recovery of visual acuity.
Huang et al. [46]	2004	25 type 2 DM (3 months)	Ginkgo biloba extract	Reduced MDA levels; decreased fibrinogen levels, promoted erythrocytes deformability, and improved blood viscosity, viscoelasticity and retinal blood flow rate.
Ribeiro et al. [57]	2006	137 type 2 DM (2 years)	Calcium dobesilate	Better activity than placebo on prevention of iBRB disruption as measured by fluorophotometry. Better results tha placebo on funduscopic hemorrhages, DR level and microaneurysms.
Steigerwalt et al. [42]	2009	46 type 2 DM (3 months)	Pycnogenol®	Reduction in retinal edema and better retinal thickness. Amelioration of the flow at the central retinal artery. Improvement of visual acuity.
Haritoglou et al. [58]	2009	635 type 2 DM (5years)	Calcium dobesilate	No reduction of the risk of development of clinically significant macular edema.
Garcia-Medina et al. [47]	2011	105 type 2 DM (5 years)	Antioxidant formulation (Vitalux Forte®)	Retardation of clinical progression in treated group. Maintainance of antioxidant plasma status levels in treated group. Plasmatic MDA decreased in treated group and increased in no treated group. No effect on visual acuity.
Haritoglou et al. [48]	2011	467 type 2 DM (2 years)	α-lipoic acid	No prevention of clinically significant macular edema. No effect on visual acuity.
Nebbioso et al. [49]	2012	32 pre-retinopathic diabetics (30 days)	α-lipoic acid + genistein + vitamins (C, E , B)	Increases of plasma antioxidant levels and ERG oscillatory potential values were observed in the group treated with antioxidants but not in the control group.

Leydhecker et al. reported that administering Pycnogenol® for six months to diabetics improved exudates in both eyes of five (of 32) patients, displaying benefits on the automated visual field [40]. Furthermore, Spadea et al. administered Pycnogenol® to 20 diabetics for two months, and 10 more patients were added to the placebo group. Retinopathy progressively worsened and visual acuity decreased in the latter group as compared to treated patients. The Pycnogenol-treated patients showed no deterioration in retinal function and they recovered their visual acuity [41]. More recently, Steigerwalt et al. studied the effects of administering Pycnogenol in 24 treated and 22 placebo type 2 diabetics for three months. A significant decrease in retinal edema was detected, as reflected in the amelioration of retinal thickness, blood flow at the central retinal artery and visual improvement [42].

A study was performed by Kähler et al. in 80 diabetics, who were divided into four groups of 20 patients each, and assigned an intake of α-lipoic acid; or selenium; or vitamin E; or nothing for three months. The MDA-TBARS serum concentrations and the urinary albumin excretion rates were significantly reduced in all the treated groups compared to non-treated participants [43]. Faure et al. also reported a significant reduction in plasmatic MDA-TBARS in 18 patients with early DR and without retinopathy. These authors also detected a significant increase in the plasmatic GSH-px activity in patients with retinopathy in comparison to those without retinopathy [44].

Vitamin E (α-tocopherol) was administered to 36 type 1 diabetics and to nine non-diabetics. The authors reported that retinal blood flow had significantly decreased in diabetics at the baseline. After treatment, diabetic retinal blood flow was comparable to that of non-diabetics [45].

Ginkgo biloba is one of the oldest living tree species, whose leaves are among the most extensively studied herbs in use. They contain flavonoids and terpenoids which are believed to have potent antioxidant properties. *Ginkgo biloba* extract was administered to 25 type 2 diabetics for three months, after which MDA levels had significantly reduced, fibrinogen levels were lower, erythrocyte deformability was promoted, while blood viscosity, viscoelasticity, and retinal blood flow rate in treated patients improved [46].

A long-lasting study by our research group evaluated antioxidant supplementation as an alternative intervention for DR patients. Initially, 105 type 2 diabetic patients with non-proliferative DR were included. Patients underwent a complete ophthalmic examination, and blood samples were drawn to determine oxidative MDA-TBARS and total antioxidant activity at the baseline and after a five year followup. Half the patient population was randomly assigned to take oral antioxidant supplementation (at nutritional doses) containing vitamins C and E, selenium, zinc and lutein. Of these patients, 97 completed the five year followup period, and the (ophthalmic and biochemical) examinations were then repeated. The variables that were compared at the beginning of the study and at the end of the followup included: best-corrected visual acuity, DR score, MDA value and TAS value. This study revealed that supplementation with a specific oral antioxidant formulation did not change best-corrected visual acuity, although the retinopathy stage did, and progression slowed among those taking the supplement; and the retinopathy stage worsened among those who did not take the antioxidant supplement. Those patients taking the supplement maintained antioxidant plasma status levels. The study concluded that oral antioxidant supplementation may be a useful adjunct long-term therapy for patients with type 2 diabetes with non-proliferative DR [47].

The results of a multicenter study on the effects of α-lipoic acid administration to 467 type 2 diabetics (235 treated and 232 untreated) over a two year period were reported in 2011. The data confirmed no prevention of clinically significant macular edema and no effect on visual acuity [48].

Nebbioso et al. evaluated the effects of a combination of α-lipoic acid, genistein and vitamins B, C, and E in 32 preretinopathic diabetics (16 treated and 16 placebo) for one month. The results demonstrate a significant increase of plasma antioxidants and the ERG oscillatory potential values in the treated group as compared to controls [49].

The role of calcium dobesilate (Ca Dob) in DR therapy is noteworthy as it consistently ranks as one of the most commonly prescribed drugs. Ca Dob (traded as Doxium® in most European, Latin American, Middle East and Asian countries) is calcium 2,5-dihydroxybenzene sulphonate, a pharmacological agent categorized as vasculo-protector and veno-tonic. It has been extensively studied, based on its physiologic functions and safety profile, for its adverse effects in the initiation and progression of DR. We searched the international literature (1970–2012) extensively to review the data on Ca Dob oral administration to diabetics for its related effects on DR patients. In fact, data from the Ca Dob postmarketing surveillance (PMS) report of OM Pharma (Geneva, Switzerland; 1974–1998) and from the safety update reports (PSUR; 1995–2003) of the 1974–1998 French Regulatory authority's pharmacovigilance database report indicate that no deaths were attributed to Ca Dob administration, and that adverse events with Ca Dob do not occur frequently. Moreover in frequency terms, the following side effects appeared: fever, gastrointestinal disorders, skin reactions, arthralgia, and agranulocytosis. The review concluded that there is a low and constant risk of adverse effects with Ca Dob given at 500–1500 mg/day over time [50,51]. Since the 1970s to the present-day, a large series of *in vitro* experiments suggest that Ca Dob might be considerably beneficial when treating DR patients. However, the results of clinical trials are ambiguous. As summarized by Farsa [51], among the activities that Ca Dob exerts in the eyes and bodies of the treated patients, we find:

1) Antioxidant and anti-ROS activity (Ca Dob activity is the result of its hydroquinone structure);
2) Angioprotective functions against ROS-induced increased capillary permeability;
3) Enhanced nitric oxide synthase (NOS) activity in endothelial cells (increased NO synthesis by the NOS isoform from its precursor L-arginine, favoring NO-dependent vasorelaxation);
4) Antiapoptotic effects in vessels and other tissues (by positively influencing the treatment of vascular disorders by down-regulating apoptosis);
5) Effects on the levels of cell adhesion molecules (vascular cell adhesion molecule: VCAM 1, and intercellular cell adhesion molecule: ICAM); and
6) Angiogenesis inhibition (mediated by the inhibition of aminopeptidases).

In 1977, Larsen et al. reported that oral administration of Ca Dob for eight months showed no positive evidence for capillary resistance in the course of DR in a double-blind crossover trial with 18 diabetics [52]. Furthermore in a controlled study, Stamper et al. reported no significant benefit from the administration of Ca Dob (750 mg/day or 1000 mg/day for one year) in 42 non-proliferative

DR patients who were evaluated by clinical examination, fluorescein angiography, angiography and fundus photography [53].

Despite the results of these studies, numerous publications on the role of Ca Dob in patients with DR have emerged over the past 40 years. Vojnikovic first studied 50 patients who had suffered from diabetes mellitus for 2–7 years, diagnosed with DR, primary open-angle glaucoma (POAG), ocular hypertension (OHT) and hyperviscosity of whole blood, plasma and aqueous humor, who were randomly assigned to two groups: 1) patients receiving Ca Dob (1500 mg/day) for three months; 2) patients receiving a placebo. At the end of the followup, retinal signs, visual acuity, and visual fields improved, while intraocular pressure and viscosity parameters significantly decreased in treated patients when compared with both the initial status and placebo patients. The data indicate that Ca Dob reduces capillary fragility, microvascular hyperpermeability and blood viscosity [54]. In 1991, the same author analyzed a sample of 79 non-insulin-dependent diabetic patients in a double-blind randomized clinical trial. They were all diagnosed with early retinopathy and POAG, and were divided into two groups: 1) patients receiving 1500mg/day of Ca Dob for six months (n=41); or 2) placebo for the same amount and period (n=38). A variety of statistically significant differences in the Ca Dob group were found when compared to the placebo patients: intraocular pressure, visual field defects, surface area of retinal hemorrhages, and whole blood and plasma viscosity reduced. The coefficients of outflow facility and serum albumin concentration increased.

The data set suggests that increased whole blood viscosity is a risk factor for DR and for POAG optic nerve damage, thus supporting the role of Ca Dob in reducing blood hyperviscosity and in lowering intraocular pressure, both of which induce a positive response in the retinal state and visual fields [55]. Moreover, Benarroch et al. reported that patients with DR receiving Ca Dob 500 mg (3 capsules/day) for three months displayed significant reductions in whole blood viscosity and capillary fragility, and significantly lowered albumin/globulin ratio, fibrinogen and cholesterol levels. These findings suggest that Ca Dob may help restore the integrity of retinal microvasculature and decrease blood viscosity, and that this could benefit DR evolution [56]. More recently, the effect of Ca Dob on the progression of early DR was evaluated in a randomized double-blind study. The agent was administrated at 2 g daily for two years. The data indicate significantly better activity than a placebo on the prevention of blood-retinal barrier disruption, independently of diabetes control [57]. In contrast, the effect of Ca Dob on occurrence of diabetic macular edema (CALDIRET study) was analyzed in a randomized, double-blind, placebo-controlled, multicenter trial carried out in 40 centers in 11 countries. The authors reported that Ca Dob does not lower the risk of developing CSME [58].

FINAL COMMENTS AND FUTURE DIRECTIONS

The experimental data discussed in this review show that different antioxidant agents may successfully prevent various biochemical and structural alterations in retinal cells cultured under hyperglycemic conditions and in experimental diabetic animals. Although the results of human trials are somewhat variable, some studies have provided promising results, especially those using a combination of different antioxidants.

Therapies addressing different targets of oxidative stress seem the most appropriate to treat this disease, when considering that ROS overproduction is a complex, continuous, and multifactorial process. In addition, antioxidant treatment should be well-tolerated for years because diabetes is a lifelong disease. Further studies into the effects of different compositions and doses of antioxidants for human supplementation are required to obtain a more effective treatment in order to prevent this blinding complication of diabetes.

SUMMARY POINTS

- Conventional treatments for DR strategies have not proved capable of halting the progression of this disease in all patients.
- The mechanisms leading to DR are not fully understood.
- Oxidative stress plays a pivotal role in the development of DR.
- Antioxidant agents may prevent damage in retinal cells cultured under hyperglycemic conditions and in the retinas of experimental diabetic animals.
- Some studies with antioxidant supplementation in patients affected by DR have provided promising results.
- Further clinical trials are needed in order to better define the compositions and dosages of antioxidant supplements needed for the treatment of DR.

References

[1a] The Diabetes Control and Complications Trial Research Group. The effect of intensive treatment of diabetes on the development and progression of long-term complications in insulin-dependent diabetes mellitus. N Engl J Med 1993;329:977–86.

[1b] UK Prospective Diabetes Study (UKPDS) Group. Intensive blood-glucose control with sulphonylureas or insulin compared with conventional treatment and risk of complications in patients with type 2 diabetes (UKPDS 33). Lancet 1998;352:837–53.

[1c] UK Prospective Diabetes Study (UKPDS) Group. Tight blood pressure control and risk of macrovascular and microvascular complications in type 2 diabetes: UKPDS 38. BMJ 1998;317:703–13.

[1d] Zhang L, Chen B, Tang L. Metabolic memory: mechanisms and implications for diabetic retinopathy. Diabetes Res Clin Pract 2012;96:286–93.

[2] Ansari NH, Zhang W, Fulep E, Mansour A. Prevention of pericyte loss by Trolox in diabetic rat retina. J Toxicol Environ Health A 1998;54:467–75.

[3] Kowluru RA, Koppolu P. Diabetes-induced activation of caspase-3 in retina: effect of antioxidant therapy. Free Radic Res 2002;36:993–9.

[3b] Kowluru RA, Koppolu P, Chakrabarti S, Chen S. Diabetes-induced activation of nuclear transcriptional factor in the retina, and its inhibition by antioxidants. Free Radic Res 2003;37:1169–80.

[4] Amano S, Yamagishi S, Inagaki Y, Nakamura K, Takeuchi M, Inoue H, et al. Pigment epithelium-derived factor inhibits oxidative stress-induced apoptosis and dysfunction of cultured retinal pericytes. Microvasc Res 2005;69:45–55.

[5] Madsen-Bouterse SA, Zhong Q, Mohammad G, Ho YS, Kowluru RA. Oxidative damage of mitochondrial DNA in diabetes and its protection by manganese superoxide dismutase. Free Radic Res 2010;44:313–21.

[6] Zeng K, Xu H, Chen K, Zhu J, Zhou Y, Zhang Q, et al. Effects of taurine on glutamate uptake and degradation in Müller cells under diabetic conditions via antioxidant mechanism. Mol Cell Neurosci 2010;45:192–9.

[7] Li J, Chen X, Xiao W, Ma W, Li T, Huang J, et al. Mitochondria-targeted antioxidant peptide SS31 attenuates high glucose-induced injury on human retinal endothelial cells. Biochem Biophys Res Commun 2011;404:349–56.

[8] Dutot M, de la Tourrette V, Fagon R, Rat P. New approach to modulate retinal cellular toxic effects of high glucose using marine epa and dha. Nutr Metab (Lond) 2011;8:39.

[9] Shen J, Shen S, Das UN, Xu G. Effect of essential fatty acids on glucose-induced cytotoxicity to retinal vascular endothelial cells. Lipids Health Dis 2012;11:90.

[10] Wu H, Xu G, Liao Y, Ren H, Fan J, Sun Z, et al. Supplementation with antioxidants attenuates transient worsening of retinopathy in diabetes caused by acute intensive insulin therapy. Graefes Arch Clin Exp Ophthalmol 2012;250:1453–8.

[11] Hammes HP, Bartmann A, Engel L, Wülfroth P. Antioxidant treatment of experimental diabetic retinopathy in rats with nicanartine. Diabetologia 1997;40:629–34.

[12] Kunisaki M, Bursell SE, Umeda F, Nawata H, King GL. Prevention of diabetes-induced abnormal retinal blood flow by treatment with d-α-tocopherol. Biofactors 1998;7:55–67.

[13] Abiko T, Abiko A, Clermont AC, Shoelson B, Horio N, Takahashi J, et al. Characterization of retinal leukostasis and hemodynamics in insulin resistance and diabetes: role of oxidants and protein kinase-C activation. Diabetes 2003;52:829–37.

[14] Jariyapongskul A, Rungjaroen T, Kasetsuwan N, Patumraj S, Seki J, Niimi H. Long-term effects of oral vitamin C supplementation on the endothelial dysfunction in the iris microvessels of diabetic rats. Microvasc Res 2007;74:32–8.

[15] Di Leo MA, Ghirlanda G, Gentiloni Silveri N, Giardina B, Franconi F, Santini SA. Potential therapeutic effect of antioxidants in experimental diabetic retina: a comparison between chronic taurine and vitamin E plus selenium supplementations. Free Radic Res 2003;37:323–30.

[16] Lin J, Bierhaus A, Bugert P, Dietrich N, Feng Y, Vom Hagen F, et al. Effect of R-(+)-α-lipoic acid on experimental diabetic retinopathy. Diabetologia 2006;49:1089–96.

[17] Obrosova IG, Minchenko AG, Marinescu V, Fathallah L, Kennedy A, Stockert CM, et al. Antioxidants attenuate early up regulation of retinal vascular endothelial growth factor in streptozotocin-diabetic rats. Diabetologia 2001;44:1102–10.

[18] Kowluru RA, Odenbach S. Effect of long-term administration of α-lipoic acid on retinal capillary cell death and the development of retinopathy in diabetic rats. Diabetes 2004;53:3233–8.

[19] Lin J, Bierhaus A, Bugert P, Dietrich N, Feng Y, Vom Hagen F, et al. Effect of R-(+)-α-lipoic acid on experimental diabetic retinopathy. Diabetologia 2006;49:1089–96.

[20] Johnsen-Soriano S, Garcia-Pous M, Arnal E, Sancho-Tello M, Garcia-Delpech S, Miranda M, et al. Early lipoic acid intake protects retina of diabetic mice. Free Radic Res 2008;42:613–7.

[21] Kowluru RA, Tang J, Kern TS. Abnormalities of retinal metabolism in diabetes and experimental galactosemia. VII. Effect of long-term administration of antioxidants on the development of retinopathy. Diabetes 2001;50:1938–42.

[22] Yatoh S, Mizutani M, Yokoo T, Kozawa T, Sone H, Toyoshima H, et al. Antioxidants and an inhibitor of advanced glycation ameliorate death of retinal microvascular cells in diabetic retinopathy. Diabetes Metab Res Rev 2006;22:38–45.

[23] Mustata GT, Rosca M, Biemel KM, Reihl O, Smith MA, Viswanathan A, et al. Paradoxical effects of green tea (Camellia sinensis) and antioxidant vitamins in diabetic rats: improved retinopathy and renal mitochondrial defects but deterioration of collagen matrix glycoxidation and cross-linking. Diabetes 2005;54:517–26.

[24] Kowluru RA, Kanwar M. Effect of curcumin on retinal oxidative stress and inflammation in diabetes. Nutr Metab (Lond) 2007;4:1–8.

[25] Padilla E, Ganado P, Sanz M, Zeini M, Ruiz E, Triviño A, et al. Calcium dobesilate attenuates vascular injury and the progression of diabetic retinopathy in streptozotocin-induced diabetic rats. Diabetes Metab Res Rev 2005;21:132–42.

[26] Leal EC, Martins J, Voabil P, Liberal J, Chiavaroli C, Bauer J, et al. Calcium dobesilate inhibits the alterations in tight junction proteins and leukocyte adhesion to retinal endothelial cells induced by diabetes. Diabetes 2010;59:2637–45.

[27] Kowluru RA, Kanwar M, Chan PS, Zhang JP. Inhibition of retinopathy and retinal metabolic abnormalities in diabetic rats with AREDS-based micronutrients. Arch Ophthalmol 2008;126:1266–72.

[28] Miranda M, Muriach M, Johnsen S, Bosch-Morell F, Araiz J, Romá J, et al. Oxidative stress in a model for experimental diabetic retinopathy: treatment with antioxidants. Arch Soc Esp Oftalmol 2004;79:289–94.

[29] Arnal E, Miranda M, Johnsen-Soriano S, Alvarez-Nölting R, Díaz-Llopis M, Araiz J, et al. Beneficial effect of docosahexanoic acid and lutein on retinal structural, metabolic, and functional abnormalities in diabetic rats. Curr Eye Res 2009;34:928–38.

[30] Sasaki M, Ozawa Y, Kurihara T, Kubota S, Yuki K, Noda K, et al. Neurodegenerative influence of oxidative stress in the retina of a murine model of diabetes. Diabetologia 2010;53:971–9.

[31] Kowluru RA, Menon B, Gierhart DL. Beneficial effect of zeaxanthin on retinal metabolic abnormalities in diabetic rats. Invest Ophthalmol Vis Sci 2008;49:1645–51.

[32] Yadav AS, Harris NR. Effect of tempol on diabetes-induced decreases in retinal blood flow in the mouse. Curr Eye Res 2011;36:456–61.

[33] Rosales MA, Silva KC, Lopes de Faria JB, Lopes de Faria JM. Exogenous SOD mimetic tempol ameliorates the early retinal changes reestablishing the redox status in diabetic hypertensive rats. Invest Ophthalmol Vis Sci 2010;51:4327–36.

[34] Obrosova IG, Minchenko AG, Vasupuram R, White L, Abatan OI, Kumagai AK, et al. Aldose reductase inhibitor fidarestat prevents retinal oxidative stress and vascular endothelial growth factor overexpression in streptozotocin-diabetic rats. Diabetes 2003;52:864–71.

[35] El-Remessy AB, Al-Shabrawey M, Khalifa Y, Tsai NT, Caldwell RB, Liou GI. Neuroprotective and blood-retinal barrier-preserving effects of cannabidiol in experimental diabetes. Am J Pathol 2006;168:235–44.

[36] Kern TS, Miller CM, Du Y, Zheng L, Mohr S, Ball SL, et al. Topical administration of nepafenac inhibits diabetes-induced retinal microvascular disease and underlying abnormalities of retinal metabolism and physiology. Diabetes 2007;56:373–9.

[37] Yoshida Y, Yamagishi S, Matsui T, Jinnouchi Y, Fukami K, Imaizumi T, et al. Protective role of pigment epithelium-derived factor (PEDF) in early phase of experimental diabetic retinopathy. Diabetes Metab Res Rev 2009;25:678–86.

[38] Pfister F, Riedl E, Wang Q, vom Hagen F, Deinzer M, Harmsen MC, et al. Oral carnosine supplementation prevents vascular damage in experimental diabetic retinopathy. Cell Physiol Biochem 2011;28:125–36.

[39] Kowluru RA, Kanwar M. Effect of curcumin on retinal oxidative stress and inflammation in diabetes. Nutr Metab (Lond) 2007;4: 1–8.

[40] Leydhecker W. Zur medicamentösen Behandlung der Diabetischen Retinopathie. Wurzburg, Germany: The Ophthalmology Department of the University Clinic of Wurzburg; 1986.

[41] Spadea L, Balestrazzi E. Treatment of vascular retinopathies with Pycnogenol. Phytother Res 2001;15:219–23.

[42] Steigerwalt R, Belcaro G, Cesarone MR, Di Renzo A, Grossi MG, Ricci A, et al. Pycnogenol improves microcirculation, retinal edema, and visual acuity in early diabetic retinopathy. J Ocul Pharmacol Ther 2009;25:537–40.

[43] Kähler W, Kuklinski B, Rühlmann C, Plötz C. Diabetes mellitus–a free radical-associated disease. Results of adjuvant antioxidant supplementation. Z Gesamte Inn Med 1993;48:223–32.

[44] Faure P, Benhamou PY, Perard A, Halimi S, Roussel AM. Lipid peroxidation in insulin-dependent diabetic patients with early retina degenerative lesions: effects of an oral zinc supplementation. Eur J Clin Nutr 1995;49:282–8.

[45] Bursell SE, Clermont AC, Aiello LP, Aiello LM, Schlossman DK, Feener EP, et al. High-dose vitamin E supplementation normalizes retinal blood flow and creatinine clearance in patients with type 1 diabetes. Diabetes Care 1999;22:1245–51.

[46] Huang SY, Jeng C, Kao SC, Yu JJ, Liu DZ. Improved haemorrheological properties by Ginkgo biloba extract (Egb 761) in type 2 diabetes mellitus complicated with retinopathy. Clin Nutr 2004;23:615–21.

[47] Garcia-Medina JJ, Pinazo-Duran MD, Garcia-Medina M, Zanon-Moreno V, Pons-Vazquez S. A 5-year follow-up of antioxidant supplementation in type 2 diabetic retinopathy. Eur J Ophthalmol 2011;21:637–43.

[48] Haritoglou C, Gerss J, Hammes HP, Kampik A, Ulbig MW an RETIPON Study Group. Alpha-lipoic acid for the prevention c diabetic macular edema. Ophthalmologica 2011;226:127–37.

[49] Nebbioso M, Federici M, Rusciano D, Evangelista M, Pescosolido N Oxidative stress in preretinopathic diabetes subjects and antioxidants. Diabetes Technol Ther 2012;14:257–63.

[50] Allain H, Ramelet AA, Polard E, Bentué-Ferrer D. Safety of calcium dobesilate in chronic venous disease, diabetic retinopathy and hemorrhoids. Drug Saf 2004;27:649–60.

[51] Farsa O. Calcium Dobesilate in Prevention and Treatment of Diabetic Retinopathy. In: Mohammad Shamsul Ola, editors. Diabeti Retinopathy; 2012. Available from: http://www.intechopen.com/books/diabetic-retinopathy/calcium-dobesilate-in-prevention-and-treatment-of-diabetic-retinopathy [accessed 24.06.13].

[52] Larsen HW, Sander E, Hoppe R. The value of calcium dobesilate in the treatment of diabetic retinopathy. A controlled clinical trial. Diabetologia 1977;13:105–9.

[53] Stamper RL, Smith ME, Aronson SB, Cavender JC, Cleasby GW, Fung WE, et al. The effect of calcium dobesilate on non-proliferative diabetic retinopathy: a controlled study. Ophthalmology 1978;85: 594–606.

[54] Vojnikovic B. Hyperviscosity in whole blood, plasma, and aqueous humor decreased by doxium (calcium dobesilate) in diabetics with retinopathy and glaucoma: a double-blind controlled study. Ophthalmic Res 1984;16:150–62.

[55] Vojnikovic B. Doxium (calcium dobesilate) reduces blood hyperviscosity and lowers elevated intraocular pressure in patients with diabetic retinopathy and glaucoma. Ophthalmic Res 1991;23: 12–20.

[56] Benarroch IS, Brodsky M, Rubinstein A, Viggiano C, Salama EA. Treatment of blood hyperviscosity with calcium dobesilate in patients with diabetic retinopathy. Ophthalmic Res 1985;17: 131–8.

[57] Ribeiro ML, Seres AI, Carneiro AM, Stur M, Zourdani A, Caillon P, et al. DX-Retinopathy Study Group. Effect of calcium dobesilate on progression of early diabetic retinopathy: a randomized double-blind study. Graefes Arch Clin Exp Ophthalmol 2006;244:1591–600.

[58] Haritoglou C, Gerss J, Sauerland C, Kampik A, Ulbig MW, CALDIRET study group. Effect of calcium dobesilate on occurrence of diabetic macular edema (CALDIRET study): randomized, double-blind, placebo-controlled, multicenter trial. Lancet 2009;373:1364–71.

CHAPTER

23

Lutein and Oxidative Stress-Mediated Retinal Neurodegeneration in Diabetes

Yoko Ozawa, Mariko Sasaki

Laboratory of Retinal Cell Biology, Department of Ophthalmology, Keio University School of Medicine, Tokyo, Japan

List of Abbreviations

AMD Age-related macular degeneration
AREDS Age-Related Eye Disease Study
AT1R Angiotensin II type 1 receptor
ATP Adenosine 5′-triphosphate
BDNF Brain-derived neurotrophic factor
DCFDA Dichlorofluorescein diacetate
DHE Dihydroethidium
ER Endoplasmic reticulum
ERG Electroretinogram
ERK Extracellular signal-regulated kinase
MPOD Macular pigment optical density
NPDR Non-proliferative diabetic retinopathy
OCT Optical coherent tomography
OP Oscillatory potential
PDR Proliferative diabetic retinopathy
RAS Renin-angiotensin system
ROS Reactive oxygen species
RPE Retinal pigment epithelium

INTRODUCTION

Oxidative stress underlies the pathogenesis of some diseases, such as diabetes, neurodegeneration, atherosclerosis, and cancer. Oxidative stress involves the accumulation of reactive oxygen species (ROS) and the cellular disorganization they cause. ROS are produced both intrinsically by mitochondrial respiration and extrinsically by cytotoxic stimuli. In diabetes, ROS are produced in response to hyperglycemia and the subsequent excessive activation of the electron transfer system [1,2]. ROS accumulate when their production exceeds the ability of biological defense systems, including antioxidative enzymes, to remove them. Under oxidative stress, damage to DNA, proteins, and lipids eventually leads to cellular dysfunction and tissue/organ dysregulation. Pathogenesis occurs when these changes exceed the thresholds of repair systems. Furthermore, because ROS can accumulate with time, oxidative stress is often involved in age-related degenerative diseases.

Diabetes causes multiple complications, such as retinopathy and nephropathy. In the later stages of this disease, retinopathy is treated by surgery (vitrectomy) and/or laser, and nephropathy by artificial dialysis. However, because these current therapies do not restore the original physiological function, a recent trend in therapeutic strategies is to slow or prevent disease progression. Moreover, the retina is part of the central nervous system, and thus regenerates poorly, if at all. Targeting oxidative stress is a promising strategy for avoiding diabetic retinopathy, and could be implemented at earlier stages in the disease than existing treatments.

In this chapter, we focus on the effects of lutein, an antioxidant, in the retina. Lutein is anticipated to be clinically applicable as a micronutrient supplement for suppressing the progression of age-related macular degeneration (AMD) [3]. Research on lutein's effects on the retinal lesions in diabetes has just begun. In this chapter, we review its effects on oxidative stress-mediated retinal pathogenesis, focusing on the results of studies in animal models of diabetes.

GENERAL INFORMATION ABOUT LUTEIN

Lutein is a xanthophyll, or hydroxycarotenoid ($C_{40}H_{56}O_2$, Figure 23.1). Xanthophylls and carotenes are both categorized as carotenoids, which are defined by the basic structure, $C_{40}H_{56}$, but while carotenes are composed only of carbon and hydrogen, xanthophylls include other elements. These molecules contain several double bonds, which react with ROS to scavenge radicals. Carotenes are

Diabetes: Oxidative Stress and Dietary Antioxidants.
http://dx.doi.org/10.1016/B978-0-12-405885-9.00023-1

transformed to vitamin A in the body, and are therefore called pro-vitamin A [4]. However, lutein's properties are considerably different from those of carotenes.

Lutein is a phytochemical, which are plant-derived compounds that are not essential nutrients for sustaining life. Because phytochemicals have pigments, fragrance, or a bitter taste, they are generally thought to help protect plants against external threats, such as ultraviolet light, pathogens, or creatures that eat them. Plant enzymes synthesize lutein from lycopene and α-carotene (Figure 23.2) [5,6].

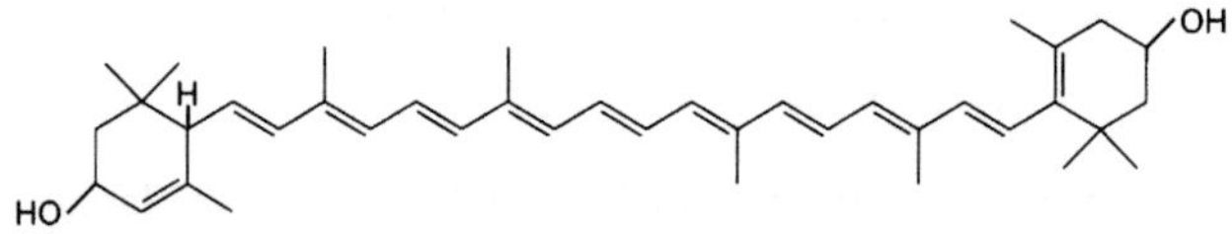

FIGURE 23.1 **Chemical structure of lutein.** Lutein is categorized as a xanthophyll carotenoid, and has the chemical composition $C_{40}H_{56}O_2$.

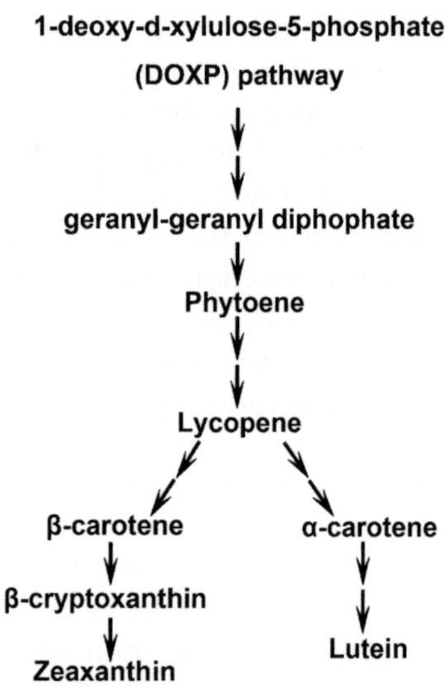

FIGURE 23.2 **Biosynthetic pathway of lutein in plants.** Overview of lutein biosynthesis. Several steps are omitted for simplification. Briefly, lutein is synthesized through a series of intermediates that include lycopene and α-carotene.

In contrast to plants, animals cannot synthesize lutein. Humans and other animals obtain lutein from foods; therefore, lutein is called a food factor. Some vegetables, such as kale, spinach, and broccoli, and the marigold flower which is used as a source for supplementary micronutrients, can provide lutein. Egg yolks also contain high levels of lutein, which is obtained by the female bird as part of her diet and deposited in the yolk.

The lutein ingested by an animal is incorporated into micelles and absorbed from the intestinal epithelium into the blood by enterocytosis. Lutein then circulates systemically to reach the liver, lung, and retina [3,7,8]. In the human retina, lutein is concentrated in the macula, the most central region (Figure 23.3), so it is called a macular pigment. The analysis of stereoisomers of this macular pigment revealed two stereoisomeric carotenoids with identical properties to lutein and zeaxanthin, another xanthophyll [4]. Lutein is also present throughout the retina, at lower concentrations then in the macula [8]. Although the concentration of both pigments is highest in the macula, there is more zeaxanthin than lutein in the macular region, while more lutein than zeaxanthin in the peripheral retina [9,10].

Within the retina, resonance Raman imaging has shown that lutein is most abundant in the neuronal network layer (the outer plexiform layer [OPL]) that connects the photoreceptor cells (the outer nuclear layer; ONL) to the secondary neurons [11]. Because lutein is a yellow-pigmented crystal, it has long been thought to act as a blue light filter, to protect retinal tissue from the high-energy end of the visible spectrum. The fact that lutein is abundant in the OPL, which is closer to the vitreous side of the retina than to the photoreceptor cell layer, is consistent with the idea that lutein filters light before it reaches the photoreceptor cells, to prevent harmful cellular events and vision loss. Lutein is also found in the photoreceptor outer segments (OSs), where light stimuli are received, and in the retinal pigment epithelium (RPE), where OSs are phagocytosed and recycled. The level of lutein in photoreceptor cells is reported to be twice that in the RPE [11,12].

Recently, a lutein-binding protein in the retina was reported [13]. This protein was identified as steroidogenic

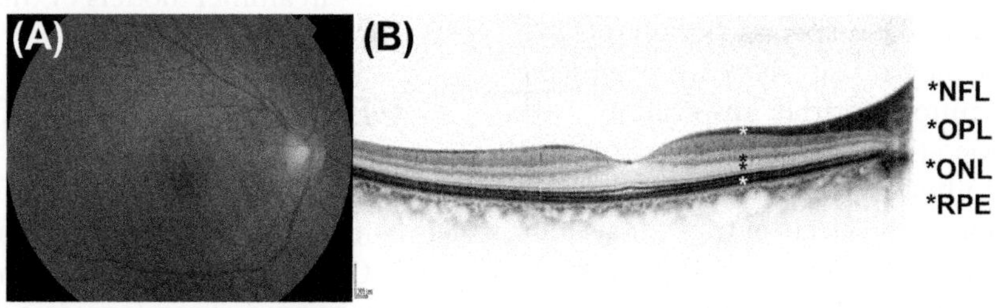

FIGURE 23.3 **Macula of the human fundus.** Human fundus photograph (A) and cross-sectional image of the macula by OCT (B). Lutein is rich in the macula but is also present in the peripheral retina. (A) The macula is the central part of the fundus. (B) * indicates NFL, OPL, ONL, and RPE, in order from top to bottom. OCT, optical coherence tomography; NFL, nerve fiber layer, consisting of the axons of retinal ganglion cells; OPL, outer plexiform layer, consisting of the synapses between photoreceptor cells and downstream neurons; ONL, outer nuclear layer, consisting of photoreceptor cells; RPE, retinal pigment epithelium.

acute regulatory domain 3 (StARD3), which is expressed in both the retina and RPE. In the monkey retina, StARD3 localizes to all the retinal neurons in the macular area, especially the cone inner segments and axons, but it is not found in Müller glial cells [13].

CLINICAL DATA FOR LUTEIN

Lutein is currently being evaluated for its limited use as a preventive therapy for AMD, a vision-threatening disease. After an inverse association between vegetable/fruit intake and AMD was reported [7], a large clinical study, the Age-Related Eye Disease Study (AREDS), was performed to examine ways to prevent AMD. The participants in AREDS with a significantly lower dietary intake of lutein/zeaxanthin were more likely to have advanced AMD (either the atrophic or exudative type) or were at a high risk of developing it [14]. Therefore, a second large-scale clinical study, AREDS2, was performed to test the effects of lutein/zeaxanthin and/or docosahexaenoic/eicosapentaenoic acids in approximately 4000 AMD patients, for their possible use in preventive therapy.

Another study showed that, in 90 patients with atrophic AMD, lutein intake increased the macular pigment optical density (MPOD) and was correlated with an increase in visual contrast sensitivity [7]. The incidence of AMD (exudative type) was low in patients who took a large amount of lutein or zeaxanthin [15] and who showed high levels of plasma carotenoids [14,16].

A study using donor eyes showed a negative association between lutein content in the retina and AMD risk [15]. Retinas from 56 donors with AMD and 56 controls were analyzed using high-performance liquid chromatography. The levels of lutein and zeaxanthin were lower in the AMD retinas in both the central retina (62% of control), including the macula, and the peripheral retina (70–80% of control). Taken together, these observations indicate that lutein obtained from the diet accumulates in the retina and may act locally to prevent disease.

The effect of different doses of a lutein supplement on serum lutein concentration and MPOD was also reported [17]. Both the serum lutein and the MPOD were positively and linearly correlated with the lutein dose.

RETINAL NEURODEGENERATION IN DIABETES

The pathogenesis of diabetic retinopathy is known to involve microangiopathy. It is well documented that occlusive changes in vessels cause retinal ischemia. Ischemia up-regulates vascular endothelial growth factor (VEGF), which promotes proliferative diabetic retinopathy and, at the end stage, leads to vision loss. However, visual impairment begins in the early stage of diabetes. Evidence for this early visual impairment was first obtained in the 1960s by electroretinogram (ERG) [18], and the details were later confirmed [19].

The implicit time of the oscillatory potentials (OPs) is slightly delayed in diabetic patients before there is any apparent retinopathy, and without a reduction in the OP amplitudes. As diabetic retinopathy progresses, the amplitudes of the OPs are reduced, and the implicit times are prolonged. As a result, the summation of the OP amplitudes decreases with advancing retinopathy. It is also reported that the implicit times of all the OPs were significantly prolonged in the moderate and severe stages of non-proliferative diabetic retinopathy (NPDR) compared with normal controls [19]. Furthermore, diabetes caused the impairment not only of the OPs, which reflect inner retinal function, but also of the photopic negative response (PhNR), which is reduced in diseases that affect the retinal ganglion cells in the inner retinal layer, such as optic nerve disease and glaucomatous optic neuropathy [19].

Recent research using optical coherence tomography (OCT) revealed that the inner retinal layer thins before the vascular lesion becomes apparent [20], consistent with the ERG response. OCT allows us to measure the thickness of each retinal layer in a cross-sectional image of the retina that is obtained non-invasively. Patients with NPDR show a thinning of the nerve fiber layer (NFL), which contains the axons of the retinal ganglion cells, compared with the NFL of control patients without retinal or optic nerve diseases.

The OP changes [18] and apoptotic changes in the inner layer of the retina, including retinal ganglion cells [21–23], have been documented in the streptozotocin (STZ)-induced diabetes model. This model enables us to investigate the underlying molecular mechanisms of clinical findings in diabetes. In the following sections, the pathological findings in the diabetic retina and their underlying mechanisms, determined from studies using this diabetes model, are presented.

ROS ACCUMULATION IN THE DIABETIC RETINA

Hyperglycemia increases ROS production by the mitochondrial electron transport chain. The most universal and critical mitochondrial function is oxidative phosphorylation, which is performed by five large multienzyme complexes, designated complexes I, II, III, IV, and adenosine triphosphate (ATP) synthase [24]. The ROS accumulation caused by hyperglycemia is avoided either by inhibiting complex II, or by overexpressing uncoupling protein-1 (UCP1) or manganese superoxide dismutase (MnSOD), a mitochondrial antioxidant enzyme. These effects established that the hyperglycemia-induced ROS are produced by the mitochondrial electron transport chain.

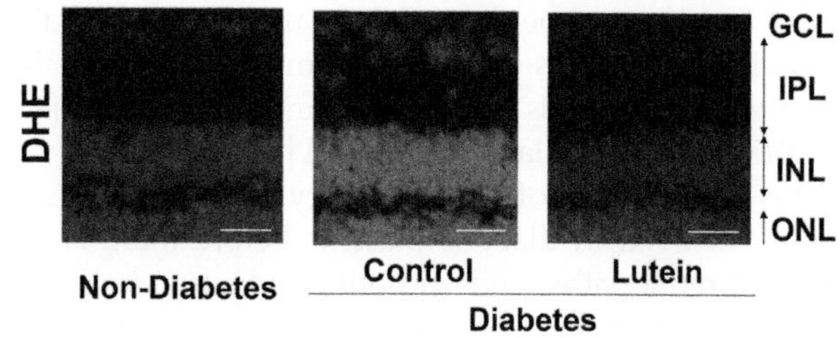

FIGURE 23.4 **Lutein's effect on ROS in the diabetic retina.** DHE staining showing the ROS level in the retina. The increased ROS level in the diabetic retina is suppressed by continuous lutein treatment. DHE, dihydroethidium; GCL, ganglion cell layer; IPL, inner plexiform layer; INL, inner nuclear layer; ONL, outer nuclear layer. *(Sasaki, Ozawa et al. Diabetologia 2010, with permission from Diabetologia).*

ROS accumulation in the presence of hyperglycemia was also shown in the retina of STZ-induced diabetes model animals by using a dihydroethidium (DHE) probe [22,25] (Figure 23.4). DHE is a superoxide indicator, although it may also detect other kinds of ROS, specifically H_2O_2 and $ONOO^-$. ROS accumulate in all the layers of the retina in diabetes. The dichlorofluorescein diacetate (DCFDA) probe, which fluoresces in response to ROS, including hydroxyl and peroxyl, also detects ROS accumulation in the diabetic retina [26].

Biological systems exist in the retina to suppress ROS accumulation. These include antioxidative enzymes, such as superoxide dismutase (SOD) 1, 2, and catalase [27,28]. In the retinal ganglion cells, one of main components of the inner retinal layer, physiologically produced ROS are processed and removed by SOD1, as shown by an accelerated reduction in retinal ganglion cells in SOD1-knockout mice [28]. However, in diabetes, the production of ROS exceeds the ability of these enzymes to control it.

Another modulator of ROS is a transcription factor that is activated under stress conditions, HIF-1α. HIF-1α is up-regulated in the diabetic retina [29], resulting in the induction of a downstream inflammatory cytokine, VEGF, along with abnormal vascular formation [30]. While HIF-1α exacerbates the disease condition in the diabetic retina by promoting cytokine expression, it also reduces oxygen consumption in the mitochondria by inhibiting the conversion of pyruvate to acetyl CoA, thereby suppressing mitochondrial biogenesis and activating the autophagy of mitochondria, concomitant with the reduction in ROS production [31].

GENERAL INFLUENCES OF ROS IN PATHOGENESIS

Excessive ROS can damage DNA, proteins, and lipids [32]. The hydroxyl radical is known to react with all components of the DNA molecule, damaging both the purine and pyrimidine bases as well as the deoxyribose backbone [33]. Elderly animals are particularly vulnerable to the DNA damage caused by accumulation of ROS, due to the age-related instability of DNA [34], which progresses diseases. ROS oxidize proteins by modifying the side chains of amino acid residues, and cysteine and methionine are particularly susceptible to oxidation [35]. ROS can also attack cellular components containing the polyunsaturated fatty acid residues of phospholipids, which are also extremely sensitive to oxidation [36]. This process is called lipid peroxidation, and it generates aldehyde products. These oxidative damages can result in abnormal conditions such as inappropriate gene expression and/or signal transduction.

In addition, ROS can act as second messengers that mediate important cellular functions, such as proliferation and programmed cell death. For example, ROS have been implicated as second messengers in the activation of NF-κB via tumor necrosis factor-α (TNF-α) and interleukin-1 [32]. In the presence of ROS, another transcription factor, STAT3, is phosphorylated and activated to influence the cellular status [36,37]. In the retina, STAT3 activation reduces rhodopsin expression, and this reduction is involved in the pathogenesis of retinal inflammatory diseases [37–39]. These studies collectively show that ROS can influence multiple pathways that affect cellular conditions.

LUTEIN'S SUPPRESSIVE EFFECTS ON ROS IN THE RETINA

Lutein is physiologically delivered to the retina, and it has been thought to protect the retina by reducing the cytotoxic influence of light stimuli by blocking blue light and by suppressing ROS as an antioxidant. However, whether lutein administration reduces ROS in the retina under disease conditions that are independent of light exposure was unclear until the report of Sasaki et al. [22].

Sasaki et al. showed that, in the STZ-induced diabetes model, including lutein as a constant component of the diet significantly reduced the intensity of DHE staining in the neural retina, without reducing the blood sugar level [22] (Figure 23.4). The authors proposed that the reduction in ROS by lutein was effected through the direct scavenging of ROS by lutein delivered to the retinal neural cells, although there might also be some effect through the activation of the retinal ROS-suppressive systems. This effect of lutein is observed independent of light stimuli. Notably, lutein's effect on ROS reduction was observed in mice, which do not have macula where lutein is concentrated; this fact encourages further investigation of lutein's effect outside the macula. In diabetes, the retinal neuronal degeneration is spread throughout the area, and is not limited to the macular region.

Lutein's suppressive effect on ROS has been reported in other retinal disease models as well. In the endotoxin-induced uveitis and retinitis model, DHE staining, as well as fluorescence of the BODIPY C-11 probe, which etects lipid peroxidation, were suppressed by lutein dministration [37]. The retina in a light exposure model lso showed increased ROS, and this increase was supressed by feeding the mice a lutein-rich diet [40]. In the etina of an acute ischemia/reperfusion model, lutein uppressed oxidative stress and retinal ganglion cell loss lue to apoptosis [41].

LUTEIN'S NEUROPROTECTIVE EFFECTS IN THE DIABETIC RETINA

A synaptic network system is spread across the inner layer of the retina, where the transmitted signals from photoreceptor cells are processed to prepare for their transfer to the brain. Thus, synaptic vesicles for neurotransmitter release are abundant in the inner layer. Interestingly, one of the synaptic vesicle proteins, synaptophysin, is decreased in the diabetic retina [22,42], in a similar way to that observed in another neurodegenerative disease, Alzheimer's disease, in which the decrease is observed in the brain [43]. The reduction in synaptophysin protein under ROS-accumulating conditions in diabetes is suppressed by lutein treatment, which reduces the ROS in the retina independent of the blood glucose level [3,22,44]. Moreover, it was shown in a neuronal cell line that the synaptophysin level is inversely correlated with ERK activation, which reduces the synaptophysin protein by accelerating its degradation through the ubiquitin proteasome system [42] (Figure 23.5).

Another influence in the diabetic retina is a decrease in brain-derived neurotrophic factor (BDNF). This is a soluble factor that is up-regulated by synaptic and neuronal activity and binds to a receptor, TrkB, to promote axonal outgrowth, synapse formation, and neuronal survival. The reduction in BDNF is also suppressed by lutein treatment [3,22,44].

The synaptic network is important not only for transmitting neuronal activity but also for neuronal survival, since the activity itself helps promote the survival of the neurons. A decrease in synaptophysin would reduce neuronal activity, thus accelerating the subsequent apoptosis of neuronal cells in the inner layer of the retina, including retinal ganglion cells [3,22,44]. The reduction in BDNF, whose receptor, TrkB, is abundantly expressed in the inner layer of the retina [45], is also likely to contribute to this retinal cell loss by apoptosis. Consistent with the effects described above, the cell loss in the inner layer of the retina is suppressed by constant lutein treatment. Consistent with these findings, the impairment of the OPs response in the ERG observed in diabetes is suppressed by continuous and long-term lutein treatment.

The reduction in synaptophysin in the diabetic retina commonly occurs downstream of the angiotensin II type 1 receptor (AT1R) through ERK activation [42], as mentioned above. AT1R is broadly expressed in the inner layer of the retina [46]. The ERK activation downstream of AT1R's activation induces ubiquitination of the synaptophysin protein, and a proteasome inhibitor suppresses the AT1R-induced synaptophysin loss [42] (Figure 23.5). A selective E3 ubiquitin ligase is induced by ERK activation. Because AT1R signaling may induce ROS by activating NADPH [47], and ROS can induce AT1R activation in an autocrine and/or paracrine manner, as shown in selective retinal ganglion cell culture [48], there should be cross-talk between the ROS and AT1R signaling in the renin-angiotensin system (RAS) [44]. Lutein treatment and the reduction of ROS may break the vicious cycle of this cross-talk and the subsequent synaptophysin change (Figure 23.6).

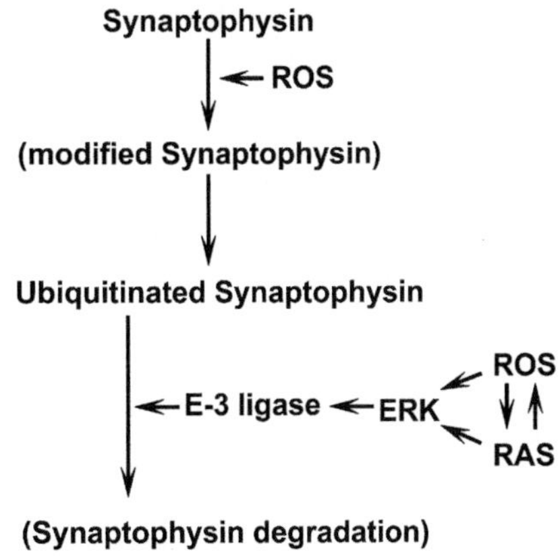

FIGURE 23.5 **Proposed model for synaptophysin reduction in the diabetic retina.** The induction of ERK activation in response to ROS may induce E3 ubiquitin ligase, which promotes the degradation of synaptophysin. ROS may also induce the ubiquitination and other modifications of synaptophysin.

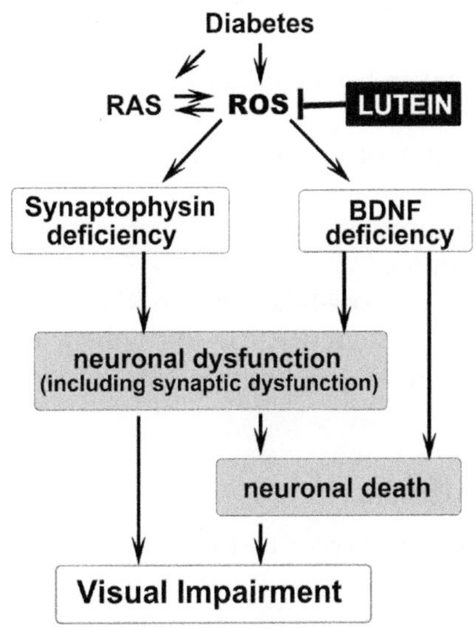

FIGURE 23.6 **Model of lutein's effects in the diabetic retina.** Lutein's neuroprotective effects in the diabetic retina involve protection of the synaptic molecule synaptophysin, the neurotrophic factor BDNF, and the suppression of subsequent retinal cell loss through apoptosis.

Other neurodegenerative influences in the diabetic retina involving ROS include ER stress [49] and altered productions of inflammatory cytokines and enzymatic factors [50]. Whether lutein can suppress all these changes, and whether the effects are applicable to the human disease, need to be resolved in future studies.

In summary, lutein, an antioxidant that cannot be synthesized in animals, can be obtained from food and delivered to the retina, where it can suppress ROS accumulation. Lutein suppresses the neurodegenerative changes in the retina of diabetic model mice (Figure 23.6), supporting the possibility that a similar effect might be anticipated in humans, although further studies are required.

SUMMARY POINTS

- Lutein is an antioxidant that cannot be synthesized in animals.
- Lutein is taken from food and delivered to the retina in animals.
- Lutein treatment suppresses ROS in the diabetic retina.
- Lutein suppresses neurodegenerative changes in the diabetic retina.
- There may be cross-talk between ROS and the rennin-angiotensin system (RAS) in the diabetic retina, and lutein treatment may suppress this pathway.

Acknowledgment

We thank all the members of the Laboratory of Retinal Cell Biology (RCB Lab).

References

[1] Schaffer SW, Jong CJ, Mozaffari M. Role of oxidative stress in diabetes-mediated vascular dysfunction: Unifying hypothesis of diabetes revisited. Vascul Pharmacol 2012;57:139–49.

[2] Nishikawa T, Edelstein D, Du XL, Yamagishi S, Matsumura T, Kaneda Y, et al. Normalizing mitochondrial superoxide production blocks three pathways of hyperglycaemic damage. Nature 2000;404:787–90.

[3] Ozawa Y, Sasaki M, Takahashi N, Kamoshita M, Miyake S, Tsubota K. Neuroprotective effects of lutein in the retina. Curr Pharm Des 2012;18:51–6.

[4] Bone RA, Landrum JT, Hime GW, Cains A, Zamor J. Stereochemistry of the human macular carotenoids. Invest Ophthalmol Vis Sci 1993;34:2033–40.

[5] Stigliani AL, Giorio G, D'Ambrosio C. Characterization of P450 carotenoid beta- and epsilon-hydroxylases of tomato and transcriptional regulation of xanthophyll biosynthesis in root, leaf, petal and fruit. Plant Cell Physiol 2011;52:851–65.

[6] Lindgren LO, Stalberg KG, Hoglund AS. Seed-specific overexpression of an endogenous Arabidopsis phytoene synthase gene results in delayed germination and increased levels of carotenoids, chlorophyll, and abscisic acid. Plant physiol 2003;132:779–85.

[7] Seddon JM, Ajani UA, Sperduto RD, Hiller R, Blair N, Burton TC, et al. Dietary carotenoids, vitamins A, C, and E, and advanced age-related macular degeneration. JAMA 1994;272:1413–20.

[8] Ziegler J, Facchini PJ, Geissler R, Schmidt J, Ammer C, Kramell R, et al. Evolution of morphine biosynthesis in opium poppy. Phytochemistry 2009;70:1696–707.

[9] Bone RA, Landrum JT, Fernandez L, Tarsis SL. Analysis of the macular pigment by HPLC: retinal distribution and age study. Invest Ophthalmol Vis Sci 1988;29:843–9.

[10] Snodderly DM, Handelman GJ, Adler AJ. Distribution of individual macular pigment carotenoids in central retina of macaque and squirrel monkeys. Invest Ophthalmol Vis Sci 1991;32:268–79.

[11] Richer S, Stiles W, Statkute L, Pulido J, Frankowski J, Rudy D, et al. Double-masked, placebo-controlled, randomized trial of lutein and antioxidant supplementation in the intervention of atrophic age-related macular degeneration: the Veterans LAST study (Lutein Antioxidant Supplementation Trial). Optometry 2004;75:216–30.

[12] Bernstein PS, Gellermann W. Measurement of carotenoids in the living primate eye using resonance Raman spectroscopy. Methods Mol Biol 2002;196:321–9.

[13] Li B, Vachali P, Frederick JM, Bernstein PS. Identification of StARD3 as a lutein-binding protein in the macula of the primate retina. Biochemistry 2011;50:2541–9.

[14] Michikawa T, Ishida S, Nishiwaki Y, Kikuchi Y, Tsuboi T, Hosoda K, et al. Serum antioxidants and age-related macular degeneration among older Japanese. Asia Pac J Clin Nutr 2009;18:1–7.

[15] Bone RA, Landrum JT, Mayne ST, Gomez CM, Tibor SE, Twaroska EE. Macular pigment in donor eyes with and without AMD: a case-control study. Invest Ophthalmol Vis Sci 2001;42:235–40.

[16] Antioxidant status and neovascular age-related macular degeneration. ; Eye Disease Case-Control Study Group Arch Ophthalmol 1993;111:104–9.

[17] Bone RA, Landrum JT. Dose-dependent response of serum lutein and macular pigment optical density to supplementation with lutein esters. Arch Biochem Biophys 2010;504:50–5.

[18] Shirao Y, Kawasaki K. Electrical responses from diabetic retina. Prog Retin Eye Res 1998;17:59–76.

[19] Kizawa J, Machida S, Kobayashi T, Gotoh Y, Kurosaka D. Changes of oscillatory potentials and photopic negative response in patients with early diabetic retinopathy. Jpn J Ophthalmol 2006;50:367–73.

[20] Park HY, Kim IT, Park CK. Early diabetic changes in the nerve fibre layer at the macula detected by spectral domain optical coherence tomography. Br J Ophthalmol 2011;95:1223–8.

[21] Barber AJ, Lieth E, Khin SA, Antonetti DA, Buchanan AG, Gardner TW. Neural apoptosis in the retina during experimental and human diabetes. Early onset and effect of insulin. J Clin Invest 1998;102:783–91.

[22] Sasaki M, Ozawa Y, Kurihara T, Kubota S, Yuki K, Noda K, et al. Neurodegenerative influence of oxidative stress in the retina of a murine model of diabetes. Diabetologia 2010;53:971–9.

[23] Martin PM, Roon P, Van Ells TK, Ganapathy V, Smith SB. Death of retinal neurons in streptozotocin-induced diabetic mice. Invest Ophthalmol Vis Sci 2004;45:3330–6.

[24] Nishikawa T, Kukidome D, Sonoda K, Fujisawa K, Matsuhisa T, Motoshima H, et al. Impact of mitochondrial ROS production on diabetic vascular complications. Diabetes Res Clin Pract 2007;77(Suppl. 1):S41–5.

[25] Pouliot M, Talbot S, Senecal J, Dotigny F, Vaucher E, Couture R. Ocular application of the kinin B1 receptor antagonist LF22–0542 inhibits retinal inflammation and oxidative stress in streptozotocin-diabetic rats. PloS one 2012;7: e33864.

[26] Santos JM, Tewari S, Kowluru RA. A compensatory mechanism protects retinal mitochondria from initial insult in diabetic retinopathy. Free Radic Biol Med 2012;53:1729–37.

[27] Kowluru RA, Kanwar M. Oxidative stress and the development of diabetic retinopathy: contributory role of matrix metalloproteinase-2. Free Radic Biol Med 2009;46:1677–85.
[28] Yuki K, Ozawa Y, Yoshida T, Kurihara T, Hirasawa M, Ozeki N, et al. Retinal ganglion cell loss in superoxide dismutase 1 deficiency. Invest Ophthalmol Vis Sci 2011;52:4143–50.
[29] Lin M, Chen Y, Jin J, Hu Y, Zhou KK, Zhu M, et al. Ischaemia-induced retinal neovascularisation and diabetic retinopathy in mice with conditional knockout of hypoxia-inducible factor-1 in retinal Muller cells. Diabetologia 2011;54:1554–66.
[30] Kurihara T, Kubota Y, Ozawa Y, Takubo K, Noda K, Simon MC, et al. von Hippel-Lindau protein regulates transition from the fetal to the adult circulatory system in retina. Development 2010;137: 1563–71.
[31] Goda N, Kanai M. Hypoxia-inducible factors and their roles in energy metabolism. Int J hematol 2012;95:457–63.
[32] Valko M, Leibfritz D, Moncol J, Cronin MT, Mazur M, Telser J. Free radicals and antioxidants in normal physiological functions and human disease. Int J Biochem Cell Biol 2007;39:44–84.
[33] Halliwell B, Gutteridge JM. Biologically relevant metal ion-dependent hydroxyl radical generation. An update. FEBS letters 1992;307:108–12.
[34] Ozawa Y, Kubota S, Narimatsu T, Yuki K, Koto T, Sasaki M, et al. Retinal aging and sirtuins. Ophthalmic Res 2010;44:199–203.
[35] Stadtman ER. Oxidation of free amino acids and amino acid residues in proteins by radiolysis and by metal-catalyzed reactions. Annu Rev Biochem 1993;62:797–821.
[36] Esterbauer H, Schaur RJ, Zollner H. Chemistry and biochemistry of 4-hydroxynonenal, malonaldehyde and related aldehydes. Free Radic Biol Med 1991;11:81–128.
[37] Sasaki M, Ozawa Y, Kurihara T, Noda K, Imamura Y, Kobayashi S, et al. Neuroprotective effect of an antioxidant, lutein, during retinal inflammation. Invest Ophthalmol Vis Sci 2009;50:1433–9.
[38] Ozawa Y, Nakao K, Kurihara T, Shimazaki T, Shimmura S, Ishida S, et al. Roles of STAT3/SOCS3 pathway in regulating the visual function and ubiquitin-proteasome-dependent degradation of rhodopsin during retinal inflammation. J biol chem 2008;283:24561–70.
[39] Ozawa Y, Kurihara T, Tsubota K, Okano H. Regulation of post-transcriptional modification as a possible therapeutic approach for retinal neuroprotection. J Ophthalmol 2011;2011:506137.
[40] Sasaki M, Yuki K, Kurihara T, Miyake S, Noda K, Kobayashi S, et al. Biological role of lutein in the light-induced retinal degeneration. J Nutr Biochem 2012;23:423–9.
[41] Li SY, Fu ZJ, Ma H, Jang WC, So KF, Wong D, et al. Effect of lutein on retinal neurons and oxidative stress in a model of acute retinal ischemia/reperfusion. Invest Ophthalmol Vis Sci 2009;50:836–43.
[42] Kurihara T, Ozawa Y, Nagai N, Shinoda K, Noda K, Imamura Y, et al. Angiotensin II type 1 receptor signaling contributes to synaptophysin degradation and neuronal dysfunction in the diabetic retina. Diabetes 2008;57:2191–8.
[43] Masliah E, Mallory M, Alford M, DeTeresa R, Hansen LA, McKeel Jr DW, et al. Altered expression of synaptic proteins occurs early during progression of Alzheimer's disease. Neurology 2001;56:127–9.
[44] Ozawa Y, Kurihara T, Sasaki M, Ban N, Yuki K, Kubota S, et al. Neural degeneration in the retina of the streptozotocin-induced type 1 diabetes model. Exp Diabetes Res 2011;2011:108328.
[45] Harada C, Guo X, Namekata K, Kimura A, Nakamura K, Tanaka K, et al. Glia- and neuron-specific functions of TrkB signalling during retinal degeneration and regeneration. Nat commun 2011;2:189.
[46] Kurihara T, Ozawa Y, Shinoda K, Nagai N, Inoue M, Oike Y, et al. Neuroprotective effects of angiotensin II type 1 receptor (AT1R) blocker, telmisartan, via modulating AT1R and AT2R signaling in retinal inflammation. Invest Ophthalmol Vis Sci 2006;47:5545–52.
[47] Chen P, Guo AM, Edwards PA, Trick G, Scicli AG. Role of NADPH oxidase and ANG II in diabetes-induced retinal leukostasis. Am J Physiol Regul Integr Comp Physiol 2007;293:R1619–29.
[48] Ozawa Y, Yuki K, Yamagishi R, Tsubota K, Aihara M. Renin-angiotensin system involvement in the oxidative stress-induced neurodegeneration of cultured retinal ganglion cells. Jpn J Ophthalmol 2012.
[49] Fu D, Wu M, Zhang J, Du M, Yang S, Hammad SM, et al. Mechanisms of modified LDL-induced pericyte loss and retinal injury in diabetic retinopathy. Diabetologia 2012;55:3128–40.
[50] Kowluru RA. Diabetic retinopathy: mitochondrial dysfunction and retinal capillary cell death. Antioxid Redox Signal 2005;7:1581–7.

CHAPTER

24

Epidemiologic Evidence on Antioxidant-related Micronutrients and Diabetic Retinopathy

Christine Lee[*], *Amanda I. Adler*[†]

[*]Department of Nutritional Sciences, University of Toronto, Toronto, ON, Canada, [†]Wolfson Diabetes & Endocrine Clinic, Cambridge University Hospitals NHS Foundation Trust, Addenbrooke's Treatment Centre, Cambridge, United Kingdom

List of Abbreviations

ARED Age-Related Eye Disease Study
NHANES National Health and Nutrition Examination Survey

INTRODUCTION

Diabetic retinopathy is a serious microvascular complication of diabetes. Some degree of retinopathy occurs in almost all individuals with type 1 diabetes and in approximately 77% of individuals with type 2 diabetes of 20–25 years of duration [1,2]. The World Health Organization has estimated that diabetic retinopathy accounts for about 5% of the 37 million cases of blindness globally [3]. The prevalence of diabetic retinopathy is likely to increase, in parallel to the growing incidence of diabetes stemming from the epidemic of obesity and aging populations.

Convincing evidence shows that optimal control of blood glucose and blood pressure delay retinopathy [4–7], and prompt treatment of retinal vascular abnormalities prevents visual loss [8]. However, all of these interventions require significant clinical resources or specialized care that imposes substantial economic costs. This highlights the need to identify adjunct therapy to prevent the development and progression of diabetic retinopathy.

Oxidative stress in the retina, which involves overproduction of superoxide in the mitochondria, is one of the pathophysiological mechanisms underlying the development of diabetic retinopathy [9,10]. Therefore, targeting oxidative stress and mitochondrial dysfunction could be a potential strategy to prevent diabetic retinopathy. Animal studies have shown that supplementing the diet of diabetic rats with vitamin C and vitamin E for 12 months inhibited the development of acellular capillaries and pericyte ghosts, early signs of diabetic retinopathy [11]. In addition, oral supplementation of micronutrients and trace minerals used in the Age-Related Eye Disease Study (AREDS) (vitamin C, vitamin E, β-carotene, zinc and copper) in diabetic rats prevented the development of diabetic retinopathy by inhibiting oxidative stress [12]. Despite experimental animal studies supporting long-term oral supplementation of antioxidants as a means to stave off diabetic retinopathy, epidemiologic evidence is needed to justify intervention studies.

This chapter focuses on existing epidemiologic evidence on the association between antioxidant-related micronutrients and diabetic retinopathy [13]. It includes observational studies with cross-sectional, case-control and prospective designs on human participants with diabetes. The exposures are antioxidant-related micronutrients, including vitamin C, vitamin E and carotenoids, measured using dietary methods or biomarkers. The outcomes are diabetic retinopathy ascertained by various diagnostic methods.

ASSOCIATION BETWEEN ANTIOXIDANT-RELATED MICRONUTRIENTS AND DIABETIC RETINOPATHY

Vitamin C

Vitamin C is a potent water-soluble antioxidant because of its electron-donating properties. By donating electrons, vitamin C prevents other compounds from being oxidized [14]. Vitamin C has been shown to protect the lens, cornea, vitreous humor and retina from oxidative damage [15].

Diabetes: Oxidative Stress and Dietary Antioxidants.
http://dx.doi.org/10.1016/B978-0-12-405885-9.00024-3

Three population-based studies have examined the association between vitamin C and diabetic retinopathy. In the San Luis Valley Diabetes Study, investigators performed a cross-sectional analysis and a longitudinal analysis on 387 participants with type 2 diabetes addressing the dietary intake of vitamin C with retinopathy. Antioxidants, including vitamin C, were measured in a single 24-hour dietary recall. The investigators assessed diabetic retinopathy by stereoscopic fundus photographs after dilating both eyes, and classified it as none, background, preproliferative or prolilferative retinopathy using the modified Airlie House criteria. Logistic regression analyses showed no association between dietary intake of vitamin C and prevalent diabetic retinopathy [16].

The Atherosclerosis Risk in Communities Study investigated the prospective association between dietary intake of vitamin C and the risk of prevalent diabetic retinopathy in 1,353 individuals with type 2 diabetes. Dietary intake of vitamin C was measured using a food frequency questionnaire. Diabetic retinopathy was ascertained by a single 45-degree non-mydriatic retinal photograph of one randomly selected eye, and was classified using the modified Airlie House criteria as one of these retinal lesions including hemorrhages, microaneurysms, hard or soft exudates, macular edema, intra-retinal microvascular abnormality or venous beading. This study reported no association between dietary intake of vitamin C at baseline and prevalent diabetic retinopathy at followup when comparing the extreme quartiles of serum vitamin C [17].

In the third National Health and Nutrition examination Survey (NHANES), investigators examined the association between serum level of vitamin C and prevalent diabetic retinopathy in 998 participants with type 2 diabetes. Diabetic retinopathy was assessed by a non-mydriatic fundus photograph of one eye chosen randomly, classified using the Airlie House criteria and the Early Treatment for Diabetic Retinopathy Study severity scale and defined as the presence or absence of any retinopathy (mild, moderate or proliferative).This cross-sectional analysis did not observe an association between serum vitamin C and prevalent diabetic retinopathy [18].

In addition to these population-based studies, five hospital-based studies have investigated the relationship between vitamin C and diabetic retinopathy [19–23]. These cross-sectional studies recruited participants with either type 1 or type 2 diabetes from hospitals or local communities. The sample sizes ranged from 82 to 199. All of these studies measured vitamin C in serum or plasma samples. Diabetic retinopathy was measured in fundoscopy [19,23], or ophthalmoscopy [20,21], and was defined as the presence or absence of retinal lesions [20,23], or the presence or absence of proliferative or non-proliferative diabetic retinopathy [19,21]. One study did not describe how it measured and defined diabetic retinopathy [22]. Despite using various methods to ascertain and define diabetic retinopathy, all of these studies reported an inverse association between serum/plasma vitamin C and diabetic retinopathy, that is, the higher the consumption of vitamin C, the lower the risk of retinopathy.

Vitamin E

Vitamin E is a fat-soluble antioxidant. It scavenges peroxyl radicals to maintain the integrity and bioactivity of long-chain polyunsaturated fatty acids in cell membranes [24]. Vitamin E has been shown to reduce epoxides in retinal epithelial cells and protect them from oxidative damage [25].

The three above-mentioned population-based studies have also investigated the association between vitamin E and diabetic retinopathy. The San Luis Valley Diabetes Study reported that dietary intake of vitamin E was not associated with prevalent diabetic retinopathy or with increased severity of diabetic retinopathy over time [16]. In the Atherosclerosis Risk in Communities Study, there was no association between dietary vitamin E and the risk of diabetic retinopathy [17]. The NHANES also showed no association between serum vitamin E and the presence of diabetic retinopathy [18]. Despite population-based studies consistently reporting null associations of vitamin E with diabetic retinopathy, hospital-based, cross-sectional studies showed conflicting results. One study reported an inverse association between serum vitamin E and diabetic retinopathy [22]; however, two studies found no significant differences in plasma vitamin E among diabetic patients with or without retinopathy and the non-diabetic controls. These two studies measured diabetic retinopathy by fluorescein angiography and classified diabetic retinopathy as the presence or absence of retinal lesions [26,27].

Carotenoids

Carotenoids play crucial roles in visual function. β-Carotene, lycopene, lutein and zeaxanthin, all present in ocular tissues, are of particular importance in protecting against oxidative stress in eyes. β-Carotenes are precursors to vitamin A and they are also antioxidants that neutralize free radicals [28]. Lycopene acts to quench singlet oxygen [29]. Lutein and zeaxanthin are highly concentrated in the retina, specifically in the macula, and act as lipid-based antioxidants to reduce the effects of light-induced oxidative damage [30].

Epidemiologic evidence on the association between carotenoids and diabetic retinopathy are scarce. The San Luis Valley Diabetes Study reported no association of dietary β-carotene with prevalent diabetic retinopathy or increased severity of diabetic retinopathy over time [16]. In a community-based, cross-sectional study, nvestigators examined the association between plasma arotenoids and diabetic retinopathy in 111 individuals vith type 2 diabetes. Diabetic retinopathy was measured y mydriatic fundus photographs, and was classified ısing the EURODIAB protocol validated against the Airlie House Classification. In this study, a higher ratio of non-provitamin A carotenoids (lycopene, lutein and eaxanthin) to provitamin A carotenoids (β-carotene, α-carotene and β-cryptoxanthin) was associated with ower risk of prevalent diabetic retinopathy. However, he authors reported a positive association between higher concentration of provitamin A carotenoids and the risk of prevalent diabetic retinopathy [31].

TABLE 24.1 Study Design of the Studies on the Association Between Antioxidant-Related Micronutrients and Diabetic Retinopathy

First Author, Year of Publication	Study Design
Ali, 1989	Cross-sectional
Brazionis, 2009	Cross-sectional
Gupta, 2005	Cross-sectional
Gurler, 2000	Cross-sectional
Martinoli, 1993	Cross-sectional
Mayer-Davis, 1998	Cross-sectional/ Longitudinal
Millen, 2003	Cross-sectional
Millen, 2004	Prospective
Rema, 1995	Cross-sectional
Sinclair, 1992	Cross-sectional
Willems, 1998	Cross-sectional

This table shows the study designs of the studies reviewed.

TABLE 24.2 Sources of Study Population of the Studies on the Association Between Antioxidant- Related Micronutrients and Diabetic Retinopathy

First Author, Year of Publication	Sources/ Case vs. Control
Ali, 1989	In- and outpatients/hospital staff
Brazionis, 2009	Communities
Gupta, 2005	Patients
Gurler, 2000	Patients with/without eye pathology
Martinoli, 1993	Outpatients/hospital staff, blood donors
Mayer-Davis, 1998	Communities
Millen, 2003	General population
Millen, 2004	Communities
Rema, 1995	Patients/spouses
Sinclair, 1992	Patients/local communities
Willems, 1998	Outpatients

This table shows the sources of study population of the studies reviewed.

DISCUSSION

This review has summarized the epidemiologic studies on the association between antioxidant-related micronutrients and diabetic retinopathy. Existing evidence does not support an association of dietary or plasma vitamin C and vitamin E with diabetic retinopathy. However, the plasma carotenoids lycopene, lutein and zeaxanthin appear to be associated with a lower risk of prevalent diabetic retinopathy. Although experimental studies suggested protective effects of antioxidants on diabetic retinopathy, these effects have not been consistently demonstrated in humans. Exploring potential sources of heterogeneity between these studies showed substantial differences which may explain, in part, the inconsistent findings in the literature.

The majority of the studies reviewed are of a cross-sectional design (Table 24.1). A cross-sectional analysis does not allow investigators to draw conclusions on the timing of the association between exposures and outcomes. For example, it does not preclude the possibility of reverse causation, e.g., an individual could have increased his or her micronutrient intake after the diagnosis of diabetic retinopathy. A prospective study, which measures exposures prior to ascertaining outcomes, could overcome the limitations of a cross-sectional study. The number of cases in cross-sectional studies and the number of participants in prospective studies were relatively small, which may not provide adequate statistical power to detect an association, if one exists.

Cases selected from hospitals' wards or clinics, by dint of receiving medical care, may have been more likely to have existing retinal lesions detected than would people from the general population who may or may not have equivalent medical attention. Such a detection bias could overestimate any association observed. In the studies reviewed, investigators selected the diabetic cases and controls from the same population, ensuring that both had similar exposure to risk factors and confounding factors. Although diabetic controls should ideally resemble the demographic characteristics of the cases, the non-diabetic controls in the hospital-based studies were selected from spouses or hospital staff, who may be more health conscious and their micronutrients may be systematically different from individuals with diabetic retinopathy (Tables 24.2 and 24.3). Furthermore, a hospital-based study may only reflect the characteristics of patients in the catchment area, and may not be generalizable to other populations. The studies measured micronutrients using either self-reported dietary methods or

TABLE 24.3 Study Sample of the Studies on the Association Between Antioxidant-Related Micronutrients and Diabetic Retinopathy

First Author, Year of Publication	Study Sample
Ali, 1989	Type 1 & 2 DM:50 with, 50 without DR; 45 non-DM control
Brazionis, 2009	111 Type 2 DM
Gurler, 2000	Type 2 DM: 25 with, 34 without DR; 24 non-DM control
Gupta, 2005	NIDDM: 20 NPDR, 22 PDR, 40 no complications
Martinoli, 1993	61 Type 1 DM, 26 non-DM control
Mayer-Davis, 1998	381 Type 2 DM
Millen, 2003	998 Type 2 DM
Millen, 2004	1353 Type 2 DM
Rema, 1995	NIDDM: 83 with, 63 without background DR; 53 non-DM control
Sinclair, 1992	Type 2 DM: 25 with, 25 without DR; 40 non-DM control
Willems, 1998	110 Type 1 DM

NIDDM = non-insulin dependent diabetes mellitus; DM = diabetes mellitus; DR = diabetic retinopathy; NPDR = non-proliferative diabetic retinopathy; PDR = proliferative diabetic retinopathy.
This table shows the study sample of the studies reviewed.

TABLE 24.4 Exposure Definition of the Studies on the Association Between Antioxidant-Related Micronutrients and Diabetic Retinopathy

First Author, Year of Publication	Exposure Definition
Ali, 1989	Plasma vitamin C
Brazionis, 2009	Plasma caroteinods
Gurler, 2000	Serum vitamin C
Gupta, 2005	Plasma vitamin C
Martinoli, 1993	Plasma vitamin E
Mayer-Davis, 1998	Dietary vitamins C and E (24-hour recall)
Millen, 2003	Serum vitamins C and E
Millen, 2004	Dietary vitamins C and E (Food frequency questionnaire)
Rema, 1995	Plasma vitamins C and E
Sinclair, 1992	Serum vitamin C
Willems, 1998	Blood vitamin E

This table shows the exposure definition of the studies reviewed.

objective biomarkers in serum or plasma samples. As participants cannot always recall dietary intake accurately or selectively report intake, self-reported information on dietary intake is prone to measurement errors and bias [32]. If the measurement errors are random and are not related to true intake, the observed association would be biased toward an absence of an effect. However, the 'flat-slope phenomenon', i.e., individuals with low intake tend to over-report and those with a high intake tend to under-report, can occur [33]. Such systematic differences in reporting would over- or underestimate the observed association. The San Luis Valley Diabetes Study [16] measured dietary intake of micronutrients in a single 24-hour recall, which may not capture the day-to-day variation of intake [34]. While a 24-hour recall is ideal for providing a snapshot of dietary intake across a population in surveys, it may not be adequate to explore a diet-disease relationship. In contrast, the Atherosclerosis Risk in Communities Study [17] measured micronutrients in a validated food frequency questionnaire which was designed to assess habitual intake in the past year [35].

Biomarkers allow a more objective measurement of dietary intake; although they are not perfect, their limitations, including physiological variations and laboratory errors, are unlikely to correlate with the errors from self-report dietary methods [36]. Most of the studies reviewed in this chapter measured micronutrients in a single serum or plasma sample (Table 24.4). Serum or plasma concentration of a nutrient reflects recent dietary intake, absorption and metabolism of foods or supplements. Such a snapshot of intake may not coincide with the window of exposures of these micronutrients in the development of diabetic retinopathy, and repeated measurements over time could better capture long-term habitual intake and explore the diet-disease relationship. Furthermore, objective measured biomarkers, when used in combination with self-reported intake, have been shown to strengthen the diet-disease analyses of prospective studies by increasing statistical power to detect associations [37].

The studies reviewed measured diabetic retinopathy using various methods, including retinal photography, fundoscopy, ophthalmoscopy, and fluorescein angiography (Table 24.5). Precise measurement of retinal lesions minimizes non-differential misclassification of outcomes. That is to say, incorrectly diagnosis of or missing diabetic retinopathy in a study participant is not related to the participant's level or intake of micronutrients. Such non-differential misclassification would underestimate the true association between exposures and outcomes. The Early Treatment for Diabetic Retinopathy Study score defined the reference standard to detect diabetic retinal lesions as stereoscopic 7-field, 30°C mydriatic fundus photographs [38]. Although direct ophthalmoscopy and indirect slit-lamp biomicroscopy performed by an ophthalmologist compared favorably to 7-field stereophotography and 2-field digital photography to

TABLE 24.5 Outcome Measurement of the Studies on the Association Between Antioxidant-Related Micronutrients and Diabetic Retinopathy

First Author, Year of Publication	Outcome Measurement
Ali, 1989	Dilated eye fundoscopy
Brazionis, 2009	Mydriatic fundus photographs
Gurler, 2000	Direct and indirect ophthalmoscopy with dilated pupils
Gupta, 2005	Direct ophthalmoscopy
Martinoli, 1993	Direct ophthalmoscopy/fluorescein angiograph
Mayer-Davis, 1998	Mydriatic retinal photos (both eyes)
Millen, 2003	Non-mydriatic fundus photos (one eye)
Millen, 2004	Non-mydriatic fundus photos (one eye)
Rema, 1995	No description
Sinclair, 1992	Fundoscopy
Willems, 1998	Fluorescein angiograph

This table shows the outcome measurement of the studies reviewed.

TABLE 24.6 Outcome Definition of the Studies on the Association Between Antioxidant-Related Micronutrients and Diabetic Retinopathy

First Author, Year of Publication	Outcome DEFINITION
Ali, 1989	Presence/absence of DR
Brazionis, 2009	EURODIAB protocol
Gurler, 2000	Presence/absence of retinal lesions
Gupta, 2005	Proliferative/non-proliferative DR
Martinoli, 1993	Presence/absence of DR
Mayer-Davis, 1998	Airlie House Criteria
Millen, 2003	Modified Airlie House Criteria
Millen, 2004	Modified Airlie House Criteria
Rema, 1995	No description
Sinclair, 1992	Presence/absence of retinal lesions
Willems, 1998	No description

DR = diabetic retinopathy; NPDR = non-proliferative diabetic retinopathy; PDR = proliferative diabetic retinopathy.
This table shows the outcome definition of the studies reviewed.

detect diabetic retinopathy, retinal photography is preferred because it provides a permanent retinal image, overcomes the limitation of the ophthalmoscope and minimizes the potential inconsistent results between ophthalmologists [39].

The classification of diabetic retinopathy varied between studies (Table 24.6). Hospital-based studies compared either the presence or absence of any retinopathy [19,20,23,26] or the presence or absence of proliferative retinopathy [21]. However, population-based studies used specific grading system, e.g., the Modified Airlie House Classification, the Early Treatment for Diabetic Retinopathy Study score and the EURODIAB protocol [16–18,31]. The difference in grading criteria made it difficult to compare results between studies. Nevertheless, the International Clinical Diabetic Retinopathy Disease Severity Scale offers a simplified clinical grading scale to classify diabetic retinopathy systematically [40].

CONCLUSION

In conclusion, the existing epidemiologic evidence does not support an association of vitamin C and vitamin E with diabetic retinopathy. However, higher plasma carotenoids lycopene, lutein and zeaxanthin appear to be associated with a lower risk of prevalent diabetic retinopathy. In part because of the methodological limitations of the studies reviewed, the evidence is inconclusive. Further prospective studies are needed to characterize the nature of the association before allocating resources for randomized controlled trial to test whether dietary intake or oral supplementation of these antioxidant-related micronutrients protect against diabetic retinopathy.

SUMMARY POINTS

- Diabetic retinopathy contributes significantly to global blindness.
- Targeting oxidative stress, one of the pathophysiological mechanisms involved, may represent an adjunct therapy to prevent the development and slow the progression of diabetic retinopathy.
- Existing epidemiologic evidence does not support an association of vitamin C and vitamin E with diabetic retinopathy.
- Some evidence suggests that the carotenoids lycopene, lutein and zeaxanthin may be associated with a lower risk of prevalent diabetic retinopathy.
- Well-designed prospective studies are needed to characterize the nature of the association between antioxidant-related micronutrients and diabetic retinopathy to justify interventional studies.

References

[1] Klein R, Klein BL, Moss SE, Davis MD, DeMetes DL. The Wisconsin Epidemiologic Study of Diabetic retinopathy. II. Prevalence and risk of diabetic retinopathy when age at diagnosis is less than 30 years. Arch Ophthalmol 1984;102:520–6.

[2] Klein R, Klein BL, Moss SE, Davis MD, DeMetes DL. The Wisconsin Epidemiologic Study of Diabetic retinopathy. III. Prevalence and risk of diabetic retinopathy when age at diagnosis is 30 or more years. Arch Ophthalmol 1984;102:527–32.

[3] Resnikoff S, Pascolini D, Etya'ale D, Kocur I, Pararajasegaram R, Pokharel GP, et al. Global data on visual impairment in the year 2002. Bull World Health Organ 2004;82:844–51.

[4] Diabetes Control and Complications Trial/Epidemiology of Diabetes Interventions and Complications (DCCT/EDIC) Study Research Group. Intensive diabetes treatment and cardiovascular disease in patients with type 1 diabetes. N Engl J Med 2005;353:2643–53.

[5] Holman RR, Paul SK, Bethel MA, Matthews DR, Neil HA. 10-year follow-up of intensive glucose control in type 2 diabetes. N Engl J Med 2008;359:1577–89.

[6] UK Prospective Diabetes Study Group. Tight blood pressure control and risk of macrovascular and microvascular complications in type 2 diabetes. UKPDS 38. BMJ 1998;317:703–13.

[7] Klein R, Klein BE, Moss SE, Cruickshanks KJ. The Wisconsin Epidemiologic Study of Diabetic retinopathy. XVII. The 14-year incidence and progression of diabetic retinopathy and associated risk factors in type 1 diabetes. Ophthalmology 1998;105:1801–15.

[8] Scanlon PH. The English national screening programme for sight-threatening diabetic retinopathy. J Med Screen 2008;15:1–4.

[9] Brownlee M. The pathobiology of diabetic complications: a unifying mechanism. Diabetes 2005;54:227–34.

[10] Santos JM, Mohammad G, Zhong Q, Kowluru RA. Diabetes retinopathy, superoxide damage and antioxidants. Curr Pharm Biotechnol 2011;12:352–61.

[11] Kowluru RA, Tang J, Kern TS. Abnormalities of retinal metabolism in diabetes and experimental galactosemia. VII. Effect of long-term administration of antioxidants on the development of retinopathy. Diabetes 2001;50:1938–42.

[12] Kowluru RA, Kanwar M, Chan PS, Zhang JP. Inhibition of retinopathy and retinal metabolic abnormalities in diabetic rats with AREDS-based micronutrients. Arch Ophthalmol 2008;126:1266–72.

[13] Lee CT, Gayton EL, Beulens JW, Flanagan DW, Adler AI. Micronutrients and diabetic retinopathy – A systematic review. Ophthalmology 2010;117:71–8.

[14] Padayatty SJ, Katz A, Wang Y, Eck P, Kwon O, Lee JH, et al. Vitamin C as an antioxidant: evaluation of its role in disease prevention. J Am Coll Nutr 2003;22:18–35.

[15] Bendich A, Machlin LJ, Scandurra O, Burton GW, Wayner DDM. The antioxidant role of vitamin C. Adv Free Radic Biol Med 1986;2:416–44.

[16] Mayer-Davis EJ, Bell RA, Reboussin BA, Rushing J, Marshall JA, Hamman RF. Antioxidant nutrient intake and diabetic retinopathy: the San Luis Valley Diabetes Study. Ophthalmology 1998;105:2264–70.

[17] Millen AE, Klein R, Folsom AR, Stevens J, Palta M, Mares JA. Relation between intake of vitamins C and E and risk of diabetic retinopathy in the Atherosclerosis Risk in Communities Study. Am J Clin Nutr 2004;79:865–73.

[18] Millen AE, Gruber M, Klein R, Klein BE, Palta M, Mares JA. Relations of serum ascorbic acid and alpha-tocopherol to diabetic retinopathy in the Third National Health and Nutrition Examination Survey. Am J Epidemiol 2003;158:225–33.

[19] Ali SM, Chakraborty SK. Role of plasma ascorbate in diabetic microangiopathy. Bangladesh Med Res Counc Bull 1989;15:47–59.

[20] Gürler B, Vural H, Yilmaz N, Oguz H, Satici A, Aksoy N. The role of oxidative stress in diabetic retinopathy. Eye (London) 2000;14:730–5.

[21] Gupta MM, Chari S. Lipid peroxidation and antioxidant status in patients with diabetic retinopathy. Indian J Physiol Pharmacol 2005;49:187–92.

[22] Rema M, Mohan V, Bhaskar A, Shanmugasundaram KR. Does oxidant stress play a role in diabetic retinopathy? Indian J Ophthalmol 1995;43:7–21.

[23] Sinclair AJ, Girling AJ, Gray L, Lunec J, Barnett AH. An investigation of the relationship between free radical activity and vitamin C metabolism in elderly diabetic subjects with retinopathy. Gerontology 1992;38:268–74.

[24] Traber MG, Atkinson J. Vitamin E, antioxidant and nothing more. Free Radic Biol Med 2007;43:4–15.

[25] Sparrow JR, Vollmer-Snarr HR, Zhou J, Jang YP, Jockusch S, Itagaki Y, et al. A2E-epoxides damage DNA in retinal pigment epithelial cells. Vitamin E and other antioxidants inhibit A2E-epoxide formation. J Biol Chem 2003;278:18207–13.

[26] Martinoli L, Di Felice M, Seghieri G, Ciuti M, De Giorgio LA, Fazzini A, et al. Plasma retinol and alpha-tocopherol concentrations in insulin-dependent diabetes mellitus: their relationship to microvascular complications. Int J Vitam Nutr Res 1993;63: 87–92.

[27] Willems D, Dorchy H, Dufrasne D. Serum antioxidant status and oxidized LDL in well-controlled young type 1 diabetic patients with and without subclinical complications. Atherosclerosis 1998;137(suppl.):S61–4.

[28] Krinsky NI. Actions of carotenoids in biological systems. Ann Rev Nutr 1993;13:561–87.

[29] Cantrell A, McGarvey DJ, Truscott TG, Rancan F, Böhm F. Singlet oxygen quenching by dietary carotenoids in a model membrane environment. Arch Biochem Biophys 2003;412:47–54.

[30] Lien EL, Hammond BR. Nutritional influences on visual development and function. Prog Retin Eye Res 2011;30:188–203.

[31] Brazionis L, Rowley K, Itsiopoulos C, O'Dea K. Plasma carotenoids and diabetic retinopathy. Br J Nutr 2009;101:270–7.

[32] Kipnis V, Midthune D, Freedman L, Bingham S, Day NE, Riboli E, et al. Bias in dietary-report instruments and its implications for nutritional epidemiology. Public Health Nutrition 2002;5(6A): 915–23.

[33] Gersovitz M, Madden JP, Smiciklas-Wright H. Validity of the 24 hr dietary recall and seven-day record for group comparisons. J Am Diet Assoc 1978;73:48–55.

[34] Beaton GH, Milner J, McGuire V, Feather TE, Little JA. Source of variance in 24-hour dietary recall data: implications of nutrition study design and interpretation. Carbohydrate sources, vitamins and minerals. Am J Clin Nutr 1983;37:986–95.

[35] Willett WC, Sampson L, Stampfer MJ, Rosner B, Bain C, Witschi J, et al. Reproducibility and validity of a semiquantitative food frequency questionnaire. Am J Epidemiol 1985;122:51–65.

[36] Potischman N. Biologic and methodologic issues for nutritional biomarkers. J Nutr 133 Supp 2003;3:875S–80S.

[37] Freeman L, Kipnis V, Schatzkin A, Tasevska N, Potischman N. Can we use biomarkers in combination with self-reports to strengthen the analysis of nutritional epidemiologic studies? Epidemiol Perspect Innov 2010;7:2.

[38] Early Treatment Diabetic Retinopathy Study Research Group. Grading diabetic retinopathy from stereoscopic color fundus photographs – an extension of the modified Airlie House classification. ETDRS report number 10. Ophthalmology 1991;98(suppl.):786–806.

[39] Scanlon PH, Malhotra R, Greenwood RH, Aldington SJ, Foy C, Flatman M, et al. Comparison of two reference standards in validating two field mydriatic digital photography as a method of screening for diabetic retinopathy. Br J Ophthalmol 2003;87:1258–63.

[40] Wilkinson CP, Ferris 3rd FL, Klein RE, Lee PP, Agardh CD, Davis M, Global Diabetic Retinopathy Project Group, et al. Proposed international clinical diabetic retinopathy and diabetic macular edema disease severity scales. Ophthalmology 2003;110: 1677–82.

CHAPTER

25

Oxidative Stress and the Lung in Diabetes: The Use of Pomegranate Juice

Gulay Eren, Zafer Cukurova, Oya Hergunsel

Bakirkoy Dr. Sadi Konuk Training and Research Hospital, Department of Anaesthesiology and Intensive Care, Istanbul, Turkey

List of Abbreviations

AGE Advanced glycosylation end-products
CAT Catalase
DM Diabetes mellitus
eNOS Endothelial nitric oxide
GSH Glutathione
GSH-Px Glutathione peroxidase
H_2O_2 Hydrogen peroxide
iNOS Inducible nitric oxide
LDL Low-density lipoprotein
MDA Malondialdehyde
NF-κB Nuclear factor-kappa B
NO Nitric oxide
$O_2{\cdot}^-$ Superoxide
OH· Hydroxyl radical
PCC Protein carbonyl content
PJ Pomegranate juice
PPR-γ Proliferator-activated receptor-γ
RAGE Receptor for advanced glycosylation end-products
ROS Reactive oxygen species
SA Sialic acid
SOD Superoxide dismutase

INTRODUCTION

Diabetes mellitus (DM) is a systemic disease that produces structural and functional alterations in various organs such as the kidneys, eyes, brain and heart. While the etiology of diabetic complications is not entirely understood, it has been proposed that several mechanisms play a role in the development and progression of these complications. Oxidative stress, non-enzymatic protein glycosylation and alteration of nitric oxide (NO) metabolism occur as a consequence of diabetes-related metabolic disorders [1].

The diabetic state itself causes oxidative stress through the autooxidation of glucose, protein glycation and lipid peroxidation [2]. In other words, hyperglycemia is thought to cause oxidative stress by means of several related mechanisms [3–5]. There are four pathways through which oxidative stress may cause the chronic complications of DM: the polyol pathway, protein kinase C activation, the hexosamine pathway and the pathway of advanced glycosylation end-products (AGE) [4]. As the blood glucose level increases, the movement of glucose through the polyol pathway increases and, as a result, sorbitol is produced. Increased sorbitol concentrations may cause osmotic stress to cells, consequently causing intracellular glutathione depletion. In the meantime, glucose activates various isomers of protein kinase C, which in turn affects the expression of nitric oxide (NO), endothelin, nuclear factor-kappa B (NF-κB), plasminogen activator inhibitor, and so on. In another mechanism, hyperglycemia increases the flux of glucose through the hexosamine pathway, again affecting inflammatory mediators and insulin resistance. Lastly, hyperglycemia increases AGE concentrations. The changes in proteins as a consequence of non-enzymatic glycosylation may alter cellular functions by binding to specific binding sites including the receptor for AGEs (RAGE). As the AGEs and other ligands bind to RAGE, signaling in generation of intracellular oxidative stress occurs, which in turn causes activation of the redox-sensitive transcription factor NF-κB. Activation of NF-κB in diabetic patients correlates with the quality of glycemic control and can be reduced by treatment with antioxidants [5].

The combined effect of the four mechanisms is a considerable overproduction of mitochondrial superoxides, causing cellular stress and damage, and a reduction in fundamental cellular antioxidant defense mechanisms, so it is wise to use either synthetic or naturally occurring antioxidants to attenuate these changes in DM.

Diabetes: Oxidative Stress and Dietary Antioxidants.
http://dx.doi.org/10.1016/B978-0-12-405885-9.00025-5

THE LUNG AS A TARGET ORGAN IN DIABETES

The extensive alveolar-capillary network constituting the huge pulmonary microvascular circulation and abundant connective tissue render the lungs highly susceptible to systemic microangiopathy, but pulmonary impairment in diabetes mellitus is under-recognized. This is because, owing to its large reserves, symptoms and disability develop later in the lung than in smaller microvasculature such as the kidney or retina, despite a comparable severity in anatomic involvement.

Pulmonary function decreases over the years in diabetic patients with impaired metabolic control, as indicated by decreases in measurements of pulmonary volume and capacity. An increasing number of studies indicate physiological and structural abnormalities in the lungs of diabetics. Structural alterations to the basal membrane of the pulmonary capillary endothelium in DM cause thickening of the alveolus-capillary membrane and a reduction in the diffusional capability [6,7]. Decreased capacity of the antioxidative defense system and increased oxidative stress were seen in the lungs of diabetic animal models [1,2,5].

As a significant complication of diabetes, basal lamina thickening has been frequently observed in various diabetic tissues such as the kidney, retina, and heart; it is the classical morphologic finding in diabetic microangiopathy. Increased non-enzymatic glycation of proteins and peptides plays a crucial role in the progression of this condition, and this may be responsible for extracellular matrix accumulation [2]. The same morphologic changes apply to the pulmonary microvasculature as well. Electron microscopic examination of diabetic lung tissue by Ozansoy and coworkers [2] revealed narrowed capillary and alveoli, expanded interstitium and extracellular matrix. They conclude that these alterations result in an increased thickness of the membrane, which may inhibit gas transport by diffusion and cause a decrease in oxygen supply to the tissue. In a similar study, Isotani et al. [8] found a significant reduction in pulmonary diffusion capacity for carbon monoxide in diabetic patients. The percentage reduction was significantly lower in subjects with proliferative retinopathy, another sign of diabetic microangiopathy, than in patients with simple diabetic retinopathy. Consistent with these findings, in another study, Guazzi et al. [9] demonstrated increased impedance to gas transfer across the alveolar-capillary membrane in type 2 DM patients; and insulin acutely improved gas exchange, possibly through facilitation of the alveolar-capillary interface conductance.

Similarly to the mechanism of damage to other organ systems, hyperglycemia affects the lungs by damaging capillaries and by the non-enzymatic glycosylation of collagen [10]. In a study of diabetes induced in hamsters, hyperglycemia to concentrations of 23–25 mmol liter^{-1} resulted in direct lung damage in which many plasmalemmal vesicles invaded the capillary endothelium, alveoli collapsed, and the lung interstitium enlarged. All these changes occurred after only six weeks of hyperglycemia [11]. The authors consider that hyperglycemia caused cellular stress which was detrimental to the lung, and they explain this damage by the aforementioned four mechanisms [4].

Some authors assume that the thickened alveolar interstitium and vascular basal lamina might be a consequence of the increased lysyl oxidase activity, an important enzyme in the formation of connective tissue [12]. Others reported that the products of oxidative modification of proteins and carbohydrates increased via these enzymes through lysyl oxidase activity [13].

A study by Eren et al. [14] revealed that diabetes caused some alterations in antioxidant capacity and structural changes in rat lungs, probably through the activation of NF-κB which was demonstrated immunohistochemically. They also showed that these disturbances could reduced by the use of pyrrolidine dithiocarbamate, a specific inhibitor of NF-κB. It is known that shear stress induced up-regulation of endothelial nitric oxide (eNOS) is mediated by NF-κB. Zhen et al. [15] confirmed this fact in their study. They have suggested that the ROS-stimulated up-regulation of eNOS expression is mediated by diminished nitric oxide (NO) availability and consequent reduction in the negative feedback regulatory effect of NO on eNOS expression, which is possibly mediated by NF-κB. Sridulyakul et al. [16] showed that eNOS expression decreased in many DM-affected organs, but not in the lungs. Consistent with these findings, Eren and coworkers [14] determined immunohistochemically that eNOS expression increased in the lungs of diabetic rats, and it could be inhibited by NF-κB antagonists.

Diabetes is also associated with an increased risk of pulmonary infections. Infections caused by certain microorganisms (*Staphylococcus aureus*, gram-negative organisms, and *Mycobacterium tuberculosis*) occur with increased frequency. Pulmonary infections due to other organisms, like influenza virus and *Streptococcus pneumonia*, are associated with increased morbidity and mortality in diabetic patients [17]. Glycosylation of immunoglobulins causes impairment in their function even only after a few hours of hyperglycemia [18]. Humoral immunity, leukocyte adherence, chemotaxis, and phagocytosis may be affected. The impairment of function can be reversed by rigorous control of glucose [19].

POLYPHENOLS AS ANTIOXIDANTS

Polyphenols are a structural class of mainly natural organic chemicals, whose structure comprises multiple phenolic units. Each particular polyphenol has a unique umber and structure of phenolic rings, which imparts s physical, chemical and biological properties.

Polyphenol antioxidants are very diverse. More than ,000 polyphenolic compounds have been identified in various plant species. All plant phenolic compounds originate from a common intermediate, phenylalanine, or a close precursor, shikimic acid. Primarily they appear in conjugated forms, with one or more sugar residues linked to hydroxyl groups, although direct linkages of the sugar (polysaccharide or monosaccharide) to an aromatic carbon also exist [20]. Polyphenols may be classified into different groups according to the number of phenol rings that they contain, or on the basis of the structural elements which bind these rings to one another. There are four broad groups: phenolic acids, flavonoids, stilbenes and lignans. Phenolic acids are abundantly present in foods and further divided into two classes: derivatives of benzoic acid and derivatives of cinnamic acid. The hydroxybenzoic acid content of edible plants is generally low, with the exception of certain red fruits. The hydroxycinnamic acids are more common. Flavonoids are the most studied group of polyphenols [21]. More than 4,000 species have been identified, many of which are responsible for the attractive colors of flowers and fruit. Flavonoids may also be subdivided – into six subclasses: flavonols, flavones, flavanones, flavanols, anthocyanins, and isoflavones. Quercetin, myricetin, catechins etc. are some of the most common flavonoids. The occurrence of stilbenes in the human diet is quite low. One of the best studied, naturally occurring polyphenol stilbenes is resveratrol, found largely in grapes. A product of grapes, red wine, also contains a significant amount of resveratrol. Lignans are diphenolic compounds that have a 2,3-dibenzylbutane structure, formed by the dimerization of two cinnamic acid residues [20].

Polyphenols are mainly provided by the diet since they are found in a wide variety of phytochemical-bearing foods. The total dietary intake of polyphenols could be as high as 1 g/d, which is much higher than that of all other phytochemicals and dietary antioxidants. To name a just few examples, fruits such as apples, blackberries, blueberries, pomegranate, grapes, cranberries, and strawberries; and vegetables such as cabbage, onion, broccoli and celery are rich in polyphenols. Fruits like grapes, apple, pear, cherries and berries contain up to 200–300 mg polyphenols per 100 grams fresh weight. The products manufactured from these fruits also contain polyphenols in significant amounts. Typically a glass of red wine or a cup of tea or coffee contains about 100 mg polyphenols. Cereals, dry legumes and chocolate also contribute to the polyphenolic intake [21,22].

There is plenty of evidence that strongly supporting the theory that polyphenols contribute to the prevention of many disorders such as cardiovascular disease, neurodegenerative diseases, cancers, osteoporosis and diabetes mellitus [20].

POMEGRANATE

The pomegranate (*Punica granatum* L.) is a small tree cultivated throughout Mediterranean region, and extracts from this plant have been used for centuries in ancient cultures for remedial purposes. The rind of the fruit and the bark of the pomegranate tree have been used as a traditional remedy for diarrhea, dysentery, intestinal infections, ulcers, hemorrhage and hemorrhoids [23,24]. Pomegranate flowers of have been used in Unani and Ayurvedic medicine [25], and they are antidiabetic [26].

Pomegranate Fruit

The fruit consists of the peel, seeds, and arils. The peel makes up about 50% of the fruit, whereas the arils and seeds make up 40% and 10%, respectively. The nutritional value of the peel is attributable to the high levels of compounds such as phenolics, flavonoids (Table 25.1), ellagitannins, and proanthocyanidin compounds, complex polysaccharides, and minerals, mainly potassium, nitrogen, calcium, magnesium, phosphorus, and sodium it contains [27], but this is not an edible part of the plant, so pharmaceuticals have been produced from it in different forms, such as pills, powders, capsules, vials, etc.

Pomegranate seeds are rich in lipids, in the form of polyunsaturated (n-3) fatty acids, such as linoleic acid and other lipids such as punicic acid, stearic acid, palmitic acid, and phytosterols. In addition to lipids, considerable amounts of protein, fiber, vitamins, minerals, polyphenols, and isoflavones are also present [28].

The arils of the pomegranate fruit contain 85% water, 10% total sugars (mainly fructose and glucose),

TABLE 25.1 Polyphenols Found in 'Pomegranate Fruit'

Flavonoids		Units (mg/100g)
Flavanols	Procyanidin dimer B1	0.13
	Procyanidin dimer B3	0.16
	(±) Catechin	0.40
	(±) Gallocatechin	0.17
	(-) Epigallocatechin	0.16
	(-) Epicatechin	0.08

Source (with permission from): *Gil M.I., Tomas-Barberan F.A., Hess-Pierce B., Holcroft D.M., Kader A.A. (2000) Antioxidant activity of pomegranate juice and its relationship with phenolic composition and processing. Journal of Agricultural and Food Chemistry 48:4581–4589.*

TABLE 25.2 The Nutritional Value of Pomegranate (Arils Only)

Nutritional value per 100 g (3.5 oz)	
Energy	346 kJ (83 kcal)
Carbohydrates	18.7 g
- Sugars	13.7 g
- Dietary fiber	4.0 g
Fat	1.2 g
Protein	1.7 g
Thiamine (vit. B1)	0.07 mg
Riboflavin (vit. B2)	0.05 mg
Niacin (vit. B3)	0.29 mg
Pantothenic acid (vit. B5)	0.38 mg
Pyridoxine (vit. B6)	0.08 mg
Folate (vit. B9)	38 μg
Vitamin C	10 mg
Calcium	10 mg
Iron	0.30 mg
Magnesium	12 mg
Phosphorus	36 mg
Potassium	236 mg
Zinc	0.35 mg

Source: US Department of Agriculture, Agricultural Research Service. 2012. USDA National Nutrient Database for Standard Reference, Release 25. Nutrient Data Laboratory Home Page, http://www.ars.usda.gov/nutrientdata.

TABLE 25.3 Showing all Polyphenols Found in 'Pomegranate, Pure Juice'

Flavonoids		Units (mg/100ml)
Anthocyanins	Cyanidin 3-O-glucoside	3.43
	Pelargonidin 3-O-glucoside	0.33
	Delphinidin 3-O-glucoside	1.36
	Cyanidin 3,5-O-diglucoside	3.39
	Delphinidin 3,5-O-diglucoside	1.56
	Pelargonidin 3,5-O-glucoside	0.06
Dihydrochalcones	Phloridzin	0.10
Flavanols	(±)Catechin	0.37
	Quercetin	0.25
PHENOLIC ACIDS		
Hydroxybenzoic acids	Ellagic acid glucoside	3.97
	Protocatechuic acid	0.08
	Gallic acid	0.45
	Ellagic acid	2.06
	Galloyl glucose	4.81
	Punicalagin	43.60
Hydroxycinnamic acids	p-Coumaric acid	5.38e-03
	Caffeic acid	0.07
	Ferulic acid	5.38e-04
	o-Coumaric acid	0.01
	5-Caffeoylquinic acid	0.12

Sources (with permissions from): **1.***Gil M.I., Cherif J., Ayed N., Artes F., Tomasbarberan F.A. (1995) Influence of Cultivar, Maturity Stage and Geographical Location on the Juice Pigmentation of Tunisian Pomegranates. Zeitschrift fuer Lebensmittel Untersuchung und Forschung 201:361–364.* **2.** *Pascual-Teresa de, S.; Santos-Buelga, C.; Rivas-Gonzalo, J.C. (2000) Quantitative analysis of flavan-3-ols in Spanish foodstuffs and beverages. Journal of Agricultural and Food Chemistry 48:5331–5337.*

and 1.5% pectin, citric acid, malic acid, vitamins and minerals, and bioactive compounds such as phenolics and flavonoids [29] (Table 25.2). The juice obtained by squeezing the arils and seeds is a rich source of antioxidants such as polyphenols, tannins, and anthocyanins, and also vitamin C, vitamin E, coenzyme Q10, and lipoic acid [28].

Anthocyanins are the most prominent group present in the arils or juice, which give the fruit or juice its color [30]. There is a wide variety of anthocyanins present in pomegranate juice (Tables 25.3 and 25.4).

TABLE 25.4 Total Polyphenol Content by Subclass for 'Pomegranate, Pure Juice'

Subclass	Total Content
Hydroxybenzoic acids	54.97 mg/100 ml
Anthocyanins	10.13 mg/100 ml
Flavanols	0.62 mg/100 ml
Hydroxycinnamic acids	0.21 mg/100 ml
Dihydrochalcones	0.10 mg/100 ml

Sources (with permissions from): **1.***Gil M.I., Cherif J., Ayed N., Artes F., Tomasbarberan F.A. (1995) Influence of Cultivar, Maturity Stage and Geographical Location on the Juice Pigmentation of Tunisian Pomegranates. Zeitschrift fuer Lebensmittel Untersuchung und Forschung 201:361–364.* **2.** *Pascual-Teresa de, S.; Santos-Buelga, C.; Rivas-Gonzalo, J.C. (2000) Quantitative analysis of flavan-3-ols in Spanish foodstuffs and beverages. Journal of Agricultural and Food Chemistry 48:5331–5337.*

Pomegranate Leaf Extract

The pomegranate leaf, like the peels, is rich in polyphenolic compounds including tannins (punicalin, pedunculagan, gallagic acid, ellagic acid and its glucose esters) and flavonoids. Among the tannins, ellagic acid and punicalgins have aroused considerable interest, and in recent years most of the health benefits of the pomegranate have been linked to these tannins [31].

Pomegranate Flower Extract

All parts of the pomegranate fruit are useful, but in the Unani and Ayurvedic systems of medicine, only the flower part has been prescribed for the treatment of diabetes [25]. The pomegranate flower contains different compounds, of which the most abundant are the polyphenols (gallic acid and ellagic acid) and triterpenes (oleanolic, ursolic, maslinic, and asiatic acids). There is also one sterol (daucosterol) and one flavonoid (punicaflavone) that can be extracted from the flower. These compounds have shown considerable biological activity and medicinal value [32].

CLINICAL EVIDENCE REGARDING POMEGRANATE

Evidence for the clinical benefits of pomegranate and its constituents has been reported in several studies: a reduction of systolic blood pressure in hypertensive patients, decreasing common carotid artery intima-media thickness [33], attenuating myocardial ischemia and improving lipid profile in diabetic patients [34,35], suppressing inflammatory cell signaling in colon cancer and inhibiting chemically induced cancerous lesion formation in mammary glands [36,37], reducing the morbidity among hemodialysis patients and preventing obesity [23].

Several studies have been performed to investigate the anti-obesity effect of pomegranate constituents (pomegranate seed extracts, leaf extracts, flower extracts and juice) [27,28,32,33,38]. Different mechanisms have been proposed to explain the effects of the different constituents. However, decreasing energy intake, inhibiting the intestinal absorption of dietary fats by inhibiting pancreatic lipase, and reduction in oxidative stress and inflammation might be the key mechanisms for the anti-obesity effects of pomegranate as a whole [23].

Pomegranate, (*Punica granatum*), is a rich source of potent polyphenolic, flavonoid antioxidants including tannins and anthocyanins. In general, epidemiological studies suggest that an intake of flavonoids, a group of polyphenolic compounds found in vegetables and fruits, is beneficial for the prevention of cardiovascular, inflammatory, and other diseases [39,40]. It is known that the prevention of free radical-related diseases depends entirely on the free radical scavenging and antioxidant activities of the compound used.

Similarly, anthocyanins, which differ structurally from other flavonoids, prevented lipid peroxidation of cell or liposome membranes. These antioxidants are more potent than many others, including vitamin C, vitamin E, coenzyme Q-10, and α-lipoic acid. In a comparative study, anthocyanins from pomegranate fruit were shown to possess higher antioxidant activity than vitamin E (α-tocopherol), ascorbic acid, and β-carotene [41]. It has also been shown that pomegranate suppresses activation of NF-κB, a transcription factor activated by ROS and therefore implicated in the pathophysiology of numerous diseases. There are plenty of studies which show that pomegranate extract inhibits NF-κB, especially in normal human cells, including chondrocytes, epidermal keratinocytes and endothelial cells [30,42]. Pomegranate juice (PJ) showed potent anti-atherogenic effects *in vivo* and *in vitro*. PJ consumption by diabetic patients resulted in anti-atherogenic effects with a significant reduction in oxidative stress in the patients' serum and macrophages [35]. Correspondingly, in an experimental study in hypercholesterolemic mice given PJ orally, the atherogenic effects induced by shear stress could be reversed by chronic administration of PJ[43]. In another clinical investigation, reduced oxidative stress in blood and decreased common carotid artery intima-media thickness, indicating a decreased atherosclerotic lesion size was demonstrated in patients with carotid artery stenosis after consumption of PJ for three years [33].

Pomegranate flower extract also exhibits an ability to scavenge ROS, as shown in a study by Kaur et al. [24]. It effectively scavenged superoxide ($O_2\cdot^-$), hydrogen peroxide (H_2O_2), hydroxyl radicals (OH·) and nitric oxide (NO·). The findings of this study can be compared with those of Noda et al. [44], who investigated the effects of pomegranate fruit extract. Pomegranate flower extract seems to possess almost equal $O_2\cdot^-$ scavenging capacity to as that reported for the fruit extract. However, pomegranate flower extract scavenges OH· radicals more potently. Noda et al. [44] reported that the fruit extract did not scavenge NO, even at concentrations of up to 2.5 mg/ml. In contrast, pomegranate flower extract was found to scavenge NO effectively [43]. Since NO plays a crucial role in the pathogenesis of inflammation, the scavenging of NO by pomegranate flower extract may explain the use of pomegranate flowers for treating inflammatory conditions in the Unani and Ayurvedic systems of medicine [25,45].

ANTIDIABETIC PROPERTIES OF POMEGRANATE

Diabetic patients usually avoid sugar-containing juices which augment their diabetic markers and other atherosclerotic complications. However, in the investigation by Rosenblat [35], PJ consumption (which contains 10% total sugars) did not increase serum glucose or blood HbA1c levels in diabetic patients, even though the glycemic index of PJ is similar to that of other fruit juices.

There are many studies describing the antidiabetic activity of pomegranate. Katz et al. [46] reported on the hypoglycemic activity of the flowers, seeds, and juice. Although the mechanisms for such effects are not clear, studies suggest that pomegranate flowers and juice may prevent diabetic complications via peroxisome proliferator-activated receptor-γ (PPAR-γ) binding and NO production [47]. Pomegranate compounds associated with antidiabetic effects include oleanolic, ursolic, and gallic acids. Gallic acid has been shown to be the component most responsible for this activity *in vitro*. Huang and coworkers [47] demonstrated a potential mechanism for the antidiabetic action of pomegranate flower extract which involved the activation of PPAR-γ. Jafri and others [26] reported that oral administration of an aqueous-ethanolic extract of pomegranate flowers had a significant blood glucose lowering effect in normal, glucose-fed hyperglycemic and alloxan-induced diabetic rats. This effect of the extract reached its maximum at 400 mg/kg. On the other hand, Parmar and Kar [48] reported that the administration of 200 mg/kg of pomegranate peel extract normalized all the adverse changes induced by alloxan, a widely used compound for inducing diabetes mellitus since it increases the serum levels of glucose and α-amylase activity and the rate of water consumption and lipid peroxidation in hepatic, cardiac, and renal tissues.

The main compounds that possess antidiabetic properties are polyphenols, which may affect glycemia through different mechanisms, including the inhibition of glucose absorption in the gut or of its uptake by peripheral tissues [22]. The hypoglycemic effects of diacetylated anthocyanins in a 10 mg/kg diet dosage given orally to 8-week-old Sprague-Dawley rats were observed when maltose was the glucose source, but not with sucrose or glucose itself [49]. This suggests that such effects are due to the inhibition of α-glucosidase in the gut mucosa. Several *in vitro* studies in cultured cells have shown that polyphenols may increase glucose uptake by peripheral tissues, which would diminish glycemia [22]. The mechanisms include inhibition of gluconeogenesis, adrenergic stimulation of glucose uptake, and stimulation of insulin release by pancreatic β-cells [27].

THE EFFECT OF POMEGRANATE ON DIABETIC LUNG INJURY

As discussed above, there is clear evidence that diabetes leads to a depletion of the cellular antioxidant defense system and increased levels of reactive oxygen species, and this is the main trigger in the development of diabetic injury in many organ systems including the lungs.

Reactive species can be eliminated by a number of enzymatic and non-enzymatic antioxidant mechanisms which yield some observable biomarkers, so these act as an indirect measurement of free radical production. These markers are the enzymatic activities of catalase (CAT), superoxide dismutase (SOD), glutathione-peroxidase (GSH-Px), and glutathione-reductase, all of which are endogenous antioxidants, as well as malondialdehyde (MDA) levels, an end-product of lipid peroxidation. Superoxide converts $O_2 \cdot^-$ to H_2O_2, which in turn is detoxified to water, either by catalase (CAT) in the lysosomes or by glutathione peroxidase in the mitochondria. Glutathione (GSH) is a major intracellular redox tampon system, which acts as a direct scavenger as well as a co-substrate for GSH-Px. Another noteworthy enzyme is glutathione reductase, which regenerates GSH, and this is used as a hydrogen donor by GSH-Px for the elimination of H_2O_2 [50].

Gumieniczek and coworkers [51] demonstrated that, in experimental DM, pulmonary oxidative stress occurs due to a reduction in antioxidant enzyme activity and increased lipoperoxidation which is revealed by a decrease in SOD activity and an increase of catalase activity. However, in a study by Ozansoy et al. [2], diabetes caused alterations to the antioxidant enzyme capacity of the lung without any change in MDA levels. Although way in which MDA levels remained normal in spite of the reduction in CAT activity and augmentation of GSH-Px is not clear, the authors explain that the lung of the diabetic rat might have slightly higher resistance to peroxidative stress. They also assert that the increase in GSH-Px activity occurred as a compensation for decreased CAT activity, relying on the fact (demonstrated by Doroshow et al.[52]) that H_2O_2 detoxification is critically dependent on the activity of GSH-Px [2].

As mentioned before, increased oxidative stress in diabetes may lead to protein oxidation, which changes the protein carbonyl content (PCC) as a result. The conversion of proteins to PCC derivatives occurs via direct oxidation by ROS with the eventual formation of oxidized amino acids [52,53]. This oxidative modification of proteins may affect a variety of cellular functions, and the best marker of intracellular damage is the PCC [53,54].

Sialic acid is a fragment of some glycoproteins and glycopeptides found hormones and enzymes, and it is reported to be a marker of microvascular complications in diabetic patients [55].

In an experimental study, streptozotocin-induced diabetic rats were treated with 100 μL/day pomegranate juice concentrate, thus maintaining 2.8 μmol total polyphenols per day for a total of 10 weeks [54]. They were compared to diabetic and control rats in regard to oxidative stress markers, antioxidant enzyme activity and structural pulmonary disturbance. PCC, a more reliable marker for intracellular oxidative stress-dependent cellular damage, and sialic acid (SA) were analyzed, along with the more frequently measured antioxidant enzyme activity indicators in diabetes, namely superoxide dismutase (SOD) and reduced glutathione (GSH). PCC and SA increased, and SOD decreased in diabetic rats, whereas GSH did not change. PJ treatment did not

·nly reverse all these changes, but it also diminished the ·istological alterations in alveolar basal membrane and ·nononuclear inflammatory cell infiltration as a consequence of these oxidative changes [54] (Figure 25.1). The ·mmunohistochemical analysis undertaken in this study ·evealed that eNOS expression increased in the lungs of ·liabetic rats, which then significantly decreased with PJ ·reatment (Figure 25.2). In a different piece of research, ·ipid peroxidation, SOD activity and distribution of ·NOS and eNOS isoforms were evaluated in diabetic ·at lung [56]. Similarly, enhanced oxidative stress and ·ncreased eNOS levels were reversed by another antioxidant, α-lipoic acid.

The antioxidative properties of pomegranate, as discussed above in detail, are ascribed to its high capability to scavenge free radicals and to inhibit lipid peroxidation. Its juice is shown also to suppress NF-κB inactivation [57]. In this situation, it is most probable that PJ treatment reduced the increased eNOS expressions through NF-κB inactivation.

This experimental data for the effects of pomegranate juice on diabetes-induced lung impairment, together with already available clinical evidence regarding other diabetic sequelae, suggests that pomegranate and its constituents may have significant potential clinical use for preventing oxidative injury to the lungs in diabetics.

SUMMARY POINTS

- Diabetes causes oxidative stress through the autooxidation of glucose, protein glycocylation and lipid peroxidation; and as a consequence, structural and functional alterations occur in the lungs of diabetics as well as other organs.
- A decreased in the capacity of the antioxidative defense system and an increase in oxidative stress were seen in the lungs of diabetic animal models. Structural alterations to the basal membrane of the pulmonary capillary endothelium in diabetes causes thickening of the alveolus-capillary membrane and a reduction in the diffusional capability.
- Many synthetic or naturally occurring antioxidants have been studied to attenuate these changes in diabetes. Pomegranate juice is a rich source of polyphenol antioxidants, which prove to be useful for this purpose.
- Pomegranate is known to suppress the activation of nuclear factor-κB, a transcription factor activated by reactive oxygen species and hence implicated in the pathophysiology of numerous diseases including diabetes. The antioxidative properties of pomegranate are ascribed to its high capability to scavenge free radicals and to inhibit lipid peroxidation.

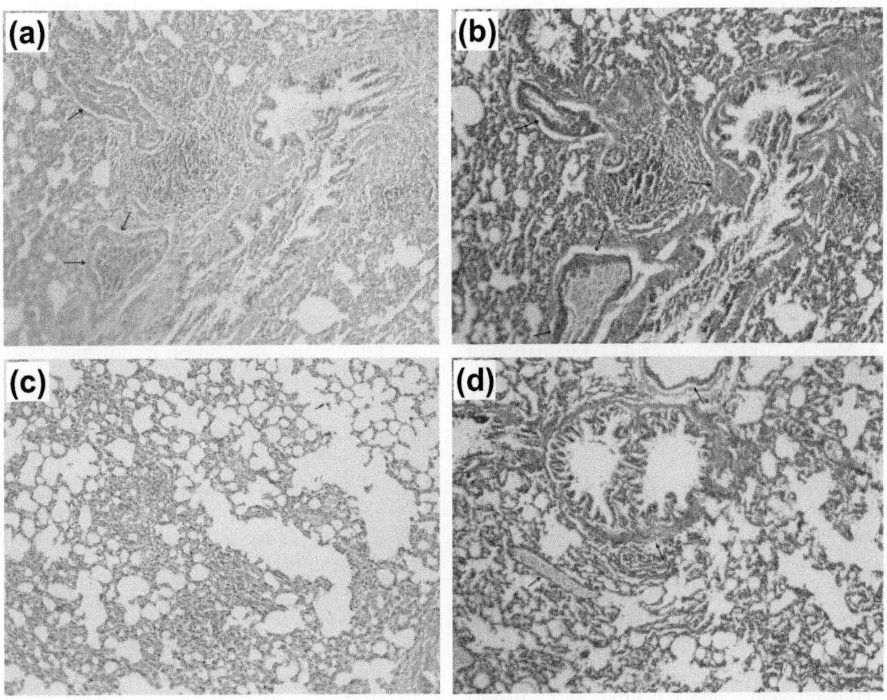

FIGURE 25.1 **Histology of the diabetic lung tissue; (a and b): without treatment, (c and d): treated with pomegranate juice (PJ).** Stainings are by Haematoxyline and Eosin in a and c; and by Periodic Acid Schiff in b and d (magnification 40x).Thickened basal membranes and intense mononuclear cell infiltration (arrows) are seen in the diabetic lung (a and b). But inflammatory reaction is less in the PJ-treated diabetic rat lung tissue (c and d). *[Pictures are taken (with permission) from the article by: Cukurova, Z., Hergunsel, O., Eren, G., Gedikbasi, A., Uhri, M., Demir, G., Tekdos, Y. (2012). The effect of pomegranate juice on diabetes-related oxidative stress in rat lung. Turkiye Klinikleri J Med Sci 2012;32(2):444–52.]* This figure is reproduced in color in the color section.

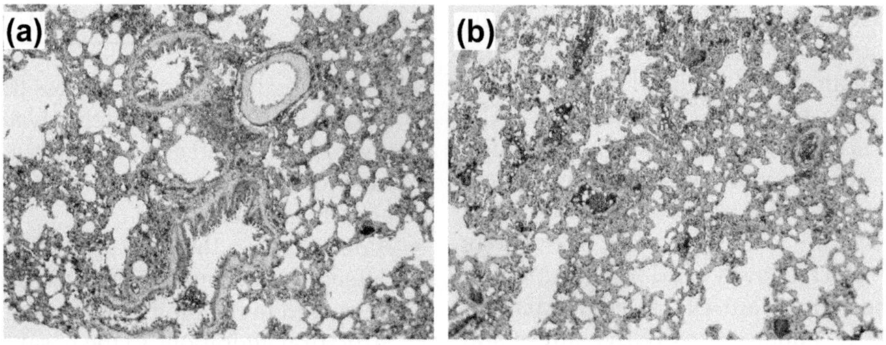

FIGURE 25.2 eNOS immunohistochemistry in lung tissue. There was intense staining demonstrating eNOS expression in diabetes (a), whereas it was significantly reduced in the pomegranate juice-treated lung (b). *[Pictures are taken from (with permission) the article by: Cukurova, Z., Hergunsel, O., Eren, G., Gedikbasi, A., Uhri, M., Demir, G., Tekdos, Y. (2012). The effect of pomegranate juice on diabetes-related oxidative stress in rat lung. Turkiye Klinikleri J Med Sci 2012;32(2):444–52.]* This figure is reproduced in color in the color section.

- Pomegranate juice is found to restore cellular defense and antioxidative capacity; and to diminish the histological alterations in alveolar basal membrane and mononuclear inflammatory cell infiltration in the lungs of diabetic rats.

References

[1] West IC. Radicals and oxidative stress in diabetes. Diabet Med 2000;17:171–80.

[2] Ozansoy G, Guven C, Ceylan A, Can B, Aktan F, Oz E, et al. Effects of simvastatin treatment on oxidant/antioxidant state and ultrastructure of streptozotocin-diabetic rat lung. Cell Biochem Funct 2005;23:421–6.

[3] Giugliano D, Ceriello A, Paolisso G. Diabetes mellitus, hypertension, and cardiovascular disease: which role for oxidative stress? Metabolism 1995;44:363–8.

[4] Brownlee M. Biochemistry and molecular cell biology of diabetic complications. Nature 2001;414:813–20.

[5] Mohamed AK, Bierhaus A, Schiekofer S, Tritschler H, Ziegler R, Nawroth PP. The role of oxidative stress and NF-κB activation in late diabetic complications. Biofactors 1999;10:157–67.

[6] Weynand B, Jonckheere A, Frans A, Rahier J. Diabetes mellitus induces a thickening of the pulmonary basal lamina. Respiration 1999;66(1):14–9.

[7] Ozsahin K, Tugrul A, Mert S, Yuksel M, Tugrul G. Evaluation of pulmonary alveolo-capillary permeability in type 2 diabetes mellitus: using technetium 99mTc-DTPA aerosol scintigraphy and carbonmonoxide diffusion capacity. J Diabetes Comp 2006;20(4): 205–9.

[8] Isotani H, Nakamura Y, Kameoka K, Tanaka K, Furukawa K, Kitaoka H, et al. Pulmonary diffusion capacity, serum angiotensin-converting enzyme activity and the angiotensin-converting enzyme gene in Japanese non-insulin dependent diabetes mellitus patients. Diabetes Res Clin Pract 1999;43:173–7.

[9] Guazzi M, Oreglia I, Guazzi MD. Insulin improves alveolar-capillary membrane gas conductance in type 2 diabetes. Diabetes Care 2002;25:1802–6.

[10] Philips B, Baker E. Hyperglycemia and the lung. Br J Anaesth 2003;90(4):430–3.

[11] Popov D, Simionescu M. Alterations of lung structure in experimental diabetes, and diabetes associated with hyperlipidaemia in hamsters. Eur Respir J 1997;10:1850–8.

[12] Ofulue F, Thurlbeck MW. Experimental diabetes and the lung. Am Rev Respir Dis 1998;138:284–9.

[13] Schleicher ED, Wagner E, Nerlic AG. Increased accumulation of glyoxidation product N(epsilon)-carboxymethyl lysine in human tissue in diabetes and aging. J Clin Invest 1997;99:457–68.

[14] Eren G, Cukurova Z, Hergunsel O, Demir; G, Kucur M, Uslu E, et al. Protective effect of the nuclear factor kappa B inhibitor pyrrolidine dithiocarbamate in lung injury in rats with streptozotocin-induced diabetes. Respiration 2010;79:402–10.

[15] Zhen J, Lu H, Wang XQ, Vaziri ND, Zhou XJ. Up-regulation of endothelial and inducible nitric oxide synthase expression by reactive oxygen species. Am J Hypertens 2008;21:28–34.

[16] Sridulyakul P, Chakraphan D, Bhattarakosol B, Patumraj S. Endothelial nitric oxide synthase expression in systemic and pulmonary circulation of streptozotocin-induced diabetic rats: comparison using image analysis. Clin Hemorheol Micro 2003;29:423–8.

[17] Joshi N, Caputo GM, Weitekamp MR, Karchmer AW. Infections in patients with diabetes mellitus. N Engl J Med 1999;341:1906–12.

[18] Hennessey PJ, Black CT, Andrassy RJ. Non-enzymatic glycosylation of immunoglobulin G impairs complement fixation. J Parenter Enteral Nutr 1991;15:60–4.

[19] Ihm SH, Yoo HJ, Park SW, Park CJ. Effect of tolrestat, an aldose reductase inhibitor, on neutrophil respiratory burst activity in diabetic patients. Metabolism 1997;46:634–8.

[20] Pandey KB, Rizvi SI. Plant polyphenols as dietary antioxidants in human health and disease. Oxid Med Cell Longev 2009;2(5): 270–8.

[21] Spencer JP, Abd El Mohsen MM, Minihane AM, Mathers JC. Biomarkers of the intake of dietary polyphenols: strengths, limitations and application in nutrition research. Br J Nutr 2008;99: 12–22.

[22] Scalbert A, Manach C, Morand C, Remesy C. Dietary polyphenols and the prevention of diseases. Crit Rev Food Sci Nutr 2005;45:287–306.

[23] Al-Muammar MN, Khan F. Obesity: The preventive role of pomegranate (*Punica granatum*). Nutrition 2012;28:595–604.

[24] Kaur G, Jabbar Z, Athar M, Alam MS. *Punica granatum* (pomegranate) flower extract possesses potent antioxidant activity and abrogates Fe-NTA induced hepatotoxicity in mice. Food Chem Toxicol 2006;44:984–93.

[25] Sivarajan VV, Balachadran I. Ayurvedic drugs and their plant sources. In: Mohan P, editor. Oxford: IBH Publishing Co Pvt. Ltd; 1994.

[26] Jafri MA, Aslam M, Javed K, Singh S. Effect of *Punica granatum* Linn. (flowers) on blood glucose level in normal and alloxan-induced diabetic rats. J Ethnopharmacol 2000;70:309–14.

[27] Viuda-Martos M, Fernandez-Lopez J, Perez-Alvarez JA. Pomegranate and its many functional components as related to human health: a review. Compr Rev Food Sci Food Saf 2010;9:635–54.

[28] Vroegrijk IO, van Diepen JA, van den Berg S, Westbroek I, Keizer H, Gambelli L, et al. Pomegranate seed oil, a rich source of punicic acid, prevents diet-induced obesity and insulin resistance in mice. Food Chem Toxicol 2011;2011(49):1426–30.
[29] Aviram M, Dornfeld L, Rosenblat M, Volkova N, Kaplan M, Coleman R, et al. Pomegranate juice consumption reduces oxidative stress, atherogenic modifications to LDL, and platelet aggregation: studies in humans and in atherosclerotic apolipoprotein E-deficient mice. Am J Clin Nutr 2000;71:1062–76.
[30] Afaq F, Saleem M, Krueger CG, Reed JD, Mukhtar H. Anthocyanin- and hydrolyzable tannin-rich pomegranate fruit extract modulates MAPK and NF-kappaB pathways and inhibits skin tumorigenesis in CD-1 mice. Int J Cancer 2005;113:423–33.
[31] Lan J, Lei F, Hua L, Wang Y, Xing D, Du L. Transport behavior of ellagic acid of pomegranate leaf tannins and its correlation with total cholesterol alteration in HepG2 cells. Biomed Chromatogr 2009;23:531–6.
[32] Lihua Zhang QF, Zhang Y. Composition of anthocyanins in pomegranate flowers and their antioxidant activity. Food Chem 2011;127:1444–9.
[33] Aviram M, Rosenblat M, Gaitini D, Nitecki S, Hoffman A, Dornfeld L, et al. Pomegranate juice consumption for 3 years by patients with carotid artery stenosis reduces common carotid intima-media thickness, blood pressure and LDL oxidation. Clin Nutr 2004;23:423–33.
[34] Esmaillazadeh A, Tahbaz F, Gaieni I, Alavi-Majd H, Azadbakht L. Concentrated pomegranate juice improves lipid profiles in diabetic patients with hyperlipidemia. J Med Food 2004;7:305–8.
[35] Rosenblat M, Hayek T, Aviram M. Anti-oxidative effects of pomegranate juice (PJ) consumption by diabetic patients on serum and on macrophages. Atherosclerosis 2006;187:363–71.
[36] Adams LS, Seeram NP, Aggarwal BB, Takada Y, Sand D, Heber D. Pomegranate juice, total pomegranate ellagitannins, and punicalagin suppress inflammatory cell signaling in colon cancer cells. J Agric Food Chem 2006;54:980–5.
[37] Kim ND, Mehta B, Yu W, Neeman I, Livney T, Amichay A, et al. Chemopreventive and adjuvant therapeutic potential of pomegranate (*Punica granatum*) for human breast cancer. Breast Canc Res Treat 2002;71:203–17.
[38] McFarlin BK, Strohacker KA, Kueht ML. Pomegranate seed oil consumption during a period of high-fat feeding reduces weight gain and reduces type 2 diabetes risk in CD-1 mice. Br J Nutr 2009;102:54–9.
[39] Graf BA, Milbury PE, Blumberg JB. Flavonols, flavonones, flavanones and human health: Epidemological evidence. J Med Food 2005;8:281–90.
[40] Arts ICW, Hollman PCH. Polyphenols and disease risk in epidemiologic studies. Am J Clin Nutr 2005;81:317–25.
[41] Youdim KA, McDonald J, Kalt W, Joseph JA. Potential role of dietary flavonoids in reducing microvascular endothelium vulnerability to oxidative and inflammatory insults. J Nutr Biochem 2002;13:282–8.
[42] Ahmed S, Wang N, Hafeez BB, Cheruvu VK, Haqqi TM. *Punica granatum* L. extract inhibits IL-1β-induced expression of matrix metalloproteinases by inhibiting the activation of MAP kinases and NF-κB in human chondrocytes *in vitro*. J Nutr 2005;135:2096–102.
[43] de Nigris F, Williams-Ignarro S, Lerman LO, Crimi E, Botti C, Mansueto G, et al. Beneficial effects of pomegranate juice on oxidation-sensitive genes and endothelial nitric oxide synthase activity at sites of perturbed shear stress. Proc Natl Acad Sci USA 2005;102(13):4896–901.
[44] Noda Y, Kaneyuki T, Mori A, Packer L. Antioxidant activities of pomegranate fruit extract and its anthocyanidins: delphinidin, cyanidin and pelargonidin. J Agric Food Chem 2002;50:166–71.
[45] Moncada S, Palmer RMJ, Higgs EA. Nitric oxide physiology, pathophysiology and pharmacology. Pharmacol Rev 1991;43:109–42.
[46] Katz SR, Newman RA, Lansky EP. Review *Punica granatum*: heuristic treatment for diabetes mellitus. J Med Food 2007;10(2):213–7.
[47] Huang TH, Peng G, Kota BP, Li GQ, Yamahara J, Roufogalis BD, et al. Anti-diabetic action of *Punica granatum* flower extract: activation of PPAR-gamma and identification of an active component. Toxicol Appl Pharmacol 2005;207(2):,160–9.
[48] Parmar HS, Kar A. Antidiabetic potential of Citrus sinensis snd *Punica granatum* peel extracts in alloxan treated male mice. Life Sci Biochem 2007;31:17–24.
[49] Matsui T, Ebuchi S, Kobayashi M, Fukui K, Sugita K, Terahara N, et al. Anti-hyperglycemic effect of diacylated anthocyanin derived from *Ipomoea batatas* cultivar Ayamurasaki can be achieved through the alpha-glucosidase inhibitory action. J Agric Food Chem 2002;50:7244–8.
[50] Johansen JS, Harris AK, Rychly DJ, Ergul A. Oxidative stress and the use of antioxidants in diabetes: Linking basic science to clinical practice. Cardiovasc Diabet 2005;4:5.
[51] Gumieniczek A, Hopkała H, Wójtowicz Z, Wysocka M. Changes in antioxidant status of lung tissue in experimental diabetes in rabbits. Clin Biochem 2002;35(2):147–9.
[52] Carrard G, Bulteau AL, Petropoulos I, Friguet B. Impairment of proteasome structure and function in aging. Int J Biochem Cell Bio 2002;34:1461–74.
[53] Stadtman ER, Levine RL. Protein oxidation. Ann NY Acad Sci 2000;899:191–208.
[54] Cukurova Z, Hergunsel O, Eren G, Gedikbasi A, Uhri M, Demir G, et al. The effect of pomegranate juice on diabetes-related oxidative stress in rat lung. Turkiye Klinikleri J Med Sci 2012;32(2):444–52.
[55] Ozben T, Nacitarhan S, Tuncer N. Plasma and urine sialic acid in non-insulin dependent diabetes mellitus. Ann Clin Biochem 1995;32(Pt 3):303–6.
[56] Hurdag C, Uyaner I, Gurel E, Utkusavas A, Atukeren P, Demirci C. The effect of alpha-lipoic acid on NOS dispersion in the lung of streptozotocin-induced diabetic rats. J Diabet Comp 2008;22(1): 56–61.
[57] Schubert SY, Neeman I, Resnick N. A novel mechanism for the inhibition of NF-kappaB activation in vascular endothelial cells by natural antioxidants. FASEB J 2002;16(14):1931–3.

CHAPTER

26

Antioxidants, Oxidative Stress and Preeclampsia in Type 1 Diabetes

Arpita Basu, Alecia L. Bryant*, Timothy J. Lyons†*

*Department of Nutritional Sciences, Oklahoma State University, Stillwater, OK, USA, †Section of Endocrinology and Diabetes, University of Oklahoma Health Sciences Center, Oklahoma City, OK, USA

List of Abbreviations

8-OHDG 8-hydroxydeoxyguanosine
AGE advanced glycation end products
CAT Catalase
Cu copper
DAPIT The Diabetes and Preeclampsia Intervention Trial
DHA Docosahexaenoic acid
EPO Erythropoietin
AOPP Advanced oxidative protein products
Fe Iron
FRAP Ferric reducing ability of plasma
GDM Gestational diabetes mellitus
GPx Glutathione peroxidase
GSH Reduced glutathione
hCG Human chorionic gonadotropin
HR Hypoxia-reoxygenation
iNOS Inducible nitric oxide synthase
LHP Lipid hydroperoxides
MDA Malondialdehyde
Mn Manganese
PAI-1 Plasminogen activator inhibitor-1
PAI-2 Plasminogen activator inhibitor-2
PE Preeclampsia
PP13 Placental protein 13
SOD Superoxide dismutase
T1DM Type 1 diabetes mellitus
TAS Total antioxidant status
TBARS Thiobarbituric acid reactive substances
TNF-α Tumor necrosis factor-alpha
UK United Kingdom
Zn Zinc

INTRODUCTION

Preeclampsia (PE), a pregnancy-specific hypertensive disorder, is a significant cause of maternal and perinatal mortality worldwide. PE has been defined as new-onset hypertension (>140/90 mmHg) after 20 weeks gestation in a previously normotensive woman, accompanied by proteinuria (>300 mg/24 hours) [1]. Women who experience PE are also at a higher risk of developing cardiovascular diseases later in life [2]. While the underlying causes of this maternal syndrome are not clearly understood, oxidative stress, especially in the placenta, is considered a biologically plausible contributor [1]. Oxidative stress, defined as an imbalance between the generation of active oxygen species and the antioxidant buffering capacity, has been shown to be elevated during pregnancy when compared to non-pregnant women [3,4]. However, oxidative stress is further enhanced in pregnancies complicated by type 1 diabetes (T1DM), and diabetes is associated with a four-fold higher prevalence of PE [5]. Few studies have addressed the role of oxidative stress and antioxidant status in the development of PE, especially prospectively, i.e., at different stages of gestational age in women with pre-gestational T1DM. Consequently, randomized controlled trials examining the effects of antioxidant supplementation as a possible treatment strategy for PE, have been reported mostly in non-diabetic pregnant women who later developed PE, while a few have examined effects in pregnant women with T1DM [6–8]. In addition to the antioxidant vitamins C and E, researchers have also identified a potential role of carotenoids, trace elements, vitamin D, and nutraceuticals such as L-arginine in the management of PE in non-diabetic pregnant women. This brief review will focus on the role of oxidative stress and antioxidant biomarkers associated with pregnancies complicated by diabetes and PE, and will discuss the potential role of antioxidants in the therapeutic management of PE based on evidence from experimental animal models and clinical trials.

Diabetes: Oxidative Stress and Dietary Antioxidants.
http://dx.doi.org/10.1016/B978-0-12-405885-9.00026-7

OXIDATIVE STRESS AND ANTIOXIDANT STATUS IN PREGNANCIES COMPLICATED BY T1DM

As summarized in Table 26.1, non-PE pregnancies complicated by T1DM have been shown to be associated with lower maternal antioxidant status and higher oxidative stress when compared to pregnancies in non-diabetic women. Most of these cross-sectional and longitudinal studies show higher levels of maternal lipid oxidation products, such as malondialdehyde (MDA), thiobarbituric acid reactive substances (TBARS) and lipid hydroperoxides (LHP) in pregnant women with T1DM compared to control groups. Interestingly, in one of these cross-sectional studies comparing pregnant versus non-pregnant women, pregnancy was shown to increase levels of lipid peroxidation and to decrease antioxidant status with advancing gestational age, and the presence of diabetes further enhanced this effect [3]. Lipid-derived products of oxidative damage, especially MDA and LHP, have also been associated with macrovascular complications in non-pregnant diabetic population [9,10]. Levels of antioxidant enzymes, such as superoxide dismutase (SOD) and glutathione peroxidase (GPx) have also been reported to be lower in diabetic patients with microvascular complications in comparison to non-diabetic controls [11]. The protective effects of SOD against inducible nitric oxide synthase (iNOS) expression and nitrosative stress have been shown in experimental models of diabetes in pregnancy [12] (Figure 26.1). These models also show protective effects of antioxidant nutrients, such as selenium and vitamins C and E, in reducing lipid peroxidation, increasing antioxidant enzyme activities, and improving fetal outcomes in diabetic rats [13,14]. In human pregnancies complicated by diabetes, observational studies correlate multivitamin use with decreased risks of birth defects [15]. In contrast, the largest clinical trial of pregnancies in women with T1DM reported that antioxidant vitamin supplementation (vitamin C and E) did not reduce the incidence of PE [8]. However, a sub-analysis in this study revealed reduced risks of PE only in women with low baseline antioxidant status. Thus, future studies of antioxidants in pregnant women with T1DM should address outcomes stratified by maternal levels of antioxidant factors, including enzymes and vitamins. Maternal circulating levels of oxidative stress and antioxidant status may serve as surrogate biomarkers to identify subgroups with higher risks of pregnancy complications, and thus the need for early intervention.

TABLE 26.1 Non-Preeclampsia Pregnancies in Women With T1DM: Effects of Pregnancy on Oxidative Stress and Antioxidant Biomarkers

Author, Year	Study Design & Duration	Subject Characteristics	Biomarkers	Significant Associations
Kinalski et al., 2001 [35]	Cross-sectional between 37 and 41 weeks of gestation	Women (n=28) with T1DM versus non-diabetic controls (n=13)	MDA, SOD, GSH	Significantly higher MDA and GSH, but lower SOD in T1DM versus controls
Peuchant et al., 2004 [36]	Cross-sectional between 26 and 32 weeks of gestation	Women (n=11) with T1DM versus non-diabetic controls (n=27)	MDA, SOD, GPx, vitamins A and E	Significantly higher MDA and lower antioxidant enzymes and vitamins in T1DM versus controls
Toescu et al., 2004 [37]	Longitudinal across 1st, 2nd and 3rd trimesters of pregnancy	Women (n=19) with T1DM versus non-diabetic controls (n=17)	Antioxidant capacity and LHP	Significantly lower antioxidant capacity and higher LHP in T1DM versus controls
Djordjevic et al., 2004 [3]	Longitudinal across 1st, 2nd and 3rd trimesters of pregnancy	Women (n=30) with T1DM versus non-diabetic controls (n=30) and non-pregnant controls (n=30)	Lipid peroxidation, SOD, CAT and GSH-Px	Significantly higher TBARS and lower antioxidant enzymes in T1DM versus pregnancies in non-diabetic women
Al- Saleh et al., 2005 [38]	Cross-sectional at term	Women (n=14) with T1DM versus non-diabetic controls (n=17)	Trace elements (copper, zinc, iron, selenium, molybdenum)	Significantly higher maternal copper and iron and copper: zinc ratio in T1DM versus controls
Escobar et al., 2012 [39]	Cross-sectional at term	Women (n=19) with T1DM; no controls	EPO, nitrotyrosine and 8-OHDG	Significant correlation between amniotic fluid EPO and nitrosative stress biomarkers suggesting chronic fetal hypoxia

The above table is a summary of key cross-sectional and longitudinal studies on the associations between oxidative stress and pregnancies complicated by type 1 diabetes.
T1DM, type 1 diabetes mellitus; MDA, malondialdehyde; SOD, superoxide dismutase; GSH, reduced glutathione; GPx, glutathione peroxidase; CAT, catalase; TBARS, thiobarbituric acid reactive substances; EPO, erythropoietin; 8-OHDG, 8-hydroxydeoxyguanosine; LHP, lipid hydroperoxides

OXIDATIVE STRESS AND ANTIOXIDANT STATUS IN PE

The prevalence of PE is significantly higher in pregnancies in women with T1DM than in non-diabetic women [5]. However, few studies address the role of oxidative stress and antioxidant status in this high-risk population. As summarized in Table 26.2, PE is associated with higher maternal lipid peroxidation and lower antioxidants, especially, vitamin C, carotenoids, and tocopherols versus women who did not develop PE. However, most of these studies are cross-sectional in nature and do not address PE in the context of T1DM. Our group has reported the first prospective study investigating the antioxidant status, defined as maternal serum carotenoids and tocopherols, as well as vitamin D, in women with T1DM who subsequently developed PE [16]. Analyses of serum samples at first, second, and third trimesters revealed significantly lower α- and β-carotenes, and generally lower vitamin D, in T1DM women who later developed PE when compared to those who remained normotensive. Interestingly, in our study, T1DM women who subsequently developed PE exhibited lower levels of α- and β-carotenes, but similar α-tocopherol levels at first trimester when compared to normotensive diabetic women. Our observational data are supported by previously reported experimental studies on the inhibitory effects of β-carotene on peroxide-induced vasoconstriction in the human placenta [17]. Thus, our prospective findings provide novel data on a potentially critical role of carotenoid deficiencies in early pregnancy in the development of PE, and thus, the need for adequate dietary intake of carotenoids

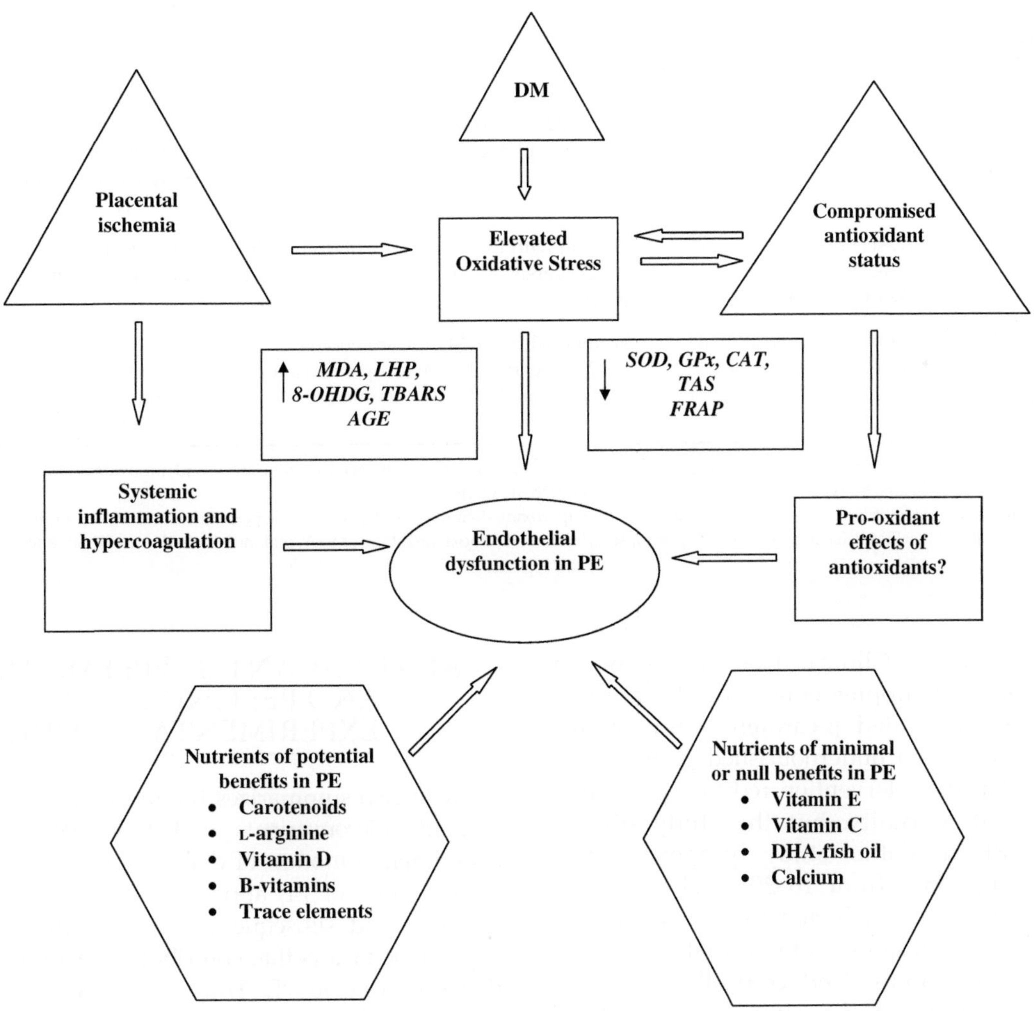

FIGURE 26.1 **Oxidative stress, diabetes mellitus and preeclampsia.** The above figure is a summary of pathways linking oxidative stress, diabetes mellitus and preeclampsia. DM, diabetes mellitus; PE, preeclampsia; MDA, malondialdehyde; LHP, lipid hydroperoxides; TBARS, thiobarbituric acid reactive substances; 8-OHDG, 8-hydroxydeoxyguanosine; AGE, advanced glycation end products; SOD, superoxide dismutase; GPx, glutathione peroxidase; CAT, catalase; TAS, total antioxidant status; FRAP, ferric reducing ability of plasma; DHA, docosahexaenoic acid.

TABLE 26.2 Pregnancies in Women With and Without T1DM: Effects of Preeclampsia on Oxidative Stress and Antioxidant Biomarkers

Author, Year	Study Design & Duration	DM?	Subject Characteristics	Biomarkers	Significant Associations with PE
Palan et al., 2001 [40]	Cross-sectional at 30–42 weeks of gestation	No	Women with PE (n=19) versus no PE (n=22)	Carotenoids	Significantly lower β-carotene and lycopene in PE versus no PE
Zhang et al., 2001 [41]	Case-control at term	No	Women with PE (n=125) versus no PE (n=179)	Carotenoids, retinol and tocopherols	Significantly higher α-tocopherol in PE versus no PE
Chappell et al., 2002 [42]	Prospective case-control from 20 weeks of gestation until delivery	No	Women with PE (n=21) versus no PE (n=17)	Antioxidant vitamins	Significantly lower ascorbic acid in PE versus no PE
Williams et al., 2003 [43]	Case-control at term	No	Women with PE (n=173) versus no PE (n=186)	Carotenoids, retinol and tocopherols	Significantly lower carotenoids, except lycopene, in PE versus no PE
Llurba et al., 2004 [44]	Cross-sectional at 32.5 weeks of gestation	No	Women with PE (n=53) versus no PE (n=30)	Lipid hydroperoxides, plasma protein-SH, SOD, GPx	Significantly higher lipid oxidation and antioxidant enzymes and lower protein-SH in PE versus no PE
Harsem et al., 2008 [45]	Cross-sectional at 33 weeks of gestation	Yes	Women with PE (n=36) versus women with T1DM and no PE (n=22) versus non-diabetic and non-PE (n=38)	AGE, 8-isoprostane, FRAP, vitamin E	Significantly higher 8-isoprostane in PE and in pregnant women withT1DM versus controls with no PE or T1DM; significantly higher AGE in pregnancies in women with T1DM versus controls
Karacay et al., 2010 [46]	Cross-sectional between 24 and 36 weeks of gestation	No	Women with PE (n=27) versus no PE (n=29)	TAS, MDA, AOPP	Significantly lower TAS and higher AOPP in PE versus no PE
Azar et al., 2011 [16]	Longitudinal across 1st, 2nd and 3rd trimesters of pregnancy	Yes	Women with T1DM (n=23) who developed PE versus no PE (n=24)	Carotenoids, tocopherols and vitamin D	Significantly lower α- and β-carotenes and generally lower vitamin D in T1DM PE versus T1DM non-PE

The above table is a summary of key cross-sectional and longitudinal studies on the associations between oxidative stress and antioxidant biomarkers and preeclampsia in pregnancies complicated by type 1 diabetes or in pregnant non-diabetic women.
PE, preeclampsia; DM, diabetes mellitus; protein-SH, protein-thiols; SOD, superoxide dismutase; GPx, glutathione peroxidase; T1DM, type 1 diabetes mellitus; AGE, advanced glycation end products; FRAP, ferric reducing ability of plasma; TAS, total antioxidant status; MDA, malondialdehyde; AOPP, advanced oxidative protein products.

throughout gestation. Clinical trials assessing the effects of carotenoid supplementation in PE are lacking. A placebo controlled β-carotene supplementation field trial in a rural undernourished population in Asia showed that the intervention reduced pregnancy-related maternal mortality, but the study did not address PE [18]. In another study, lycopene supplementation (2 mg/day) from 16–20 weeks gestation until delivery has been reported to reduce the incidence of PE in a small sample of non-diabetic women [19]. Thus, larger randomized controlled trials are needed to define the role of carotenoids in PE development in the high risk pregnancies of women with T1DM.

ANTIOXIDANT SUPPLEMENTATION AND PE: FINDINGS FROM EXPERIMENTAL STUDIES

Table 26.3 summarizes the mechanistic effects of antioxidant micronutrients and bioactive compounds in experimental models of diabetic pregnancy and PE. The pathogenesis of PE appears to be caused by placental ischemia and subsequent release of inflammatory and angiogenic factors that contribute to endothelial dysfunction occurring in PE. Thus, researchers have attempted to identify the safety and efficacy of dietary or pharmacological agents that target these pathways in diabetic animal models of PE. The teratogenic effects of diabetes

TABLE 26.3 Pre-Clinical Studies: Effects of Antioxidants and Micronutrients in Experimental Models of Preeclampsia and Diabetic Pregnancy

Author, Year	Study Design & Duration	Cell/Animal Model	Treatment	Primary Outcomes
Nash et al., 2005 [23]	Animals treated and outcomes evaluated at 20 days of gestation	Normal and streptozotocin-induced **diabetic rats**	Vitamin E-enriched diet ((DL-α-tocopherol hydrogen succinate;5% weight)	Significant improvements in oxidative stress, placental blood flow and blood pressure in vitamin versus control groups
Zabihi et al., 2007 [24]	Animals treated and outcomes evaluated at 10 and 11 days of gestation	Normal and streptozotocin-induced **diabetic rats**	Folic acid injections (15mg/kg body weight)	Significant improvements in oxidative stress and CuZnSOD in diabetic rats
Hung et al., 2010 [26]	Cells treated for 48 hours	Human term placentas	Ascorbic acid (50 μM) and α-tocopherol (50 μM) or vehicle	Significant reduction in apoptotic and autophagic changes at normoxia (8% oxygen) but increase in these pathways during HR in the vitamin versus vehicle
Orendi et al., 2010 [47]	Cells treated for 48 or 72 hours	Several choriocarcinoma cell lines to mimic the villous trophoblast cells	Ascorbic acid (30–200 μM) versus controls	Significant dose-dependent increase in PP13 in the vitamin versus control groups
Singh et al., 2011 [25]	Animals treated and outcomes evaluated at 10 days of gestation	Normal and streptozotocin-induced **diabetic rats**	Resveratrol (100 mg/kg body weight) by gavage feeding	Significant reduction in oxidative stress and apoptosis in diabetic embryos
Williams et al., 2011 [48]	Cells treated for 6 days	Placental explants from 7 weeks' gestational age	Folic acid at concentrations of 10^{-6} M, 10^{-8} M, and 10^{-10} M versus controls	Significant up regulation of trophoblast invasion and placental development in the folic acid versus control groups
Watson et al., 2012 [49]	Cells treated for 24 hours	Human trophoblast cell lines (BeWo and JEG-3)	Inorganic sodium selenite (NaSe; 25 nM, 50 nM, 100 nM, 200 nM, 300 nM, 400 nM and 800 nM) or organic selenomethionine (SeMet; 250 nM, 500 nM, 1000 nM and 1500 nM) or no selenium	Significant up regulation of endogenous antioxidant enzymes (thioredoxin reductase and glutathione peroxidase) following selenium treatment versus controls

The above table is a summary of key experimental studies showing the effects of antioxidants and micronutrient supplementation in pathogenic mechanisms underlying preeclampsia or pregnancy complicated by diabetes.
CuZnSOD, copper-zinc containing superoxide dismutase; HR, hypoxia-reoxygenation; PP13, placental protein 13.

during pregnancy were identified and reported more than three decades ago. These studies showed growth retardation and organ malformation in diabetic rat embryos, and abnormal maternal and fetal accumulation of trace elements, such as zinc, copper and manganese in pregnant diabetic rats compared to non-diabetic pregnant groups [20–22]. Similar toxic effects of diabetes in pregnant rats have also been associated with elevated oxidative stress and consequent placental dysfunction, decreased placental blood flow, and elevated maternal blood pressure, features resembling human PE [23]. In several animal models of PE in the presence of diabetes, treatment with nutrients such as vitamin E and folic acid, and food bioactive compounds such as resveratrol was shown to improve oxidative stress and placental blood flow, to restore the activities of antioxidant enzymes, and to reduce apoptosis in embryos [23–25]. The authors of these studies reported no significant toxic effects of these dietary agents in the experimental animals or embryos. In contrast, in a study reported by Hung et al., cultured human placental cells treated with a combination of vitamins C (50 μM) and E (50 μM) revealed increased apoptosis and autophagy under conditions of hypoxia-reoxygenation (HR) that mimics insufficient placentation in human PE [26]. Similarly, and also in cell culture, Aris et al. reported adverse effects of antioxidant vitamins C (50 and 100 μM) and E (25 and 50 μM) on human trophoblast cells (increased production of pro-inflammatory tumor necrosis factor-α (TNF-α) and decreased secretion of human chorionic gonadotropin (hCG) [27]. Thus, the effects of antioxidant vitamins, especially C and E, in ameliorating placental oxidative stress and dysfunction as salient features of human PE are unclear. Further studies must address their dose-dependent as well as synergistic effects with other nutrients and dietary factors in PE.

ANTIOXIDANT SUPPLEMENTATION AND PE: FINDINGS FROM CLINICAL TRIALS

The summary of studies in Table 26.4 shows the effects of supplementation with vitamins C and E on the development of PE in pregnant women with and without T1DM. The role of vitamin E as an essential nutrient for normal reproduction in rats led to its discovery by Evans and Bishop in 1922 [28]. In spite of this historical association of vitamin E with pregnancy, studies provide conflicting evidence on the ability of vitamin E, alone or in combination with vitamin C, to reduce the risk of PE in pregnancies in women with and without T1DM. However, most of the reported clinical trials on antioxidant vitamin supplementation have been conducted in non-diabetic pregnant women, and only a few examine the effects in pregnancies complicated by T1DM. The main findings of the largest clinical trial, the Diabetes and Preeclampsia Intervention Trial (DAPIT), in pregnant women with T1DM showed no benefit from supplementation with vitamins C and E [8]. In this prospective study, 762 women with pre-pregnancy T1DM (mean gestational age 14.3 weeks) were recruited at 25 clinics in the UK and randomly assigned to receive vitamin supplement (1,000 mg vitamin C + 400 IU vitamin E) or matched placebo until delivery. At baseline, the placebo group had a higher percentage of women with previous history of PE, hypertension, and microalbuminuria than the vitamin-treated group. The overall study findings revealed no significant difference in the rates of PE between vitamin and placebo groups, and also no adverse maternal and fetal effects of vitamin use. The study also showed no significant differences in PAI-1:PAI-2 ratio, a biomarker of inflammation and hypercoagulability associated with risks of PE. However, this landmark study provides evidence on significantly lower incidence of PE in women with baseline plasma vitamin C less than 10 μmol/L and baseline serum tocopherol (adjusted for serum cholesterol) between 3 and 5 μmol/mmoL when compared to higher levels in the cohort. Thus, baseline vitamin deficiencies in these high-risk pregnant women with T1DM might be associated with more pronounced oxidative stress that responds more favorably to antioxidant supplementation. Supplementation may lead to improvements in endothelial dysfunction not seen among those with adequate levels at baseline. Other reported clinical trials in pregnant women with T1DM also show no significant reduction in incidence of PE with similar antioxidant composition of vitamins C and E as used in the DAPIT [6,7,29].

In contrast to the DAPIT findings, which showed no adverse effects of vitamins C and E supplementation, two other studies showed a significant increase in risks of low birth weight infants, perinatal deaths, and preterm rupture of membranes in the vitamin group compared to those assigned to placebo [6,7]. It should also be noted that in comparison to the DAPIT, some of these studies did not examine the effects of vitamins C and E supplementation according to baseline antioxidant status. Furthermore they only included a small number of women with pregestational diabetes in combination with other high-risk pregnancies, and they did not report maternal levels of inflammatory and/or coagulation biomarkers which might explain the observed discrepancies. These observations from clinical trials also conform to the reported data from mechanistic studies showing adverse effects of high dose vitamin C and E supplementation [26,27]. Thus, future studies must address the dose-response effects of vitamins C and E in PE, especially among high-risk pregnant women with T1DM and low baseline antioxidant status.

Several other groups aiming to find optimal treatment strategies for PE have also identified roles for L-arginine, a combination of vitamins B, C, E and trace minerals, and vitamin D in reducing risks of PE (Table 26.5). Some of these agents have been associated with physiological functions other than antioxidant effects. For example, L-arginine has been shown to improve endothelial function as a substrate for the synthesis of vasodilator nitric oxide, and vitamin D supplementation has been shown to reduce maternal inflammatory responses [30,31]. On the other hand, in line with findings from vitamins C and E trials, studies also show no significant reduction in risks of PE following administration of high dose calcium, selenium, or DHA-enriched fish oil when compared to those receiving placebo [32–34]. Thus, keeping in view the fact that PE is a multi-factorial condition associated with several aberrations in pathways involving oxidative stress, inflammation, coagulation, and angiogenesis, effective forms of intervention may need to demonstrate functions beyond antioxidant effects. Thus, future studies should address the safety and efficacy of these nutrients and dietary factors, in different doses and forms, especially in pregnant women at high risk of PE, such as those with T1DM and those with low baseline antioxidant levels.

SUMMARY POINTS

- The prevalence of preeclampsia is higher in pregnant women with type 1 diabetes than in non-diabetic pregnant women.
- Pregnancies complicated by type 1 diabetes exhibit higher oxidative stress and lower levels of antioxidant enzymes and vitamins when compared to pregnancies in non-diabetic women.
- Antioxidant carotenoid deficiencies, specifically of α- and β-carotenes, in early gestation may be associated with later development of preeclampsia in type 1 diabetes.

TABLE 26.4 Clinical Trials: Effects of Antioxidant Vitamin Therapy in Preeclampsia

Author, Year	Study Design & Duration	DM?	Subject Characteristics	Intervention	Primary Outcomes
Chappell et al., 1999 [50]	Randomized placebo controlled trial From 18–22 weeks' gestation until delivery; high-risk women randomized at 16 weeks	No	Women (n=283) with abnormal uterine-artery doppler screening or previous history of PE	1000mg vitamin C and 400 IU α-tocopherol or matched placebo (soya-bean oil) capsules	Significant risk reduction of PE and decrease in PAI-1/PAI-2 ration in the vitamin group versus placebo
Rumbold et al., 2006 [51]	Randomized placebo controlled trial From 14 and 22 weeks' gestation until delivery	No	Women (n=1877) with singleton pregnancies; no documentation of pre-gestational diabetes in enrolment criteria	1000mg vitamin C and 400 IU α-tocopherol or matched placebo (microcrystalline cellulose) capsules	No significant reduction in risks of PE in the vitamin group versus placebo
Poston et al., 2006 [6]	Randomized placebo controlled trial From 14 and 22 weeks' gestation until delivery	Yes	Women (n=2,410) with risk factors for PE including history of PE and T1DM	1,000 mg vitamin C and 400 IU α-tocopherol or matched placebo (sunflower seed oil) capsules	No significant reduction in risks of PE; increased rates of low birth weight babies in the vitamin group versus placebo
Villar et al., 2009 [29]	Randomized placebo controlled trial From 14 and 22 weeks' gestation until delivery	Yes	Women (n=1,365) with risk factors for PE including history of PE and pre-gestational diabetes	1,000 mg vitamin C and 400 IU α-tocopherol or matched placebo (sunflower seed oil) capsules	No significant reduction in risks of PE in the vitamin group versus placebo
Xu et al., 2010 [7]	Randomized placebo controlled trial From 12 and 18 weeks' gestation until delivery	Yes	Women (n=2,647) with risk factors for PE including history of PE and pre-gestational diabetes including T1DM	1,000 mg vitamin C and 400 IU α-tocopherol or matched placebo capsules	No significant reduction in risks of PE in the vitamin group versus placebo; increased risks of perinatal death and preterm rupture of membranes in the vitamin versus placebo
McCance et al., 2010 [8]	Randomized placebo controlled trial From 8 and 22 weeks' gestation until delivery	Yes	Women (n=762) with pre-pregnancy T1DM, singleton pregnancy, ≥16 years	1,000 mg vitamin C and 400 IU α-tocopherol or matched placebo (olive oil) capsules	No significant reduction in risks of PE; subgroup analysis showed reduced risks of PE among women with low antioxidant status at baseline
Roberts et al., 2010 [52]	Randomized placebo controlled trial From 9 and 16 weeks' gestation until delivery	No	Women (n=9969) with singleton pregnancy, gestational age <16 weeks; pre-gestational hypertension and diabetes among exclusion criteria	1,000 mg vitamin C and 400 IU α-tocopherol or matched placebo (mineral oil) capsules	No significant reduction in risks of PE in the vitamin group versus placebo
Kalpdev et al., 2011 [53]	Randomized placebo controlled trial From 8 and 22 weeks' gestation until delivery	No	Women (n=50) with pre-pregnancy hypertension	1,000 mg vitamin C and 400 IU α-tocopherol or no supplementation	No significant reduction in risks of superimposed PE in the vitamin versus no treatment group
Vadillo-Ortega et al., 2011 [30]	Randomized placebo controlled trial From 14 and 32 weeks' gestation until delivery	No	Women (n=672) with history of PE or incidence of PE in first degree relative; pre-gestational hypertension and diabetes among exclusion criteria	Two medicinal bars (6.6g L-arginine, 500 mg vitamin C, 400 IU vitamin E, 50 mg niacin, 4 mg vitamin B6), antioxidant bar (500 mg vitamin C, 400 IU vitamin E, 50 mg niacin, 4 mg vitamin B6) or placebo bar	Significant risk reduction of PE in L-arginine plus vitamin group when compared to placebo; vitamins alone showed a decreasing trend

The above table is a summary of key clinical trials on the effects of antioxidant vitamin supplementation in reducing risks of preeclampsia in pregnancies complicated by diabetes or in non-diabetic pregnant women.
PE, preeclampsia; DM, diabetes mellitus; T1DM, type 1 diabetes mellitus; PAI-1, plasminogen activator inhibitor-1; **PAI-2,** plasminogen activator inhibitor-2.

TABLE 26.5 Clinical Trials: Effects of Micronutrients and Nutraceutical Supplementation in Preeclampsia

Author, Year	Study Design & Duration	DM?	Subject Characteristics	Intervention	Primary Outcomes
Levine et al., 1997 [32]	Randomized placebo controlled trial From 13 to 21weeks' gestation until delivery	No	Women (n=4589) with gestational age between 11 and 21 weeks; pre-existing diseases among exclusion criteria	2 g of elemental calcium or placebo	No significant decrease in incidence of PE or pregnancy-associated hypertension in calcium versus placebo
Rumiris et al., 2006 [54]	Randomized placebo controlled trial From 8 to 12 weeks' gestation until delivery	No	Women (n=60) between 8 and 12 weeks' gestation; history of medical complications among exclusion criteria	Antioxidant group [vitamins A (1000 IU), B6 (2.2 mg), B12 (2.2 μg), C (200 mg), and E (400 IU), folic acid (400 μg), N-acetylcysteine (200 mg), Cu (2 mg), Zn (15 mg), Mn (0.5 mg), Fe (30 mg), calcium (800 mg), and selenium (100 μg) or control group received Fe (30 mg) and folic acid (400 μg).	Significant reduction in risks of PE in the antioxidant micronutrient group when compared to the control group
Haugen et al., 2009 [31]	Prospective study Vitamin D intake (food and supplements) data collected at 15, 22 and 30 weeks' gestation	No	Women (23,423) with singleton pregnancies; no documentation of pre-gestational diabetes	Vitamin D intakes (5–20 μg/day) versus no supplement	Vitamin D intake from supplements associated with a significant decrease in risks of PE
Tara et al., 2010 [33]	Randomized controlled trial From 12 weeks' gestation until delivery	No	Women (n=166) with gestational age ≤12 weeks; pre-gestational hypertension and diabetes among exclusion criteria	Selenium (100 μg selenium yeast) or placebo yeast tablets	No significant decrease in incidence of PE; significant increase in serum selenium versus placebo
Wibowo et al., 2012 [55]	Randomized placebo controlled trial From 8 to 12 weeks' gestation until 2 weeks' postpartum	No	Women (n=110) with singleton pregnancy between 8 and 12 weeks' gestation; history of medical complications including diabetes among exclusion criteria	Antioxidant-fortified milk [Cu (2 mg), Zn (15 mg), Mn (1 mg), Fe (30 mg), vitamin B6 (2.2 mg), B12 (2.2 mg), C (200 mg), E (400 mg), selenium (100 μg), and calcium (800 mg)] versus control milk	Significant reduction in the incidence of PE in the antioxidant versus control group
Zhou et al., 2012 [34]	Randomized controlled trial From 20 weeks' gestation until delivery	No	Women (n=2399) with gestational age <21 weeks and singleton pregnancies; none had pre-gestational DM	DHA-enriched fish oil (800 mg/d) or vegetable oil capsules	No significant decrease in incidence of PE or GDM in fish oil versus placebo

The above table is a summary of key clinical trials on the effects of micronutrients and nutraceutical supplementation in reducing risks of preeclampsia and oxidative stress.
PE, preeclampsia; Cu, copper; Zn, zinc; Mn, manganese; Fe, iron; DHA, docosahexaenoic acid; GDM, gestational diabetes mellitus

- Experimental models using human placental cells show adverse effects of high dose treatment with antioxidants vitamins C and E.
- Clinical trials on vitamin C (1,000 mg) and vitamin E (400 IU) mostly show no effects in reducing incidence of preeclampsia in pregnant women with and without type 1 diabetes.
- The largest clinical trial in pregnant women with type 1 diabetes (conducted in the UK) shows significant reduction in rates of preeclampsia, but only in a subgroup of women with low baseline vitamin C and E levels.
- Clinical trials in pregnant non-diabetic women show vitamins C and E in combination with other nutrients and bioactive compounds, such as L-arginine, B vitamins and trace minerals, significantly reduces incidence of preeclampsia.
- Combinations of antioxidant nutrients may be more useful than a single agent in the prevention of preeclampsia in high-risk pregnant women with type 1 diabetes, especially when stratified by baseline antioxidant status and/or other metabolic risk factors.

References

[1] Roberts J, Pearson G, Cutler J, Lindheimer M. Summary of the NHLBI working group on research on hypertension during pregnancy. Hypertens Pregnancy 2003;22:109.

[2] Chambers JC, Fusi L, Malik IS, Haskard DO, De Swiet M, Kooner JS. Association of maternal endothelial dysfunction with preeclampsia. JAMA 2001;285:1607–12.

[3] Djordjevic AA, Spasic SS, Jovanovic-Galovic AA, Djordjevic RR, Grubor-Lajsic GG. Oxidative stress in diabetic pregnancy: SOD, CAT and GSH-Px activity and lipid peroxidation products. J Matern Fetal Neonatal Med 2004;16:367–72.

[4] Makedou K, Kourtis A, Gkiomisi A, Toulis KA, Mouzaki M, Anastasilakis AD, et al. Oxidized low-density lipoprotein and adiponectin levels in pregnancy. Gynecol Endocrinol 2011;27:1070–3.

[5] Hanson U, Persson B. Outcome of pregnancies complicated by type 1 insulin-dependent diabetes in Sweden: acute pregnancy complications, neonatal mortality and morbidity. Am J Perinatol 1993;10:330–3.

[6] Poston LL, Briley AL, Seed PT, Kelly FJ, Shennan AH. Vitamins in Pre-eclampsia (VIP) Trial Consortium. Vitamin C and vitamin E in pregnant women at risk for pre-eclampsia (VIP trial): randomised placebo-controlled trial. Lancet 2006;367:1145–54.

[7] Xu H, Perez-Cuevas R, Xiong X, Reyes H, Roy C, Julien P, et al. INTAPP study group. An international trial of antioxidants in the prevention of preeclampsia (INTAPP). Am J Obstet Gynecol 2010;202(239); e1–239.e10.

[8] McCance DR, Holmes VA, Maresh MA, Patterson CC, Walker JD, Pearson DM, et al. Vitamins C and E for prevention of preeclampsia in women with type 1 diabetes (DAPIT): a randomised placebo-controlled trial. Lancet 2010;376:259–66.

[9] Martín-Gallán P, Carrascosa A, Gussinyé M, Domínguez C. Biomarkers of diabetes-associated oxidative stress and antioxidant status in young diabetic patients with or without subclinical complications. Free Radic Biol Med 2003;34:1563–74.

[10] Cighetti G, Fermo I, Aman CS, Ferraroni M, Secchi A, Fiorina P, et al. Dimethylarginines in complicated type 1 diabetes: roles of insulin, glucose, and oxidative stress. Free Radic Biol Med 2009;47:307–11.

[11] Hartnett ME, Stratton RD, Browne RW, Rosner BA, Lanham RJ, Armstrong D. Serum markers of oxidative stress and severity of diabetic retinopathy. Diabetes Care 2000;23:234–40.

[12] Weng H, Li X, Reece E, Yang P. SOD1 suppresses maternal hyperglycemia-increased iNOS expression and consequent nitrosative stress in diabetic embryopathy. Am J Obstet Gynecol 2012;206(448):e1–7.

[13] Cederberg J, Simán CM, Eriksson UJ. Combined treatment with vitamin E and vitamin C decreases oxidative stress and improves fetal outcome in experimental diabetic pregnancy. Pediatr Res 2001;49:755–62.

[14] Guney M, Erdemoglu E, Mungan T. Selenium-vitamin E combination and melatonin modulates diabetes-induced blood oxidative damage and fetal outcomes in pregnant rats. Biol Trace Elem Res 2011;143:1091–102.

[15] Correa A, Gilboa SM, Botto LD, Moore CA, Hobbs CA, Cleves MA, et al. National Birth Defects Prevention Study. Lack of periconceptional vitamins or supplements that contain folic acid and diabetes mellitus-associated birth defects. Am J Obstet Gynecol 2012;206(218); e1218.e13.

[16] Azar M, Basu A, Jenkins AJ, Nankervis AJ, Hanssen KF, Scholz H, et al. Serum carotenoids and fat-soluble vitamins in women with type 1 diabetes and preeclampsia: a longitudinal study. Diabetes Care 2011;34:1258–64.

[17] Cueto SM, Romney AD, Wang Y, Walsh SW. Beta-carotene attenuates peroxide-induced vasoconstriction in the human placenta. J Soc Gynecol Investig 1997;4:64–71.

[18] West KP, Katz J, Khatry SK, LeClerq SC, Pradhan EK, Shrestha SR, et al. Double blind, cluster randomised trial of low dose supplementation with vitamin A or beta carotene on mortality related to pregnancy in Nepal. The NNIPS-2 study group. BMJ 1999;318:570–5.

[19] Sharma JB, Kumar A, Kumar A, Malhotra M, Arora R, Prasad S, et al. Effect of lycopene on pre-eclampsia and intra-uterine growth retardation in primigravidas. Int J Gynaecol Obstet 2003;81:257–62.

[20] Eriksson UJ, Tydén O, Berne C. Development of phosphatidyl glycerol biosynthesis in the lungs of fetuses of diabetic rats. Diabetologia 1983;24:202–6.

[21] Eriksson UJ, Lewis NJ, Freinkel N. Growth retardation during early organogenesis in embryos of experimentally diabetic rats. Diabetes 1984;33:281–4.

[22] Eriksson UJ. Diabetes in pregnancy: retarded fetal growth, congenital malformations and feto-maternal concentrations of zinc, copper and manganese in the rat. J Nutr 1984;114:477–84.

[23] Nash P, Olovsson M, Eriksson U. Placental dysfunction in Suramin-treated rats: impact of maternal diabetes and effects of antioxidative treatment. J Soc Gynecol Investig 2005;12:174–84.

[24] Zabihi S, Eriksson UJ, Wentzel P. Folic acid supplementation affects ROS scavenging enzymes, enhances VEGF-A, and diminishes apoptotic state in yolk sacs of embryos of diabetic rats. Reprod Toxicol 2007;23:486–98.

[25] Singh CK, Kumar A, Hitchcock DB, Fan D, Goodwin R, LaVoie HA, et al. Resveratrol prevents embryonic oxidative stress and apoptosis associated with diabetic embryopathy and improves glucose and lipid profile of diabetic dam. Mol Nutr Food Res 2011;55:1186–96.

[26] Hung TH, Chen SF, Li MJ, Yeh YL, Hsieh TT. Differential effects of concomitant use of vitamins C and E on trophoblast apoptosis and autophagy between normoxia and hypoxia-reoxygenation. PLoS. One 2010;5:1–2.

[27] Aris A, Leblanc S, Ouellet A, Moutquin JM. Detrimental effects of high levels of antioxidant vitamins C and E on placental function: considerations for the vitamins in preeclampsia (VIP) trial. J Obstet Gynaecol Res 2008;34:504–11.

[28] Vaisrul S. Target for tocopherol. JAMA 1971;217:1545.

[29] Villar JJ, Purwar MM, Merialdi MM, Zavaleta NN, Ngoc N, Anthony J, et al. World Health Organisation multicenter randomised trial of supplementation with vitamins C and E among pregnant women at high risk for pre-eclampsia in populations of low nutritional status from developing countries. BJOG 2009;116:780–8.

[30] Vadillo-Ortega F, Perichart-Perera O, Espino S, Avila-Vergara M, Ibarra I, Ahued R, et al. Effect of supplementation during pregnancy with L-arginine and antioxidant vitamins in medical food on pre-eclampsia in high risk population: randomised controlled trial. BMJ 2011;342:1193.

[31] Haugen M, Brantsaeter A, Trogstad L, Alexander J, Roth C, Magnus P, et al. Vitamin D supplementation and reduced risk of preeclampsia in nulliparous women. Epidemiology 2009;20:720–6.

[32] Levine RJ, Hauth JC, Curet LB, Sibai BM, Catalano PM, Morris CD, et al. Trial of calcium to prevent preeclampsia. N Eng J Med 1997;337:69–76.

[33] Tara F, Maamouri G, Rayman M, Ghayour-Mobarhan M, Sahebkar A, Yazarlu O, et al. Selenium supplementation and the incidence of preeclampsia in pregnant Iranian women: a randomized, double-blind, placebo-controlled pilot trial. Taiwan J Obstet Gynecol 2010;49:181–7.

[34] Zhou SJ, Yelland L, McPhee AJ, Quinlivan J, Gibson RA, Makrides M. Fish-oil supplementation in pregnancy does not reduce the risk of gestational diabetes or preeclampsia. Am J Clin Nutr 2012;95:1378–84.

[35] Kinalski MM, Sledziewski AA, Telejko BB, Kowalska II, Kretowski AA, Zarzycki WW, et al. Lipid peroxidation, antioxidant defense and acid-base status in cord blood at birth: The influence of diabetes. Horm. Metab Res 2001;33:227–31.

[36] Peuchant E, Brun JL, Rigalleau V, Dubourg L, Thomas MJ, Daniel JY, et al. Oxidative and antioxidative status in pregnant women with either gestational or type 1 diabetes. Clin Biochem 2004;37:293–8.
[37] Toescu VV, Nuttall SL, Martin UU, Nightingale PP, Kendall MJ, Brydon PP, et al. Changes in plasma lipids and markers of oxidative stress in normal pregnancy and pregnancies complicated by diabetes. Clin Sci (Lond) 2004;106:93–8.
[38] Al-Saleh E, Nandakumaran M, Al-Shammari M, Makhseed M, Sadan T, Harouny A. Maternal-fetal status of copper, iron, molybdenum, selenium and zinc in insulin-dependent diabetic pregnancies. Arch Gynecol Obstet 2005;271:212–7.
[39] Escobar J, Teramo K, Stefanovic V, Andersson S, Asensi MA, Arduini A, et al. Amniotic fluid oxidative and nitrosative stress biomarkers correlate with fetal chronic hypoxia in diabetic pregnancies. Neonatology 2012;103:193–8.
[40] Palan PR, Mikhail MS, Romney SL. Placental and serum levels of carotenoids in preeclampsia. Obstet Gynecol 2001;98:459–62.
[41] Zhang C, Williams MA, Sanchez SE, King IB, Ware-Jauregui S, Larrabure G, et al. Plasma concentrations of carotenoids, retinol, and tocopherols in preeclamptic and normotensive pregnant women. Am J Epidemiol 2001;153:572–80.
[42] Chappell LC, Seed PT, Briley AL, Kelly FJ, Hunt BJ, Charnock-Jones DS, et al. A longitudinal study of biochemical variables in women at risk of preeclampsia. Am J Obstet Gynecol 2002;187: 127–36.
[43] Williams MA, Woelk GB, King IB, Jenkins L, Mahomed K. Plasma carotenoids, retinol, tocopherols, and lipoproteins in preeclamptic and normotensive pregnant Zimbabwean women. Am J Hypertens 2003;16:665–72.
[44] Llurba E, Gratacos E, Martin-Gallan P, Cabero L, Dominguez C. A comprehensive study of oxidative stress and antioxidant status in preeclampsia and normal pregnancy. Free Radic Biol Med 2004;37:557–70.
[45] Harsem NK, Braekke K, Torjussen T, Hanssen K, Staff AC. Advanced glycation end products in pregnancies complicated with diabetes mellitus or preeclampsia. Hypertens Pregnancy 2008;27:374–86.
[46] Karacay O, Sepici-Dincel A, Karcaaltincaba D, Sahin D, Yalvac S, Akyol M, et al. A quantitative evaluation of total antioxidant status and oxidative stress markers in preeclampsia and gestational diabetic patients in 24–36 weeks of gestation. Diabetes Res Clin Pract 2010;89:231–8.
[47] Orendi KK, Gauster MM, Moser GG, Meiri HH, Huppertz BB. Effects of vitamins C and E, acetylsalicylic acid and heparin on fusion, beta-hCG and PP13 expression in BeWo cells. Placenta 2010;31:431–8.
[48] Williams PJ, Bulmer JN, Innes BA, Pipkin F. Possible roles for folic acid in the regulation of trophoblast invasion and placental development in normal early human pregnancy. Biol Reprod 2011;84:1148–53.
[49] Watson MM, van Leer LL, Vanderlelie JJ, Perkins AV. Selenium supplementation protects trophoblast cells from oxidative stress. Placenta 2012;33:1012–9.
[50] Chappell LC, Seed PT, Briley AL, Kelly FJ, Lee R, Hunt BJ, et al. Effect of antioxidants on the occurrence of pre-eclampsia in women at increased risk: a randomised trial. Lancet 1999;354:810–6.
[51] Rumbold AR, Crowther CA, Haslam RR, Dekker GA, Robinson JSACTS Study Group. Vitamins C and E and the risks of preeclampsia and perinatal complications. N Engl J Med 2006;354: 1796–806.
[52] Roberts JM, Myatt L, Spong CY, Thom EA, Hauth JC, Leveno KJ, Eunice Kennedy Shriver National Institute of Child Health and Human Development Maternal-Fetal Medicine Units Network, et al. Vitamins C and E to prevent complications of pregnancy-associated hypertension. N Engl J Med 2010;362:1282–91.
[53] Kalpdev A, Saha SC, Dhawan V. Vitamin C and E supplementation does not reduce the risk of superimposed PE in pregnancy. Hypertens Pregnancy 2011;30:447–56.
[54] Rumiris D, Purwosunu Y, Wibowo N, Farina A, Sekizawa A. Lower rate of preeclampsia after antioxidant supplementation in pregnant women with low antioxidant status. Hypertens Pregnancy 2006;25:241–53.
[55] Wibowo N, Purwosunu Y, Sekizawa A, Farina A, Idriansyah L, Fitriana I. Antioxidant supplementation in pregnant women with low antioxidant status. J Obstet Gynaecol Res 2012;38:1152–61.

Index

Note: Page numbers with "f" denote figures; "t" tables; "b" boxes.

D

H

W

X

Z

Color Plates

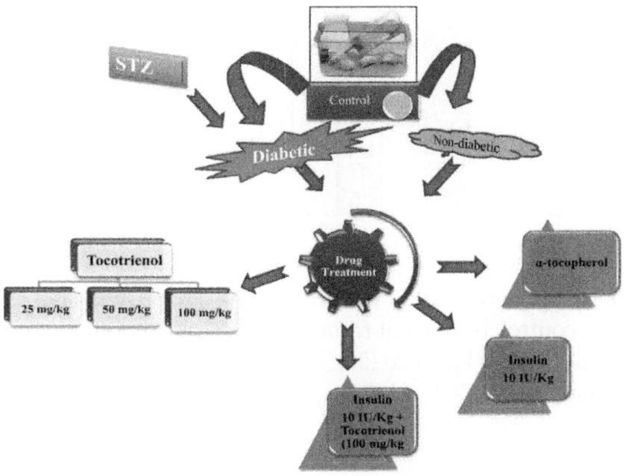

FIGURE 14.1 **Study design.**

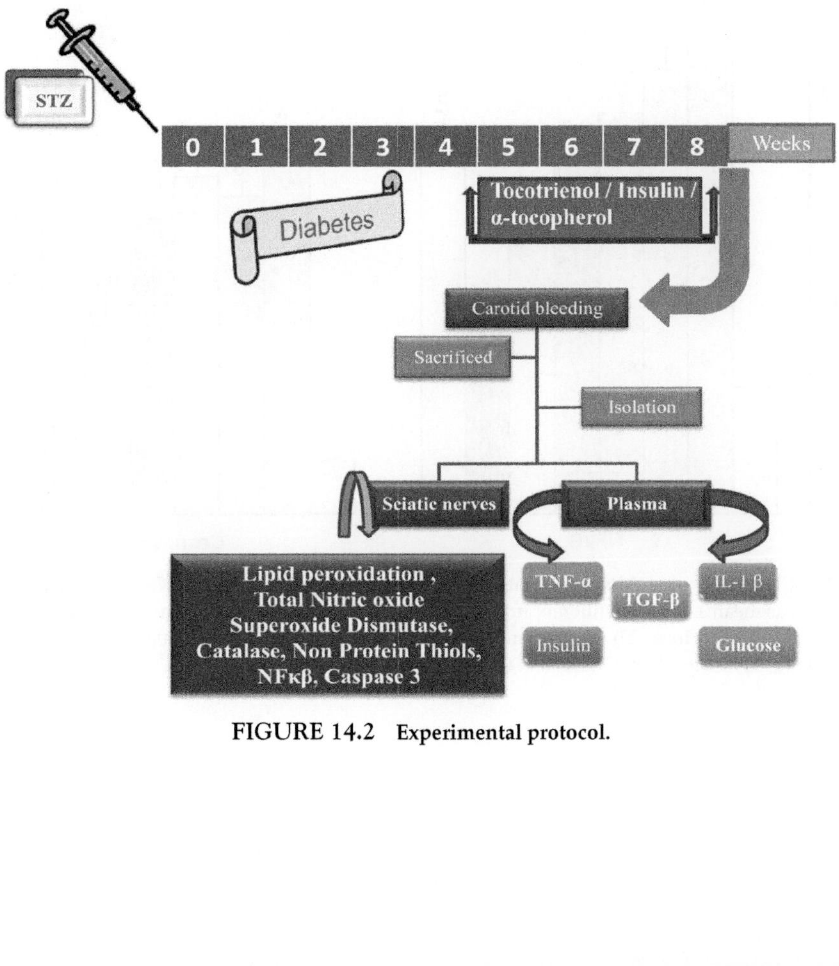

FIGURE 14.2 **Experimental protocol.**

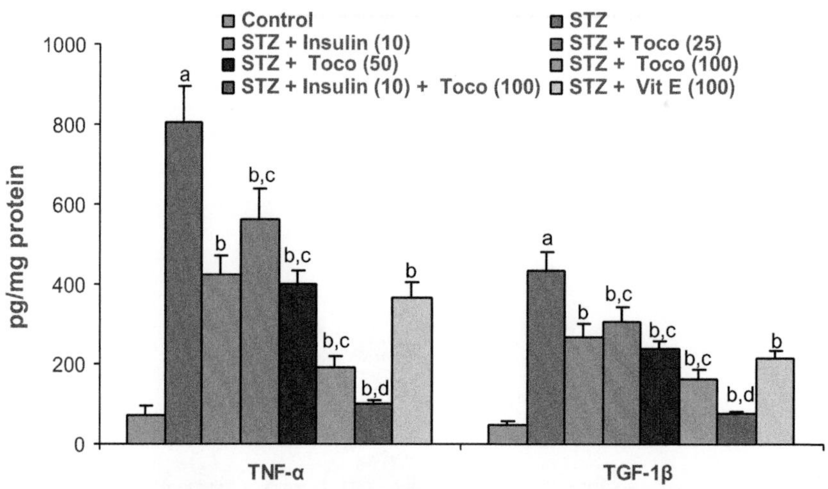

FIGURE 14.3 Effect of tocotrienol (Toco) and its combination with insulin on TNF-α and TGF-β1 levels in the kidneys of diabetic rats. Data are expressed as mean ± S.E.M. a different from control; b different from diabetic group; c different from one another; d different from tocotrienol and insulin per se groups. Toco (25) = Tocotrienol 25mg/kg, Toco (50) = Tocotrienol 50mg/kg, Toco (100) = Tocotrienol 100mg/kg, Vit E (100) = α-Tocopherol 100 mg/kg. *Adapted from Kuhad and Chopra (2009) [34].*

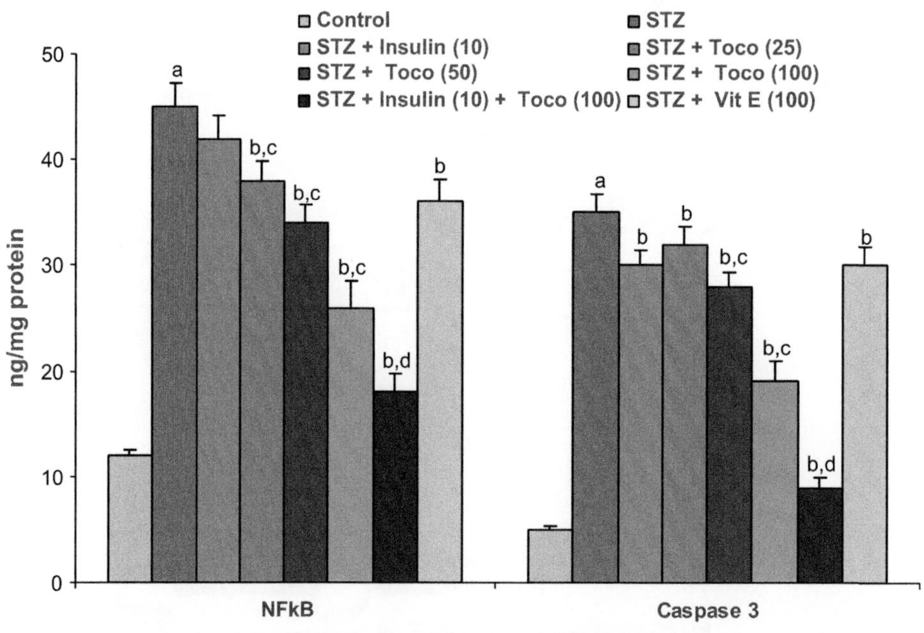

FIGURE 14.4 Effect of tocotrienol (Toco) and its combination with insulin on p65 subunit of NFκβ and caspase-3 levels in the kidneys of diabetic rats. Data are expressed as mean ± S.E.M. a different from control; b different from diabetic group; c different from one another; d different from tocotrienol and insulin per se groups. Toco (25) = Tocotrienol 25mg/kg, Toco (50) = Tocotrienol 50mg/kg, Toco (100) = Tocotrienol 100mg/kg, Vit E (100) = α-Tocopherol 100 mg/kg. *Adapted from Kuhad and Chopra (2009) [34].*

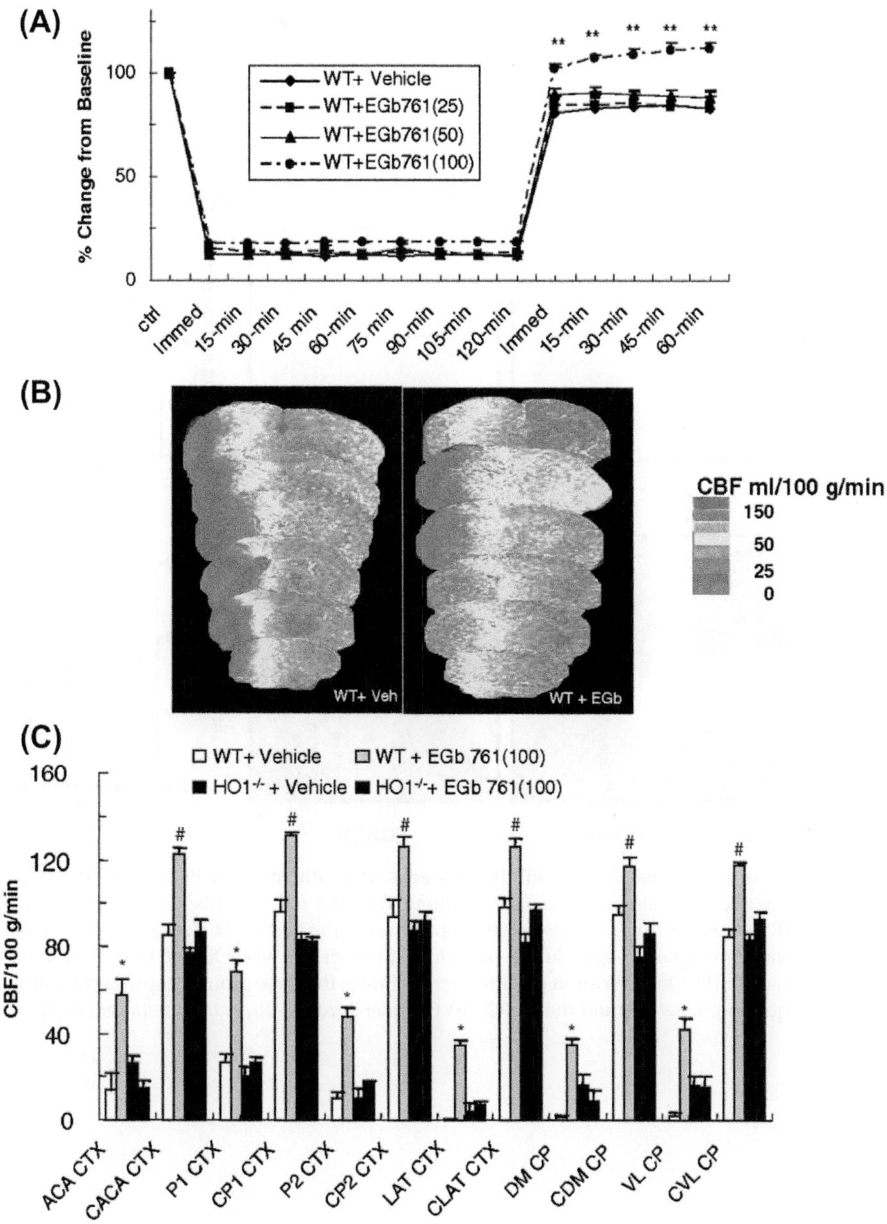

FIGURE 17.2 **Effects of EGb761 on cerebral blood flow.** (A) Relative cerebral blood flow (CBF) was recorded at baseline, at the induction of ischemia and at 15-min intervals during ischemia and 1 h of reperfusion. **$p < 0.01$. (B) 14C-IAP autoradiographic images of a wild-type (WT) mouse and an EGb761-treated mouse. Red represents areas of higher blood flow whereas blue represents areas of lower blood flow. (C) Mean CBF of each mouse group; *$p < 0.05$; #$p < 0.01$. Key: ACA CTX, anterior cerebral artery cortex; CACA, contralateral anterior cerebral artery; P1, parietal 1; CP1&2, contralateral parietal 1&2; LAT CTX, lateral cortex; CLAT CTX, contralateral lateral cortex; DM, dorsomedial; CDM, contralateral dorsomedial; VL, ventrolateral; CVL, contralateral ventrolateral; CP, caudate putamen. *Reproduced with permission from Saleem et al. [69].*

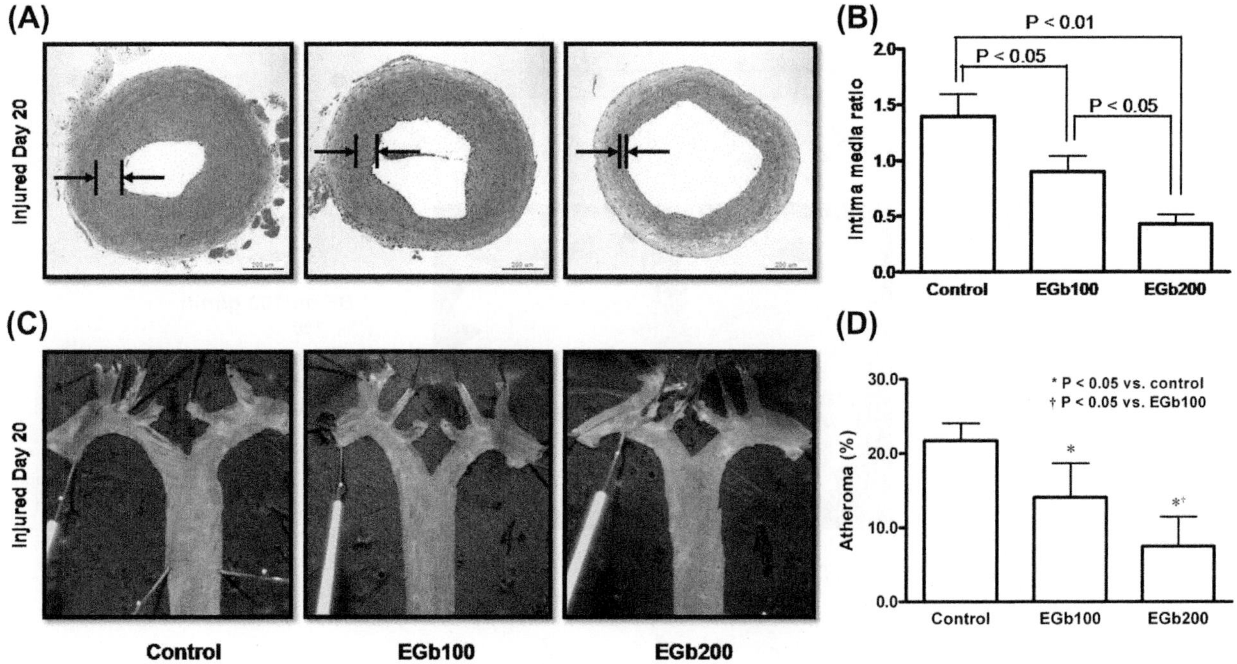

FIGURE 17.3 ***In vivo* inhibition of neointimal formation after 6 weeks of treatment with EGb761 (EGb100 group, 100mg/kg; EGb200 group, 200mg/kg).** (A) Haematoxylin and eosin-stained sections. (B) Intima-to-media ratios (IMRs; n=10 in each group) are shown. Treatment with EGb761 produced a lower IMR than in controls in a dose-dependent manner (the higher the dose of EGb761, the lower the IMR; $p < 0.05$). (C) Representative examples of aortas from ApoE−/−gene knock-out mice stained *en-face* with Oil Red O. Red staining indicates the aortic arch where plaque accumulation is the highest. (D) Quantification of aortic arch plaque in the three groups, expressed as the mean ± SEM (percentage). A dose-dependently decreased plaque volume was found in the EGb761 treatment groups. *Reproduced with permission from Lim et al. [22].*

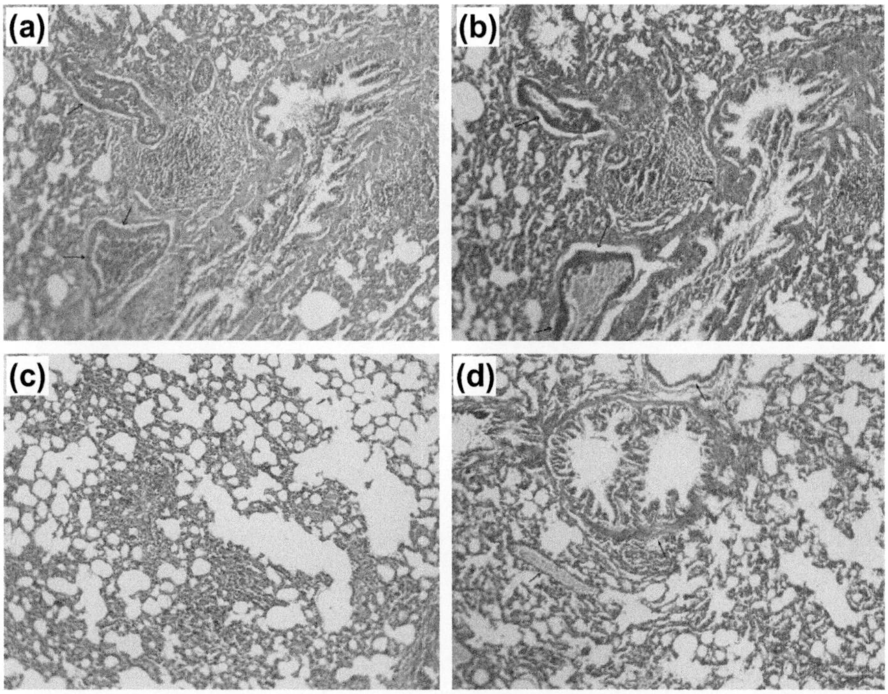

FIGURE 25.1 **Histology of the diabetic lung tissue; (a and b): without treatment, (c and d): treated with pomegranate juice (PJ).** Stainings are by Haematoxyline and Eosin in a and c; and by Periodic Acid Schiff in b and d (magnification 40x).Thickened basal membranes and intense mononuclear cell infiltration (arrows) are seen in the diabetic lung (a and b). But inflammatory reaction is less in the PJ-treated diabetic rat lung tissue (c and d). *[Pictures are taken (with permission) from the article by: Cukurova, Z., Hergunsel, O., Eren, G., Gedikbasi, A., Uhri, M., Demir, G., Tekdos, Y. (2012). The effect of pomegranate juice on diabetes-related oxidative stress in rat lung. Turkiye Klinikleri J Med Sci 2012;32(2):444–52.]*

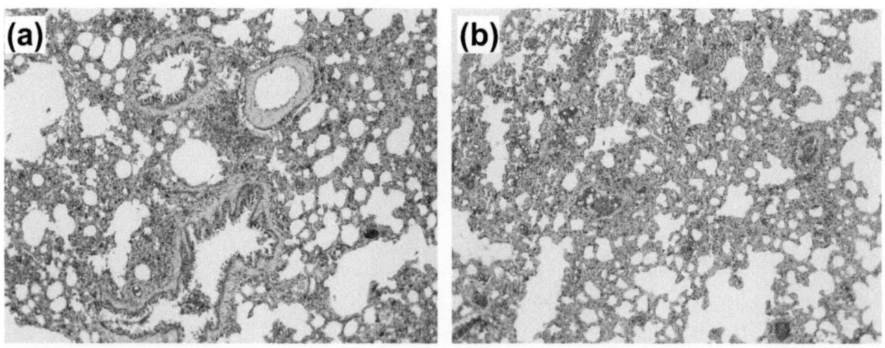

FIGURE 25.2 **eNOS immunohistochemistry in lung tissue.** There was intense staining demonstrating eNOS expression in diabetes (a); whereas it was significantly reduced in the pomegranate juice-treated lung (b). *[Pictures are taken from (with permission) the article by: Cukurova, Z., Hergunsel, O., Eren, G., Gedikbasi, A., Uhri, M., Demir, G., Tekdos, Y. (2012). The effect of pomegranate juice on diabetes-related oxidative stress in rat lung. Turkiye Klinikleri J Med Sci 2012;32(2):444–52.]*

Printed and bound by CPI Group (UK) Ltd, Croydon, CR0 4YY
08/05/2025
01865025-0001